普通高等教育“十三五”规划教材
全国高等医药院校规划教材

英文原版改编版

EMERGENCY MEDICINE

急诊医学

留学生与双语教学用

Rosen's Emergency Medicine : Concepts and Clinical Practice (eighth edition)

［美］约翰·A.马克思 ［美］罗伯特·S.霍克伯格 ［美］罗恩·M.沃尔斯 著
John A. Marx　Robert S. Hockberger　Ron M. Walls　Original Editors

柴艳芬　主编
CHAI Yanfen　Chief Editor of Adaptation Edition

清華大學出版社
北　京

ELSEVIER

ELSEVIER
Elsevier (Singapore) Pte Ltd.
3 Killiney Road, #08-01 Winsland House I, Singapore 239519
Tel: (65) 6349-0200; Fax: (65) 6733-1817

Rosen's Emergency Medicine: Concepts and Clinical Practice, 8/E
Copyright © 2014 by Saunders, an imprint of Elsevier Inc.
Copyright © 2010, 2006, 2002, 1998, 1992, 1988, 1983 by Mosby, Inc., an affiliate of Elsevier Inc.
ISBN-13: 9781455706051

This English Adaptation of Rosen's Emergency Medicine: Concepts and Clinical Practice, 8/E, by John A. Marx, Robert S. Hockberger & Ron M. Walls was undertaken by Tsinghua University Press and is published by arrangement with Elsevier (Singapore) Pte Ltd.

Rosen's Emergency Medicine: Concepts and Clinical Practice, 8/E, by John A. Marx, Robert S. Hockberger & Ron M. Walls 由清华大学出版社进行改编，并根据清华大学出版社与爱思唯尔（新加坡）私人有限公司的协议约定出版。

急诊医学（柴艳芬主编）
ISBN: 9787302449836

图书在版编目（CIP）数据

急诊医学：英文原版改编版：英文 /（美）约翰 · A. 马克思（John A. Marx）等著，柴艳芬主编．—北京：清华大学出版社，2016（2020.4重印）
（普通高等教育“十三五”规划教材．全国高等医药院校规划教材．留学生与双语教学用）
ISBN 978-7-302-44983-6

Ⅰ.①急… Ⅱ.①约… ②柴… Ⅲ.①急救医学—高等学校—教材—英文 Ⅳ.① R459.7

中国版本图书馆 CIP 数据核字（2016）第 216214 号

责任编辑：李 君 王 华
封面设计：戴国印
责任校对：刘玉霞
责任印制：杨 艳

出版发行：清华大学出版社
网 址：http://www.tup.com.cn, http://www.wqbook.com
地 址：北京清华大学学研大厦A座 **邮 编：**100084
社 总 机：010-62770175 **邮 购：**010-62786544
投稿与读者服务：010-62776969, c-service@tup.tsinghua.edu.cn
质量反馈：010-62772015, zhiliang@tup.tsinghua.edu.cn
印 装 者：三河市铭诚印务有限公司
经 销：全国新华书店
开 本：185mm×260mm **印 张：**36.25 **插 页：**2 **字 数：**1135千字
版 次：2016年11月第1版 **印 次：**2020年4月第4次印刷
定 价：138.00元

产品编号：056588-01

Notice

注　意

由于医学科技的发展，该领域的理论知识和临床实践在不断变化。随着新的研究与经验不断扩充我们的知识结构，在实践、治疗和用药方面做出适当的调整是必要或适宜的。建议读者检查相关操作的最新信息，或检查每一用药生产厂家所提供的最新产品信息，在临床执业医师的指导下确定药物的推荐剂量、服用方法、服用时间以及相关禁忌证。经治医师根据对患者的了解和相关经验，确立诊断，确定每一位患者的服药剂量和最佳治疗方法，并采取适当的安全预防措施，是其职责所在。不论是出版商还是著作者，对于在本出版物使用过程中出现的任何个人损伤和(或)财产损失，均不承担任何责任。

临床医学专业
留学生教材建设专家指导委员会委员名单

（按姓氏拼音排序）

改编者名单

主　　编　柴艳芬

主　　审　崔书章

副 主 编　寿松涛　陈玉国　陈晓辉

编　　委（以姓氏拼音排序）

曹　钰　四川大学华西医院
柴艳芬　天津医科大学总医院
陈晓辉　广州医科大学第一附属医院
陈玉国　山东大学齐鲁医院
崔书章　天津医科大学总医院
韩继媛　华中科技大学同济医学院附属协和医院
黄　亮　南昌大学第一附属医院
靳　衡　天津医科大学总医院
李　莉　郑州大学第一附属医院
李惠萍　温州医科大学第二附属医院
李丽君　西安交通大学第二附属医院
刘　志　中国医科大学第一附属医院
刘晨燕　天津医科大学总医院
彭　鹏　新疆医科大学第一附属医院
寿松涛　天津医科大学总医院
田英平　河北医科大学第二附属医院
王　沛　天津医科大学总医院
王力军　天津医科大学总医院
王秀杰　哈尔滨医科大学第一附属医院
杨立山　宁夏医科大学总医院
余慕明　天津医科大学总医院
袁志明　天津医科大学总医院
翟建华　天津医科大学总医院
张　泓　安徽医科大学第一附属医院
张剑锋　广西医科大学第一附属医院
张劲松　南京医科大学附属医院

编写秘书　么　颖　天津医科大学总医院
焦丽娜　天津医科大学总医院

Contributors of Adaptation Edition

CAO Yu	West China Hospital, Sichuan University
CHAI Yanfen	Tianjin Medical University General Hospital
CHEN Xiaohui	First Affiliated Hospital of Guangzhou Medical University
CHEN Yuguo	Qilu Hospital of Shandong University
CUI Shuzhang	Tianjin Medical University General Hospital
HAN Jiyuan	Union Hospital Tongji Medical College Huazhong University of Science and Technology
HUANG Liang	First Affiliated Hospital of Nanchang University
JIN Heng	Tianjin Medical University General Hospital
LI Li	First Affiliated Hospital of Zhengzhou University
LI Huiping	Second Affiliated Hospital & Yuying Children's Hospital of Wenzhou Medical University
LI Lijun	Second Affiliated Hospital of Xi'an Jiaotong University
LIU Zhi	First Hospital of China Medical University
LIU Chenyan	Tianjin Medical University General Hospital
PENG Peng	First Affiliated Hospital of Xinjiang Medical University
SHOU Songtao	Tianjin Medical University General Hospital
TIAN Yingping	Second Hospital of Hebei Medical University
WANG Lijun	Tianjin Medical University General Hospital
WANG Pei	Tianjin Medical University General Hospital
WANG Xiujie	First Affiliated Hospital of Harbin Medical University
YANG Lishan	General Hospital of Ningxia Medical University
YU Muming	Tianjin Medical University General Hospital
YUAN Zhiming	Tianjin Medical University General Hospital
ZHAI Jianhua	Tianjin Medical University General Hospital
ZHANG Hong	First Affiliated Hospital of Anhui Medical University
ZHANG Jianfeng	First Affiliated Hospital of Guangxi Medical University
ZHANG Jinsong	Jiangsu Province Hospital

General Foreword
总序言

随着中国政治、经济、文化的快速发展，中国软实力和国际影响力的不断提升，“留学中国计划”的逐步实施，越来越多的外国人认识到留学中国的未来价值，来华留学生规模不断扩大。2013 年，有来自 200 个国家和地区的 346 499 名外国留学生在我国 746 所高等院校和科研机构学习或进修，我国已经成为亚洲最大的留学目的地国家。

近年来，来华学习医学的留学生人数增长尤为迅猛，目前来华学习医学的留学生人数已位居来华留学生人数的首位，2013 年占比高达 21.76%，为 29 048 名。

为了维护我国高等教育的国际声誉，教育部高度重视来华医学留学生教育教学质量，不断加强对医学留学生教育教学的规范和管理，多种措施付诸实施。2007 年教育部即制定了《来华留学生医学本科教育（英语授课）质量控制标准暂行规定》，要求招生院校严格落实执行。2013 年 7 月，教育部国际合作与交流司下达了《关于对招收本科临床医学专业（英语授课）来华留学生的高等学校进行专项工作检查的通知》，委托中国高等教育学会外国留学生教育管理分会组成专家组对招生院校进行专项工作检查。2013 年 8 月，全国性的“来华留学生（医学）教学专业委员会”成立大会暨第一次学术研讨会在天津医科大学成功召开。2014 年上半年，教育部国际合作与交流司又组织专家组对部分医学院校实施了飞行检查。2014 年 6 月，“来华留学医学教育 2014 学术研讨会暨首届医学院校国际教育学院院长论坛”在安徽医科大学举办。

来华留学生的教学质量是来华留学教育事业可持续发展的核心保障，来华留学生教育的教材建设是保障和提升教学质量非常重要的手段。适合来华医学留学生使用的教材的需求越来越迫切，临床医学专业的教材长期匮乏和不足，教材编写、教材内容、教材形式、教材版权等都需要进行整合和改进完善。

在教育部国际合作与交流司的指导和中国高等教育学会外国留学生教育管理分会的支持下，众多医学院校的领导和专家经过多次讨论、磋商，决定成立“来华医学留学生教育教材建设专家指导委员会”，委托天津医科大学和清华大学出版社共同承担全国性临床医学专业英文版立体化教材编写和出版的具体组织工作。

天津医科大学有近 17 年的英语授课培养外国留学生的历史，在来华医学留学生教育的实践方面开始较早，是教育部指定的第一批计划招生全英文临床医学专业的 30 余所院校之一，也是教育部首批批准的“来华留学教育示范基地”，设有教育部来华留学英语教学师资培训中心（医学），至今已举办 6 期培训班，为全国 52 所医科院校培训英语授课教师 364 人，所编教材在全国 30 余所西医院校教学中被借鉴或使用，在全国医学高等院校来华留学生教育教学领域里具有代表性和很大的影响力。

清华大学出版社在高等教育综合出版领域里，排名我国第二位，是以出版全方位、多学科、立体化的高等教育教材为主的大社；上级主管单位为教育部，主办单位是清华大学，高质量、创新型、探究型的特色教材是其出版的重点任务，也是其肩负的社会职责所在，其所具有的强烈的社会责任感、主动性和积极性值得肯定。

据悉，该套教材近50种，主要供临床医学留学生、七年制或八年制医学生、医学本科生英语或双语教学使用。部分教材由我国长期从事医学留学生教育的教授、学者编写，其余大部分教材由清华大学出版社从多家国外出版社引进，改编出版，以适应我国临床医学专业留学生课堂教学和临床实习所需。

该套教材的陆续出版，是我国对高校来华留学生教育教材系列化、专门化的首次探索。希冀其会对全面提升来华医学留学生教育质量水平，对规范来华医学留学生教育的教材建设，甚至对其他学科的留学生教材建设，起到积极的示范效应和引领性作用。

这是一个良好的开端，希望该套教材在今后教学中经过不断探索、不断总结，得到修订，日臻完善。

中国高等教育学会外国留学生教育管理分会

副会长兼秘书长 贺向民

2014年10月

Preface

前　言

Emergency Medicine is a newborn speciality that consists of nearly all aspects of medicine. Emergency Medicine is a recognized board certified medical specialty, out of emergency medical specialty have grown numerous subspecialies. Nowadays, with the vigorous development of medicine and technology, emergency medicine as a grade-2 subject has gained more progress. The emergency physicians of Tianjin Medical University General Hospital have been devoted to emergency medicine education since 1980s.For the purpose of international communication, this textbook was written upon Rosen's Emergency Medicine (8th ed)for students of both foreign and domestic.

There are eight sections in this text .The chapters of this book follow an outline format and are divided by organ-system (i.e., cardiovascular emergencies, pulmonary emergencies, and gastrointestinal emergencies, etc), as well as special topics (i.e., environmental emergencies, trauma, toxicology).The common emergency diseases and conditions encountered in ED were elaborated in this book, ranging from epidemiology, etiology, principle, clinical feature, differential diagnose, to emergency room management of disease.

Although this edition was primarily designed for foreign medical students, we believe it is also available for emergency physicians, intensivists, and emergency nurses. It is our hope that this edition will be useful to you.

In compiling the book, we received assistance from many sources, and would like to thank those people for their invaluable support.

Editors

March. 09. 2016

Abbreviations
缩略语

AAA	abdominal aortic aneurysm
ABG	arterial blood gas
ACEI	angiotensin-Converting Enzyme Inhibitor
Ach	acetylcholine
ACPE	acute cardiogenic pulmonary edema
ACS	acute coronary syndrome
AED	automated external defibrillator
Af	atrial fibrillation
AF	atrial flutter
AG	anion gap
AIDS	acquired immunodeficiency syndrome
AKI	acute kidney injury
ALI	acute lung injury
AMI	acute myocardial infarction
ARB	angiotensin receptor blocker
ARDS	acute respiratory distress syndrome
ARF	acute renal failure
ATN	acute tubular necrosis
AV	atrioventricular
AVB	atrioventricular Block
BNP	B-type natriuretic peptide
BP	blood pressure
BUN	blood ureanitrogen
CABG	coronary artery bypass grafting
CAD	coronary artery disease
cAMP	cyclic adenosine monophosphate
CBC	complete blood count
CBF	cerebral blood flow
CCB	calcium channel blocker
CHB	complete heart block
CHF	congestive heart failure
CI	cardiac index
CK	creatine kinase
CNS	central nervous system
CO	cardiac output
CO_2	carbon dioxide
COPD	chronic obstructive pulmonary disease
CPAP	continuous positive airway pressure
CPB	cardiopulmonary bypass
CPK	creatine phosphokinase
CPR	cardiopulmonary resuscitation
Cr	creatinine
CRP	C-reactive protein
CSF	cerebrospinal fluid
CT	computed tomography
CTA	computed tomography angiography
CVA	cerebrovascular accident
CVP	central venous pressure
CXR	chest x-ray
DBP	diastolic blood pressure
DCM	dilated cardiomyopathy
DIC	disseminated intravascular coagulation
DKA	diabetic ketoacidosis
DM	diabetes mellitus
DVT	deep venous thrombosis
ECG	electrocardiogram
ED	emergency department
EEG	electroencephalography
eFAST	extended focused abdominal sonography in trauma
EICU	emergency intensive care unit
EMS	emergency medical services
ESR	erythrocyte sedimentation rate
$ETco_2$	end-tidal carbon dioxide
ETT	endotracheal tube
FAST	focused assessment with sonography for trauma
FEV_1	forced expiratory volume in 1 second
FFP	fresh frozen plasma
FRC	functional residual capacity
GABA	γ-aminobutyric acid
GCS	Glasgow Coma Scale
GFR	glomerular filtration rate
HCO_3^-	bicarbonate ion.

HF	heart failure
HIV	human immunodeficiency virus
HR	heart rate
HTN	hypertension
ICH	intracerebral hemorrhage
ICP	intracranial pressure
ICU	intensive care unit
iPEEP	intrinsic positive end-expiratory pressure
ITP	idiopathic thrombocytopenic purpura
JT	junctional tachycardia
JVD	jugular venous distention
LBBB	left bundle branch block
LDH	lactate dehydrogenase
LMWH	low-molecular-weight heparin
LP	lumbar puncture
LV	left ventricule
LVA	left ventricular aneurysm
LVH	left ventricular hypertrophy
MAP	mean arterial pressure
MDCT	multidetector computed tomography
MI	myocardial infarction
MOF	multiorgan failure
MRA	magnetic resonance angiography
MRI	magnetic resonance imaging
NMBA	neuromuscular blocking agent
NO	nitric oxide
NP	natriuretic peptide
NSAID	nonsteroidal anti-inflammatory drug
NTG	nitroglycerin
NT-proBNP	amino-terminal pro-B-type natriuretic peptide
P_ACO_2	partial pressure of carbon dioxide in alveolus
P_aCO_2	partial pressure of carbon dioxide in arterial blood
P_aO_2	partial pressure of oxygen in the arterial blood
PCI	percutaneous coronary intervention
PE	pulmonary embolism
PEA	pulseless electrical activity
PEFR	peak expiratory flow rate
PPV	positive-pressure ventilation
PRBC	packed red blood cells
PTH	parathyroid hormone
PVC	premature ventricular contraction
RAAS	renin-angiotensinaldosterone system
RBBB	right bundle branch block
RBC	red blood cell
ROSC	return of spontaneous circulation
RSI	rapid sequence intubation
RV	right ventricle
SA	sinoatrial
SAH	subarachnoid hemorrhage
SaO_2	arterial oxygen saturation
SBO	small bowel obstruction
SBP	systolic blood pressure
SCD	sudden cardiac death
$ScvO_2$	central venous oxygen saturation
SIRS	systemic inflammatory response syndrome
SLE	systemic lupus erythematosus
SNS	sympathetic nervous system
STEMI	ST segment elevation MI
SV	stroke volume
SVT	supraventricular tachycardia
TB	tuberculosis
TEE	transesophageal echocardiography
TIA	transient ischemic attack
TTP	thrombotic thrombocytopenic purpura
UA	unstable angina
Vf	ventricular fibrillation
VILI	ventilator-induced lung injury
V_T	tidal volume
VT	ventricular tachycardia
WBC	white blood cell
WHO	World Health Organization

Contents
目 录

Pulmonary Emergencies

Gastrointestinal Emergencies

Renal Emergency

Hematologic Emergency

Metabolic Emergencies

Neurologic Emergencies

SECTION 3 Surgical Emergencies

SECTION 6 Toxinlogy Emergency

SECTION 7 Other Emergencies

SECTION 8 Pharmacotherapy of selected emergencies

SECTION 1

Selected Diagnosic and Therapeutic Techniques of Emergency Medicine

Dignostic Techniques

Chapter 1

Emergency Ultrasound

KEY CONCEPTS

EUS is the simultaneous performance and interpretation of a focused sonographic examination at the bedside of the patient for the diagnosis, resuscitation, monitoring, guidance, and treatment of emergency medical conditions.

The most common uses of EUS in decreasing order are trauma, cardiac (cardiac arrest and pericardial effusion), abdominal aortic aneurysm, pelvic, biliary, procedural, renal, and DVT.

FAST examination, originally focused on the detection of dependent peritoneal fluid and pleural effusion.

EUS guidance can assist many percutaneous procedures, such as vascular access, torso cavities evacuation,arthrocentesis, LP, abscess drainage, nerve blocks, and others.

PERSPECTIVE

Emergency ultrasound(EUS) is the simultaneous performance and interpretation of a focused sonographic examination at the bedside of the patient for the diagnosis, resuscitation, monitoring, guidance, and treatment of emergency medical conditions.

Not all pathologic processes will be detected by such examinations.

APPLIED ULTRASOUND PHYSICS AND INSTRUMENTATION

By definition,US is sound with frequencies higher than 20,000 Hz. US is kinetic energy, a longitudinal, mechanical, and directional wave.

US waves are characterized by their amplitude, wavelength, and frequency. Lower frequencies penetrate deeper tissue at the expense of resolution, whereas higher frequencies improve resolution but cannot penetrate deeper structures.

M-mode or motion mode displays received waves over both time and distance and is used to calculate rates, speeds, and distances by sending a steered one-dimensional line across tissue. The most familiar display is B-mode or brightness mode, which graphs the amplitude of reflected US waves as shades of gray from black to white on a monitor screen.

US resolution can be described as axial, in the long axis of the transducer, or lateral, perpendicular to the long axis of the transducer.The area from the probe to the focus is called the near field, and that from the focus to the end of the image is called the far field. The best imaging with maximum reduction in artifacts occurs at the focus.

Focal zones can be increased for more resolution, but frame rate will decrease, causing a slow-motion image that is poor for imaging of moving tissues.

Harmonics listens for multiples of the frequency sent out and often cleans up images near the screen, such as in the gallbladder, apex of the heart, or soft tissue of skin.

Doppler US shows the velocity of moving structures, typically red blood cells, thus representing flow. Color flow Doppler shows direction (by red or blue colors representing flow in opposite directions) and velocity of flow (by degrees of brightness of the color, where lighter is higher velocity). Power Doppler or power angiography describes only the presence of flow and not direction.

Other US terms and artifacts commonly used are listed in Box 1-1.

Box 1-1 Common Definitions

Window: soft tissue where transducer is placed to interrogate tissue in the body
Anechoic: without sounds (black)
Echogenic: with sounds (white)
Hyperechoic: with more reflected sounds than adjacent tissue(more echogenic)
Hypoechoic: with less sound than adjacent tissue (less echogenic)
Shadowing: sound blocked by a reflective barrier
Enhancement: more echogenicity due to increased velocity of sound, typically behind a fluid-filled structure, such as the bladder or gallbladder
Reverberation: an artifact that results from multiple reflections at a given interface, often in parallel
Mirror image: a propagation speed artifact that repeats images that are beyond a strong reflector (e.g., diaphragm), creating a mirror image
Lateral cystic shadowing: a refraction artifact seen on the edge of cystic structures, causing an artificial shadow
Beam width artifact: a volume-averaging artifact causing artifactual echoes in the inferior aspect of anechoic structures or spaces

EQUIPMENT AND SAFETY

A variety of US machines are available, including palm size, laptop, cart based, and combination devices.

Probe design and footprints can be divided into three categories: flat linear array probes, curved linear array probes, and phased array probes.Transesophageal echocardiographic, three-dimensional, and biplanar probes are recently being used in emergency US, creating new imaging venues.

The ALARA (as low as reasonably achievable) principle suggests that the least amount of energy be used to produce satisfactory imaging. Doppler modes should be minimized over sensitive tissue, including early gestation, germinal tissue, and mucosal or neural tissue. The thermal index should be kept below 2.0, and the mechanical index should be kept below 1.9.

APPLICATIONS AND CATEGORIZATION

Grouping of these US applications into categories of resuscitative, diagnostic, symptom or sign based, procedural guidance, and monitoring and therapeutic helps describe the relationship between the uses of US in emergency medicine (Table 1-1).

The most common uses of emergency US in decreasing order are trauma, cardiac (cardiac arrest and pericardial effusion), AAA, pelvic, biliary, procedural, renal, and DVT.

Table 1-1 Classification of Emergency Ultrasound Applications

RESUSCITATIVE	DIAGNOSTIC	SYMPTOM OR SIGN BASED	PROCEDURAL GUIDANCE	MONITORING AND THERAPEUTIC
Cardiac	Cardiac	Hypotension	Any emergency medicine procedure	Central vein size
Trauma	FAST	Dyspnea		Fluid collections
Abdominal aorta	Pregnancy	Chest pain		Cardiac contractility
Pregnancy	AAA	Abdominal pain		Fetal heart rate
Thoracic	Biliary	Extremity pain		Low-frequency clot dissolution
Procedural	Urinary tract			
	DVT			
	Soft tissue and musculoskeletal			
	Thoracic			
	Ocular			
	Advanced uses			
	New uses			

Trauma Ultrasound

The trauma US examination , also called the FAST examination, originally focused on the detection of dependent peritoneal fluid and pleural effusion. Newer versions include the EFAST (extended FAST) for the evaluation of potential pneumothorax and FAST for evaluation of the extremities.

The volume of fluid required for a positive US study depends on the site of injury and site of sonographic detection, but 250 mL or more is generally visible, and nearly 600 mL of fluid is necessary to cause a positive flank stripe when fluid is infused from the pelvis.

In general, 50 mL of pericardial fluid is required to cause hemodynamic compromise in a patient without prior pericardial inflammation. However, tears in the pericardium that communicate with the pleural space or even the peritoneum can cause false-negative examination findings.

Pleural fluid can be detected by US, but this depends on the position of the body. Pneumothorax detection is based on the absence of the normal sonographic sliding of the visceral and parietal pleurae.

Typically, fluid in the peritoneum, pericardium, and pleural cavity is anechoic, but it can have echogenicity with clotting, depending on the age of the clot or bowel contents.

The FAST technique uses a low- to middle-frequency probe (2-5 MHz). Within the peritoneum, dependent spaces include the following, grouped by tissue window: the right flank, which evaluates the hepatorenal space (also called Morison's pouch; Fig. 1-1), the right subphrenic space, and the right costophrenic angle; the left flank, which evaluates the perisplenic space between the diaphragm and spleen, the splenorenal space, the perirenal space, and the left subphrenic space; and the suprapubic view, which is performed by placement of the transducer superior to the pubic bone with a full bladder to visualize the pouch of Douglas in women and the retrovesical space in men. Extra views include the paracolic gutters inferior from the flank views and medial from the iliac spine to visualize free fluid surrounding the bowel.

The typical cardiac views include the transverse subcostal images, which visualize the four cardiac chambers and pericardial space, and the sagittal subcostal view to assess the pericardial space and the collapsibility and diameter of the IVC, indicating right-sided heart pressures.

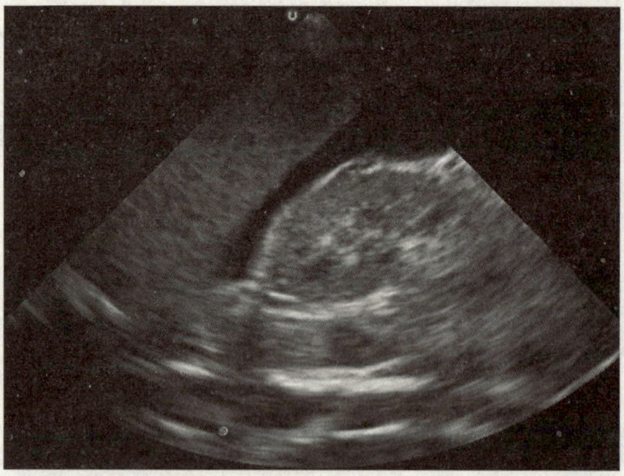

Fig. 1-1 Free fluid in the peritoneum in Morison's pouch seen from right flank.

For pleural fluid, the superiorly angled flank views allow visualization of the costophrenic angles. The evaluation for pneumothorax uses either a low-frequency probe at a shallow depth or, more typically, a high-frequency probe for better resolution, placed at the anterior chest in the second intercostal space for anterior pneumothorax and at the axilla for large pneumothoraces and pleural effusion. Diaphragm injuries have been described with dislocation of typical organ patterns.

The sensitivity of the FAST examination ranges from 60% to 99%, and its specificity ranges from 80% to 99%.

US can diagnose pneumothorax with excellent sensitivity and specificity compared with plain chest radiography and variable accuracy compared with CT scanning.

There are certain populations of patients in whom FAST evaluation has limited benefit.In patients with purely anterior penetrating trauma to the abdomen, the sensitivity of trauma US is poor because bowel injuries can occur without significant hemoperitoneum.

With pelvic fractures, the sensitivity ranges from 20% to 80%. More important, the detection of free fluid in an unstable patient with a pelvic fracture may be due to uroperitoneum from bladder injury rather than hemoperitoneum from vascular injury.In addition, retroperitoneal injuries to the genitourinary tract are not assessed with four-quadrant FAST examination.

Pelvic Ultrasound

Typically, pelvic US is used to confirm intrauterine pregnancy, which indirectly excludes ectopic pregnancy in most patients. Another use during pregnancy is the detection of fetal viability, incomplete abortion, ectopic pregnancy, and molar pregnancy. Pelvic US is used in nonpregnancy states to detect tubo-ovarian abscesses, masses, and hemoperitoneum in the hemodynamically unstable patient.

Indications for sonographic evaluation of the first-trimester pregnant patient include symptoms or signs that suggest an ectopic pregnancy, molar pregnancy, or fetal demise and dating of the pregnancy. Intrauterine pregnancy is confirmed with a gestational sac with a yolk sac or fetal pole within the fundus of the uterus (Fig. 1-2). An embryonic or fetal demise has US findings of a fetal pole measuring more than 5 mm without fetal heart rate or a gestational sac of more than 20 mm in diameter without a fetal pole. A molar pregnancy appears as an echogenic, cystic uterus with disorganized echoes and is associated with high β-human chorionic gonadotropin concentrations without the sonographic finding of intrauterine pregnancy. Findings of an ectopic pregnancy include a chorionic ring or gestational sac with evidence of a yolk sac or fetal pole outside the uterus or in an abnormal location in the uterus, such as the cornu or cervix.In addition, there is a class called indeterminate, which may account for 20% of pregnant patients presenting to the ED in the first and early second trimesters. Heterotopic pregnancies can occur at a rate of 1/5000 and be detected by the same techniques and definitions.

Pelvic US is performed by transabdominal or endovaginal techniques. The transabdominal technique uses a low-frequency transabdominal transducer placed over the lower abdomen suprapubically. Ideally, the patient has a full bladder, which provides a sonographic window, but this may not be necessary if the uterus is large or the patient is thin. In the endovaginal technique, the transducer is placed in the vagina, optimally with an empty bladder to visualize the same structures. Endovaginal transducers are high frequency, providing excellent axial resolution but poor penetration of distant structures with more accuracy. Endovaginal US can detect small (7 mL) amounts of peritoneal fluid. Endovaginal US in the hemodynamically compromised patient has replaced culdocentesis for detection of ruptured ectopic pregnancy.

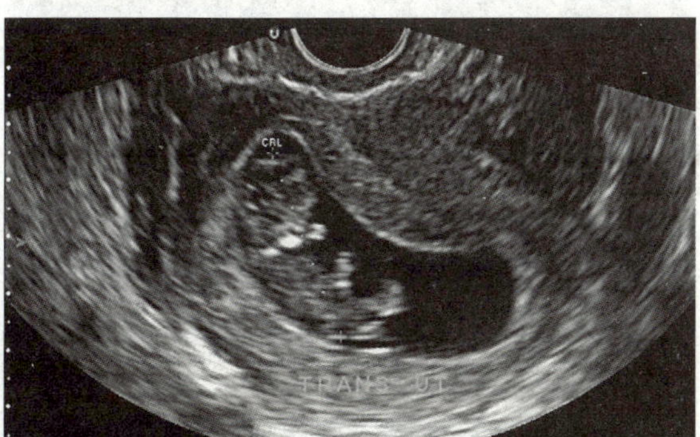

Fig. 1-2 Intrauterine pregnancy with fetus on endovaginal scanning.

The gynecologic differential diagnosis of significant free fluid in a pregnant woman, in addition to ectopic pregnancy, should include uterine rupture and ruptured corpus luteum pregnancy. Pelvic US in nonpregnancy states has shown good accuracy for tuboovarian abscess and improved decision-making for female patients with right lower abdominal pain.

Cardiac Ultrasound

The use of cardiac US by emergency physicians is presentation and symptom specific and focused in nature. Indications include cardiac arrest, possible pericardial effusion, trauma, chest pain, hypotension, and procedural guidance. Cardiac US is often included in algorithms and protocols for certain symptoms or signs, such as dyspnea or hypotension.

Cardiac US is performed through the transthoracic and transabdominal windows with use of small curvilinear or phased array transducers. Typical views include the subcostal four-chamber and long-axis views, parasternal long-axis view, parasternal short-axis view, and apical four-chamber view. In addition, the apical four-chamber view provides excellent comparison of the right and left ventricles in terms of size and function. The long-axis subcostal view shows some of the right side of the heart but highlights the IVC, including size and respiratory variation.

Cardiac US shows good accuracy in detection of pericardial effusion (Fig. 1-3), assessment of left ventricular function, and evaluation of patients with undifferentiated shock. In addition, aspects of cardiac US are being used for the assessment of intravascular volume status and cardiac output and in the

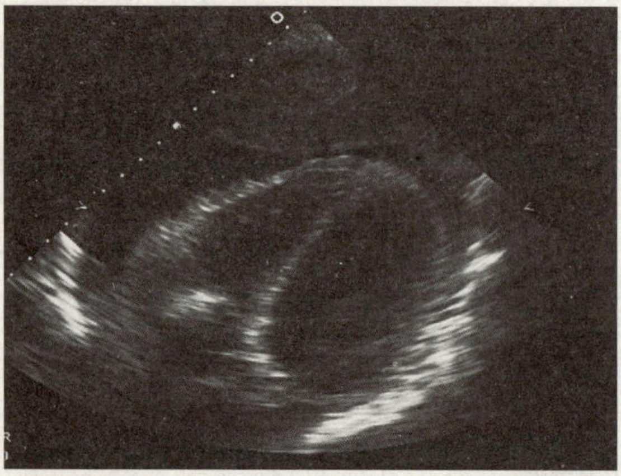

Fig. 1-3 Pericardial effusion in subcostal view.

evaluation of dyspnea.

In cardiac arrest, US can detect ventricular motion in both asystole and PEA.In asystole, the prognosis is poor in the absence of sonographic ventricular activity. Cardiac US can detect pseudoasystole by revealing Vf or coordinated cardiac contractions without a palpable pulse. Use of cardiac US in PEA and near-PEA states can be diagnostic for pericardial effusion. Cardiac US can detect ventricular capture when the patient is paced, transcutaneously or by a transvenous pacer. US can also identify pneumothorax, another treatable cause of cardiac arrest. Cardiac US is feasible during pulse checks and prehospital life support, as advanced cardiac life support guidelines suggest minimizing non-cardiopulmonary resuscitation intervals.

Emergency cardiac US is diagnostic for both medical and traumatic pericardial effusions with excellent accuracy.

Cardiac US is used for detection of pericardial effusions, chamber enlargement, and global activity in chest pain syndromes for the evaluation of pericardial tamponade, pulmonary embolus, cardiogenic shock, aortic dissection, pneumothorax, and bony chest wall fracture.

US protocols have been developed to evaluate undifferentiated hypotension. Cardiac US windows with the addition of abdominal views can assess for effusion, global ventricular activity, ventricular chamber size, IVC size and respiratory change, peritoneal fluid, and AAA to narrow the differential diagnosis. Sepsis is the most common diagnosis for patients with hyperdynamic ventricular activity.

Central pressures can be estimated by examination of the IVC size and collapsibility. This technique has good accuracy in assessment of blood loss, hypovolemia, and CHF.

Cardiac US is also a procedural guide for placement of transvenous pacer wires and for pericardiocentesis.

Abdominal Vascular Ultrasound

Emergency physicians use abdominal US to detect AAA, another silent disease in patients with flank, abdominal, or back pain, and to evaluate unexplained hypotension in the older patient. The use of US to detect aortic dissection and occlusion is described as well.

The technique involves imaging of the aorta from the subxiphoid space to the umbilicus to evaluate for dilation above a diameter of 3 cm (Fig. 1-4). For the detection of infrarenal aneurysms, the technique should visualize the aorta from the diaphragm to the aortic bifurcation. Fusiform aneurysms are more common, but detection of saccular aneurysms requires both the transverse and longitudinal planes. If an aneurysm is found, a peritoneal view of Morison's pouch is performed to detect intraperitoneal fluid. Proximal iliac arteries may be followed if it is technically feasible or time allows.

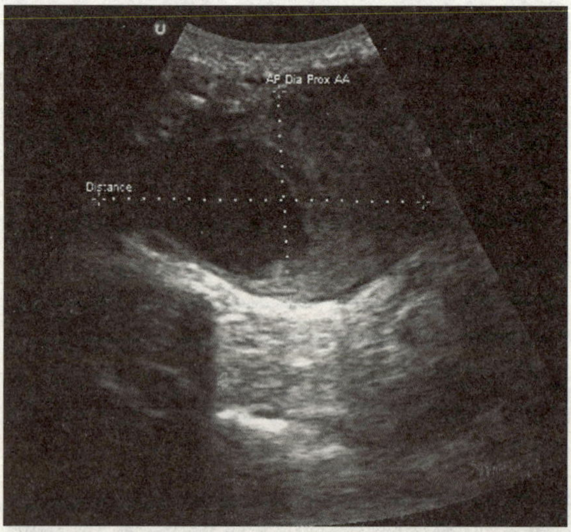

Fig. 1-4 Large AAA with echogenic intraluminal clot.

Emergency physician use of US for AAA detection has shown good accuracy compared with other imaging modalities and laparotomy.

Aortic dissection may be detected by a combination of abdominal and cardiac scanning. A linear echogenic flap, anywhere across the lumen of the aorta, is suggestive of dissection, sometimes with the detection of different flows on either side of the flap by color Doppler scanning. The cardiac US examination can show unexplained pericardial effusion; a dilated aortic root; aortic insufficiency; and a linear echogenic flap seen in the ascending aorta, aortic arch , or descending aorta.

Aortic occlusion is another condition that may be detected by US. Echogenic thrombus may fill the aorta and disrupt perfusion below the diaphragm. Clear identification of the borders and lack of Doppler flow in the abdominal aorta are characteristic of the syndrome.

Biliary Ultrasound

Biliary US to detect gallstones and associated cholecystitis was one of the early applications of US in emergency medicine. The sonographic technique involves a modified biplanar approach to the right upper quadrant. A complete evaluation includes visualization of the common bile duct. The diagnosis of cholelithiasis is made after identification of echogenic foci within the gallbladder lumen with shadowing (Fig. 1-5). Other image patterns include stones that will not shadow, sludge, and the wall echo sign of a gallbladder full of gallstones. Signs of cholecystitis include a dilated gallbladder, increased gallbladder wall thickness, sonographic Murphy's sign, and pericholecystic fluid. A nonmobile stone in the gallbladder neck is highly suggestive of eventual cholecystitis. Biliary US is fast and accurate, with a sensitivity of 87% to 94% and a specificity of 82% to 96% in detection of gallstones, comparable to radiology ultrasonography. Biliary US has replaced nuclear medicine testing.

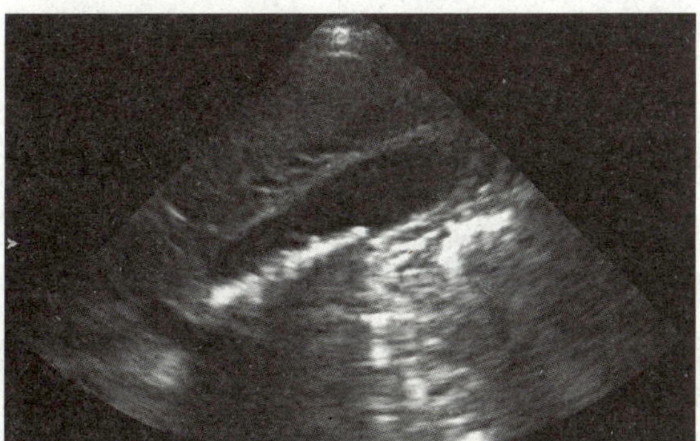

Fig. 1-5 Echogenic layering gallstones seen in gallbladder with posterior shadowing.

Urinary Tract Ultrasound

Renal or urinary tract US can detect hydronephrosis or urinary retention.

Renal US includes biplanar views of the kidneys with emphasis on dilation of the calyceal system and pelvis of the respective kidney (Fig. 1-6). In addition, visualization of the bladder can diagnose secondary hydronephrosis from an obstructed bladder stone and may demonstrate nonobstructive bladder jets through the use of Doppler US. The windows for the two kidneys are similar to those of the trauma flank series, with the exception that the patient may be rolled on the opposite side so that the transducer may be placed more posteriorly on the back if necessary. The bladder view is performed suprapubically, and calculations of volume may be made with on-machine calculators or by formula.

Renal US has a sensitivity of 83% and a specificity of 92% in detection of hydronephrosis (Fig. 1-6). Bladder US is useful for detection of a full bladder and the presence of a Foley catheter and for guidance during suprapubic aspiration or Foley placement.

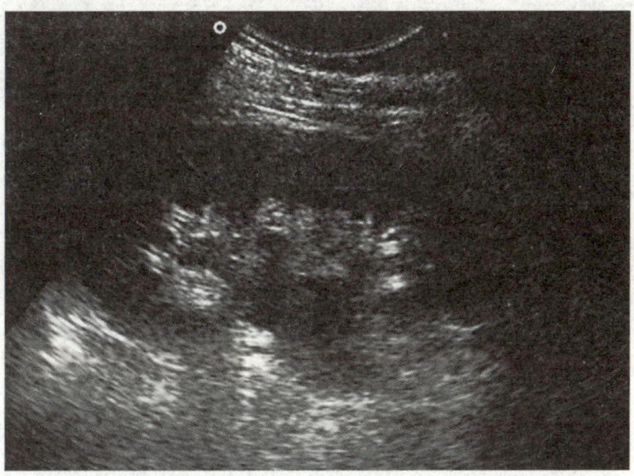

Fig. 1-6 Hydronephrosis in renal pelvis and calyces.

Deep Venous Thrombosis Ultrasound

The swollen extremity often requires sonographic imaging to assess for DVT. Emergency physicians commonly use compression US to rule out DVT. The two-level compression technique involves visualization of the compressibility of the common femoral and popliteal veins. The three-level technique adds the junction of the superficial femoral and deep femoral veins (Fig. 1-7). Use of upper extremity veins is less common because Doppler US is needed for the subclavian vein, which is not compressible under the clavicle.The accuracy of this technique ranges from 70% to 99%, depending on operator experience.

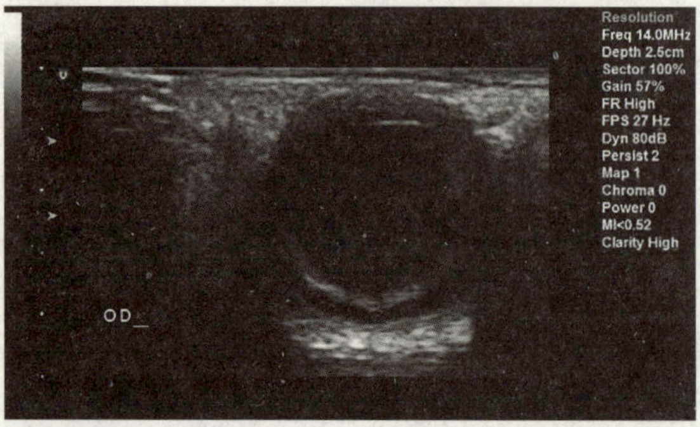

Fig. 1-7 DVT with layering clot in popliteal vein seen on compression US examination.

Thoracic and Tracheal Ultrasound

Thoracic applications include the detection of pleural effusion, pneumothorax, pneumonia, and interstitial edema. The technique of thoracic US uses a low-frequency probe to survey for pleural effusions and a high-frequency probe to detect pleurallines and related artifacts. Pleural fluid appears as an anechoic collection above the diaphragm (Fig. 1-8). In addition, a collapsed lung may be visualized as an echogenic floating structure. Normally, the parietal and visceral pleural lines slide against each other, and lack of sliding is the finding most consistent with pneumothorax (on M-mode, called the seashore sign). Additional findings of pneumothorax include the presence of horizontal artifacts called A-lines (on M-mode, called the stratosphere sign) and the absence of B-lines (vertical white lines from reverberation of air with fluid) at the parietal-visceral pleural line (Fig. 1-9). Confounding factors include adhesions of the pleura, COPD, prior pneumothorax, and mainstem bronchus intubation. A lung point sign is the edge of the pneumothorax where the lung is still adherent to the parietal pleura, and part of the image shows no sliding until the lung moves into the interspace with respirations. The accuracy of US for detection of pneumothorax (sensitivity 100%, specificity 98%) is better than that of plain chest radiography in the acute setting, but there may be reduced accuracy after 24 hr.

Severe pneumonia is visualized as echogenic "liver-like" echogenicity as the lung accumulates fluid with consolidation. Peripneumonic collections are common and may indicate inflammation. The

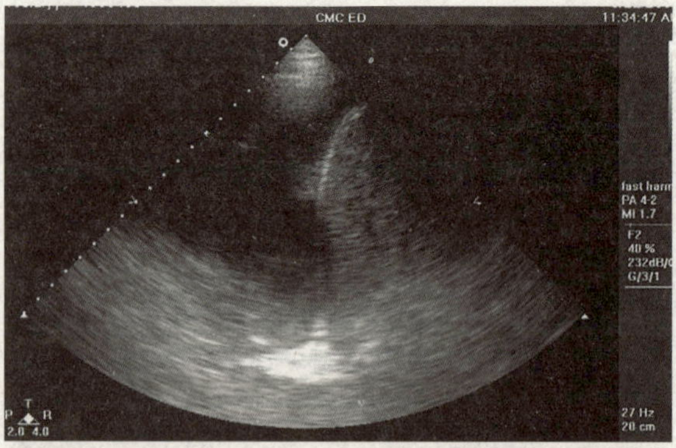

Fig. 1-8 Large pleural effusin.

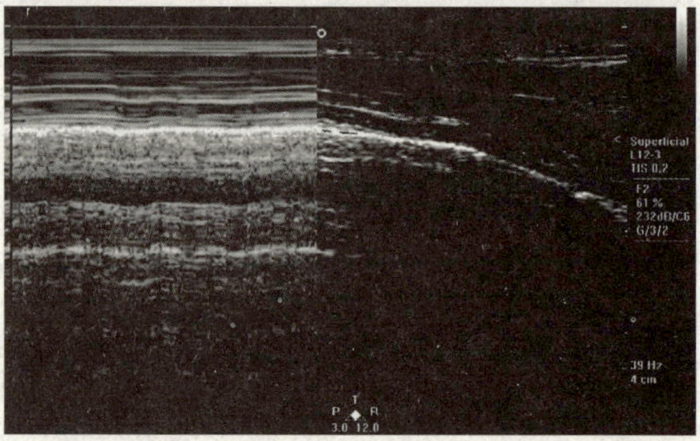

Fig. 1-9 M-mode image of normal lung sliding.

dynamic air bronchogram, hyperechoic areas within bronchi that move with respiration, usually within "heparinized" lung, has been described as another sign of alveolar consolidation. Pulmonary edema is indicated by the presence of comet tails (B-lines), which are reverberation artifacts that reflect from the parietal pleural interface into the lung. Normally found in dependent areas of the lung, the widespread distribution of these artifacts in an apical lung may indicate increased lung congestion. Dynamic tracheal US for the confirmation of endotracheal intubation has relatively good sensitivity and specificity, but static US seems to lack accuracy. This technique may have a role in patients in cardiac arrest or with equivocal $ETco_2$ levels.

Ocular Ultrasound

The eye is an excellent acoustic window, and short-duration gray scale US over a closed eyelid can visualize both the anterior and the posterior chamber well. Ocular US has been described for intraocular disease, such as retinal detachment, retinal hemorrhage,vitreal hemorrhage, intraocular foreign body, dislocated lens, and retro-orbital hemorrhage. The sensitivity of ocular US for retinal detachment by emergency physicians is 100%, and the specificity is 83% to 92%. In addition, the optic nerve sheath diameter can be measured behind the eye, reflecting intracranial pressure. The sensitivity of such measurements ranges from 83% in children to 100% in adults.

Soft Tissue Ultrasound

Soft tissue US is used to differentiate cellulitis from abscess,to detect foreign bodies and hernias,and to evaluate other soft tissue pathologic processes, including masses, pseudoaneurysms, and glands. A high-frequency linear transducer moves from normal skin to the abnormal area. Cellulitis or edema will cause an echogenic pattern with cobblestoning between fat lobules (Fig. 1-10). Abscesses are irregular hypoechoic to anechoic collections within the subcutaneous layer but may connect with the surface (Fig. 1-11). US is diagnostic in soft tissue disease for cellulitis, abscess, and necrotizing fasciitis.

US can differentiate peritonsillar abscess from cellulitis and can be used for guidance of peritonsillar aspiration. It can also detect early Ludwig's angina

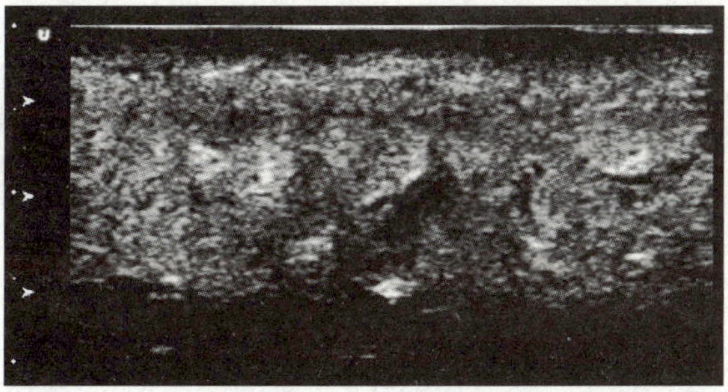

Fig. 1-10 Sonographic cellulitis with echogenic subcutaneous tisse.

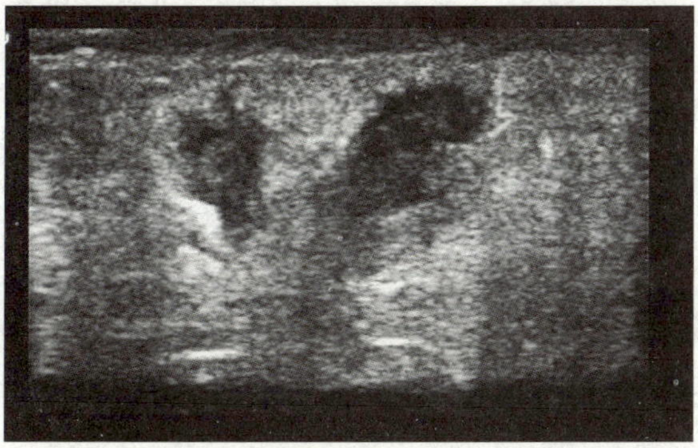

Fig. 1-11 Sonographic subcutaneous abscess.

with abscess, dental abscess, epiglottitis, glandular abnormalities, and pseudoaneurysm in soft tissues and fascia of the face. US has also been used in various body areas, including the penis and scrotum, for signs of disruption or infection.

Detection of foreign bodies is characterized by variable echogenicity in the tissue with shadowing beneath the foreign body. Metal foreign bodies, such as bullets and intrauterine devices, have characteristically high-reflective echogenicity and ring-down artifacts.

Musculoskeletal Ultrasound

US has been particularly useful for joint effusion and muscle, tendon, and bone injury. US is excellent for detection of fluid in joints, confirmation of effusions, and guidance of drainage procedures. Joint effusions typically are anechoic or echogenic, depending on type and age.

Diagnosis of ligamentous injuries and muscle avulsion and hemorrhage has also been reported. Muscle and tendon abnormalities are detected by anechoic and heterogeneous abnormalities.

Fractures are seen as a defect in the bony cortex.

US is accurate in the detection of fractures, joint effusions, bursitis, cysts, and hematomas.

Transcranial Doppler Ultrasound

Transcranial Doppler US has been used for detection of abnormal flow patterns in the brain and for detection and treatment of middle cerebral artery strokes.

Testicular Ultrasound

Testicular scanning is an advanced US application that requires visualization of the normal and symptomatic testicle with a high-frequency probe. Absent or decreased flow on the affected side indicates possible torsion, whereas increased flow indicates epididymitis.

Abdominal Bowel Ultrasound

The use of bedside US for evaluation of appendicitis, diverticulitis, and other bowel disease is an area of increasing interest. There has been variable experience with the use of graded compression US to detect appendicitis (>6 mm), with reported sensitivity of 67% and specificity of 92% (Fig. 1-12).In women, endovaginal US can be used to rule out adnexal

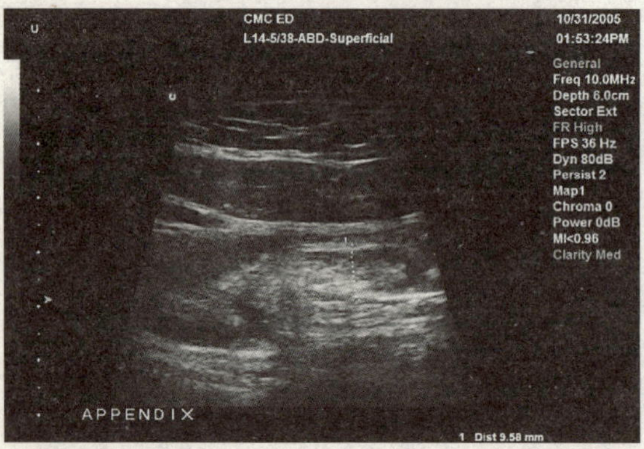

Fig. 1-12 Image of noncompressible appendix compatible with appendicitis.

disease.

The use of US for diverticulitis, intussusception, volvulus, and SBO has been reported. Thickening of the bowel, dilated bowel with fluid-filled loops, and changes invascularity suggest disease.

Hernias, described in the soft tissue section, may also be detected as masses in the ventral, inguinal, paramedian, femoral, and scrotal areas.

Ultrasound for Procedural Guidance

The use of US for procedural guidance has expanded for many emergency procedures, especially vascular access, and is advocated for error reduction.

Procedural guidance can be static or dynamic. Static guidance suggests that US has been placed over the anatomic area, and the area is marked while angle and distance information is noted. Dynamic guidance describes procedures performed with real-time US visualization of the needle entering the anatomic area on the monitor as well as on the patient.

There are two common axis approaches to vein cannulation: transverse, in which the vein appears as a circular structure on the screen; and longitudinal, in which the vein appears as a tubular structure along the width of the screen. In the transverse approach, the probe's long axis is centered transverse to the long axis of the anatomic area, guiding the needle to bisect the probe at its center, which gives centering and depth information (Fig. 1-13). In the longitudinal axis , the probe is placed along the long axis of the anatomic area, and the needle is introduced in the long axis of the probe, giving depth and trajectory information (Fig. 1-14). Finally, an oblique axis has been described, essentially approaching the vessels at 45 degrees but visualizing the target vessels and surrounding structures.

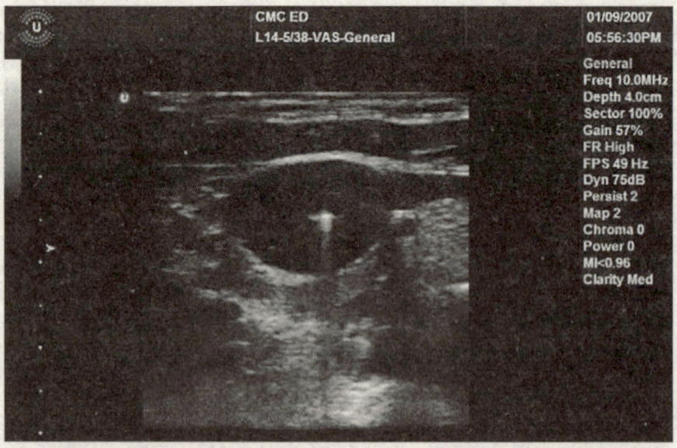

Fig. 1-13 Transverse image of internal jugular vein for procedural guidance.

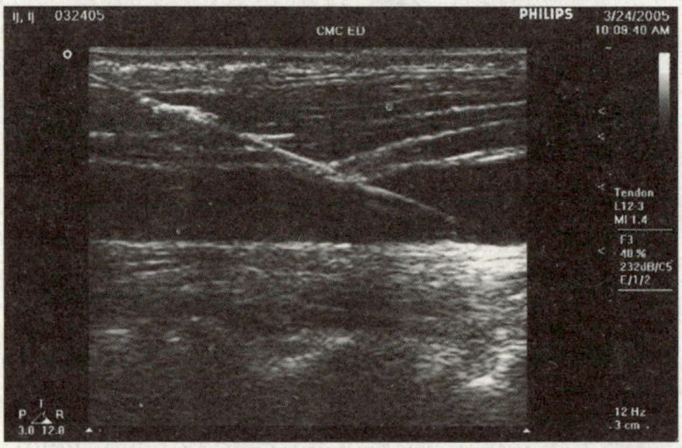

Fig. 1-14 Longitudinal image of the needle in an internal jugular vein for procedural guidance.

The most studied and most advocated use of US procedural guidance is for central line insertion. US guidance for internal jugular central line insertion can be recommended as a safe and best practice.

US permits the physician to assess the internal jugular for overlap with the carotid artery, vessel diameter, and presence of luminal clot or vessel obliteration.

US does not prevent posterior vein wall penetration as reported in case reports and simulated models. Adverse events (hematoma, arterial cannulation, pneumothorax, and unsuccessful placement) can occur in up to 20% of patients having US-guided internal jugular catheterization.

Femoral vein insertion has been studied in cardiac arrest patients, and improved cannulation rate and reduced complications have been reported.

US does not contribute to procedural success in subclavian vein cannulation because of the lack of a convenient window for the subclavian vein under the clavicle.The supraclavicular fossa is a window for central line insertion.

Emergency physicians are able to use US to insert peripheral intravenous catheters in patients with difficult access with high success rates. Veins that are large in width (0.4 cm) or at moderate depth (0.3-1.5 cm) have a higher success rate.

Sonographic confirmation of intraosseous placement has also been described with detection of Doppler flow outside the bone and inside the marrow. Numerous other procedures using US guidance have been described in emergency practice (Table 1-2).

Table 1-2 Ultrasound-Guided Emergency Procedures

ULTRASOUND	PROCEDURE
Vascular access	Central venous access Internal jugular vein Subclavian near axillary vein Subclavian with supraclavicular approach Femoral vein Peripheral vein Basilic Brachial Cephalic Forearm veins Intraosseous needle Arterial cannulation Radial artery Arterial sampling
Torso fluid collections	Paracentesis Thoracentesis Pericardiocentesis
Cardiac	Pacer placement
Musculoskeletal	Arthrocentesis Hip Knee Other joints Fracture reduction Foreign body removal Tendon sheath injection
Soft tissue	Abscess drainage Hernia reduction
Anesthesia	Interscalene Peripheral nerves Axillary Femoral nerve Hematoma block
Airway	Endotracheal tube placement
Urinary bladder	Suprapubic aspiration and cystostomy Foley guidance
Neurologic	LP

Out-of-Hospital Ultrasound: Disasters and Remote Settings

US has been used in the out-of-hospital, military battlefield, disaster, and international medicine settings. The use of US has been described in European and other settings by physicians in the out-of-hospital arena, including ground, helicopter, air, and space, and by paramedics for FAST and abdominal aorta examinations.

INTEGRATION INTO EMERGENCY MEDICINE PRACTICE

US has been integrated into emergency medicine practice because of the need for effective, noninvasive, nonpainful, portable imaging techniques. US is a skill that requires constant attention with hands-on practice and interpretation. Emergency US, the performance and interpretation of ultrasonographic examination at the bedside in the emergency setting, has enhanced many aspects of emergency care, making diagnosis and treatment more rapid, efficient, safe, and accurate.

(CHAI Yanfen LIU Chenyan)

Chapter 2

Monitoring the Emergency Patient

KEY CONCEPTS

Monitoring modalities, when used appropriately, help to identify the effectiveness of interventions, predict deterioration, track the patient's clinical course, and inform clinical decision-making.

Capnography supplements oximetry by providing useful information regarding pathologic conditions and response to therapy.

Continuous monitoring can advance patient safety in select patients. Alarm limits should be adjusted to ensure reasonable warnings are delivered, optimally reducing the number of false alarms.

PERSPECTIVE

Monitoring is a routine part of ED care. From vital sign measurement to the provision of critical care, monitoring physiologic function provides clinicians with potentially relevant clinical information as a "snapshot" in time.

This chapter focuses on the following monitoring modalities: noninvasive BP measurement, pulse oximetry, and ventilation monitoring and the use of $ETco_2$ measurement.

NONINVASIVE BLOOD PRESSURE MEASUREMENT

BP measurement by sphygmomanometer is the most common method of noninvasively measuring arterial pressure by indirectly measuring SBP, DBP, MAP, and pulse pressure. Therefore BP closely represents the interplay of CO and overall systemic vascular resistance, making it an important screening and monitoring tool in ED patients.

Traditional BP measurement by sphygmomanometer can be obtained by Doppler, palpation, auscultation, and oscillometric methods. Palpation allows for only BP determination ,and generally is used only in noisy environments (such as EMS transport). Doppler is particularly helpful in identifying the presence of a systolic pulse in hypotensive individuals or in internally or externally (i.e., compartment syndrome) flow-limited extremities. Auscultation, otherwise known as "manual" BP measurement, remains a common, reliable, and reproducible method of BP measurement 100 yr after the Korotkoff technique was discovered.

This method relies on placing the stethoscope at the antecubital fossa, inflating the BP cuff, and recording the pressure at which auscultation of the pulse returns (SBP) and when it disappears (DBP). Auscultation is generally considered to underestimate the SBP and overestimate DBP. The oscillometric technique measures oscillations in the pressure during deflation of the cuff; the maximal point of oscillation represents MAP. This is the most common noninvasive method of measuring BP in the ED, commonly called the "automatic" BP. The quality of the device, cuff size, body positioning, and arm positioning are all components of Cuff-based BP measuring technique that can affect the accuracy. Clinical circumstances such as obesity, dysrhythmias, and extremes of age (young children and elderly) may also affect the accuracy.

Newer continuous, noninvasive BP monitors have the advantage of providing additional advanced hemodynamic measures, such as SV and CO.

The gold standard, and the most accurate method of measuring BP, remains the intra-arterial catheter. Common situations in which invasive arterial monitoring may be of benefit include (1) anticipated hemodynamic instability, (2) monitoring of conditions or treatments that result in large fluid or BP shifts, (3) frequent arterial blood sampling, and (4) expected inaccuracies in noninvasive BP management (e.g., because of obesity or dysrhythmias).

PULSE OXIMETRY

Pulse oximetry provides a real-time assessment of the effectiveness of interventions and disease progression as related to oxygenation. Its use has become so widespread as both a screening and monitoring tool that it is frequently regarded as the "fifth vital sign."

Pulse oximetry measures the percentage of arterial hemoglobin that is in the oxyhemoglobin state. It reflects the amount of oxygen that hemoglobin is carrying as a percent of the maximum it can carry; this is commonly referred to as the percent SaO_2. SaO_2 represents by far the larger reservoir of blood. The relationship between SaO_2 and P_aO_2 is described by the oxyhemoglobin dissociation curve. Although the two measures correlate well, their relationship is nonlinear. Users should be aware that large changes in the SaO_2 occur with small changes in the P_aO_2 in hypoxic patients, pulse oximeters are generally accurate between 80% and 100%. Measurements can be made on the ears or fingers, although the fingers are generally better in patients with poor perfusion.

Pulse oximetry is largely used in initial triage of patients, particularly those with cardiopulmonary complaints, or in the monitoring and management of patients who are sedated or critically ill, particularly with respiratory distress or during endotracheal intubation. SaO_2 values at or below 96% have been shown to be 100% sensitive for detection of hypoxia (P_aO_2 < 70 torr), but such a cutoff can be different in patients with obstructive lung disease.

Pulse oximetry has several important clinical limitations. By design, pulse oximetry measures only two wavelengths. At these wavelengths, traditional pulse oximeters are unable to distinguish oxyhemoglobin and deoxyhemoglobin from two other important dyshemoglobinemias: methemoglobin (MetHb) and carboxyhemoglobin (COHb). Multiwavelength CO-oximeters are now available that can distinguish the four wavelengths. Oxygen saturation by pulse oximetry will be equivalent to actual saturation, presuming insignificant amounts of MetHb and COHb exist in the blood.In heavy smokers, COHb levels of 3% to 15% can commonly be found, but this has little impact on the accuracy of the SaO_2.Averaging saturation measurements over several seconds limits the impact of motion artifact and improves the accuracy.

SaO_2 does not aid in determining the adequacy of ventilation when significant hypercapnia may precede hypoxia and supplemental oxygen may mask hypoventilation. For this situation, one needs ventilation monitoring through $ETco_2$ measurement.

END-TIDAL CARBON DIOXIDE MONITORING

The concentration of CO_2 in an exhaled breath is intrinsically linked to tissue metabolism, systemic circulation, and ventilation. Capnography is the graphic record, represented as a waveform, or capnogram, of the instantaneous CO_2 concentrations in respired gases during a respiratory cycle. Capnography provides continuous, real-time, breath-to-breath feedback on the clinical status of the patient, allowing the clinician to determine the baseline ventilatory status and to track changes over time. Although the concentrations of CO_2 can be displayed continuously throughout the respiratory cycle, by convention only the maximum CO_2 concentration at the end of each tidal breath, the $ETco_2$, is ordinarily displayed. Capnometry is the quantitative measurement of $ETco_2$ displayed as a number without a waveform. Colorimetric detectors use color scales to estimate ranges of $ETco_2$ but are not sufficiently accurate to give quantitative measurements. Their use is therefore limited to confirmation of correct ETT placement and its continuous location in the trachea.$ETco_2$ monitoring has now become a standard monitoring modality in the ED and nonhospital medical setting.

CO_2 monitors are configured as either sidestream or mainstream, depending on the location of the photoelectric detector or sensor. Mainstream devices measure CO_2 directly from the airway, with the sensor attached directly to the ETT. Sidestream devices, more commonly used by EMS personnel and in the ED, aspirate a sample of gas through tubing into a sensor located inside the monitor and are used for both intubated and nonintubated patients.

In patients with normal cardiopulmonary function, there is a close correlation between P_ACO_2 and P_aCO_2. The $ETco_2$ is usually 2 to 5 mmHg less than the P_aCO_2 because of the dilution of the end-tidal gases by physiologic dead space gas. Conditions that affect ventilation-perfusion ratios, cardiac arrest, hypovolemia, obstructive lung disease, and the lateral decubitus position can widen the Pa-$ETco_2$ gradient. Although $ETco_2$ may not accurately reflect the absolute P_aCO_2 in critically ill patients, it is still valuable in detecting ventilatory trends and identifying sudden airway events.

A normal capnogram has four phases (Fig. 2-1A). Phase 1-2 represents a CO_2-free portion of the respiratory cycle. Most often this is the inspiratory phse.

Phase 2-3, the rapid upstroke of the curve, represents the transition from inspiration to expiration and the mixing of dead space and alveolar gas. Prolongation of phase 2-3 (Fig. 2-1B) occurs with obstruction to expiratory gas flow (e.g., obstructive lung disease, bronchospasm, kinked ETT) or leaks in the breathing system.

Phase 3-4, the alveolar plateau, represents the predominance of CO_2-rich alveolar gas in the breath stream and tends to slope gently upward with the uneven emptying of alveoli. Point 4 (the $ETco_2$) represents the maximum CO_2 concentration in each breath and is the number that appears on the monitor. The slope of this phase can be increased by the same obstructive factors that increase the slope of phase 2-3 and is also a normal physiologic variation in pregnancy.A dip in the plateau indicates a spontaneous respiratory effort during mechanical ventilation, as in hypoxia, hypercarbia, or inadequate anesthesia (Fig. 2-1C).

Phase 4-5, the inspiratory downstroke, is a nearly vertical drop to baseline. This slope can be prolonged and blend in with the expiratory phase in endotracheal cuff leaks (Fig. 2-1D). Abnormal respiratory patterns that are fast or chaotic limit the usefulness of $ETco_2$ monitoring because characteristic waveform patterns are difficult to discern.

Capnography is an extremely valuable monitoring modality for intubated patients, providing information regarding respiratory function and immediate notification of accidental extubation. It can be used to confirm ETT placement in the trachea, continuously monitor tube position in the trachea during transport, provide qualitative and quantitative methods of

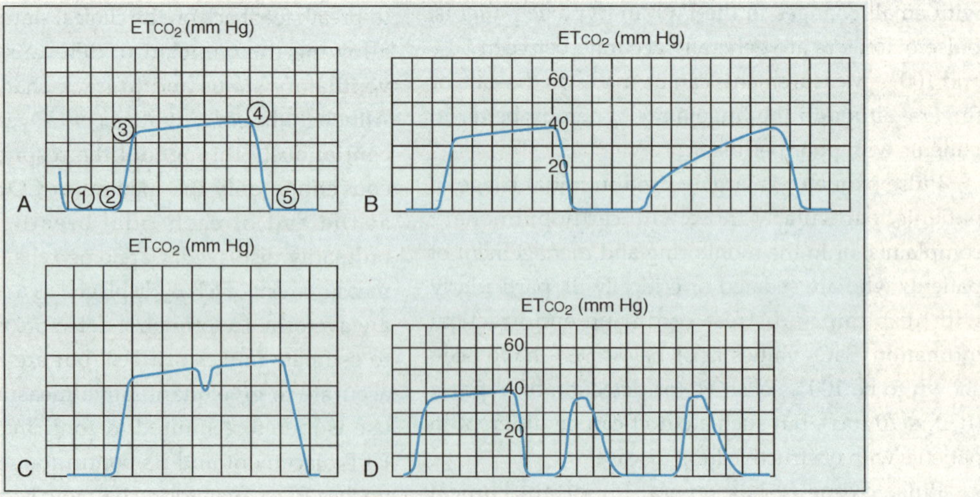

Fig. 2-1 A. Four phases of a normal capnogram. 1-2, The carbon dioxide–free portion of the respiratory cycle. 2-3, The rapid upstroke of the curve, representing the transition from inspiration to expiration and the mixing of dead space and alveolar gas.The alveolar plateau, representing the alveolar gas rich in carbon dioxide and tending to slope gently upward with the uneven emptying of the alveoli. 4-5, The respiratory downstroke, which is a nearly vertical drop to baseline. B. C and D. See text for explanation.

assessing CO, gauge effectiveness of CPR during cardiac arrest, determine prognosis in CPR and in trauma, maintain appropriate $ETco_2$ levels in patients with elevated ICP, estimate P_aCO_2 in patients with normal lung function, assess response to treatment in patients with ARDS, determine adequacy of ventilation in patients with altered mental status, assess ventilatory status of actively seizing patients, and help detect metabolic acidosis.

Along with visualizing tracheal rings on bronchoscopy, capnography is the other gold standard used to confirm intubation of the trachea. Misleading $ETco_2$ readings can occur with esophageal intubation after bag or mask ventilation and ingestion of carbonated beverages or antacids. However, detection of $ETco_2$ usually ceases after six breaths, and if capnography is used, the waveform, which initially appears normal, progressively becomes smaller, losing height until it disappears (flatline) by the sixth breath. $ETco_2$ is also falsely elevated for 5 to 10 min after injection of sodium bicarbonate. Capnography can confirm intubation of the trachea but may give falsenegative results in cardiac arrest if delivery of CO_2 from the periphery to the lungs is sufficiently diminished. In these situations, it is difficult to determine whether the absence of the waveform is a result of esophageal intubation or poor pulmonary blood flow. In nonarrest settings the $ETco_2$ has 100% sensitivity and specificity in confirming correct tube placement and is also useful for monitoring for accidental tube dislodgement.

Airway, breathing, and circulatory assessment of critically ill or injured patients can be rapidly determined through use of $ETco_2$ values and the capnogram. The presence of a normal capnogram denotes a patent airway and spontaneous breathing, and normal $ETco_2$ levels indicate adequate ventilation and perfusion. Capnography can therefore be used to assess critically ill patients and patients who are actively seizing. Capnographic measurement also provides reliable readings in low-perfusion states.

$ETco_2$ is a useful noninvasive measurement that is highly correlated with CO and is the earliest indicator of ROSC in CPR. ROSC is heralded by an almost immediate increase in $ETco_2$ from baseline.$ETco_2$ has prognostic value in terms of mortality during CPR. No patient with a mean $ETco_2$ less than 10 mm Hg after 20 min of CPR has survived.

Capnography is the only ventilation monitoring modality that is accurate and reliable in patients with active, generalized seizures.

Capnography can also rapidly detect the common airway, respiratory, and CNS complications associated with the nerve agents in chemical terrorism, including apnea, upper airway obstruction, laryngospasm, bronchospasm, and respiratory failure.

Capnography provides dynamic monitoring of ventilatory status in patients with acute respiratory distress, such as from asthma, bronchiolitis, COPD, CHF, and cystic fibrosis.

Bronchospasm in obstructive lung disease leads to upward slanting of the expiratory plateau of the capnogram (Fig. 2-2, middle panel). Changes in $ETco_2$ over time and the slope of this phase of the capnogram have been shown to correlate well with spirometric measurements (FEV_1 and PEFR). Capnography can also be used to distinguish obstructive from restrictive lung disease. Characteristic capnographic patterns associated with restrictive and obstructive lung disease are shown in Figure 2-2 (bottom pael).

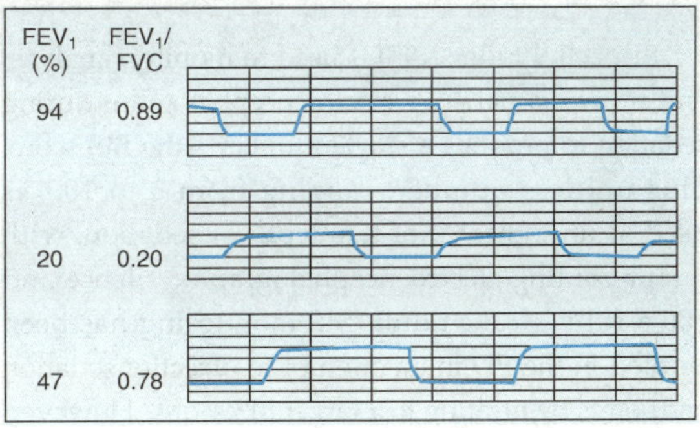

Fig. 2-2 Capnogram shape in normal subjects (top panel), patients with bronchospasm (middle panel), and those with obstructive and restrictive (bottom panel) lung disease.

Capnography is the earliest indicator of airway or respiratory compromise and displays an abnormally high or low $ETco_2$ 5 to 240 s before pulse oximetry detects a falling oxyhemoglobin saturation, especially in patients receiving supplemental oxygen.

Obtunded or unconscious patients, including those with alcohol intoxication, intentional or unintentional drug overdose, and postictal patients (especially those treated with benzodiazepines), may have impaired ventilation.

In addition to its established uses for assessment of ventilation and perfusion, capnography is a valuable tool for assessing metabolic status(Figs. 2-3 and 2-4, respectively).As a patient becomes acidotic, HCO_3 decreases and a compensatory respiratory alkalosis develops with an increase in minute ventilation and a resultant decrease in $ETco_2$. The more acidotic the patient, the lower the HCO_3; the higher the respiratory rate, the lower the $ETco_2$.

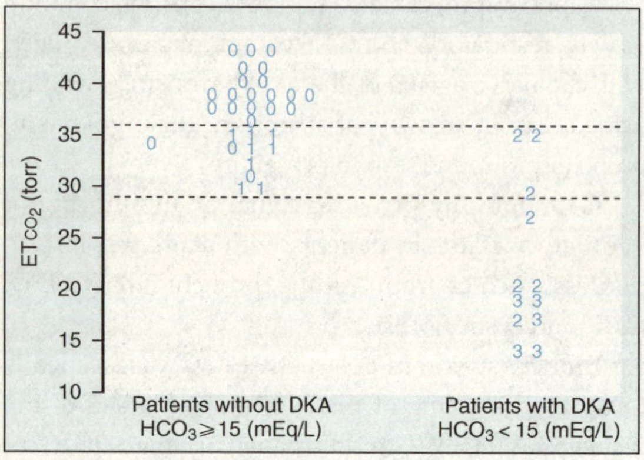

Fig. 2-3 Predictive value of $ETco_2$ in detecting metabolic acidosis in diabetics.

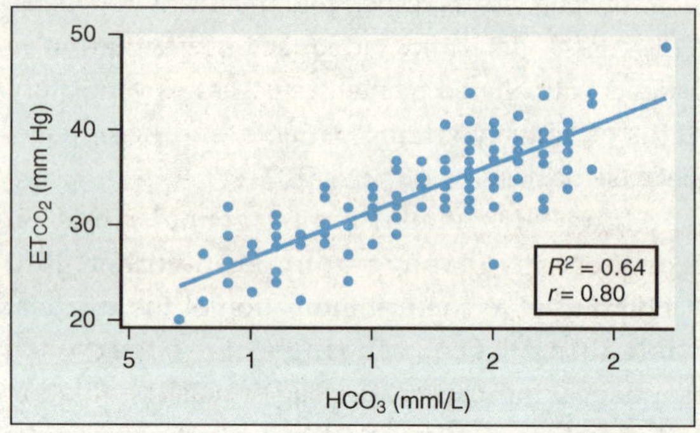

Fig. 2-4 $ETco_2$/serum HCO_3^- correlation in gastroenteritis. r, correlation coefficient; R^2, coefficient of determination for multivariate analysis.

CEREBRAL FUNCTION MONITORING

Bispectral Index (BIS) is used to monitor, analyze, and process a patient's electroencephalogram during sedation to produce a single number—the BIS score. This unitless number, ranging from 0 to 100, is used as an indicator of the depth of sedation, with 0 representing electroencephalographic silence and 100 a fully awake adult. BIS monitoring has been studied in the ED in an attempt to objectify sedation endpoints by titrating to a target BIS score. However, the evidence of its ability to reliably reflect depth of sedation is conflicting. More important, the threshold beyond which ventilatory compromise occurs has not been determined, further limiting the usefulness of routine BIS monitoring for sedation in the ED. BIS monitoring reliably distinguished patients undergoing procedural sedation and analgesia who were sedated to the point of general anesthesia from those with lesser degrees of sedation but did not discriminate mild-tomoderate sedation from moderate-to-deep sedation.

Another technology that monitors cerebral function is cerebral oximetry. Cerebral tissue oxygenation (i.e., regional SaO_2) is measured by near-infrared spectroscopy monitoring of the nonpulsatile signal component, reflecting tissue circulation of cerebral vasculature.

MONITOR ALARMS AND LIMITS

Continuous vital sign monitoring has become a routine part of ED care. Continuous monitoring in select patient populations has limited usefulness. A multidisciplinary team-based approach that focuses on identifying optimal application of monitoring, standardizing alarm limits and the staff response, and using improved alarm technology has the potential to improve patient safety and enhance workplace efficiency and satisfaction.

(SHOU Songtao)

Therapeutic Techniques

Chapter 3

Airway

KEY CONCEPTS

Knowledge of the clinical course of the patient's condition and anticipation of possible deterioration are crucial to the decision to intubate.

Assessment of the patient for potential difficulty with intubation, BMV, ventilation using an EGD, and cricothyrotomy is an essential step before neuromuscular blockers are administered. The mnemonics LEMON, MOANS, and RODS can serve as useful aids.

In the absence of a "crash" patient (agonal, unresponsive to laryngoscopy) or a difficult airway, RSI is the airway management method of choice for ED patients.

Tube placement confirmation using $ETco_2$ is essential after intubation, and failure to detect adequate quantities of exhaled CO_2 is evidence of esophageal intubation until proved otherwise.

Videolaryngoscopy is transforming intubation by eliminating the traditional anatomic barriers to direct laryngoscopy.

Cricothyrotomy is indicated in the "can't intubate, can't oxygenate" failed airway and should be performed without hesitation once this situation has been identified.

PERSPECTIVE

Airway management is the cornerstone of resuscitation and is a defining skill for the specialty of emergency medicine. RSI with direct laryngoscopy is the most commonly used method for emergency intubation, but emergency airway management includes various intubation maneuvers, use of ancillary devices and rescue techniques when intubation fails.

PATHOPHYSIOLOGY

Decision to Intubate

A decision to intubate should be based on careful assessment of the patient with respect to three essential criteria: (1) failure to maintain or protect the airway, (2) failure of ventilation or oxygenation, and (3) the patient's anticipated clinical course and likelihood of deterioration.

CLINICAL FEATURES

Identification of the Difficult Airway

In most patients,intubation is technically easy and straightforward.Preintubation assessment should evaluate the patient for difficult intubation, difficult bag-mask ventilation (BMV), difficult ventilation with an extraglottic device(EGD), and difficult cricothyrotomy. Knowledge of all four domains is crucial to successful planning. Neuromuscular paralysis generally should be avoided in patients for whom a high degree of intubation difficulty is predicted, unless the administration of the NMBA is part of a planned approach to the difficult airway.

Difficult Direct Laryngoscopy: LEMON

When direct laryngoscopy is planned, a standard screening process for difficulty should be undertaken with every patient. One such approach uses the mnemonic LEMON (Box 3-1).

Box 3-1 LEMON Approach for Evaluation of Difficult Direct Laryngoscopy

Look externally for signs of difficult intubation (by gestalt)
Evaluate the "3-3-2 rule"
Mallampati
Obstruction or obesity
Neck mobility

L-Look Externally. The patient first should be examined for external markers of difficult intubation. For example, the severely bruised and bloodied face of a combative trauma patient, immobilized in a cervical collar on a spine board, might (correctly) invoke an immediate appreciation of anticipated difficult intubation.

E-Evaluate 3-3-2. The second step in the evaluation of the difficult airway is to assess the patient's anatomy to determine his or her suitability for direct laryngoscopy. Direct laryngoscopy requires the ability to visualize the glottis by direct vision through the mouth, using alignment of the oral, pharyngeal, and laryngeal axes.The "3-3-2 rule" is an effective summary of these geometric evaluations. The 3-3-2 rule requires that the patient be able to place 3 of his or her own fingers between the open incisors, 3 of his or her own fingers along the floor of the mandible beginning at the mentum, and 2 fingers from the laryngeal prominence to the floor of the mandible (Fig. 3-1). A patient with a receding mandible and high-riding larynx can be impossible to intubate using direct laryngoscopy.

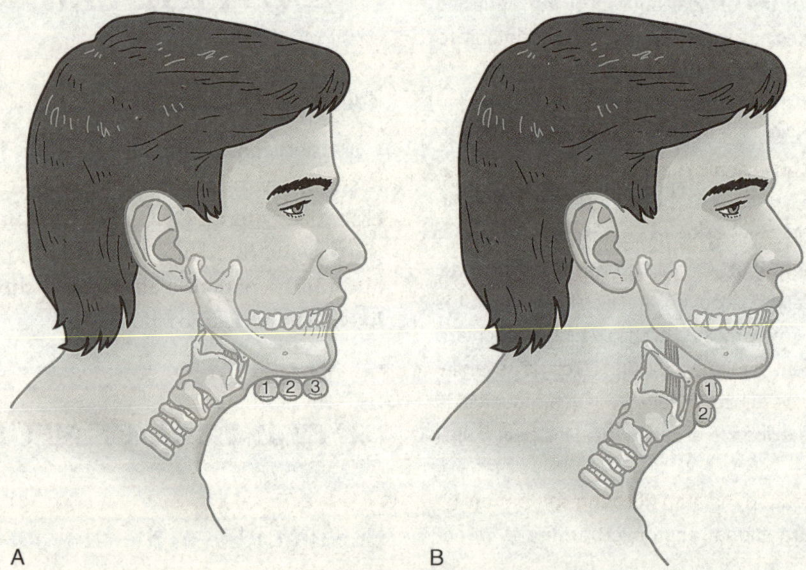

Fig. 3-1 Final two steps of the 3-3-2 rule. A, Three fingers are placed along the floor of the mouth beginning at the mentum. B, Two fingers are placed in the laryngeal prominence.

M-Mallampati Scale. Oral access is assessed using the Mallampati scale (Fig. 3-2). Visibility of the oral pharynx ranges from complete visualization, including the tonsillar pillars (class Ⅰ), to no visualization at all, with the tongue pressed against the hard palate (class Ⅳ). Class I and class Ⅱ predict adequate oral access, class Ⅲ predicts moderate difficulty, and class IV predicts a high degree of difficulty. A Mallampati score may have to be improvised with the direct laryngoscope blade as a tongue depressor in obtunded or uncooperative patients.

O-Obstruction or Obesity. Upper airway (supraglottic) obstruction may make visualization of the glottis, or intubation itself, mechanically impossible. Conditions such as epiglottitis, laryngeal tumor, Ludwig's angina, neck hematoma, or glottic polyps can compromise laryngoscopy, passage of ETT, BMV, or all three.Obese patients generally are more difficult to intubate.

N-Neck Mobility. Neck mobility is assessed by having the patient flex and extend the head and neck through a full range of motion. Modest limitations of motion do not seriously impair laryngoscopy, but severe loss of motion, as can occur in ankylosing spondylitis or rheumatoid arthritis, may render laryngoscopy impossible. Cervical spine immobilization in trauma artificially reduces

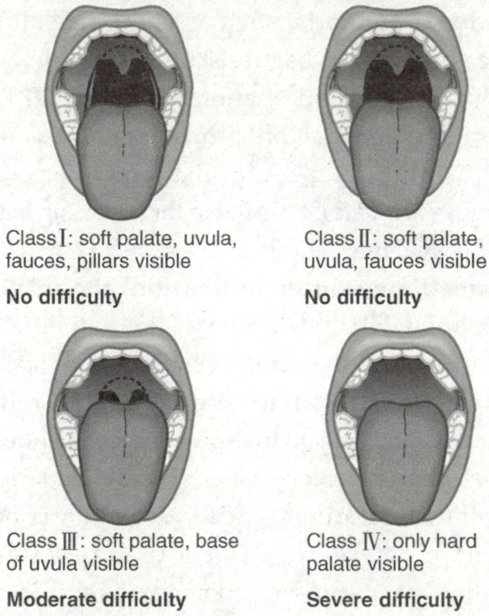

Fig. 3-2 The Mallampati scale assesses oral access for intubation.

cervical spine mobility and predicts a more difficult laryngoscopy, but direct laryngoscopy is still highly successful in this group of patients.

Identification of a difficult intubation does not preclude use of an RSI technique. The crucial determination is whether the clinician judges that the patient has a reasonable likelihood of intubation success, despite the difficulties identified, and that ventilation with a bag and mask or an EGD will be successful in the event that intubation fails.

Difficult Bag-mask Ventilation: MOANS

Attributes of difficult BMV have largely been validated and can be summarized with the mnemonic MOANS (Box 3-2).

Box 3-2 MOANS Mnemonic for Evaluation of Difficult Bag-Mask Ventilation

*M*ask seal
*O*bstruction or obesity
*A*ged
*N*o teeth
*S*tiffness (resistance to ventilation)

Mask seal compromise or difficulty; Obstruction (particularly supraglottic obstruction, but it can be present anywhere in the airway) or Obesity (because of redundant upper airway tissues,chest wall weight, and resistance of abdominal mass); advanced Age; edentulousness ("No teeth"), which independently interferes with mask seal; and "Stiffness" or resistance to ventilation (e.g., asthma, COPD, pulmonary edema, restrictive lung disease, term pregnancy) may each contribute to increased difficulty with BMV.A new approach involves placing the mask inside the patient's lower lip. This may limit air leak in patients without teeth and eliminates the risk of aspiration associated with dental prosthetics or rolled gauze (Fig. 3-3).

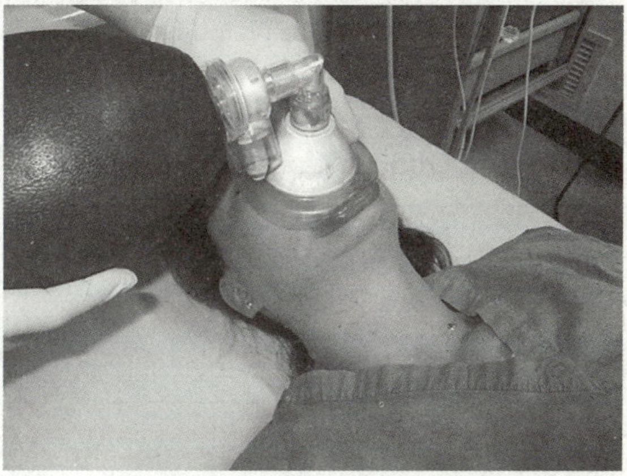

Fig. 3-3 Mask ventilation in edentulous patients can be performed by placing the lower rim if the mask on the inside of the patient's lower lip to improve mask seal.

Difficult Extraglottic Device Placement: RODS

Placement of an EGD, such as a laryngeal mask airway (LMA), often can convert a "can't intubate, can't oxygenate" situation to a "can't intubate, can oxygenate" situation, which allows time for rescue of a failed airway.Difficulty achieving placement or ventilation with an EGD is predicted by the mnemonic RODS. Fortunately, if the clinician has already performed the LEMON and MOANS assessments, only the D for distorted anatomy remains to be evaluated (Box 3-3). EGD are placed blindly and have either a mask or a balloon structure that, when inflated, obstructs the oropharynx proximally and the esophageal inlet distally, permitting indirect ventilation. Distorted upper airway anatomy can result in a poor seal and ineffective ventilation.

Box 3-3 RODS Mnemonic for Evaluation of Difficult Extraglottic Device Placement

*R*estricted mouth opening
*O*bstruction or obesity
*D*istorted anatomy
*S*tiffness (resistance to ventilation)

Difficult Cricothyrotomy: SMART

Difficult cricothyrotomy can be anticipated

whenever there is disturbance of the ability to locate and access the landmarks of the anterior airway via the neck and is remembered by the SMART mnemonic (Box 3-4). Prior surgery; hematoma, tumor, or abscess; scarring; local trauma; obesity; edema; or subcutaneous air each has the potential to make cricothyrotomy more difficult. Perform an examination for the landmarks needed to perform cricothyrotomy as part of the preintubation difficult airway assessment of the patient.

Box 3-4 SMART Mnemonic for Evaluation of Difficult Cricothyrotomy

*S*urgery
*M*ass (abscess, hematoma)
*A*ccess/anatomy problems (obesity, edema)
*R*adiation
*T*umor

Measurement and Incidence of Intubation Difficulty

The most widely used system for grading laryngoscopic view of the glottis is that of Cormack and Lehane (CL), which grades laryngoscopy according to the extent to which laryngeal and glottic structures can be seen. In grade 1 laryngoscopy, all or nearly all of the glottic aperture is seen. Grade 2 laryngoscopy visualizes only a portion of the glottis (arytenoid cartilages alone or arytenoid cartilages plus part of the vocal cords). Grade 3 laryngoscopy visualizes only the epiglottis. In grade 4 laryngoscopy, not even the epiglottis is visible.

Emergency adult inpatient intubations, as many as 10% were considered difficult.The incidence of difficult ED intubations is likely much higher, with some estimates between 4% and 26%.A grade 1 view is associated with virtually 100% intubation success.

Confirmation of Endotracheal Tube Placement

The most serious complication of endotracheal intubation is unrecognized esophageal intubation with resultant hypoxic brain injury. Although direct visualization of the ETT passing through the vocal cords generally is a reliable indicator of tracheal intubation, such clinical anatomic observations are fallible, and additional means are required to ensure correct placement of the tube within the trachea. Traditional methods, such as chest auscultation, gastric auscultation, bag resistance, exhaled volume, visualization of condensation within the ETT, and chest radiography, all are prone to failure as means of confirming tracheal intubation.Other clinical techniques are readily available for detecting tracheal or esophageal intubation.

Immediately after intubation, the intubator should apply ETco$_2$ detection device to the ETT and assess it through six manual ventilations. Disposable, colorimetric ETco$_2$ detectors are highly reliable, convenient, and easy to interpret, indicating adequate CO_2 detection by color change (Fig. 3-4 and Fig. 3-5, see color illustrations). ETco$_2$ detection is highly reliable in determining tracheal and esophageal intubation in patients with spontaneous circulaton.

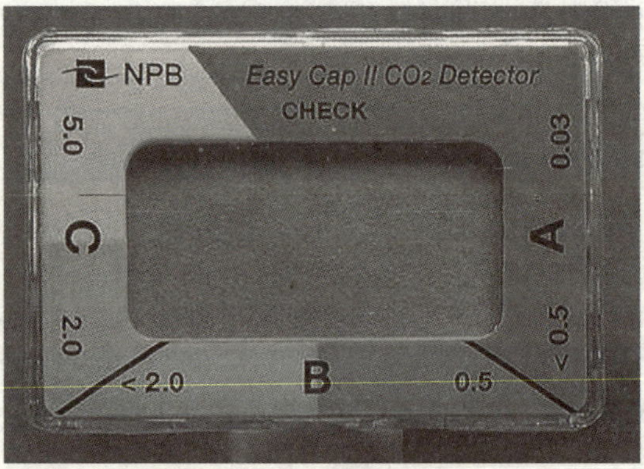

Fig. 3-4 ETco$_2$ detector before application. The indicator is purple, which indicates failure to detect CO_2. This also is the appearance when the esophagus is intubaed.

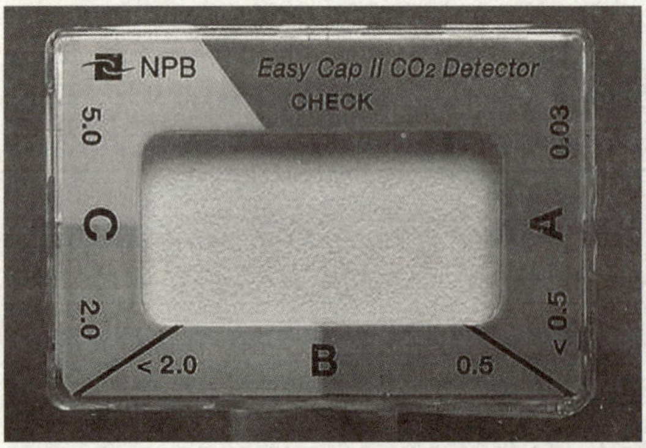

Fig. 3-5 Positive detection of CO_2 turns the indicator yellow, indicating tracheal placement of the endotracheal tube.

ETco$_2$ detection should be considered the primary means of ETT placement confirmation. Secondary means include physical examination findings, oximetry, and radiography. The examiner should auscultate both lung fields and the epigastric area. Pulse oximetry is useful in detecting esophageal intubation but may not show a decreasing SaO_2 for several minutes after a failed intubation.The primary purpose of chest radiography is to ensure that the tube is well positioned below the cords and above the carina.In cases in which doubt persists, a fiberoptic scope can be passed through the ETT to identify tracheal rings.

MANAGEMENT

Approach to Intubation

After it is determined that the patient requires intubation, an approach must be planned.

The approach is predicated on two key determinations that must be made before active airway management is begun (Fig. 3-6). The first determination is whether the patient is in cardiopulmonary arrest or a state of near arrest and is predicted to be unresponsive to direct laryngoscopy. Such a patient is treated with the crash airway algorithm by an immediate intubation attempt without use of drugs, supplemented by a single, large dose of succinylcholine if the attempt to intubate fails and the patient is thought not to be sufficiently relaxed (Fig. 3-7). Next, it must be determined whether the patient represents a difficult intubation as determined by the LEMON, MOANS, RODS, and SMART evaluations, and if so, the difficult airway algorithm is used (Fig. 3-8).

RSI provides the safest and quickest method of achieving intubation for patients who require emergency intubation but who have neither a crash airway nor a difficult airway. After administration of the RSI drugs, intubation attempts are repeated until the patient is intubated or a failed intubation is identified. If more than one intubation attempt is required, SaO_2 is monitored continuously, and if SaO_2 falls to 90% or less, BMV is performed until SaO_2 is recovered for another attempt. If the clinician cannot maintain SaO_2 despite optimal use of BMV or an EGD, a failed airway exists. This is referred to as a "can't intubate, can't oxygenate" situation. In addition, if three attempts at laryngoscopy have

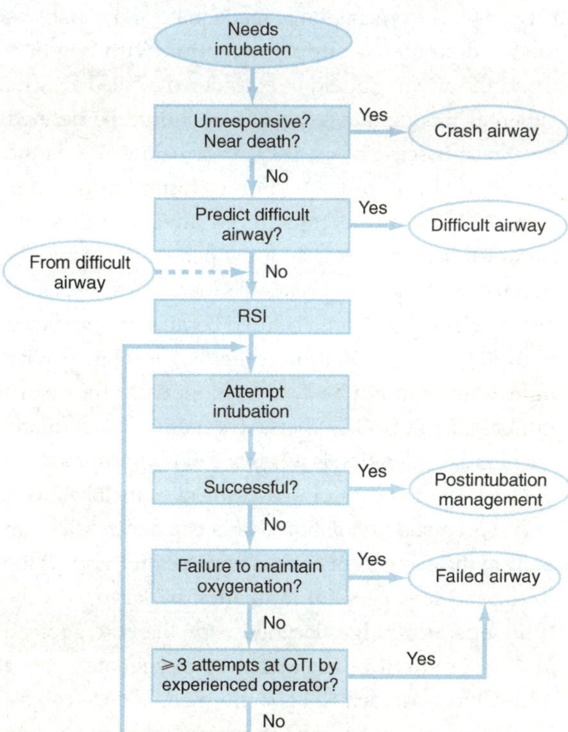

Fig. 3-6 Main emergency airway management algorthm.

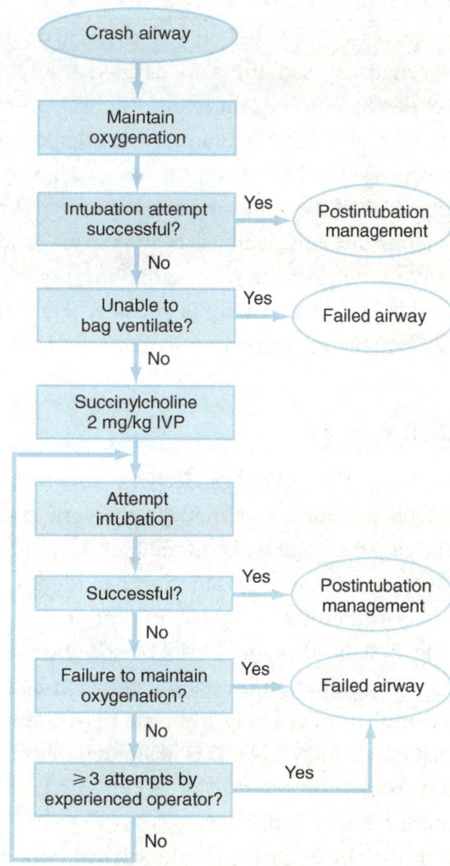

Fig. 3-7 Crash airway algorthm.

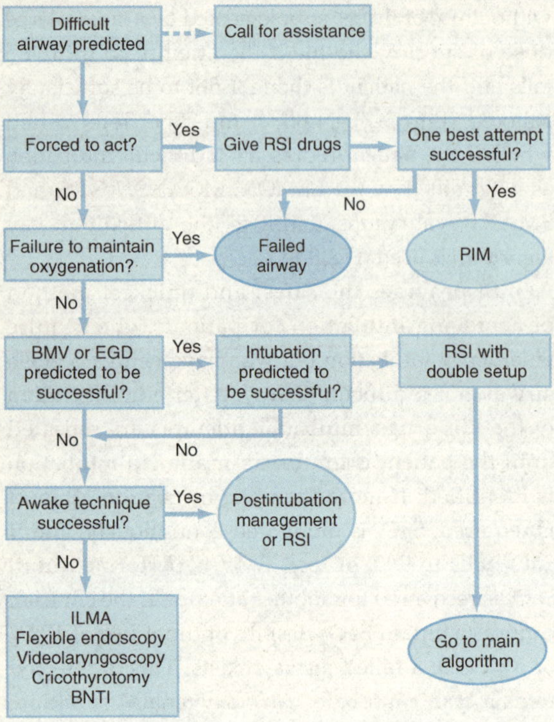

Fig. 3-8 Difficult airway algorihm.

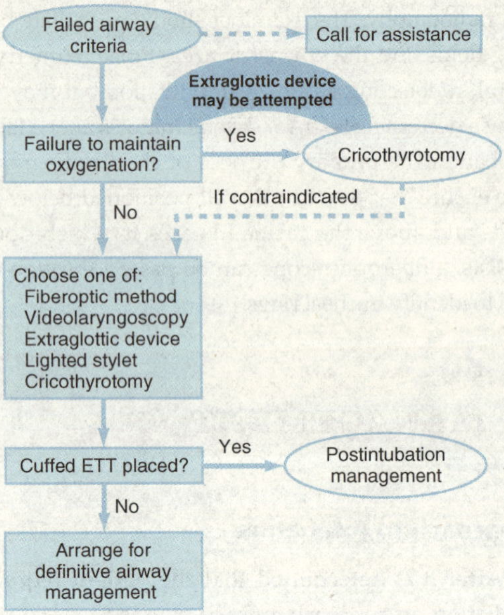

Fig. 3-9 Failed airway algorithm.

been unsuccessful, a failed airway exists. The three failed laryngoscopy attempts are defined as attempts by an experienced clinician using the best possible patient positioning and technique. If available, video laryngoscopes should be used for one or all of these attempts. Also, if the clinician ascertains after even a single attempt that intubation will be impossible , and no alternative laryngoscope (e.g., video laryngoscope) is available, a failed airway is present. The failed airway is managed according to the failed airway algorithm (Fig. 3-9).

Difficult Airway

The LEMON, MOANS, RODS, and SMART assessments provide a systematic framework to assist in identifying the potentially difficult airway.

When preintubation evaluation has identified a potentially difficult airway, a different approach is used (Fig. 3-8), NMBA should not be administered to a patient for intubation unless the clinician believes that (1) intubation is likely to be successful and (2) oxygenation via BMV or EGD is likely to be successful if a first intubation attempt does not succeed and oxygenation is required.

In the difficult airway algorithm, the first determination is whether the operator is "forced to act." If so, RSI drugs are given and, if intubation is not successful, the airway is considered failed and the operator moves immediately to the failed airway algorithm. In the vast majority of difficult airway situations, however, the operator is not forced to act, and the first step is to ensure that oxygenation is sufficient to permit a planned, orderly approach (Fig. 3-8). If oxygenation is inadequate and cannot be made adequate by supplementation with bag and mask, the airway should be considered a failed airway. Whereas inadequate oxygenation should be defined on a case-by-case basis, SaO_2 at or below 90% is the accepted threshold. Oxyhemoglobin saturations in the 80s might be considered adequate in some circumstances, particularly if the patient is chronically hypoxemic. When oxygenation is inadequate, the failed airway algorithm should be used because the predicted high degree of intubation difficulty, combined with failure to maintain SaO_2, is analogous to the "can't intubate, can't SaO_2. When oxygenation is adequate, the next consideration is whether RSI is appropriate, on the basis of the operator's assessment of the likelihood of (1) successful ventilation with a bag and mask or an EGD in the event intubation is unsuccessful, and (2) the likelihood of successful intubation by laryngoscopy. If the operator judges laryngoscopy likely to succeed and is confident of the ability to oxygenate even if intubation fails, then RSI is performed. In such cases a double setup can be used in which RSI is performed and preparations simultaneously are undertaken for rescue cricothyrotomy or another rescue technique. If RSI is not advisable and time allows, an awake technique can be used.Usually the technique involves sedation and topical anesthesia. The awake technique often is direct or flexible or rigid videolaryngoscopy, assisted by topical anesthesia and sedation (comparable to that for a painful procedure). If the glottis is adequately visualized, the patient can be intubated at that time, or, in a stable difficult airway situation, the clinician may proceed with planned RSI, now assured of intubation success. If the awake laryngoscopy is unsuccessful, the patient is intubated with any of numerous techniques shown in the last box in Fig. 3-8. For each of these methods, the patient is kept breathing but variably sedated and anesthetized, and each of the methods results in placement of a cuffed ETT in the trachea.

Failed Airway

Management of the failed airway is dictated by an assessment of whether the patient can be oxygenated. If adequate oxygenation cannot be maintained, the rescue technique of first resort is cricothyrotomy (Fig. 3-9). If an alternative device (i.e., an EGD such as a LMA or Combitube) is readily at hand, however, an attempt can be made to use it simultaneously with preparations for immediate cricothyrotomy, as long as initiation of cricothyrotomy is not delayed.Only a single attempt with the EGD is recommended in this circumstance.

If adequate oxygenation is possible, several options are available for the failed airway. The fundamental difference in philosophy between the difficult airway and the failed airway is that the difficult airway is planned for, and the standard is to place a cuffed ETT in the trachea. The failed airway is *not* planned for, and the standard is to achieve an airway that provides adequate oxygenation to avert the immediate problem of hypoxic brain injury. Some of the devices used in the failed airway are temporary and do not provide airway protection.

THERAPEUTIC MODALITIES

Methods of Intubation

Four methods are most common for intubation of the emergency patient, with RSI being the most frequently used in nonarrested patients.

Rapid Sequence Intubation

RSI is the cornerstone of modern emergency airway management and is defined as the virtually simultaneous administration of a potent sedative (induction) agent and an NMBA, usually succinylcholine, for the purpose of endotracheal intubation. The central concept of RSI is to take the patient from the starting point (e.g., conscious, breathing spontaneously) to a state of unconsciousness with complete neuromuscular paralysis, then to achieve intubation *without* interposed assisted ventilation. The purpose of RSI is to avoid PPV until the ETT is placed correctly in the trachea with the cuff inflated. This requires a preoxygenation phase, during which the nitrogen reservoir in the functional residual capacity in the lungs is replaced with oxygen, permitting at least several minutes of apnea in the normal adult before oxygen desaturation to 90% ensues (Fig. 3-10, see color illustration).

Use of RSI also facilitates successful endotracheal intubation by causing complete relaxation of the patient's musculature, allowing better access to the airway. Finally, RSI permits pharmacologic control of

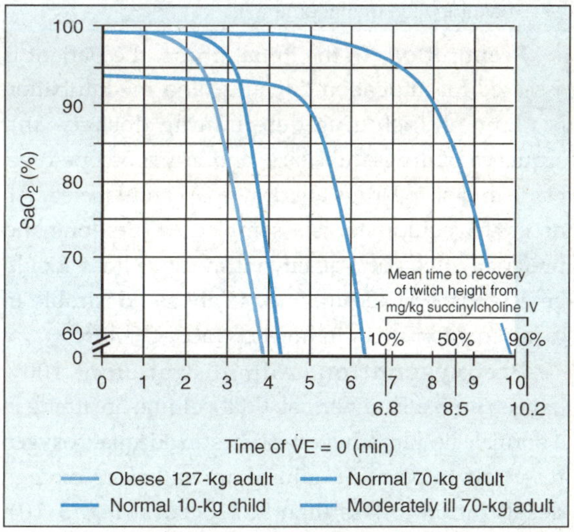

Fig. 3-10 Desaturation time for apneic, fully preoxygenated patients. Children, patients with comorbidity, and obese patients desaturate much more rapidly than healthy, normal adults. The box on the lower right side of the graph depicts time to recovery from succinylcholine, which in almost all cases exceeds safe apnea time. Note also the precipitous decline of oxygen saturation from 90% to 0% for all groups.

the physiologic responses to laryngoscopy and intubation, mitigating potential adverse effects. These effects include further ICP increase in response to the procedure and to the sympathetic discharge resulting from laryngoscopy (Box 3-5). RSI is a series of discrete steps, and every step should be planned (Box 3-6).

Box 3-5 Pretreatment Agents for RSI

Reactive airways disease: Lidocaine 1.5 mg/kg IV, to mitigate bronchospasm. Albuterol 2.5 mg by nebulizer (if time permits and not already given).

Cardiovascular disease: Fentanyl 3 μg/kg to mitigate sympathetic discharge.

Elevated ICP: Lidocaine 1.5 mg/kg IV to mitigate ICP increase in response to airway manipulation. Fentanyl 3 μg/kg to mitigate sympathetic discharge and attendant rise in ICP

Box 3-6 The Seven Ps of RSI

1. *P*reparation
2. *P*reoxygenation
3. *P*retreatment
4. *P*aralysis with induction
5. *P*ositioning
6. *P*lacement of tube
7. *P*ostintubation management

Preparation. In the initial phase, the patient is assessed for intubation difficulty, and the intubation is planned, including determining dosages and sequence of drugs, tube size, and laryngoscope type, blade and size. Drugs are drawn up and labeled. All necessary equipment is assembled.At least one and preferably two good-quality intravenous lines should be established. Redundancy is always desirable in case of equipment or intravenous access failure.

Preoxygenation. Administration of 100% oxygen for 3 min of normal, tidal volume breathing in a normal, healthy adult establishes an adequate oxygen reservoir to permit 8 min of apnea before oxygen desaturation to less than 90% occurs (Fig. 3-10). Oxygen saturation monitors permit earlier detection of desaturation during laryngoscopy, but preoxygenation remains an essential step in RSI.

Pretreatment. During this phase, drugs are admin istered 3 min before administration of the succinylcholine and induction agent to mitigate the effects of laryngoscopy and intubation on the patient's presenting or comorbid conditions. Pretreatment focuses on three main objectives, in certain at-risk patients. The three groups of patients at risk are those with reactive airways disease, elevated ICP, or a cardiovascular or neurovascular condition for which an acute elevation in BP and HR might be hazardous (Box 3-5).

Paralysis with Induction. In this phase, a potent sedative agent is administered by rapid intravenous push in a dose capable of rapidly producing unconsciousness. This is immediately followed by rapid administration of an intubating dose of an NMBA, usually succinylcholine. It is usual to wait 45 s from the time the succinylcholine is given to allow sufficient paralysis to occur.

Positioning. The patient should be positioned for intubation as consciousness is lost. Usually, positioning involves head extension, often with flexion of the neck on the body.Accordingly, Sellick's maneuver(application of firm backward-directed pressure over the cricoid cartilage)should be considered optional, applied selectively, and released or modified to improve laryngeal view or tube passage, as indicated. During this phase after administration of the induction agent and NMBA, although the patient becomes unconscious and apneic, BMV should not be initiated unless the oxygen saturation falls to 90%.

Placement of Tube. Approximately 45 s after the administration of succinylcholine, the patient is relaxed sufficiently to permit laryngoscopy. The ETT is placed under direct visualization of the glottis. If the first attempt is unsuccessful, but oxygen saturation remains high, it is not necessary to ventilate the patient with a bag and mask between intubation attempts. If the oxygen saturation is approaching 90%, the patient may be ventilated briefly with a bag and mask between attempts to reestablish the oxygen reservoir. When BMV is performed, Sellick's maneuver is advisable to minimize passage of air into the stomach.

Postintubation Management. Obtain a chest radiograph to confirm that mainstem intubation has not occurred and to assess the lungs. In general, long-acting NMBA(e.g., pancuronium, vecuronium) are avoided and the focus is on optimal management using opioid analgesics and sedative agents to facilitate mechanical ventilation. An adequate dose of a benzodiazepine (e.g., midazolam 0.1-0.2 mg/kg intravenous) and an opioid analgesic (e.g., fentanyl 3-5 μg/kg intravenous, or morphine 0.2-0.3 mg/kg intravenous) is given to improve patient comfort and decrease sympathetic response to the ETT. Propofol infusion (5-50 μg/kg/min intravenous) with supplemental analgesia is an effective method for managing intubated patients without hypotension or ongoing bleeding and is especially helpful for management of neurologic emergencies, as its clinical duration of action is very short (<5 min), allowing frequent neurologic examinations. An NMBA is added only if appropriate use of sedation and analgesia fail to adequately control the patient. Table 3-1 presents a sample RSI protocol using etomidate and succinylcholine. "Zero" refers to the time at which the induction agent and succinylcholine are pushed.

Table 3-1 Sample Rapid Sequence Intubation Using Etomidate and Succinylcholine

TIME	STEP
Zero minus 10 min	Preparation
Zero minus 5 min	Preoxygenation
	100% oxygen for 3 min *or* eight vital capacity breaths
Zero minus 3 min	Pretreatment
	As indicated
Zero	Paralysis with induction
	Etomidate, 0.3 mg/kg
	Succinylcholine, 1.5 mg/kg
Zero plus 30 sec	Positioning
	Sellick' s maneuver optional
Zero plus 45 sec	Placement
	Laryngoscopy and intubation
	$ETco_2$ confirmation
Zero plus 2 min	Postintubation management
	Sedation and analgesia as indicated
	Initiate mechanical ventilation
	NMBA only if needed after adequate sedation/analgesia

Blind Nasotracheal Intubation

Historically, blind nasotracheal intubation (BNTI) was used extensively in the ED and out-of-hospital setting, but has fallen out of favor largely because of the superiority of RSI. BNTI remains a valid method of intubation in the out-of-hospital setting, where it occasionally is used. In the ED, BNTI rarely, if ever, should be used and is reserved for patients in whom the presence of a narrowly defined type of difficult airway makes RSI undesirable or contraindicated and alternatives (e.g., flexible endoscope) are not available.

Awake Oral Intubation

Awake oral intubation is a technique in which sedative and topical anesthetic agents are administered to permit management of a difficult airway without neuromuscular blockade. Sedation and analgesia are achieved in a manner analogous to that for painful procedures in the ED. Topical anesthesia may be achieved by spray, nebulization, or local anesthetic nerve block. After the patient is sedated and topical anesthesia has been achieved, gentle direct, video, or flexible endoscopic laryngoscopy is performed to determine whether the glottis is visible and intubation possible. If the glottis is visible, the patient may be intubated during initial laryngoscopy, or the operator,confident that the glottis can be visualized, may opt to perform RSI to gain benefit from pretreatment, induction, and paralysis, as might be the case in a head-injured patient.

Oral Intubation without Pharmacologic Agents

The arrested or near death patient may not require pharmacologic agents for intubation.If the glottis is not adequately visualized, administration of a single dose of succinylcholine alone may facilitate laryngoscopy.

Pharmacologic Agents

Neuromuscular Blocking Agents

The NMBA are divided into two main classes. The *depolarizing* agent, succinylcholine, exerts its effects by binding noncompetitively with ACh receptors on the motor endplate and causing sustained depolarization of the myocyte. The other major class of NMBA comprises the *competitive*, or *nondepolarizing*, agents, which bind competitively to ACh receptors, preventing access by ACh and preventing muscular activity. The competitive agents are of two pharmacologically distinct types, steroid-based agents (aminosteroid compounds) and benzylisoquinolines. Each of these basic chemical types has distinct properties, but only the aminosteroid compounds are used in the ED.

Induction Agents

A patient who presents with any degree of clinical responsiveness, requires a sedative or induction agent at the time of administration of any NMBA. Patients who already are deeply unconscious and unresponsive may not require a full dose of an induction agent.Patients who are unconscious because of CNS insult should receive an induction agent to attenuate adverse responses to airway manipulation. Induction agents also enhance the effect of the NMBA and improve intubation conditions because the intubation is done at the earliest phase of neuromuscular blockade, and the relaxation effects of the induction agent are additive to those of the NMBA.

Evolution of Airway Devices

Direct Laryngoscopy

Historically, orotracheal intubation by direct laryngoscopy has been the standard mode of emergency airway management, principally because few alternatives for tracheal intubation existed.Since 2001, there has been an explosion of new intubation devices, capitalizing principally on video technology but also on fiberoptic and other optical innovations.

Videolaryngoscopes

Modern laryngoscopes incorporate video imaging into specially designed laryngoscope blades to provide glottic visualization superior to that of a direct laryngoscope without the need to create a straight-line visual axis through the mouth (Fig. 3-11 and Fig. 3-12).

Fiberoptic and Video Intubating Stylets

Several semirigid fiberoptic and video intubating stylets also are available (Fig. 3-13 and Fig. 3-14)

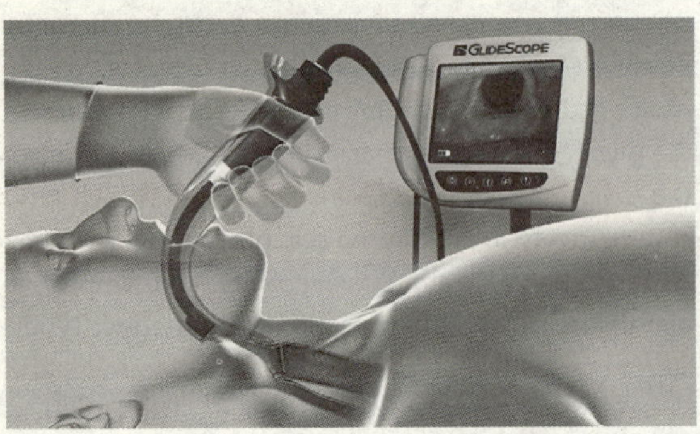

Fig. 3-11 Glide Scope AVL uses a high-resolution digital display; includes single-use Stats (blade sheaths) that cover the video baton; and has the ability to record still images and video clips through internal and removable storage devices.

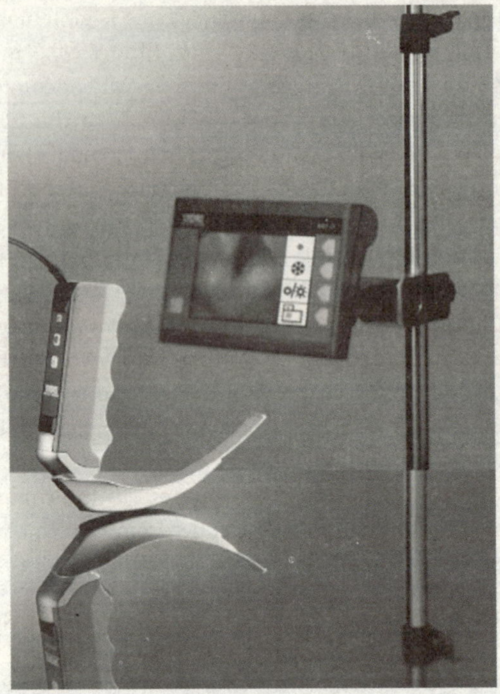

Fig. 3-12 The C-MAC video laryngoscope uses an integrated complementary metal oxide semiconductor (CMOS) video chip to capture a video image from near the distal tip of an otherwise conventional laryngoscope blade.

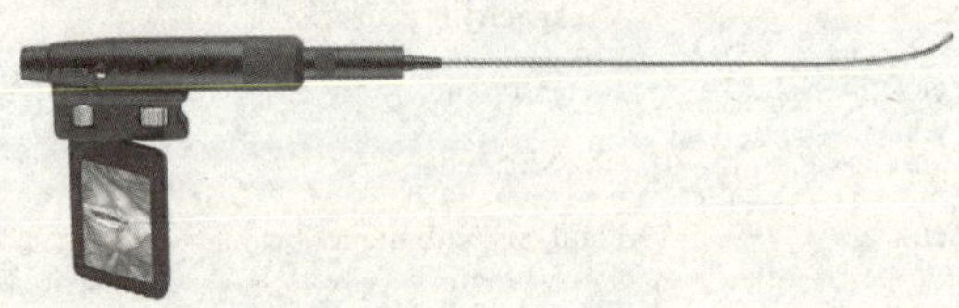

Fig. 3-13 The Clarus Video System (Clarus Medical) incorporates a curved fiberoptic stylet surrounded by a malleable but rigid protective metal sheath.

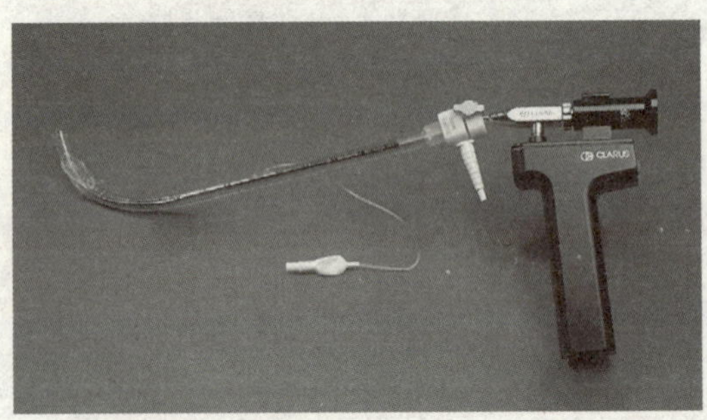

Fig. 3-14 The Shikani optical stylet (SOS; Clarus Optical) with endotracheal tube mounted. The eyepiece and battery pack are at the right.

Flexible Intubating Scopes

Intubation using a flexible endoscope is an important option for certain difficult airways, particularly in those with distorted upper airway anatomy, such as angioedema or blunt anterior neck trauma.

Extraglottic Devices

LMA collectively include a number of commercially available ovoid, silicone mask devices designed to seal above the glottis and permit ventilation through a central channel with a standard bag. The most widely used is the original LMA, shown in Fig. 3-15. A new form of noninflatable LMA, the i-gel, has a viscous gel cuff and does not require inflation (Fig. 3-16). In addition, the intubating laryngeal mask airway (ILMA) is designed to facilitate intubation through the mask after correct placement (Fig. 3-17).

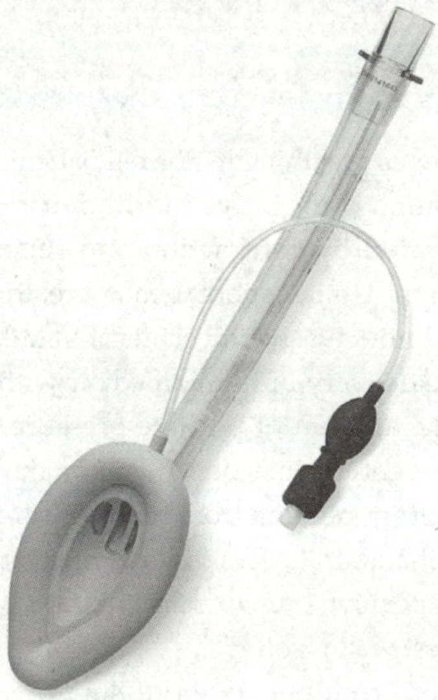

Fig. 3-15 The standard laryngeal mask airway (LMA Classic) is available in sizes from infant to large adult.

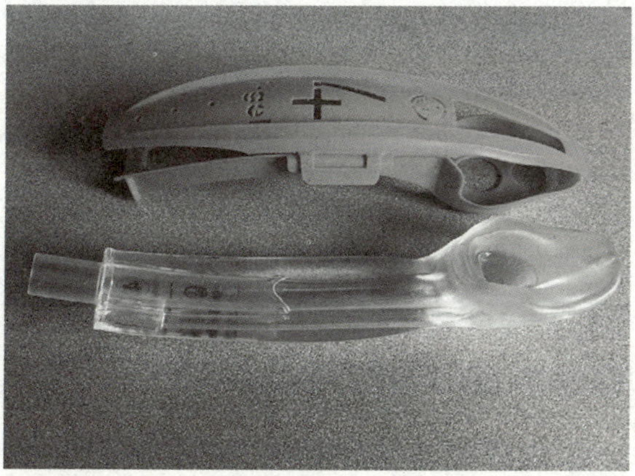

Fig. 3-16 The i-gel mask airway does not have an inflatable cuff and is available in sizes from infant to adult.

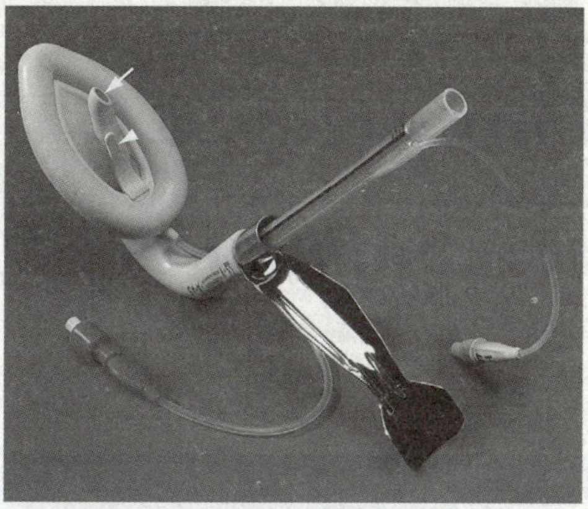

Fig. 3-17 The intubating laryngeal mask airway is modified to facilitate insertion of an endotracheal tube after placement and ventilation have been achieved.

Surgical Airway Management

Needle Cricothyrotomy with Transtracheal Jet Ventilation

When upper airway obstruction is present in adults, percutaneous or surgical cricothyrotomy is recommended. The primary indication for transtracheal ventilation in the ED is the initiation of emergency oxygenation for a pediatric patient who is apneic and in whom intubation and BMV are impossible because of supraglottic obstruction or disruption.

Cricothyrotomy

Cricothyrotomy is the creation of an opening in the cricothyroid membrane through which a cannula, usually a cuffed tracheostomy tube, is inserted to permit ventilation. When surgical airway management is required, cricothyrotomy is the procedure of choice in the emergency setting, where it is faster, more straightforward, and more likely to be successful than tracheotomy (Fig. 3-18).

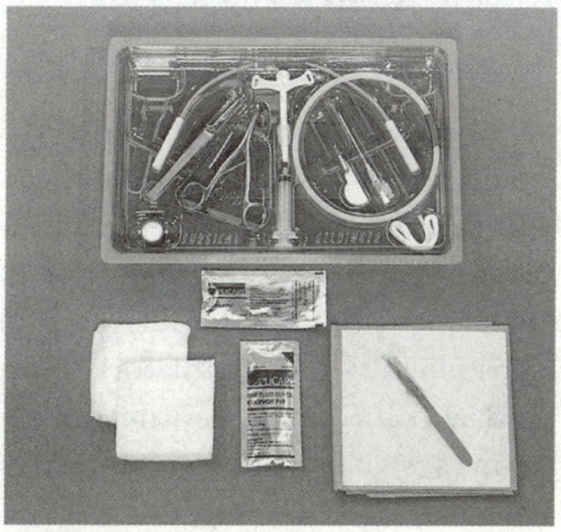

Fig. 3-18 Melker universal cricothyrotomy kit.

(ZHANG Jinsong)

Chapter 4

Mechanical Ventilation and Noninvasive Ventilatory Support

KEY CONCEPTS

Primary goals of mechanical ventilation are improved gas exchange and decreased work of breathing while maximizing patient comfort and minimizing the potential for complications.

Noninvasive ventilatory support is often adequate for reversal impending respiratory failure and should considered as the first-line therapy for patients with exacerbations of COPD and ACPE in whom immediate intubation is not required.

After intubation, ABG should be performed to confirm appropriate ventilation and provide correlation with noninvasive monitoring modalities. Hemodynamic consequences as a result of positive pressure should be anticipated.

Sudden difficulty in the treatment of patients receiving mechanical ventilation should prompt a quick and systematic evaluation for life-threatening conditions, followed by assessment of the ventilator settings, the ventilator circuit, airway pressures, and physiologic problems.

PERSPECTIVE

Invasive and noninvasive ventilation are essential components in the management of critically ill patients. Some patients require support for respiratory failure, whereas other patients require assistance primarily for airway protection. The reasons for initiating ventilatory support are varied and will influence ventilation strategy, hemodynamics, sedation strategy, and subsequent clinical course.

PRINCIPLES OF MECHANICAL VENTILATION

Physiology of Positive Pressure Breathing

Spontaneous breathing in normal patients is based on the initiation of negative intrathoracic pressure and is mediated by contraction and relaxation of the diaphragm. Unlike spontaneous breathing, both invasive and noninvasive mechanical ventilation are based on the delivery of humidified air with positive pressure. The amount of positive pressure required for adequate ventilation is dependent on the patient's respiratory effort, ranging from mild assistance to full support. "Inhalation" occurs by driving air into the lungs under positive pressure; air is passively exhaled owing to chest wall recoil.

Transition from negative pressure breathing to positive pressure breathing affects cardiovascular and pulmonary physiology. Pressure changes in the thoracic cavity directly affect pressures in the chambers of the heart. During spontaneous inspiration, venous return and preload are augmented, CO is increased, and there is an increased pressure gradient between the LV and the aorta. With the initiation of PPV, venous return is diminished, CO falls, and there is a decreased pressure gradient between the left ventricle and the aorta. Relative hypotension can occur after ventilatory support has been initiated, and this may be exaggerated in patients with clinical hypovolemia or vasodilatory states.

Invasive Mechanical Ventilation

How the ventilator defines a breath is referred

to as the control variable. The ventilator can give breaths based on delivery of a set pressure or a set volume, referred to as pressure-controlled ventilation (PCV) and volume-controlled ventilation (VCV), respectively. The amount of time over which the breath is delivered is defined as the inspiratory time, and the rate at which air travels through the circuit is defined as inspiratory flow.

In PCV, a set amount of pressure is applied to the airway to expand the lungs. When the target pressure is reached, gas delivery ends and passive exhalation is permitted. During PCV, target pressure and inspiratory time are set, whereas the delivered V_T and inspiratory flow vary as functions of dynamic lung compliance and airway resistance. Ability to control the pressure delivered to the lungs is particularly useful to prevent barotraumas. In addition, because inspiratory flow is not fixed, PCV may improve ventilator synchrony in intubated patients with a high respiratory drive. A significant disadvantage of PCV is that V_T cannot be guaranteed or limited and can change with acute changes in lung compliance. PCV offers advantages over VCV in clinical conditions in which control of airway pressure is strictly mandated. This includes patients with the potential to develop dynamic hyperinflation and iPEEP, such as patients with severe asthma or those with respiratory failure from COPD.

In VCV, a breath is defined by delivery of a set V_T to the lungs. Inspiratory flow is fixed, and inhalation ends when a preset V_T has been delivered; PIP and end-inspiratory alveolar pressures vary based on lung compliance and set V_T. The main benefit to VCV is the ability to control V_T and minute ventilation, but it may be problematic by causing high peak pressures when the compliance of the respiratory system is poor. Clinically, poor respiratory system compliance occurs in conditions including pulmonary edema, ALI or ARDS, pneumothorax, and obesity.

PCV versus VCV, it is important to consider the underlying reason for mechanical ventilation. VCV should be used when strict control of V_T is mandated. Specifically, this includes patients with known ALI or ARDS, in whom low-V_T strategies have been proven to reduce mortality. In addition, patients with decreased chest wall compliance should be placed on VCV to ensure that adequate V_T is delivered. This includes patients with morbid obesity or severe chest wall burns. Conversely, in conditions in which strict control of airway pressure is desired, PCV should be used. As detailed earlier, this includes patients with asthma or COPD. In addition, because inspiratory flow is not limited in pressure-cycled ventilation, this strategy may be preferred to VCV in patients with a high respiratory drive, such as patients with salicylate overdose. For patients who do not require strict control of either pressure or volume, similar ventilation mechanics can generally be achieved with either PCV or VCV (Table 4-1).

Table 4-1 Features of Pressure Control versus Volume Control

	SET PARAMETERS	VARIABLE PARAMETERS	CLINICAL IMPLICATIONS	CLINICAL CONDITIONS
PCV	Peak pressure target, inspiratory time, respiratory rate (RR), PEEP	V_T, inspiratory flow	Controls airway pressure, but V_T becomes a function of lung compliance(no guaranteed V_T or minute ventilation) Allows estimation of end-inspiratory alveolar pressure based on ventilator settings Variable inspiratory flow helpful for patients with high respiratory drive	Severe asthma COPD Salicylate toxicity
VCV	VT, RR, inspiratory flow pattern, inspiratory time	PIP, end-inspiratory alveolar pressure	Guaranteed delivery of V_T,but may result in high or injurious lung pressures End-inspiratory alveolar pressure cannot be reliably estimated and must be measured (Pplat)	ALI ARDS Obesity Severe burns

Newer ventilators are able to deliver breaths that combine volume and pressure strategies, referred to as dual-control ventilation. A common dual-control method of ventilation is pressure release volume control (PRVC). A variation of volume control, PRVC is set to deliver a specific V_T while simultaneously minimizing airway pressure. Unlike with strict volume control, pressure is measured and modulated by the ventilator with each breath to ensure the delivery of the preset V_T . In addition, a pressure limit is set, and the ventilator sounds an alarm when that pressure has been exceeded. Theoretically, this combines the advantages of pressure and volume control to ensure the delivery of a specific V_T while the airway pressure is monitored. This mode of ventilation has not been specifically studied but likely does not offer significant advantage over traditional VCV or PCV, particularly if strict parameters for airway pressure are desired.The most common ventilator modes can be categorized on the basis of how often the ventilator will initiate a breath for the patient and can be divided broadly into continuous mechanical ventilation (CMV), intermittent mechanical ventilation (IMV), and continuous spontaneous ventilation (CSV). CMV and IMV can be delivered via pressure-control or volume-control methods. In CSV, no mandatory breaths are delivered to a patient; the size of the breath is determined by the effort of the patient and can be augmented with applied pressure to the airway. These methods are compared in Table 4-2. Other, more complex modes of ventilation include proportional-assist ventilation (PAV)and airway pressure release ventilation (APRV), though these generally are not used in the ED.

Table 4-2 Selecting Ventilator Strategy: Features of Potential Options

MODE	PARAMETERS SET BY PROVIDER	CLINICAL SCENARIO
CMV		
A/C	Pressure or volume control, RR	Paralyzed or deeply sedated patient, sedated patients with intermittent spontaneous respiratory effort;can lead to hyperventilation
IMV		
SIMV	Pressure or volume control, RR (backup rate)	Patients with regular but poor spontaneous respiratory effort; if used in deeply sedated patients, set RR will need to be higher
CSV		
PSV	Level of pressure support, PEEP	Spontaneously breathing patients with good respiratory effort requiring minimal ventilatory support
CPAP	Level of CPAP	Alert, spontaneously breathing patients with immediately reversible causes of respiratory distress; COPD and ACPE are classic indications for noninvasive ventilation
BL-PAP	IPAP and EPAP	Similar to CPAP

CMV is intended to provide full ventilatory support for patients with little or no spontaneous respiratory activity. CMV, also referred to as assist-control (A/C) ventilation, provides a preset number of breaths per minute. In addition to preset breaths, A/C will also deliver a breath in response to patient effort. In this mode, patients can trigger a breath at any rate but will always receive at least the preset number of breaths. For the promotion of ventilator synchrony, a spontaneous patient-initiated breath will take priority over a preset breath, meaning that if the ventilator is set to deliver 12 breaths/min, a breath is provided every seconds in the absence of spontaneous inspiratory effort. When the patient makes a spontaneous effort, the ventilator provides an additional breath and the timer resets for another 5 s. A/C ventilation is the most useful initial mode of mechanical ventilation in ED patients. One of the biggest challenges with A/C ventilation, however, is that patient-initiated breaths are not proportional to patient effort.Clinically, this requires adequate sedation of patients when ventilated in A/C mode to prevent spontaneous respiratory efforts that will result in hyperventilation, air trapping, hypotension, and poor ventilator synchrony.

Synchronized intermittent mandatory ventilation (SIMV) provides intermittent ventilatory support to patients by delivering both mandatory and spontaneous breaths. In SIMV, a mandatory breath is given at a preset rate, but the breath is synchronized as much as possible with spontaneous patient effort. Much as with A/C, the patient will receive at least the minimum number of preset mandatory breaths; if the patient provides no effort, the preset number of breaths will be given. If a patient has a rate of spontaneous respirations lower than the set rate, the ventilator will provide the preset number of full breaths but will deliver as many as possible in synchrony with patient effort. In these scenarios there is little difference between A/C and SIMV. If a patient has a rate of spontaneous respirations higher than preset rate, the patient receives all preset full breaths at the set rate, but additional breaths generated by the patient will be commensurate with his or her respiratory effort. Additional breaths can be given via pressure support. SIMV is useful in patients who are sedated.

CSV, in contrast to A/C or SIMV, delivers a breath only on patient-initiated trigger. Pressure-support ventilation(PSV) is designed to support patients'spontaneous respiratory effort by delivering an applied pressure to the airway on the trigger of a breath. The amount of pressure required to support a full breath is variable and depends on the patient's ability to overcome the work of breathing. When inspiratory flow stops, signaling the end of inhalation, pressure support ceases and exhalation is allowed to proceed spontaneously. The level of pressure support is the only parameter determined by ventilator settings: inspiratory flow, inspiratory time, and V_T are determined by the patient effort. This mode of ventilation most closely resembles normal spontaneous breathing and for this reason promotes patient control and comfort. In the ED, PSV is rarely used for intubated patients. PSV may prove most useful in awake and interactive patients who have been intubated for temporary airway protection rather than for respiratory failure.

Positive End-Expiratory Pressure

PEEP is often used during invasive mechanical ventilation. During acute respiratory failure, lung volumes are typically decreased; application of PEEP increases FRC, improves oxygenation, and decreases intrapulmonary shunt. Potential adverse effects of PEEP include decreased CO, lung overdistention, and pneumothorax.

Applied PEEP must be differentiated from intrinsic PEEP (iPEEP, or auto-PEEP).

Noninvasive Techniques

Noninvasive positive-pressure ventilation (NPPV) is the delivery of CSV via sealed mask . As with PSV, the ventilator is set to provide a defined level of pressure when a patient takes a breath; inspiratory flow and inspiratory time are completely patient mediated. The most common types of noninvasive ventilation in the ED are CPAP and Bi-level positive airway pressure (BL-PAP). BiPAP, a term commonly used for BL-PAP, is the proprietary name of a portable device. Inspiratory positive airway pressure (IPAP) augments patient respiratory effort by decreasing the work of breathing during inspiration, whereas expiatory positive airway pressure (EPAP) acts as PEEP to maintain FRC and alveolar recruitment. Notably, although PEEP, CPAP, and EPAP all represent positive airway pressure at the end of expiration, PEEP by convention refers to pressure applied during invasive mechanical ventilation, whereas CPAP is the application of positive pressure (invasively or noninvasively) during spontaneous breathing.

MANAGEMENT

General Approach: Noninvasive versus Invasive Ventilation

NPPV is an appealing option for patients requiring ventilatory assistance with potentially reversible conditions when tracheal intubation is not immediately necessary, or as a therapeutic adjunct for patients with "do-not-intubate" directives. Need for emergency intubation is a contraindication to NPPV, except as a means to improve preoxygenation in preparation for intubation. Other relative contraindications include decreased level of consciousness, lack of respiratory drive, increased secretions, hemodynamic instability, and conditions, such as facial trauma, that would prevent an adequate mask seal.

Patients most likely to respond to NPPV in the ED are those with more readily reversible causes of their distress, such as COPD exacerbation or ACPE. Notably, though helpful in most patients with COPD exacerbation, NPPV has been shown to have the largest benefit for patients with hypercapnic acidosis and pH below 7.3. Treatment failure, defined as subsequent need for intubation, is predicted by a Glasgow Coma Scale score of less than 11, a sustained arterial pH less than 7.25, and tachypnea greater than 30 breaths/min.

Approach to Initial Ventilator Settings

The first consideration in the use of NPPV is whether to provide support in the form of CPAP or BL-PAP. Support will be given by a full-face (oronasal) mask or nasal mask; this choice is determined by patient comfort, feelings of claustrophobia, and the need for the patient to effectively cough or speak. Inspiratory support (IPAP) can be initiated at 10 cm H_2O, and expiratory support (EPAP) can be initiated at 5 cm H_2O. Subsequent titration of these parameters is based on the patient's clinical response, particularly pressure tolerance, respiratory rate, and oxyhemoglobin saturation. Though blood gas analysis is confirmatory, improvement inclinical condition can be observed by decrease in work of breathing, good patient-ventilator synchrony, and patient report. If required, EPAP and IPAP can be adjusted by 1 to 2 cm H_2O at a time based on clinical response. If work of breathing is unchanged, increases in IPAP and EPAP reduce hypercarbia by increasing V_T and minute ventilation while increasing oxygenation by combating atelectasis and promoting alveolar recruitment. IPAP greater than 20 cm H_2O can be uncomfortable and can cause gastric insufflation and should be avoided.

For the intubated patient, initial ventilator settings should facilitate ventilation that improves gas exchange, promotes ventilatory synchrony, and minimizes the potential for complications. Reasonable initial ventilator settings should deliver a V_T of 6 to 8 mL/kg of estimated ideal body weight (IBW) at rate of 12 to 14 breaths/min. If VCV is used, V_T can be set directly, and if PCV is used, V_T is determined by adjusting the targeted pressure to be delivered; initial pressure targets should not exceed 30 cm H_2O. Initial F_iO_2 should be set at 1.0 but generally can be adjusted down quickly to maintain an oxygen saturation of 90% or greater. PEEP is routinely given and is set initially at 5 cm H_2O.

Ongoing Management

Mechanical ventilation requires monitoring and regular adjustment to ensure appropriate gas exchange, safe delivery of desired V_T, and prevention of metabolic derangement. Changes to ventilator settings are guided dynamically by multiple factors, including pulse oximetry,$ETco_2$ monitoring, ventilation pressures, and ABG. For the adequacy of ventilation to be monitored, capnography may be used; ABG should be measured 15 to 20 min after initiation of ventilatory support to correlate $ETco_2$ with Pco_2.Minute ventilation can subsequently be altered by adjusting V_T or respiratory rate. To avoid oxygen toxicity, F_iO_2 should be reduced to the lowest level that provides acceptable (>90%) oxygen saturation.

Maintenance of adequate gas exchange is the primary goal of invasive ventilation. Peak inspiratory pressure(PIP) and plateau pressure (Pplat) are the main measurements of pressure during ventilation. PIP, sometimes referred to as peak airway pressure, measures the maximum amount of pressure in the ventilator circuit during a breath cycle. It reflects lung compliance and airway resistance. In PCV, PIP can be estimated as the sum of the set pressure target and PEEP. PIP also generally reflects the amount of pressure in the alveoli at the end of inspiration, an important determinant in the development of VILI. In VCV, PIP is influenced greatly by airway resistance and therefore is not reflective of end-inspiratory alveolar pressure. Alveolar pressure at end inspiration in VCV is approximated by the Pplat.

Acute increases in PIP indicate increased airway resistance or changes in compliance of the respiratory system and can indicate potentially dangerous clinical deterioration. Decreases in PIP, conversely, indicate decreased resistance or decreased air flow in the ventilatory circuit and should prompt investigation of the ventilator circuit for leaks. Large or sudden decreases in PIP suggest disconnection of the ventilator circuit or unintended extubation. For patients with underlying respiratory failure secondary to increased airway resistance, such as in asthma or COPD, more gradual decreases in PIP are associated with clinical improvement.

Other Management Considerations

Aside from specific ventilator management, considerations in the care of the intubated patient include analgesia and sedation, potential neuromuscular paralysis, and secretion management. After intubation, the primary goals of care in the ED are sustained effective ventilation and patient comfort. Sedation should be maintained at the highest RASS score at which the patient is comfortable (between 0 and −5) and should be serially readdressed. Any paralyzed patient should remain deeply sedated (Table 4-3).

Table 4-3 The Richmond Agitation-Sedation Scale(RASS)

SCORE	TERM	DESCRIPTION
+4	Combative	Overtly combative, violent, immediate danger to staff
+3	Very agitated	Pulls or removes tube(s) or catheter(s),aggressive
+2	Agitated	Frequent nonpurposeful movement, fights ventilator
+1	Restless	Anxious, but movements not aggressive or vigorous
0	Calm	Alert and calm
−1	Drowsy	Not fully alert, but has sustained awakening (>10 s)
−2	Light sedation	Briefly awakens with eye contact to voice (<10 s)
−3	Moderate sedation	Movement or eye opening to voice but no eye contact
−4	Deep sedation	No response to voice but movement or eye opening with physical stimulation
−5	Unarousable	No response to voice or physical stimulation

After rapid sequence intubation, additional NBMA should generally be used only when poor ventilator synchrony interferes with ventilation sedation and analgesia.With proper sedation and analgesia, however, neuromuscular blockade usually is not required. If needed, longer-acting agents such as rocuronium and vecuronium should be used; note that impaired hepatic or renal function may increase duration of paralysis.

Analgesia is achieved by generous doses of opioid medications; fentanyl and morphine remain the most commonly used agents for analgesia in critically ill patients. Both morphine and fentanyl can be used for analgesia. Fentanyl may be preferred in patients with renal insufficiency.

Sedation after intubation can be accomplished via multiple pharmacologic modalities, lorazepam and midazolam are the most commonly used agents in the ICU.

Other medications for the sedation of ventilated patients in the ED include dexmedetomidine and haloperidol.It is administered as a loading dose followed by a continuous infusion and can precipitate bradycardia and relative hypertension.

Haloperidol can also be used as an adjunct to traditional sedation regimens in mechanically ventilated patients. The use of haloperidol may be particularly useful in patients who remain acutely agitated after large doses of other sedative medications, especially because it does not affect hemodynamics. Notably, however, haloperidol does not have any analgesic or amnestic properties and cannot be used as a single therapy for sedation in critically ill patients.

Other ED considerations in the care of the ventilated patient include secretion management and steps to reduce potential ventilator-associated pneumonia(VAP). Management of secretions is achieved via regular endotracheal suctioning, recognizing a balance between secretion clearance and the disruption of ventilation. In addition, a nasogastric or orogastric tube should be placed for gastrointestinal decompression. Finally, evidence demonstrates benefit in the prevention of VAP from placing the patient in the semirecumbent position by elevating the head of the bed. Use of VAP care "bundles," including elevation of the head of the bed, have decreased incidence of VAP in the ICU.

Complications of Positive-Pressure Ventilation

Initiation of PPV and elevated intrathoracic pressure can be associated with relative hypotension, and any subsequent changes in end-inspiratory alveolar pressures or PEEP during the management of ventilation may have hemodynamic consequences.

PPV also has a direct impact on the lungs. Injuries from elevated lung volume or lung pressure are known as volutrauma and barotrauma, respectively, and contribute to the development of VILI. Current data support that maximum "safe" end-inspiratory alveolar pressures are 30 to 32 cm H_2O. Barotrauma can also manifest overtly with pneumothorax or pneumomediastinum.

Another potential complication of PPV is the development of iPEEP. iPEEP results in unexpectedly high PIP, difficulty in ventilation, hypotension, and potential circulatory collapse. Ventilation difficulty caused by iPEEP can be improved by decreasing the respiratory rate or decreasing the inspiratory time.

Troubleshooting the Ventilator

When a patient's condition suddenly deteriorates during mechanical ventilation, a systematic approach should be applied to immediately assess for life-threatening conditions (Fig. 4-1). The first step in evaluating the ventilated patient who has a change in clinical status is to assess vital signs. Patients with acute hemodynamic compromise or acute hypoxia should be removed from the ventilator and bagged manually on 100% oxygen. Tension pneumothorax, increased iPEEP, and accidental extubation are the most life-threatening concerns in this situation.Changes in breath sounds may indicate a pneumothorax or a migration of the ETT. Clinical examination, SO_2, and $ETco_2$ monitoring can be used as surrogates for tube placement.Acute hypotension can be precipitated by extreme elevations in intrathoracic pressure.

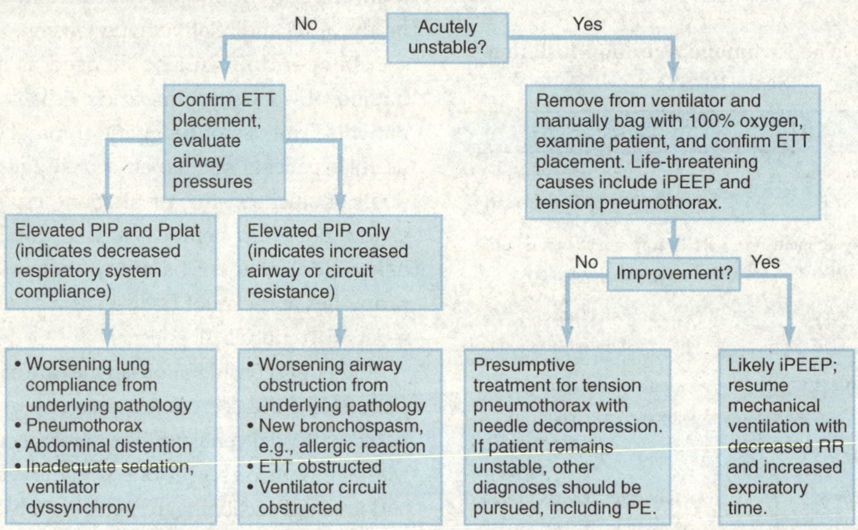

Fig. 4-1 Algorithm for evaluation of the distressed patient on mechanical ventilation.

Acute distress without hemodynamic changes can be precipitated by multiple factors, both mechanical and physiologic (Table 4-4). Again, the initial evaluation should begin by confirming position and patency of the ETT, including evaluation of the tracheal balloon.

Table 4-4 Troubleshooting the Ventilator:Potential Causes of Acute Respiratory Distress

With Hemodynamic Compromise: Immediately Discontinue Mechanical Ventilation	
Increased iPEEP	
Tension pneumothorax	
Massive pulmonary embolus	
Without Hemodynamic Compromise: Search for Underlying Cause	
MECHANICAL	**PHYSIOLOGIC**
Endotracheal tube migration into bronchus	Worsening lung compliance
Endotracheal tube obstruction	Worsening airway obstruction
Endotracheal tube cuff leak	Abdominal distention
Inadvertent extubation	Pulmonary embolus
Discontinuity in ventilator circuit	Pain or inadequate sedation

The next step in evaluation of ventilator-related causes of distress should focus on airway pressures. Acute decreases in PIP indicate discontinuity in the ventilator circuit.Patients with increased PIP can be considered in two categories: those with concomitant increases in Pplat, and those with unchanged Pplat. If both PIP and Pplat acutely increase, this suggests decreased compliance of the respiratory system. Elevated PIP with unchanged Pplat indicates problems with increased airway resistance, either in the lungs or the ventilator circuit. Specific conditions that cause decreased respiratory system compliance or increased airway resistance are detailed in Fig.4-1.

Special Clinical Circumstances

Acute Exacerbation of COPD

Strategies for managing intubated patients with COPD focus on improving gas exchange while minimizing iPEEP. Reduction of iPEEP is achieved by decreasing airway resistance with bronchodilators and corticosteroids and ensuring adequate expiratory time during mechanical ventilation. Adequate expiratory time is achieved by decreasing respiratory rate, V_T, and inspiratory time. Adequate oxygenation (saturation of 90%) is achieved while minimizing barotrauma by deliberately reducing minute ventilation, so-called "permissive hypercapnia." The ideal ratio of inspiratory-to-expiratory time (I/E ratio) is variable, but the ratio should initially be set at 1 : 4. iPEEP can also result in poor patient ventilator synchrony, causing inadequate gas exchange. Initially, deep sedation and analgesia (or sometimes paralysis) are required to prevent ventilator asynchrony and permit effective ventilation. Corticosteroids often are indicated.

Status Asthmaticus

In acute asthma, respiratory failure is both a result of airway obstruction and airway inflammation.In addition, acute inflammatory changes throughout the lung contribute to decreased lung compliance. Recommendations for ventilator settings include VCV with V_T of 6 to 8 mL/kg IBW, respiratory rate of 10 to 15 breaths/min, and no PEEP. Decreased inspiratory time allows greater expiratory time and is achieved by increasing the inspiratory flow rate.

ALI and ARDS

Strictly, the difference between these conditions is defined by P_aO_2/F_iO_2, with ALI being less severe than ARDS. ALI and ARDS can be caused by pulmonary or extrapulmonary inflammation, including VILI. Decreased V_T are of clear benefit in the management of patients with ALI and ARDS. Therefore in patients with ALI or ARDS ($P_aO_2/F_iO_2 < 300$), low-V_T ventilation strategy should be used. Initial ventilator settings should be volume cycled, with V_T based on 6 mL/kg of IBW.

(SHOU Songtao YU Muming)

Chapter 5

Adult Resuscitation

KEY CONCEPTS

CPR quality, including minimization of chest compression pauses, is critical to successful resuscitation from cardiac arrest.

Restoration of adequate cardiac function is the defining factor of ROSC. Restoration of normal brain function is the defining factor of successful resuscitation.

Resuscitation of a cardiac arrest victim does not end with ROSC. Rapid diagnosis and proper management of the pathologic conditions which precipitated and resulted from the arrest as well as goal-directed hemodynamic management can improve the outcome.

Induced prolonged hypothermia (32-34℃ for 12-24 hr) is the first and only post-ROSC intervention which can improve survival and functional outcome of comatose cardiac arrest survivors.

PERSPECTIVE

Epidemiology

It is estimated that 236,000 to 325,000 patients are treated for out-of-hospital cardiac arrest each year in the United States. The proportion of EMS-treated cardiac arrest patients with an initial rhythm of Vf has declined over time to 1/3 or less in recent U.S. studies. However, the number of patients receiving bystander CPR remains low, averaging only 26% in the home and 45% in public locations. Bystander AED is applied in 1% of home arrests and 8% of arrests in public settings.

There is tremendous variability in survival to hospital discharge after EMS-treated cardiac arrest, ranging from 3% to 16.7% with a median of 7.9%. For the subset of patients who achieved ROSC long enough to be admitted to the hospital, there is significant interinstitutional variability in survival, ranging from 19% to 59%. Of patients surviving to hospital discharge, one third have persistent neurologic deficits, and less than half return to prearrest function. In patients meeting the inclusion criteria for clinical therapeutic hypothermia trials, favorable outcome has been reported in approximately 50% of comatose cardiac arrest survivors treated with hypothermia. It is important to recognize that the entire system of care affects patient outcomes, and the variability in outcomes across the country likely reflects variability in how well these systems function.

PRINCIPLES OF DISEASE

Etiology

Understanding the causes of cardiac arrest helps direct therapy and diagnostic testing during resuscitation and in the immediate post-cardiac arrest period (Table 5-1). Cardiac arrest from a primary cardiac origin typically manifests as Vf or much less often as pulseless VT. CAD is the most common pathologic condition found in patients who die suddenly from Vf. Autopsy studies showed a 75% incidence of previous MI and a 20%-30% incidence of AMI. Other anatomic abnormalities associated with SCD caused by Vf or VT include myocardial hypertrophy, cardiomyopathy, and specific structural abnormalities. PEA and asystole are less common presenting rhythms in patients with a cardiac cause of arrest. These rhythms most often occur as a deterioration of Vf or VT, or develop in response to resuscitation treatments, such as defibrillation.

Table 5-1 Common Causes of Nontraumatic Cardiac Arrest

GENERAL	SPECIFIC	DISEASE OR AGENT
Cardiac		CAD Cardiomyopathies Structural abnormalities Valve dysfunction
Respiratory	Hypoventilation	CNS dysfunction Neuromuscular disease Toxic and metabolic Encephalopathies
	Upper airway obstruction	CNS dysfunction Foreign body Infection Trauma Neoplasm
	Pulmonary dysfunction	Asthma COPD Pulmonary edema Pulmonary embolus Pneumonia
Circulatory	Mechanical obstruction	Tension pneumothorax Pericardial tamponade Pulmonary embolus
	Hypovolemia Vascular tone	Hemorrhage Sepsis Neurogenic
Metabolic	Electrolyte abnormalities	Hypokalemia Hyperkalemia Hypermagnesemia Hypomagnesemia Hypocalcemia
Toxic	Prescription medications	Antidysrhythmics Digitalis beta-blockers CCB Tricyclic antidepressants
	Drugs of abuse	Cocaine Heroin
	Toxins	Carbon monoxide Cyanide
Environmental		Lightning Electrocution Hypothermia or hyperthermia Drowning or near drowning

Followed by hypotension and bradycardia, primary respiratory failure generally causes initial hypertension and tachycardia and progresses to PEA, Vf or asystole. Circulatory obstruction (e.g., tension pneumothorax, pericardial tamponade) and hypovolemia generally manifest with initial tachycardia and hypotension, progressing through bradycardia to PEA, but also may deteriorate to Vf or asystole.

The most common metabolic cause of cardiac arrest is hyperkalemia, which is most frequently in patients with renal failure. Hyperkalemia results in progressive widening of the QRS complex, which can deteriorate to VT, Vf, asystole or PEA. Other electrolyte abnormalities (e.g., hypomagnesemia, hypermagnesemia, hypokalemia) may lead to significant dysrhythmias, but the frequency with which they cause cardiac arrest is not documented.

Cardiac arrest from drug toxicity has specific characteristics depending on the drugs involved. Specific therapy directed at drug toxicity is essential but may not be immediately effective. Prolonged resuscitation efforts involving a method that provides adequate perfusion may be needed.

Electrocution causes cardiac arrest through primary dysrhythmias or apnea. Alternating current in the range of 100 mA to 1 A generally causes Vf. Currents greater than 10 A can cause ventricular asystole. Lightning produces a massive direct current electrocution that can result in asystole and prolonged apnea. Hypothermia-induced cardiac arrest can manifest with any ECG rhythm, and successful resuscitation depends on rapid rewarming, which often requires aggressive and invasive measures (e.g., intravascular rewarming, peritoneal lavage, CPB (cardiopulmonary bypass), open-chest cardiac massage). Drowning, as a form of asphyxia, usually results in bradyasystolic arrest. Because drowning is often accompanied by hypothermia, the victim may benefit from prolonged resuscitation efforts similar to those for hypothermia.

CLINICAL FEATURES AND MANAGEMENT

Most cardiac arrest cases managed in the ED initially occured outside the hospital. An increasing number of first responders, nontraditional providers and public venues are being equipped with AED. Dramatic resuscitation rates have been achieved when these programs enable providers and the lay public to deliver defibrillation within the first few minutes of arrest. If these programs fail to enable the patients to be defibrillated within this critical time window, there will be limited or no effect on survival.

Advanced life support units staffed by paramedics often have standing orders to follow advanced protocols. Because quality of CPR and the time of defibrillation are the two most important determinants of outcomes, there is no evidence to interrupt properly performed advanced measures to transport a patient who is still in cardiac arrest. In cases of cardiac arrest refractory to properly performed advanced measures, the patients may be pronounced dead at the scene if appropriate protocols have been outlined within the system.

History and Physical Examination

Historical information from the patient's family, bystanders and EMS personnel provides key information regarding causes and prognosis. Information surrounding the event includes whether the arrest was witnessed, the time of arrest, what the patient was doing (e.g., eating, exercising, trauma), the possibility of drug ingestion, time of initial CPR, initial ECG rhythm, and interventions by EMS providers. Important past medical history includes baseline health and mental status; previous heart, lung,renal or malignant diseases; hemorrhage; infection; and risk factors for CAD and PE. If possible, the patient's current medications and allergies should also be obtained.

Physical examination of a cardiac arrest patient is necessarily focused on a few key goals: (1) ensure adequacy of airway maintenance and ventilation, (2) confirm the diagnosis of cardiac arrest, (3) find evidence of the cause, and (4) monitor for complications of therapeutic interventions. This examination occurs in descending order of importance, simultaneously with therapeutic interventions. And it is repeated frequently to assess for response to therapy and occurrence of complications (Table 5-2).

Table 5-2 Physical Examination Findings Indicating Potential Cause of Cardiac Arrest and Complications of Therapy

PHYSICAL EXAMINATION	ABNORMALITIES	POTENTIAL CAUSES
General	Pallor	Hemorrhage
	Cold	Hypothermia
Airway	Secretions, vomitus, or blood	Aspiration Airway obstruction
	Resistance to PPV	Tension Pneumothorax Airway obstruction Bronchospasm
Neck	Jugular venous distention	Tension pneumothorax Cardiac tamponade Pulmonary embolus
	Tracheal deviation	Tension pneumothorax
Chest	Median sternotomy scar	Underlying cardiac disease
Lungs	Unilateral breath sounds	Tension pneumothorax Right mainstem intubation Aspiration
	Distant or no breath sounds or no chest expansion	Esophageal intubation Airway obstruction Severe bronchospasm
	Wheezing	Aspiration Bronchospasm Pulmonary edema
	Rales	Aspiration Pulmonary edema Pneumonia

Continued

PHYSICAL EXAMINATION	ABNORMALITIES	POTENTIAL CAUSES
Heart	Audible heart tones	Hypovolemia Cardiac tamponade Tension pneumothorax Pulmonary embolus
Abdomen	Distended and dull	Ruptured AAA Ruptured ectopic pregnancy
	Distended and tympanitic	Esophageal intubation Gastric insufflation
Rectal	Blood, melena	Gastrointestinal hemorrhage
Extremities	Asymmetrical pulses	Aortic dissection
	Arteriovenous shunt or fistula	Hyperkalemia
Skin	Needle tracks or abscesses	Intravenous drug abuse
	Burns	Smoke inhalation Electrocution

Cardiopulmonary arrest is defined by the triad of unconsciousness, apnea, and pulselessness. The pulse is palpated in a large artery (carotid or femoral). If any question exists as to the diagnosis of pulselessness, CPR should be initiated. With sudden onset of cardiac arrest, as in Vf, loss of consciousness occurs within 15 s, but agonal gasping respirations persist for several minutes. A brief seizure may result from cessation of cerebral blood flow. Primary respiratory arrest results in transient tachycardia and hypertension that progress to loss of consciousness, bradycardia and pulselessness.

After the initial minutes of cardiac arrest, physical examination may provide little evidence of the duration of arrest. Pupils dilate within 1 minute but constrict if CPR is initiated immediately and performed effectively. Dependent lividity and rigor mortis develop after hours of cardiac arrest. Temperature is an unreliable predictor of duration of cardiac arrest because it does not decrease significantly during the first hour of arrest. Moderate to severe hypothermia may cause cardiac arrest or may be caused by prolonged arrest, with opposite prognostic implications.

Monitoring

Traditional monitoring during CPR relies on evaluation of the ECG in one or more leads and palpation of carotid or femoral artery pulses. Absence of palpable pulse during CPR may indicate inadequate forward flow. But the degree of forward flow cannot be estimated accurately in the presence of a palpable pulse, because pressures generated during CPR may be transmitted equally to the venous and the arterial vasculatures. In addition, myocardial blood flow does not depend on the palpated arterial pressure during chest compression (CPR systole) but on the CPP, which is the difference between aortic and right atrial pressure during relaxation (CPR diastole). ECG monitoring during cardiac arrest indicates the presence or absence of electrical but not the mechanical activity. Although these two monitoring modalities may be the best attainable in certain circumstances, they do not provide reliable information regarding the effectiveness of CPR and interventions or prognosis.

Unfortunately, there is no ideal monitoring technique providing all the information that might be desired during resuscitation. Even the modalities discussed below are often difficult or impossible to establish or interpret during CPR. A brief overview of CPP, ETco_2 and ScvO_2 monitoring will be provided, which if available can be used to detect inadequate CPR with high specificity (Table 5-3).

Table 5-3 Indicators of Inadequate Blood Flow During Cardiopulmonary Resuscitation

MONITORING TECHNIQUE	INDICATOR
Carotid or femoral pulse	Not palpable
CPP	<15 mm Hg

Continued

MONITORING TECHNIQUE	INDICATOR
Arterial relaxation (diastolic) pressure	<40 mm Hg
$PETco_2$	<10 mm Hg (before vasopressor)
$ScvO_2$	<40%

Resuscitation

Restoration of adequate cardiac function is the defining factor of ROSC, and restoration of normal brain function is the defining factor of successful resuscitation. Interventions are performed rapidly and efficiently to maximize the chances of a good neurologic outcome. The quality of CPR is perhaps the most underappreciated component of the resuscitation effort. Important quality performance measures include compression rate (at least 100 per minute), compression depth (>5 cm), duty cycle (CPR being performed at >50% of pulseless interval) full relaxation, and minimum pauses, especially before and after defibrillation. Furthermore, hyperventilation has been shown to be common and it reduces cardiac output during CPR. Currently, health care professionals recommend a 30:2 compression-to-ventilation ratio in all adult resuscitation scenarios until an advanced airway has been established. Once the airway has been secured, CPR should be performed continuously without pausing, while providing six to eight ventilations every minute. In addition to monitoring specific CPR performance parameters, physiologic monitoring, if available, can help optimize CPR quality for the individual patient (Table 5-3). Fig. 5-1 is an algorithm for management of cardiac arrest. Interventions specific to each rhythm are discussed in the following sections.

Post-Cardiac Arrest

Resuscitation of a cardiac arrest victim does not end with ROSC. Management includes rapid diagnosis ,treatment of the disorders which cause the arrest and the complications of prolonged global ischemia. Simultaneous management of these entities makes caring for a post-cardiac arrest patient particularly challenging. A comprehensive goal-driven program of post-cardiac arrest care is the most successful in affecting survival and neurologic status.

Induction of prolonged therapeutic hypothermia in comatose survivors of cardiac arrest has been shown to improve survival and functional outcome. Hypothermia is maintained for 12 to 24 hr, followed by gradual rewarming over 12 to 24 hr. Effective application of therapeutic hypothermia in comatose cardiac arrest survivors requires a coordinated interdisciplinary effort. And it is best carried out through the use of a predetermined goal-directed algorithm developed with input from emergency medicine, cardiology and critical care physicians and nurses.

A simultaneous immediate concern in a comatose cardiac arrest survivor is whether the patient has ACS. Diagnosing ACS in an unconscious patient after cardiac arrest presents a unique challenge. A standard 12-lead ECG should be obtained as soon as feasible after ROSC, with additional right-sided and/or posterior leads as indicated. Immediate PCI is indicated in post-ROSC patients with STEMI or new LBBB, or high clinical suspicion of AMI, and it can be performed during therapeutic hypothermia.

If there is no evidence of hemorrhage and profound hypertension, antiplatelet and anticoagulant therapies should be administered to all patients after ROSC, whether or not therapeutic hypothermia is induced.

Resuscitation of a cardiac arrest victim does not end with ROSC. Rapid diagnosis and proper management of the pathologic conditions which result from the arrest as well as the goal-directed hemodynamic management can improve the outcome (Fig. 5-2).

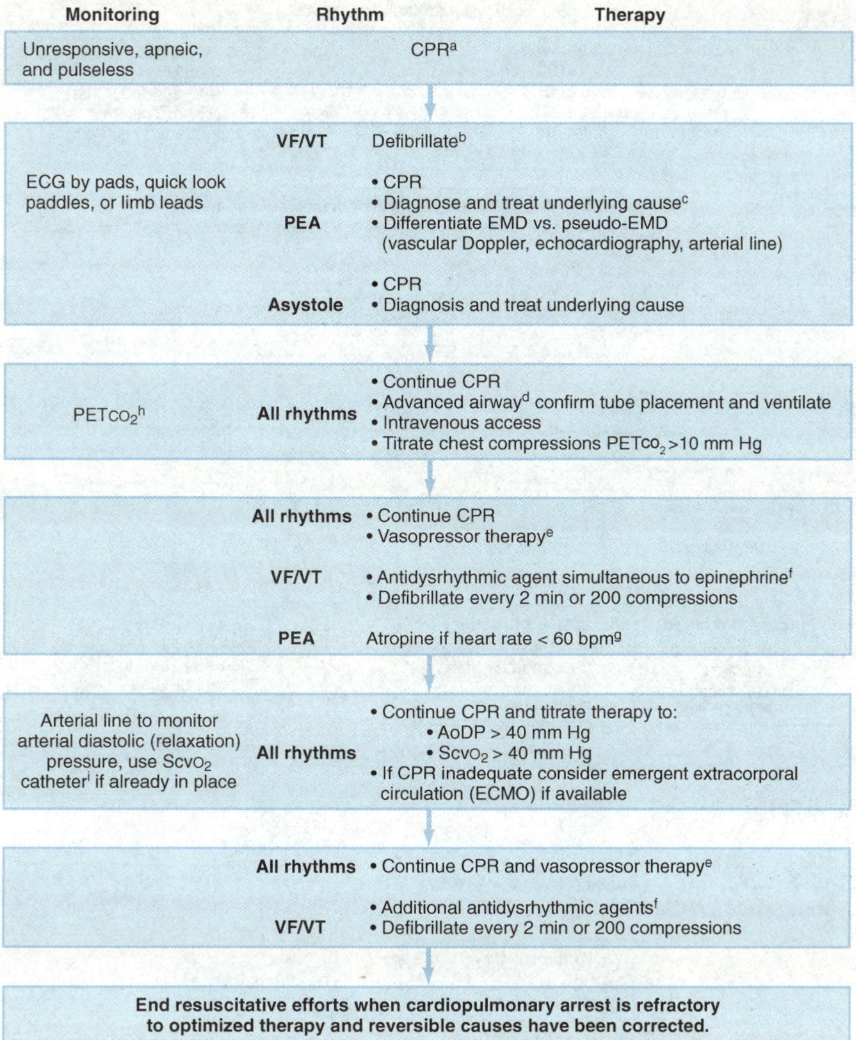

Fig. 5-1 Emergency treatment algorithm for treatment of cardiac arrest. [a]If cardiac arrest is witnessed and known to be of short duration, immediate rhythm assessment and defibrillation of VF/VT precede CPR. In cases of prolonged untreated VF/VT, 1 to 2 min of CPR before defibrillation may enhance the ability to achieve ROSC. [b]Biphasic defibrillation should use manufacturer-recommended energy versus monophasic defibrillation (360 J). [d]Endotracheal intubation or supraglottic airway when feasible with minimal interruption in chest compressions. [e]Epinephrine, initial dose of 1 mg IV or intraosseously (IO) or 2.5 mg by ETT. Repeat every 3 to 5 min. Subsequent doses may be increased up to 0.1 mg/kg. An alternative to epinephrine is vasopressin, 40 U via intravenous push. Vasopressin is potentially more effective if the presenting rhythm is asystole. The dose (40 U) can be repeated once in 3 min, followed by administration of epinephrine every 3 to 5 min. [f]Amiodarone, 300 mg via intravenous push followed by 150 mg every 30 min. Lidocaine is an alternative antidysrhythmic if amiodarone is not available. Magnesium sulfate, 1 to 2 g via intravenous push in torsades de pointes or known hypomagnesemia. [g]Atropine, 1 mg via intravenous push or 2.5 mg by ETT. Repeat dose every 3 to 5 min to a total dose of 0.04 mg/kg. [h]Changes in the $PETco_2$ may not be predictive of myocardial blood flow in the setting of high-dose vasopressor therapy. [i]Invasive monitoring should be performed only if adequate personnel are available and if it would not delay therapeutic interventions.

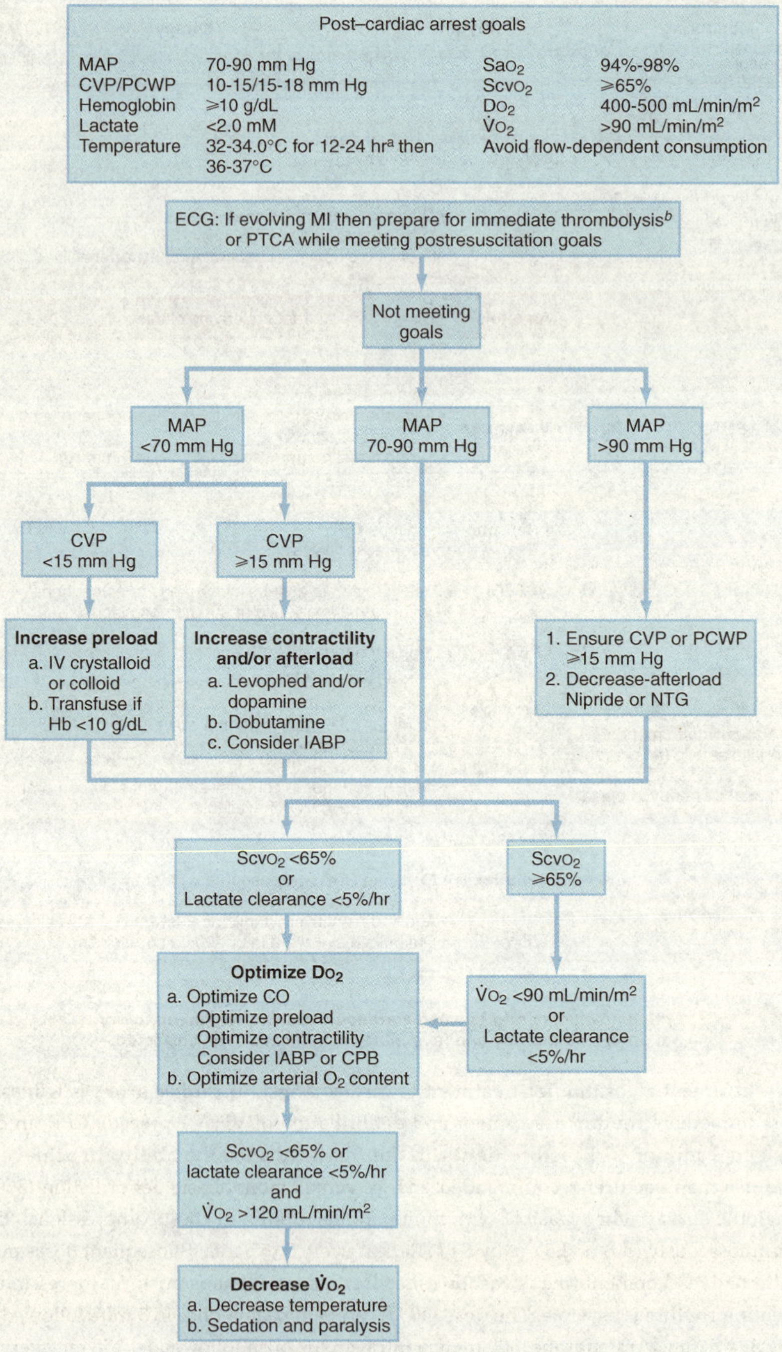

Fig. 5-2 Goal-directed post-arrest treatment algorithm. [a]Therapeutic hypothermia is indicated in comatose survivors of witnessed cardiac arrest who has a presenting rhythm of Vf. It may also be effective in patients resuscitated from other cardiac arrest presentations. Relative contraindications include an unwitnessed cardiac arrest, severe cardiogenic shock, life-threatening dysrhythmias, uncontrolled bleeding, preexisting coagulopathy, pregnancy, another obvious reasons for coma (e.g., drug overdose or status epilepticus), known end-stage terminal illness, and a preexisting do-not-resuscitate status. [b]Initiation of therapeutic hypothermia is not a contraindication to thrombolytic therapy.

(ZHANG Jinsong)

Chapter 6

Brain Resuscitation

KEY CONCEPTS

Neuronal injury is a dynamic process that continues for hours or days after an ischemic insult to the brain.

Hypotension, hypoperfusion, and hypoxia must be avoided during brain resuscitation.

Hyperthermia, hyperglycemia, and seizures should be treated promptly during brain resuscitation.

Comatose survivors of out-of-hospital cardiac arrest should be rapidly cooled in the ED and maintained at 33°C in EICU setting for 12 to 24 hr after resuscitation.

PERSPECTIVE

Recognition of the dominant role of the brain in determining the quality of human life dates back to the dawn of recorded medical history. Until recently, however, medical efforts after cardiac arrest have focused exclusively on cardiac resuscitation. Recent advances in the understanding of the pathophysiologic mechanisms of brain ischemia have encouraged attention to cerebral resuscitation as a critical component of what is now recognized as a complex multisystem pathophysiologic state called post–cardiac arrest syndrome. This chapter reviews the pathophysiology of postischemic encephalopathy and discusses therapies for improving neurologic recovery after cardiac arrest.

PATHOPHYSIOLOGY

The human brain consists of 10 billion neurons, each with multiple connections to other cells, totaling an estimated 500 trillion synapses. Although the brain constitutes only 2% of body weight, it receives 15% of the body's cardiac output and accounts for 20% of the body's overall oxygen use because of its high metabolic activity. Although no mechanical or secretory work is performed by the brain, energy expenditures include the synthesis of cellular constituents (e.g., an estimated 2000 mitochondria are reproduced each day by each cell) and neurotransmitter substances, the axoplasmic transport of these substances, and the transmembrane pumping of ions.

When the brain is deprived of adequate blood flow, the resulting ischemia is characterized by a bewildering array of inter-related physiologic and cellular responses that ultimately result in neuronal cell death (Fig. 6-1). Although this complex cascade of events can be triggered by periods of ischemia lasting only a few minutes, the resulting neuronal death is usually delayed by hours or days. Furthermore, the biology of cerebral cell death after global cerebral ischemia follows (with slight variations) the pattern of delayed cerebral cell death that follows stroke, traumatic brain injury, and other forms of hypoxic or toxic brain injury. Increased understanding of the brain's response to injury during the period between insult and neuronal cell death will eventually allow more specific brain resuscitation therapis.

MANAGEMENT

Standard Strategies

Return of Spontaneous Circulation

Cardiac resuscitation is the first priority in cerebral resuscitation. The degree of brain injury after cardiac arrest depends on both the duration of complete cerebral ischemia (the "downtime," or time before the initiation of CPR) and the duration of relative ischemia that occurs

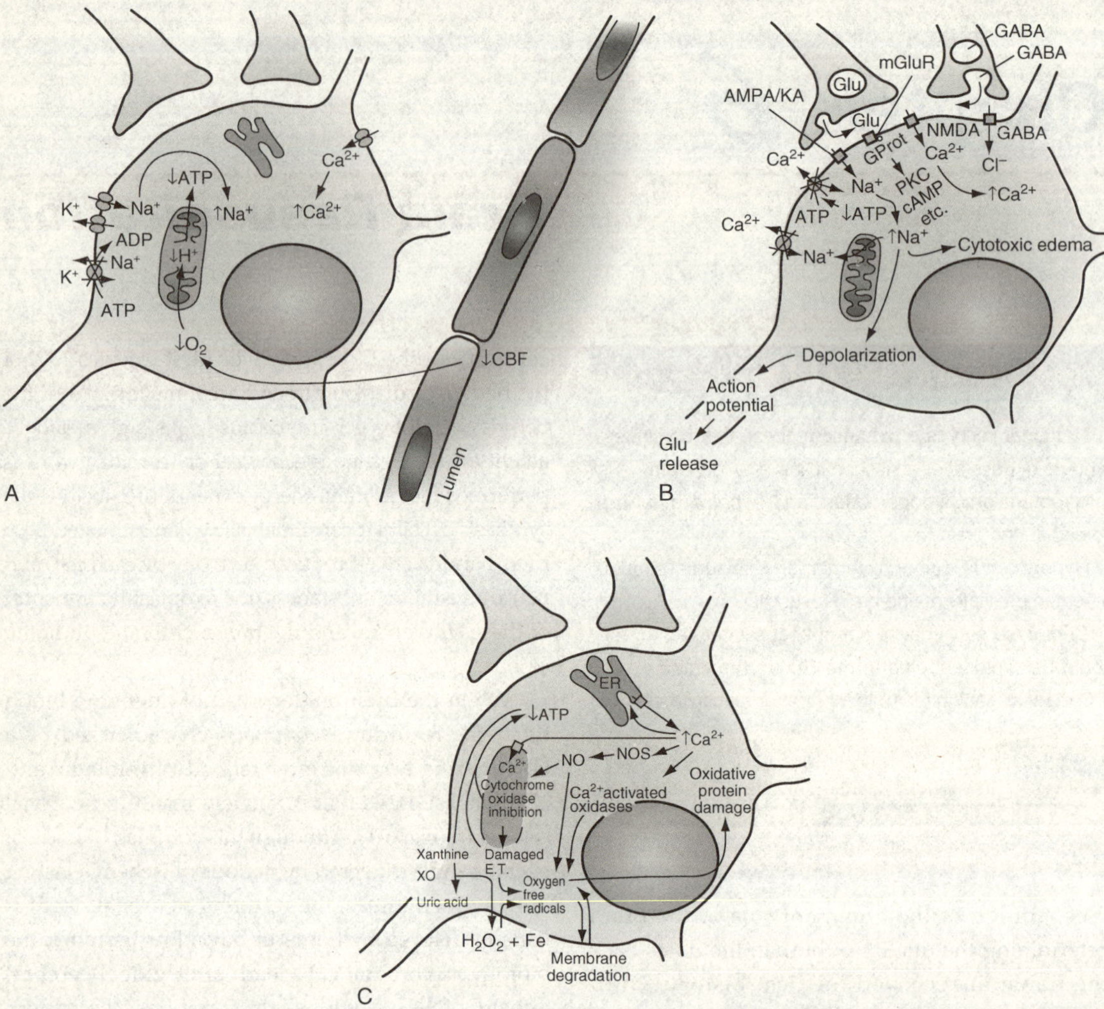

Fig. 6-1 Synopsis of events contributing to neuron cell death cascade after ischemia. A. Decreased *CBF* and arterial oxygen content during ischemia cause decreased *ATP* production, failure of ATP-driven ion pump efflux of potassium ions (K^+), and influx of sodium ions (Na^+) and calcium ions (Ca^{2+}) through voltage-gated channels. B. Na^+ influx causes depolarization and glutamate release, opening Glu receptor α-amino-3-hydroxy-5-methyl-4-isoxazolepropionate (AMPA) and kainate (KA) channels and exacerbating intracellular Na^+ ($[Na^+]i$)overload. Increased $[Na^+]i$ leads to cytotoxic edema.Glu-mediated *N*-methyl-Daspartate (NMDA) channels allow intracellular Ca^{2+} overload. Insufficient ATP causes failure of energy-dependent Ca^{2+} pumps, and high $[Na^+]i$ prevents removal of Ca^{2+} by Na^+/Ca^{2+} exchange pumps. *GABA* release can attenuate excitatory changes by opening a receptor-gated Cl^-. C. Increased $[Ca^{2+}]i$ is amplified by calcium-induced release of Ca^{2+} from the endoplasmic reticulum (ER). Mitochondria may be injured attempting to buffer increasing $[Ca^{2+}]i$, resulting in further metabolic failure and diminished ATP. Ca^{2+} activates nitric oxide synthase(NOS), *transforming it to* NO, which is amplified by NO activation of NOS. NO contributes to the formation of damaging oxygen free radicals and inhibits mitochondrial cytochrome oxidase function. ATP degradation to xanthine and then uric acid by xanthine oxidase (XO) yields H_2O_2, which reacts with iron to form dangerous oxygen radicals. Oxygen free radicals react with lipids in the cell membrane, which produces membrane degradation and more free radicals. Oxygen free radicals also can damage proteins. D. Ca^{2+} also activates kinase transcription factors, such as mitogen-activated protein kinase (MAPK). Oxygen radicals trigger NF-κB, another transcription factor. Many genes, including *IEG*, *HSP* genes, genes for caspases, and the Bax/Bcl-2 systems, are activated. IEG products include AP-1, which is another transcription factor. Mitochondrial release of cytochrome c, existing and newly formed caspases, and other factors trigger apoptosis. DNA is damaged by oxygen free radicals and by endonucleases formed in apoptosis. DNA damage activates poly(ADP-ribose) polymerase (PARP), which further depletes ATP stores. E. Ca^{2+} and apoptosis activate calpains, proteases that degrade a variety of structural elements (e.g., cytoskeletal and membrane proteins), signaling elements (e.g., G proteins, kinases), and PARP. F. Transcription and NO contribute to neuronal expression of cytokines, chemokines, and growth factors. These intercellular signals activate complement, epithelial cells, leukocytes, and microglia. Complement can amplify chemotactic signals, activate microglia directly, or cause cellular damage by creation of the membrane attack complex (MAC). Leukocyte integrins, epithelial cell selectins, and intercellular adhesion molecules (ICAM) allow demargination. Activated leukocytes cause neuronal injury by releasing potent oxidants and protease. Cerebrovascular resistance may be affected by epithelial release of NO and endothelin and by leukocyte clumping.

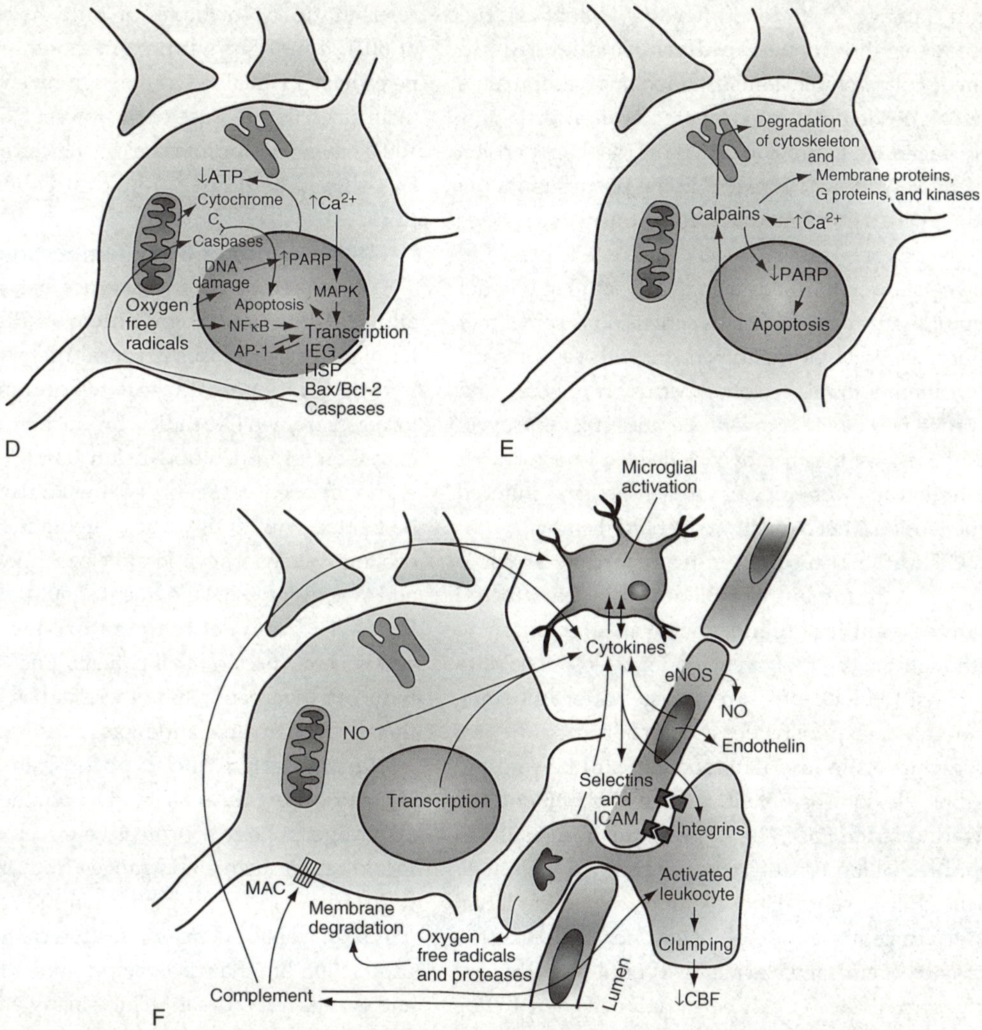

(Fig. 6-1, cont'd.)

during CPR and that may occur from cardiogenic shock preceding or subsequent to the period of cardiac arrest. Extensive clinical evidence on hospital discharge rates and neurologic recovery rates supports the concept first proposed nearly 100 yr ago that success in resuscitation is inversely proportional to the duration of cardiac arrest.Although duration of arrest generally predicts outcome in the population of patients with sudden cardiac death, it cannot be used reliably to predict the outcome of individual patients. The epidemiology of neurologic outcome of survivors is described in detail in the following section and is influenced by patient comorbidity and other individual characteristics. Depending on their timing and severity, low-flow states, hypotension, or hypoxia preceding cardiac arrest may provide protective preconditioning or may increase the risk of poor neurologic outcome.

Treatment of Hypotension, Hypoperfusion, and Hypoxia

Maintaining cerebral oxygen delivery after cardiac resuscitation is a mainstay of therapy. Oxygen delivery requires a sufficiently high cerebral perfusion pressure, a sufficiently low cerebrovascular resistance (CVR), and adequate blood oxygen saturation.

Hypotension in the postarrest period can dangerously lower cerebral perfusion pressure. Although CBF is normally independent of perfusion pressure over a wide range of arterial blood pressure, such autoregulation is often lost in the injured brain. As a result, perfusion of ischemic tissue becomes passively dependent on arterial pressure, and hypotension can compromise CBF and result in significant additional brain damage. Therefore, after ROSC, low arterial pressures should be rapidly normalized, with intravascular volume administration and vasopressors used as needed. Because elevated arterial pressures may be needed to provide sufficient CBF, hypertension usually should not be treated in the postresuscitation period. Very high BP may require treatment, but specific cutoffs are controversial. In general, diastolic pressures may be allowed to run as high as 120 mm Hg without requiring treatment. In fact, hypertension is sometimes induced clinically or experimentally with vasopressors in an attempt to raise cerebral perfusion pressure and improve neurologic recovery. Because it is unproved, and the risks of this therapy include blood-brain barrier disruption and worsening of vasogenic edema, induced hypertension is not currently a standard therapy.

CVR after resuscitation from cardiac arrest is another determinant of CBF and may be affected by hyperventilation and microvascular patency. Although the cerebral circulation may lose its ability to adjust to blood pressure changes after ischemia, attenuated responsiveness to carbon dioxide and oxygen levels in arterial blood can still be present. Carbon dioxide is a potent vasoactive agent, and the lowering of the P_aCO_2 by hyperventilation results in rapid reduction of CBF. Because reductions in CBF reduce total cerebral blood volume, hyperventilation may transiently abort brainstem herniation in the presence of critically elevated ICP until osmotherapy or ventriculostomy can be initiated. When ICP is not elevated, however, the vasoconstriction and increased CVR caused by hyperventilation can cause potentially dangerous reductions in CBF. Although controversy surrounds whether increases in ICP are clinically significant after global ischemia, the measurement of ICP is generally not recommended in the management of adult cardiac arrest survivors. In general, ventilation to maintain a P_aCO_2 of 35 to 40 mm Hg is safe and appropriate, and inadvertent hyperventilation should be avoided.

Normal arterial oxygen saturation should be maintained after resuscitation from cardiac arrest. Because the injured brain may not be able to compensate for hypoxia by augmenting CBF, cerebral oxygen delivery may diminish rapidly as the oxygen content of blood decreases. Hyperoxia secondary to the use of 100% oxygen in the immediate postarrest period, however, has also been shown to increase oxidative brain injury in animal models of cardiac arrest and resuscitation. Normoxia or mild hyperoxia (P_aO_2 of 80-120 mm Hg with oxyhemoglobin saturation percentage maintained in the high nineties) should be maintained through use of the lowest F_iO_2. The use of 100% oxygen is appropriate during cardiac arrest, but F_iO_2 should be titrated downward shortly after the ROSC.

Maintenance of Body Temperature

Hyperthermia (or fever) exacerbates brain injury and worsens neurologic outcome. Elevated body temperature increases cerebral metabolic demand by 8% to 13% per ℃, escalates glutamate release, increases oxygen free radical production, and increases cytoskeletal and blood-brain barrier breakdown with increased vasogenic edema.Hyperthermia may be treated with antipyretics, circulating air or water cooling systems, or evaporative cooling via water mist and fans. Aggressive treatment should, at a minimum, be used to prevent temperature increases in the postischemic period in all patients, and the practice of inducing therapeutic hypothermia has emerged as a therapy for comatose survivors of cardiac arrest.

Resuscitative Mild Hypothermia

Hypothermia was first reported more than 50 yr ago to have a protective effect in global and focal brain ischemia and ranges from mild (32-34℃) to profound (5℃). Hypothermia reduces glutamate release, metabolic demand, free radical formation, and production of inflammatory cytokines. Cell-signaling and genetic responses to cellular injury are also affected by hypothermia, and hypothermia may protect the brain from programmed neuronal cell death.

Mild hypothermia is easier to achieve and has fewer adverse effects than lower temperatures and has consistently been found to be neuroprotective in experimental cerebral ischemia.It is recommended cooling unconscious adult patients after cardiac arrest to 33℃ for 12 to 24 hr.

Techniques used to induce hypothermia in comatose survivors of cardiac arrest, including traditional and advanced surface cooling, administration of ice-cold saline, and endovascular cooling, are discussed. The optimal method of cooling patients resuscitated from cardiac arrest has not been established.

The rate of cooling needed for effective neuroprotection, the optimal duration of cooling, and the best process for rewarming after hypothermia are all unknown. Animal experimentation and the consensus recommendations suggest that cooling should be initiated as early and as rapidly as possible. Cooling may begin during the out-of-hospital phase of resuscitation and may even be initiated before ROSC. Patients were then allowed to rewarm passively or with a combination of passive and active rewarming.

Cooling of comatose survivors of out-of-hospital cardiac arrest requires a multidisciplinary hospital policy and should be initiated as early as possible (Box 6-1). In hospitals capable of hypothermic resuscitation, cooling is optimally started in the field or the ED and maintained in the ICU. Regardless of cooling technique, patients cooled after cardiac arrest require pharmacologic therapy to prevent shivering because shivering effectively warms the patient. When paralysis is not clinically desirable, it may be possible to sufficiently lower the shivering threshold in awake patients with meperidine, buspirone, dexmedetomidine, or a combination of these. Shivering can sometimes also be reduced in a patient cooled by an endovascular catheter even when the core temperature is 33℃ by applying a warming blanket, because surface temperature receptors control thermoregulation to a much greater extent than core temperature receptors. Other pharmacologic treatments that may be used during induced hypothermia include antipyretics. Neurotensin is an endogenous neuropeptide involved in thermoregulation that can induce hypothermia and neuroprotection in experimental models of cerebral ischemia.

Box 6-1 Abbreviated Protocol for Induced Hypothermia after Cardiac Arrest

For access to a wide variety of detailed post–cardiac arrest care and hypothermia protocols collected by the University of Pennsylvania

Hypothermia is most effective as part of an institutional comprehensive post–cardiac arrest critical care program that begins in the ED and continues into the ICU and into recovery and rehabilitation.

Early resuscitation, excellent CPR, rapid ROSC, and quick transport to definitive care are fundamental. The value of prehospital cooling is unproven, but if cooling is initiated by EMS, transport should be to an institution capable of maintaining hypothermia on arrival and avoiding any early (even transient) rewarming.

Skeleton Protocol (Abstracted from University of Michigan Protocol)

- Evaluate adult survivors of cardiac arrest by following institutional criteria for appropriateness of induced hypothermia.
- Begin cooling by rapidly infusing 2 L of cold (4℃) intravenous saline immediately after arrival or ROSC.
- Expose patient; avoid external warming—no blankets and no heated ventilator circuit.
- Place temperature-sensing urinary catheter and esophageal temperature probe. (Redundant monitoring allows esophageal temperature probe connection to cooling device, and bladder temperature probe to patient monitoring system.)
- Initiate definitive cooling by endovascular temperature-control device at maximal rate to target temperature of 33℃.
- Prevent shivering with sedation and nondepolarizing paralytic. Bolus in ED. Bolus or drip in ICU.
- Avoid hypotension and hypoxia.
- Most ED diagnostic workup, if needed, should follow initiation of cooling. (In patients with AMI] who are going to primary coronary intervention, cooling should not delay door-to-balloon time. Cooling is initiated in the ED if there is time before the catheterization laboratory is ready; otherwise, cooling is initiated in the laboratory.)
- Admit to ICU.
- Continuous EEG monitoring for occult status epilepticus recommended. Treat seizures if present.
- Manage ABG in a consistent manner (may choose pH-stat or alpha-stat).
- At 24 hr after initiation of cooling, initiate rewarming to a target temperature of 36.5℃ at a rate of 0.15℃/hr.
- Discontinue paralytics at the onset of warming. Control shivering with sedation, narcotics, and surface counter warming.
- Lighten sedation as tolerated as rewarming progresses.
- Discontinue endovascular temperature control device after 48 hr. (May use the device to maintain normothermia after rewarming is complete until it is removed.)
- Remove or minimize sedation to allow neurologic evaluation before 72 hr to allow the best possible clinical prognostication at that time point. Neurology consultation recommended.

Treatment of Hyperglycemia

Postischemic hyperglycemia has detrimental effects on CBF, metabolism, edema formation, and neurologic outcome. Increased neuronal damage from hyperglycemia in global cerebral ischemia may also be glutamate mediated. Active treatment of hyperglycemia after global brain ischemia, and the administration of glucose should be avoided except in verified hypoglycemia.

Seizure Management

Seizures may result from global cerebral ischemia and may exacerbate the underlying brain injury. Seizure activity can increase brain metabolism by 300% to 400%, worsening the mismatch between oxygen delivery and demand in the postarrest period, with greater metabolic failure and neuronal loss and worsened neurologic outcome. The prophylactic use of anticonvulsant drugs in patients resuscitated from cardiac arrest is controversial and is not standard care. Common therapeutic agents include benzodiazepines, phenytoin, and barbiturates. Each of these anticonvulsant drugs has also been considered as specific therapy for cerebral ischemia because of the antagonism of excitatory amino acids, sodium channel blockade, or effects on cerebral metabolism.

Immobilization, Sedation, and Head Position

The comatose brain responds to external stimuli (e.g., physical examination, airway suctioning) with increases in cerebral metabolism. This elevation of regional brain metabolism requires increased regional CBF at a time when the oxygen demand/perfusion ratios may be precariously balanced. Protection from afferent sensory stimuli with administration of titrated doses of sedative-anesthetic drugs and muscle relaxants may prevent oxygen supply/demand imbalance and improve the chances for neuronal recovery.

All activity that increases ICP (e.g., straining, coughing) should be restricted, and tracheal suction should be performed only when necessary and with care. Torsion or compression of neck veins should be avoided by eliminating compressive dressings and not rotating or flexing the head.

CLINICAL OUTCOMES

Global cerebral ischemia resulting from a period of cardiac arrest is a frequently fatal and highly morbid condition, but the prognosis for its victims is not universally poor. An increasing body of data is providing more complete and precise estimates of the functional outcomes and quality of life of survivors of cardiac arrest, and the results are better than many physicians assume.

(ZHANG Jinsong)

Chapter 7

Implantable Cardiac Devices

KEY CONCEPTS

Pacemaker malfunction soon after implantation (within 6-8w) is usually a result of a lead problem, such as a lead displacement, or a pacemaker programming failure, such as a pacing rate too slow for the patient's needs.

Pacemaker malfunction arises in a limited number of ways: failure to pace, oversensing, undersensing, and pacing at an inappropriate rate (too fast or too slow).

If a patient with a pacemaker has a fever of unclear cause,pacemaker lead infection and endocarditis should be considered.

Because paced ventricular complexes are conducted with a LBBB pattern, a paced rhythm obscures the electrocardiographic diagnosis of AMI. A right bundle branch pattern is abnormal and suggests lead displacement.

Defibrillation is safe in patients with a pacemaker or ICD.

PERSPECTIVE

Electrical cardiac pacing for the management of bradyarrhythmias was first described in 1952, and permanent transvenous pacing devices were introduced into clinical practice in the early 1960s. The first devices for endocardial defibrillation were implanted in surviving victims of SCD in 1980. Implanted electrical devices for the management of cardiac dysrhythmias have changed rapidly over the years, with both increasing complexity and miniaturization.

Implantable cardioverter-defibrillator (ICD) significantly improves survival for the prevention of SCD resulting from ventricular dysrhythmias.

INDICATIONS FOR PERMANENT PACEMAKERS AND ANTIARRHYTHMIA DEVICES

With use of an evidence-based approach, recommendations are categorized as class Ⅰ, Ⅱ, or Ⅲ. Class Ⅰ includes conditions for which there is general agreement that a device should be implanted. A class Ⅱ recommendation includes conditions for which these devices are frequently used but for which there is disagreement about their need or benefit. Class Ⅲ is reserved for conditions for which there is general agreement that a device is not needed.

Class I indications for a permanent pacemaker or ICD are listed in Box 7-1 and Box 7-2. In general, pacing is recommended for patients with symptomatic heart block, symptomatic sinus bradycardia, and Af with a symptomatic bradycardia (low ventricular response rate) in the absence of medications that affect AV conduction. Controversial indications include pacing in patients with syncope, heart block, or fatigue in the presence of some conduction disease or bradycardia. The likelihood of a patient's improvement after pacing can be assumed only if the symptoms can be closely correlated with inadequate rate.

Box 7-1 Class I Indications for Permanent Pacing in Adults

1. Third-degree and advanced second-degree AVB at any anatomic level associated with any of the following:
   - Symptomatic bradycardia (including HF) or ventricular dysrhythmia presumed to be a result of AVB

- Symptomatic bradycardia secondary to drugs required for dysrhythmia management or other medical condition
- Documented periods of asystole lasting more than 3 s or an escape rate of less than 40 beats/min or an escape rhythm originating below the AV node in an awake, asymptomatic patient in sinus rhythm
- Awake, asymptomatic patients with Af and bradycardia a documented pause of 5 s or longer
- After catheter ablation of the AV node
- Postoperative AVB that is not expected to resolve
- Neuromuscular disease with AVB (e.g., the muscular dystrophies)

2. Symptomatic bradycardia resulting from second-degree AVB regardless of type or site of block
3. Asymptomatic, persistent third-degree AVB with awake ventricular rate over 40 beats/min with cardiomegaly or left ventricular dysfunction or if block is below AV node
4. Chronic bifascicular or trifascicular block with intermittent third-degree AVB or type II second-degree AVB
5. Second or third-degree AVB with exercise in the absence of myocardial ischemia

Box 7-2 Class I Indications for Implantable Cardioverter-Defibrillator Therapy

1. Cardiac arrest resulting from Vf or VT not caused by a transient or reversible event
2. Spontaneous sustained VT
3. Syncope of undetermined origin with clinically relevant, hemodynamically significant sustained VT or Vf induced at electrophysiologic study when drug therapy is ineffective, not tolerated, or not preferred
4. Nonsustained VT with coronary artery disease, prior MI, left ventricular dysfunction, and inducible Vf or sustained VT at electrophysiologic study that is not suppressible by a class I antiarrhythmic drug

Pacemaker Terminology

A letter code standardizes nomenclature for pacemakers. Table 7-1 includes an explanation of the five-letter code scheme and the standard abbreviations in each category. The first three code letters are used most commonly.The codes of a permanent pacemaker that are used most frequently and the indications, advantages, and disadvantages of each are listed in Table 7-2. Detailed algorithms for matching a patient with a pacemaker exist. The majority of permanent pacemakers are dual chamber and often rate adaptive.

Table 7-1 Five-Letter Pacemaker Code

Letter 1	Letter 2	Letter 3	Letter 4	Letter 5
CHAMBER PACED	CHAMBER SENSED	SENSING RESPONSE	PROGRAMMABILITY	ANTITACHYCARDIA FUNCTIONS
A = atrium	A = atrium	T = triggered	P = simple	P = pacing
V = ventricle	V = ventricle	I = inhibited	M = multiprogrammable	S = shock
D = dual	D = dual	D = dual (A and V inhibited)	R = rate adaptive	D = dual (shock pace)
O = none	O = none	O = none	C = communicating O = none	

Table 7-2 Common Permanent Pacemakers

CODE	INDICATION	ADVANTAGES	DISADVANTAGES
VVI	Intermittent backup pacing; inactive patient	Simplicity; low cost	Fixed rate; risk of pacemaker syndrome
VVIR	Af	Rate responsive	Requires advanced programming
DDD	Complete heart block	Atrial tracking restores normal physiology	No rate responsiveness; requires two leads and advanced programming
DDDR	Sinus node dysfunction; for rate responsiveness AVB and need	Universal pacer; all options available by programming	Complexity, cost, programming, and followup evaluation

Pacemaker Components

All pacemaker systems have three basic components: the pulse generator, which houses the power source (battery); the electronic circuitry; and the lead system, which connects the pulse generator to the endocardium.

Nearly all implanted pacemakers are lithium powered. Lithium powered pulse generators function normally for 4 to 10 or more years, depending on the pacemaker features, such as single versus dual chamber, pacing threshold, and rate adaptiveness.

Permanent pacemakers have endocardial leads that are positioned in contact with the endocardium of the RV and, in the case of a dual-chamber device, the right atrium, with a subclavian or cephalic vein approach used for insertion. Despite pacemaker leads are continuously improved, problems with the electrical circuitry remain the most common cause of pacemaker malfunction.

The Standard Electrocardiogram during Normal Cardiac Pacing

The modern pacemaker has two basic functions: to stimulate the heart electrically and to sense intrinsic cardiac electrical activity.

The two basic functions of a pacemaker can be easily recognized and confirmed on a standard 12-lead ECG or rhythm strip. The normal function of a single-chamber VVI pacemaker is most easily recognized (Fig. 7-1).The pacer spike is a narrow deflection that is usually less than 5 mm in amplitude with a bipolar lead configuration and usually 20 mm or more in amplitude with a unipolar lead. A wide QRS complex appears immediately after the stimulus artifact. Depolarization begins in the right ventricular apex, and the spread of excitation does not follow normal conduction pathways. Characteristically, a LBBB conduction pattern is seen. A right bundle branch pattern is abnormal and suggests lead displacement. In VVI pacing the paced QRS complexes are independent of intrinsic atrial depolarization if present (AV dissociation).

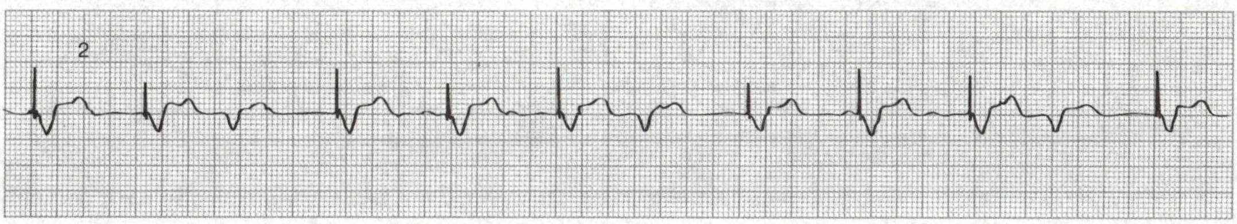

Fig. 7-1 Normal VVI pacemaker (rhythm strip). This rhythm strip was recorded in a patient with a VVI pacemaker implanted for the treatment of symptomatic CHB. The pacing rate is approximately 75 beats/min (determined by measuring the time between consecutive pacemaker spikes). Each pacemaker spike is followed by a paced QRS complex. The third QRS from the left has a slightly different morphology than the paced QRS complexes. It is an intrinsic QRS complex that is sensed by the pacemaker, and a paced beat does not occur again until the programmed rate of the pacemaker is exceeded. The time interval between the spontaneous QRS and the next paced beat is approximately the same as the interval between consecutive pacemaker spikes. This sequence is subsequently repeated twice on this strip.

The recognition of normal dual-chamber pacing is more complex owing to the interactive sensing and pacing of the right atrium and ventricle (Fig. 7-2). Dual-chamber devices are typically used in patients with nonfibrillating atria coupled with intact AV conduction. A normal-appearing QRS complex may follow an intrinsic "P" wave as a result of normal sinoatrial node discharge if the intrinsic atrial depolarization is conducted to the ventricles. The intrinsic p wave and QRS complex inhibit the atrial and ventricular circuitry. A normal QRS complex follows a paced p wave if the paced atrial beat is conducted through the AV node and the programmed AV delay period is not exceeded. If it is not conducted to the ventricles (AV delay period exceeded), the pacemaker stimulates the ventricle, resulting in a paced p wave and a wide, paced QRS complex with LBBB configuration.

Recognition of the interactivity of the paced chambers is important. A paced p wave may be mistaken for failure to sense or pace, and malfunction may be diagnosed when it is not present (pseudomalfunction). In addition, if the programmed rate of the pacemaker approximates the patient's intrinsic heart rate, fusion of paced and native beats may occur and represents another common type of pseudomalfunction (Fig. 7-3).

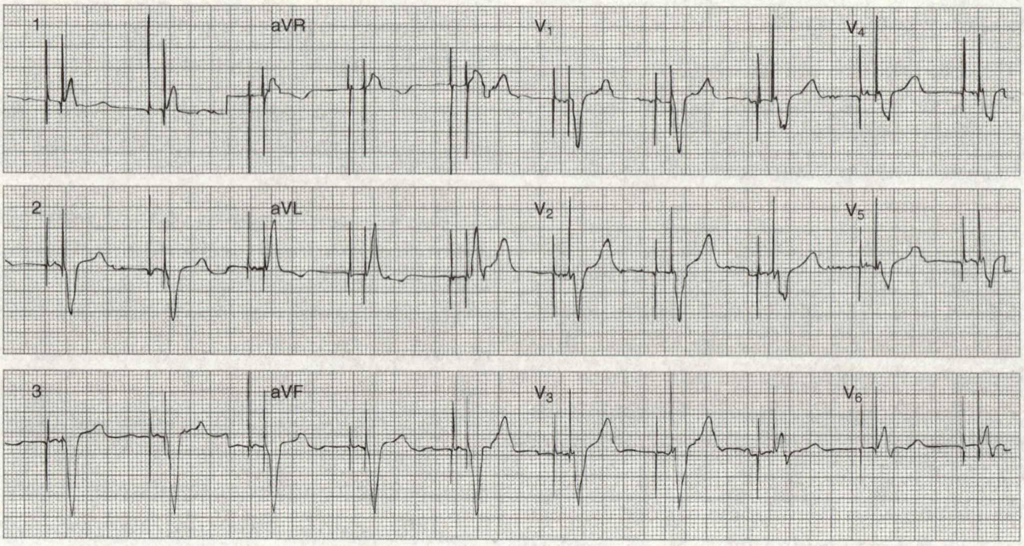

Fig. 7-2 Normal DDD pacemaker (12-lead ECG). Each QRS complex is preceded by two pacemaker spikes. The first spike results in atrial depolarization, and the second produces a wide QRS complex. The QRS complex is conducted with a left bundle branch morphology, which is expected with endocardial pacing at the right ventricular apex.

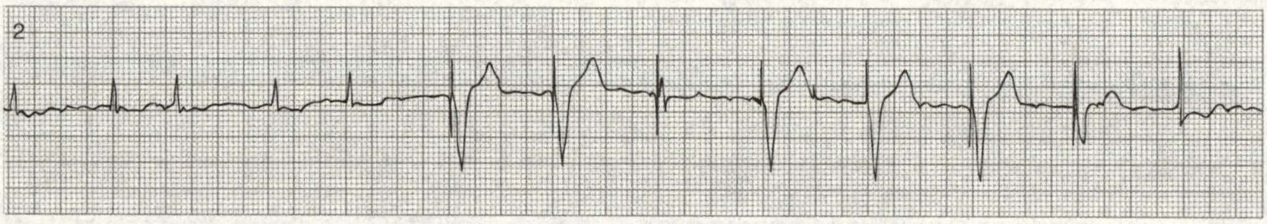

Fig. 7-3 VVI pacemaker with fusion beats (pseudomalfunction). This VVI pacemaker was implanted in a patient with Af and intermittent symptomatic CHB. In the lead Ⅱ rhythm strip, the first five QRS complexes are normal in morphology and irregular,as would be expected in Af. The next two QRS complexes are wide and preceded by a pacemaker spike. This represents normal sensing and pacing. The eighth QRS complex is narrow but preceded by a pacemaker spike. The spikes occur at a fixed and regular interval. In this instance, spontaneous ventricular depolarization had begun at approximately the time the pacemaker discharged. The 12th QRS complex in the sequence represents a fusion beat. Within the QRS complex of the 13th beat, a pacemaker spike is visible. Again, this represents nearly simultaneous conduction of a supraventricular beat and pacemaker electrical discharge. At first glance, this may appear to be failure to sense; however, the pacemaker is functioning normally and competing with the underlying rhythm.

Complications of Implantation

Infection

Pacemaker implantation carries a risk of infection. The incidence of infection is small.

Pain and local inflammation at the site of the pacemaker are the first manifestations of a wound infection, cellulitis, or pocket infection.

Thrombophlebitis

Thrombosis of varying degrees can involve the axillary, subclavian, and innominate veins or the superior vena cava (SVC). The site of insertion does not appear to affect the incidence of this complication. Chronic thrombosis of the veins of the upper arm is common and usually asymptomatic owing to extensive venous collateral circulation.

Patients develop symptoms usually indicative of acute thrombosis. These patients typically have edema, pain, and venous engorgement of the arm ipsilateral to the site of lead insertion. Although rare, SVC syndrome resulting from pacemaker lead-induced thrombosis occurs.

The "Pacemaker Syndrome"

After pacemaker implantation, a patient may develop new complaints or report a worsening of the symptoms that prompted evaluation and eventual pacemaker therapy. Such complaints often include syncope or near-syncope, orthostatic dizziness,fatigue, exercise intolerance, weakness, lethargy, chest fullness or pain, cough, uncomfortable pulsations in the neck or abdomen, right upper quadrant pain, and other nonspecific symptoms. Elevated levels of BNP and diuresis are considered markers for the syndrome in its more severe form.

These symptoms are termed the pacemaker syndrome. The cause of this syndrome is the loss of AV synchrony and the presence of ventriculoatrial conduction, and it is most commonly encountered in the setting of VVI pacing. It is also described with the DDI mode.

Treatment usually requires replacing a VVI pacemaker with a dual-chamber pacemaker or lowering the pacing rate of the VVI unit. If symptoms occur in a patient paced in the DDI mode, optimizing the timing of atrial and ventricular pacing is usually required. Persistence or worsening of symptoms of CHF may also be caused by the altered ventricular activation sequence inherent with stimulation of the RV. Biventricular pacing may be required in selected patients.

The same symptoms may be observed in patients with true pacemaker malfunction,which may necessitate pacemaker reprogramming or replacement of the pulse generator or pacemaker lead.

Pacemaker Malfunction

The term pacemaker malfunction refers specifically to problems with the circuitry or power source of the pulse generator, the pacemaker lead (most commonly displacement or fracture), or the interface between the pacing electrode and the myocardium (pacing or sensing threshold).In addition, environmental factors, such as extracardiac or extracorporeal electrical signals, may interfere with normal pacemaker function. With use of the standard ECG, pacemaker malfunction can be separated into three broad categories: (1) failure to capture, (2) inappropriate sensing, or (3) inappropriate pacemaker rate.Malfunction is most commonly a result of inappropriate sensing, followed by failure to capture.Typical presentations and causes of pacemaker malfunction are listed in Box 7-3.

Box 7-3 Causes of Pacemaker Malfunction

Failure to Capture

- Lead disconnection, break, or displacement
- Exit block
- Battery depletion

Undersensing

- Lead displacement
- Inadequate endocardial lead contact
- Low-voltage intracardiac P waves and QRS complexes
- Lead fracture

Oversensing

- Sensing extracardiac signals: myopotentials
- T wave sensing

Inappropriate Rate

- Battery depletion
- Ventriculoatrial conduction with pacemaker-mediated tachycardia
- 1 : 1 response to atrial dysrhythmias

In the context of suspected pacemaker malfunction, knowledge of the pacing modalities (Table 7-1) and what is normal for a given pacing modality are critical when the ECG is reviewed. Fortunately, patients are provided with important identifying information, usually in the form of a wallet card, after pacemaker implantation. The most important information is provided in the five-letter code. If this information is not available, a standard posteroanterior and a lateral chest radiograph can provide critical information. A single lead in the apex of the right ventricle indicates a VVI pacemaker. With VVI pacing, only one stimulus artifact or spike is seen with each stimulated ventricular depolarization (Fig. 7-1). If sinus node activity is present, the paced QRS complex is dissociated from the intrinsic P waves.If separate leads are identified in the right atrium and right ventricle, the pacing modality is most often DDD or DVI, and paced P waves and QRS complexes (two spikes for each QRS complex) are seen (Fig.7-2). Although DDD and DVI units are capable of pacing both the right atrium and the RV, only one spike may be seen (Fig. 7-4). Failure to identify two spikes with a DDD or DVI unit can represent normal pacemaker function.

A magnet placed externally over the pulse generator is frequently used in the assessment of pacemaker function.The technique is most commonly used when the patient's intrinsic heart rate exceeds the pacemaker's set rate and pacemaker function is inhibited. Magnet application then allows pacing to occur, despite the patient's native cardiac activity, and pacing rate and the presence of capture can be determined. Magnets are made by each manufacturer, but any cardiac pacemaker magnet will typically activate the reed switch within any of the devices.

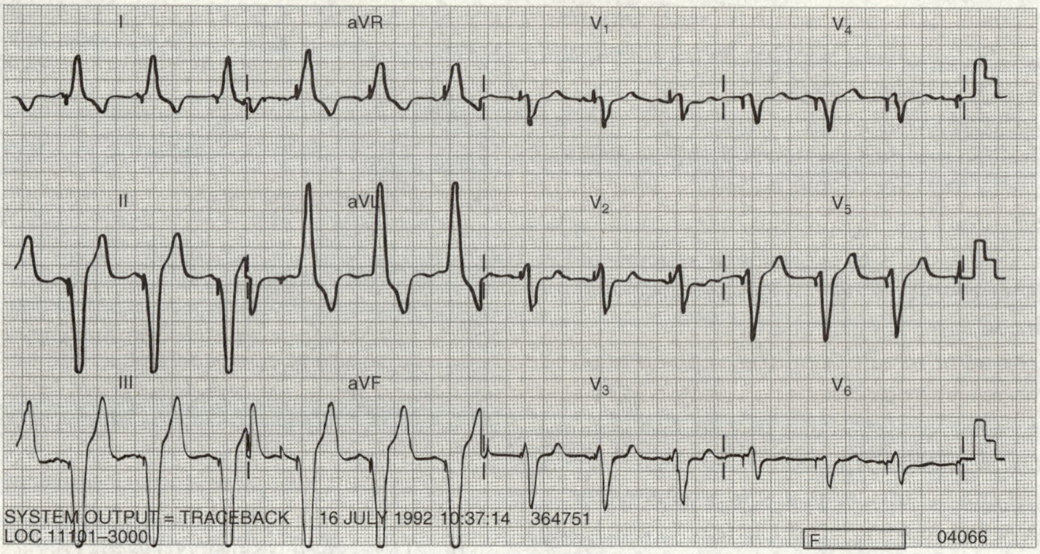

Fig. 7-4 Normal DDD pacemaker (half-standard 12-lead ECG). Three paced QRS complexes preceded by a stimulus artifact or spike are evident in leads Ⅰ, Ⅱ, and Ⅲ. Paced QRS complexes occur after spontaneous or intrinsic P waves are sensed and AV conduction delay exceeds the pacemaker's programmed AV interval. The first QRS complex in the augmented leads, best seen in lead aVF, demonstrates both a paced P wave and a paced QRS complex. Although the pacemaker is a dual-chamber device, two spikes may not always be seen preceding every QRS complex, and the presence of only one spike, or no spikes, should not be interpreted as evidence of pacemaker malfunction. Also evident on this ECG are the different amplitudes of the pacemaker spikes from lead to lead. When a single-lead rhythm strip is recorded, the selected lead should be the one in which the pacemaker spikes are most easily identified.

Failure to Capture

Failure to capture may range from the complete absence of pacemaker spikes to spikes not followed by a stimulus-induced complex (Fig. 7-5). A complete absence of pacemaker spikes may result from battery depletion, fracture of the pacemaker lead, or disconnection of the lead from the pulse generator unit.

Current lithium-iodine batteries are not subject to sudden power failure, and they display typical end-of-life functional changes over a period of months to a year before complete depletion.As a result, urgent or emergent battery replacement is rare.

Lead displacement is the most common cause and is most likely to occur within the first month of pacemaker insertion. The chest radiograph may demonstrate the tip of the pacing catheter displaced from the right ventricular apex.The atrial leads of dual-chamber devices are commonly displaced into the body of the right atrium, resulting in loss of contact between the

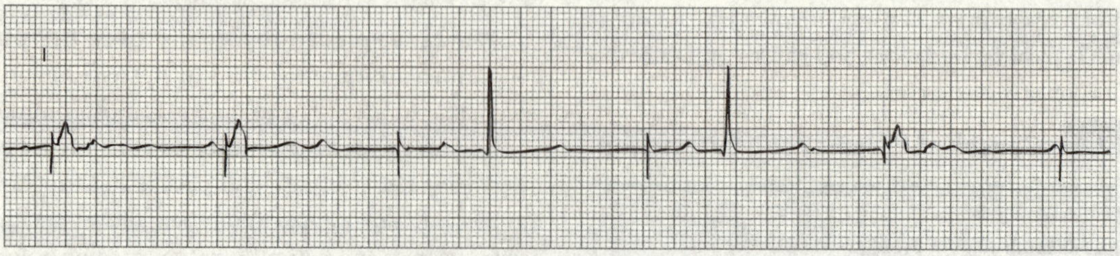

Fig. 7-5 Intermittent failure to capture and slow pacing rate (lead Ⅰ). This lead Ⅰ rhythm strip demonstrates intermittent failure to capture of a VVI pacemaker. The first and second pacemaker spikes are followed by wide-paced QRS complexes; the third and fourth spikes are not. The pacemaker spikes occur at a rate of approximately 50/min. The device was programmed to pace at a rate of 75/min. This is a typical example of "end-of-life" pacing characteristics of a depleted battery.

pacing lead and the atrial endocardium.

Lead fracture produces an insulation break, resulting in failure to capture as a result of current leakage. It can be detected as a change in pacing threshold during pacemaker interrogation. Lead fractures occur at predictable locations, usually at the site of attachment to the pulse generator or at abrupt angulations that serve as stress points. Inadequate contact of the lead with the pulse generator can mimic a lead fracture.Loss of lead-pulse generator contact can be detected on the chest radiograph with close inspection of the pulse generator.

Exit block can also result in failure to pace. Exit block should be considered when the preprogrammed pacing stimulus output fails to result in capture in the presence of a normally functioning pulse generator and an intact lead system. This problem is most commonly a result of changes in the endocardium in contact with the pacing system. Causes include ischemia or infarction of the endocardium in contact with the electrodes; systemic hyperkalemia; and the use of class III antiarrhythmic drugs, such as amiodarone, which affect ventricular depolarization.

Inappropriate Sensing

For a pacemaker to function in a noncompetitive mode, it must be capable of sensing the intrinsic or "native" electrical activity of the heart. The electrical activity that is sensed is determined by the pacing modality (Table 7-1). Sensing parameters are determined at the time of pacemaker insertion on the basis of the signal size of the intracardiac ECG and can be changed or fine-tuned externally at a later time if needed.

Undersensing

Failure to sense may be complete or intermittent. It may result from a change in the sensing parameters selected at the time of insertion. This is most commonly encountered after acute right ventricular infarction or during the progressive fibrosis that accompanies many cardiomyopathies, causing intracardiac signals to decrease in amplitude. Lead displacement, fracture, and poor contact with the endocardium may also cause undersensing.

Undersensing is typically recognized electrocardiographically as the appearance of pacemaker spikes occurring earlier than the programmed rate. The spike may or may not be followed by a paced complex, depending on when it occurs during the cardiac refractory period (Fig. 7-6). Failure of a stimulus spike to produce a complex when it occurs during the atrial or ventricular refractory period should not be interpreted as failure to pce.

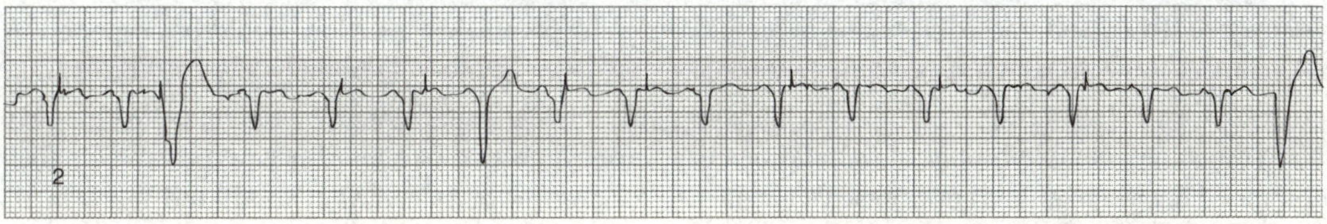

Fig.7-6 Failure to sense or undersensing (lead II). Pacemaker spikes are evident during inscription of the ST segment on this rhythm strip. These spikes do not produce QRS complexes because they occur during the ventricular refractory period of the preceding spontaneous QRS complex. The third QRS complex on the strip is a paced QRS complex. The device is capable of capture but is undersensing the spontaneous rhythm.

Oversensing

In rare instances the pacemaker may detect electrical activity that is not of cardiac origin. The result may be intermittent, irregular pacing or an apparent complete absence of pacemaker function. Myopotentials produced by the pectoralis muscle (Fig. 7-7) and extracorporeal electrical signals are frequently oversensed when a unipolar lead system is used. T waves that follow an intrinsic ventricular depolarization are the most common oversensed cardiac signals. Common medical sources of electrical interference include electrocautery, which can cause temporary pacemaker inhibition, and magnetic resonance imaging, which can alter pacemaker circuitry and result in fixed-rate or asynchronous pacing. Electromagnetic interference resulting from close proximity to a microwave oven should not cause pacemaker problems with currently implanted pacemaker units. Interference can be caused by the use of a digital cellular phone. These devices may cause pacemaker inhibition, inappropriate ventricular tracking, or asynchronous pacing. Malfunction is

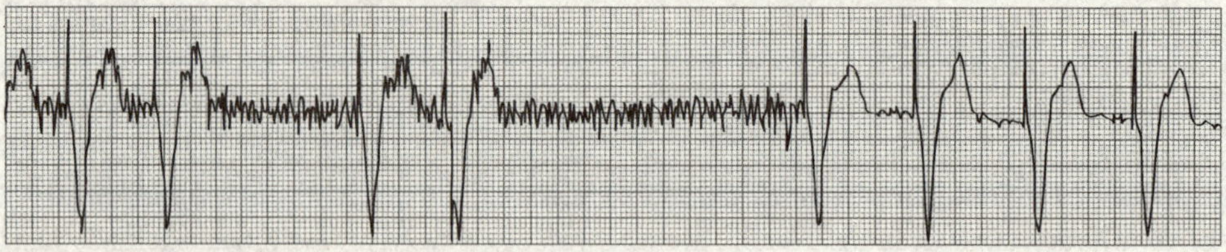

Fig. 7-7 Oversensing (lead Ⅱ). This VVI unipolar lead pacemaker is oversensing myopotentials produced by contraction of the pectoralis major. Myopotentials result in the undulating and irregular baseline seen in the middle of the strip. After muscular contraction ceases, normal pacing resumes (last four complexes on the strip).

most commonly seen when the phone is within 10 cm of the pulse generator and often occurs when the phone is applied to the ear ipsilateral to the site of the pacemaker pocet.

Inappropriate Pacemaker Rate

A pacing rate below the programmed rate is a typical finding in pulse generator depletion and does not occur abruptly with lithium-iodine batteries. An extreme increase in pacing rate, the so-called "runaway pacemaker," is rarely, if ever, encountered with current pacemaker technology and circuitry in which upper rate limits are set (typically 140 beats/min). An "endless loop" tachycardia may develop during dual-chamber pacing when ventriculoatrial conduction occurs, and the resulting retrograde atrial depolarization results in a stimulated or paced ventricular depolarization. If AF develops during dual-chamber pacing, flutter waves may be sensed and tracked, resulting in a rapid, paced ventricular rate. In both instances, the ventricular rate does not exceed its set upper limit. Patients with such rhythms may complain only of palpitations or symptoms of hemodynamic compromise.When such rhythms are detected, magnet application usually converts the pacemaker to a fixed rate in a competitive mode and terminates the tachyarrhythmia.

Management

History

The patient should be asked for the pacemaker identification card. The information on the card explains why a pacemaker was placed and the pacing modality used.

Most patients with pacemaker malfunction have symptoms reminiscent of those that prompted pacemaker therapy: syncope,near-syncope, orthostatic dizziness, lightheadedness, dyspnea, or palpitations.

The majority of pacemaker complications and most instances of pacemaker malfunction occur within the first few weeks or months of pacemaker implantation. A wound infection or pocket infection typically arises with localized pain. Bacteremia secondary to infection of the pacing catheter may arise only with fever and without other manifestations of the SIRS. Pain in the arm ipsilateral to the site of insertion should suggest acute thrombophlebitis.

Patients who develop the pacemaker syndrome secondary to the loss of AV synchrony may have nonspecific complaints of easy fatigability, generalized weakness, dyspnea, or an uncomfortable fluttering or "pounding" sensation in the neck or abdomen. Syncope or near-syncope may also occur, but these complaints should prompt an evaluation for true pacemaker malfunction. The pacemaker syndrome should be a diagnosis of exclusion.

Physical Examination

A pacemaker infection should be suspected in the presence of fever. Extremely low (<60 beats/min) or high (>100 beats/min in the resting patient) pulse rates are suggestive of altered pacing parameters (battery depletion or pacemaker-mediated tachycardias). Hypotension may be present in either instance. Cannon "A" waves on inspection of the jugular venous pulse wave indicate AV asynchrony. Auscultation of lungs may reveal bibasilar rales if CHF is present.

During pacing, the first heart sound may vary in intensity as a result of AV dissociation (VVI mode), and the second heart sound may be paradoxically split when ventricular pacing occurs (the right ventricle is activated first). A pericardial friction rub may also be heard if the tip of the pacing catheter has perforated the wall of the right ventricle. Perforation, however, usually occurs at the time of pacemaker implantation and is usually recognized at that time. Although the pacing catheter traverses the tricuspid valve, tricuspid regurgitation is rarely heard unless there is myocardial disease such as right ventricular dilation, which is common in the cardiomyopathies. Pedal edema may be present and is important if it is a new symptom or if chronic edema has recently worsened.

Chest Radiograph

A chest radiograph should be obtained to define pacing catheter tip position and to determine the number of pacing leads, unless this information is available from another source. A ventricular pacing catheter tip in the right ventricular outflow tract or an atrial catheter tip in the SVC or right ventricle is abnormal. The pulse generator site should also be examined on the radiograph.

12-Lead Electrocardiogram

A standard ECG and a long rhythm strip should be obtained in all patients. With bipolar pacing systems, the stimulus artifact may be extremely small and difficult to recognize in some leads (Fig. 7-4). Inspection of the rhythm strip may reveal failure to sense or pace, a low pacing rate, or an abnormally rapid rhythm, suggesting a pacemaker-mediated tachycardia.

Disposition of the Emergency Departmentent Patient with a Pacemaker

Most instances of malfunction are subtle and difficult to recognize without interrogation of the pacemaker with manufacturer-specific devices by someone skilled in the technique. In all instances of suspected pacemaker malfunction, the patient's cardiologist should be consulted.

Advanced Cardiac Life Support Interventions

Electrical defibrillation at recommended shock strengths (200J, 300J, and 360 J) can be safely performed in the patient with a pacemaker. If the sternal paddle is placed adjacent to the sternum, it is at a safe distance (>10 cm) from the pulse generator. Alternatively, defibrillation electrodes can be placed in an anteroposterior configuration. A cardiologist or technician should ensure that the pacing parameters of the unit are not altered if the resuscitation is successful. A chest radiograph should also be obtained after resuscitation to ensure that the pacing catheter was not displaced during chest compression.

Immediate return of pacing (capture) may not occur after defibrillation; this is commonly the result of global myocardial ischemia and increased pacing threshold and is not an indication of pacemaker malfunction. Temporary transcutaneous pacing may be needed if the pacemaker cannot be reprogrammed or normal pacing does not resume spontaneously. Transcutaneous pacing can also be safely used because the anterior and posterior pacing electrodes, if properly positioned, are distant from the pulse generator. Attempting temporary transvenous pacing is usually not necessary and is unlikely to be successful, especially if undertaken without fluoroscopic guidance. Chronic venous thrombosis, which is common and most often asymptomatic after pacemaker insertion, may preclude temporary catheter insertion through the neck veins. Insertion through the femoral vein is also difficult because the permanently implanted catheter may prevent entry into the RV. Blind insertion may also dislodge the permanent catheter.

IMPLANTABLE CARDIOVERTER DEFIBRILLATORS

The ICD was first used clinically in 1980.Generally accepted indications for ICD implantation are noted in Box 7-2. Many patients still require drug therapy after ICD implantation to suppress ventricular dysrhythmias, minimize the frequency of ICD shocks, improve patients' tolerance, and decrease energy use, which prolongs ICD life.

Terminology and Components

The majority of ICD are now placed percutaneously in a manner similar to that of the standard pacemaker. A transvenous electrode system has largely replaced epicardial lead placement.

The typical modern ICD consists of components similar to those in the standard permanent pacemaker—namely, a power source, electronic circuitry, and lead system. In addition, the standard ICD has a high-voltage capacitor and complex microprocessor memory. The power source is lithium chemistry based with a battery life of 5 to 10 yr. The longevity is largely determined by the frequency of shocks. All ICD are also ventricular pacemakers, providing pacing for bradyarrhythmias.

The right ventricular lead is used for sensing and pacing, and shocks are typically delivered between a coil in the right ventricular lead and the pulse generator. If dual-chamber pacing is required, a second lead is placed in contact with the endocardium of the right atrium.

The diagnostic and treatment functions of the ICD are determined at the time of implantation. In most instances, the cardioversion and defibrillation thresholds are determined at the time of ICD insertion by inducing VT and Vf and adjusting the shock strength at a level above the minimum required to terminate the induced rhythm. Optimally, the required shock strength for defibrillation is less than half the maximum output (approximately 30 J) of the device. VT is typically managed with use of either low-energy shocks or programmed pacing that interrupts the VT reentrant circuit. Programmed pacing is less likely to have proarrhythmic effects and requires less energy, thereby extending battery life. In the setting of Vf, ICD are capable of delivering up to five additional discharges if the first shock fails.

The patient with an ICD should have close follow-up monitoring by a cardiologist familiar with ICD programming. This allows the cardiologist to determine the frequency of ICD activation (programmed antitachycardia pacing or shocks) and to confirm the programmed functions of the device. The majority of patients with ICD have underlying heart disease, most commonly extensive atherosclerotic coronary artery disease, which is complicated by a low ejection fraction and congestive heart failure. The patient's medications and metabolic status, such as electrolyte disorders that accompany diuretic usage, may also affect ICD function.

Complications of Implantation

Complications of ICD implantation are nearly identical in type and frequency to those of permanent pacemaker implantation. They include infection of the wound, the subcutaneous pouch fashioned for the device, and the lead system as well as acute thrombophlebitis and chronic thrombosis of the veins traversed for lead insertion. Management of these complications is similar to that for patients with permanent pacemakers.

Malfunction

Patients with ICD malfunction usually come to the ED with a limited number of specific symptoms (Box 7-4).

Box 7-4 Causes of Implantable Cardioverter-Defibrillator Malfunction

Increase or abrupt change in shock frequency

- Increased frequency of Vf or VT (consider ischemia, electrolyte disorder, or drug effect)
- Displacement or break in ventricular lead
- Recurrent nonsustained VT
- Sensing and shock of supraventricular tachyarrhythmias
- Oversensing of T waves
- Sensing noncardiac signals

Syncope, near-syncope, dizziness

- Recurrent VT with low shock strength (lead problem,change in defibrillation threshold)
- Hemodynamically significant SVT
- Inadequate backup pacing for bradyarrhythmias (spontaneous or drug induced)

Cardiac arrest

- Assume malfunction, but probably caused by Vf that failed to respond to programmed shock parameters

In contrast to patients with a permanent pacemaker, ICD patients are aware of when the ICD discharges to terminate VT or Vf. The most common complaint of ICD patients is the occurrence of frequent shocks. An increasing shock rate may be appropriate and not indicative of ICD malfunction if the patient is experiencing an increase in the frequency of VT or Vf episodes. An increase in the frequency of episodes may occur in the setting of hypokalemia, hypomagnesemia, ischemia (with or without infarction) related to underlying CAD, or the proarrhythmic effect of drugs administered to decrease the frequency of ventricular tachyarrhythmias. Many ICD patients, particularly those to whom the technology is new, report that their device discharged, but subsequent device interrogation reveals that no discharge occurred.

An increase in the shock frequency is a manifestation of ICD sensing malfunction if (1) a supraventricular tachyarrhythmia is inappropriately sensed as VT, (2) shocks are delivered for nonsustained VT, or (3) intracardiac T waves detected by the ICD system are sensed as QRS complexes and the ICD interprets this as an increased heart rate. Temporary ICD deactivation with magnet application may be necessary if oversensing is the problem. Syncope, near-syncope, dizziness, or lightheadedness in the patient with an ICD may indicate undersensing of sustained

VT or inappropriately low shock strength to terminate the rhythm. An approach to the evaluation of ICD malfunction is shown in Fig. 7-8.

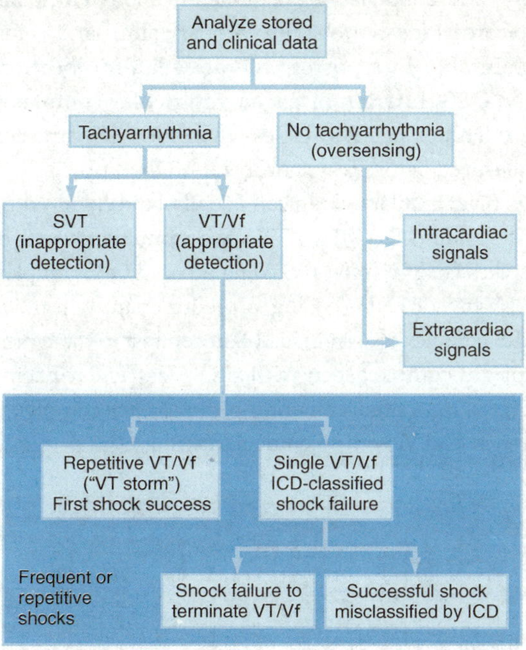

Fig. 7-8 Approach to the patient with shocks.

Advanced Cardiac Life Support Interventions

An ICD does not prevent sudden death in all patients at risk, and a patient with an ICD may arrive in cardiac arrest (2% annual incidence in patients with implanted devices). Cardiac arrest is not necessarily an indication of ICD malfunction. Appropriate repeated shocks may have been delivered but were ineffective. Alternatively, the ICD may not have sensed Vf or the ventricular ectopic activity that typically precedes Vf. Resuscitation efforts in the patient with an ICD should be undertaken in accordance with current recommendations. Transthoracic defibrillation can be performed in the standard manner with a monophasic or biphasic defibrillator if Vf is the arrest rhythm. The sternal electrode or paddle should be placed in a parasternal location approximately 10 cm from the ICD subcutaneous pouch if the device has been implanted in the right deltopectoral area. If it has been implanted in the left deltopectoral region, this recommended safety distance is usually exceeded.

ICD discharge during manual chest compressions poses no risk to providers, although the rescuer may feel a weak shock. Although this generally is not indicated, the device can be deactivated with magnet application during resuscitation efforts. Deactivation is probably more important in the immediate postresuscitation period because recurrent ventricular dysrhythmias are common at this time after prolonged global myocardial ischemia during the arrest period, reperfusion, and the hyperadrenergic state, which is worsened by the use of intravenous epinephrine during resuscitation. ICD malfunction should be assumed, and these postresuscitation rhythms treated with standard pharmacologic agents (lidocaine and amiodarone). Although class 1 antidysrhythmic agents may raise the defibrillation threshold of the ICD, their impact on the defibrillation threshold during transthoracic countershock is clinically inconsequential owing to the high shock strengths that are used.

Disposition of the Emergency Department Patient with an Implantable Cardioverter-Defibrillator

As a result of the difficulty in documenting or excluding ICD function or malfunction in the patient with transient symptoms,the device should be interrogated to guide further evaluation and therapy. In cases in which the patient reports a single ICD shock, an assessment for acute cardiac ischemia, worsening of chronic CHF, symptoms of new-onset HF, and electrolyte abnormalities should be performed. In the absence of a change in clinical status, such patients can be discharged in consultation with the managing or consulting cardiologist after timely follow-up is ensured. For patients reporting multiple shocks, interrogation is essential, because in many of these cases the defibrillator has not discharged and the patient is experiencing hiccoughs, diaphragmatic twitching, or other nonelectrical phenomena. In such cases, discharge home is the rule. When multiple defibrillator discharges are confirmed by interrogation, immediate consultation is required along with admission to a monitored setting for extended telemetric observation. If frequent ventricular ectopy is noted, intravenous amiodarone should be given. ICD interrogation allows assessment of ICD function and preceding dysrhythmia episodes. Reprogramming may be necessary. If a lead problem is detected, reimplantation is required. A magnet can be placed over the ICD to inactivate the defibrillator. This should be done only if the emergency physician is confident that the ICD is delivering inappropriate shocks, such as a SVT.

Biventricular Pacing

Biventricular pacing, also known as cardiac resynchronization therapy, is a therapy for patients with left-sided HF and ventricular dyssynchrony. It is beneficial for patients with NYHA class Ⅲ or Ⅳ HF despite optimal medical therapy, a left ventricular ejection fraction of 35% or less, and sinus rhythm with QRS duration of 120 ms or greater. LBBB causes an altered sequence of depolarization of the LV such that the interventricular septum contracts before the left ventricular free wall, leading to inefficient mechanical pumping. Biventricular pacing "resynchronizes"the ventricles by simultaneously pacing the left and right ventricles, eliminating the delay in left ventricular free wall contraction and improving systolic function. Right atrial and right ventricular leads are positioned as for conventional atrial and univentricular pacing. The left ventricular lead is positioned in a left ventricular epicardial location via the coronary sinus and veins, preferably in a posterolateral or lateral location. The QRS duration of paced ventricular complexes is often but not always less than the QRS duration measured before resynchronization therapy.

Biventricular pacing can usually be recognized on the standard ECG (Fig. 7-9). Two stimulus artifacts or "spikes" may be seen preceding a paced QRS complex. With biventricular pacing, a predominantly negative QRS complex is seen in lead I, in contrast to the typical upright complex seen with right ventricular pacing (Fig. 7-2). A predominantly positive QRS complex is seen in lead V_1 with biventricular pacing.

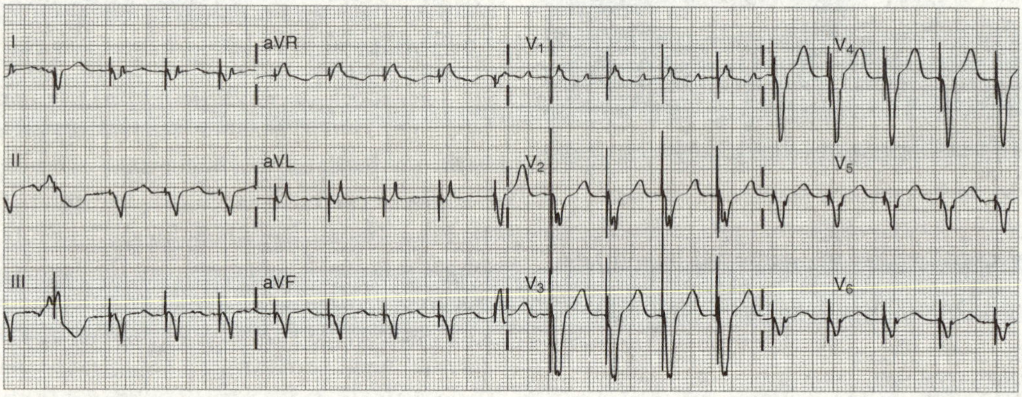

Fig. 7-9 Biventricular pacemaker. This 12-lead ECG demonstrates an atrial sensed, biventricular pacemaker in a patient with CRT and ICD system (CRT-D). The PR interval is 350 ms and represents the programmed AV delay for this patient. The paced QRS complexes have an S wave in lead I and an R wave in lead V_1 that are distinctly different from the morphology and axes seen with right ventricular apical pacing. The second beat from the left is a PVC. There is a pacemaker "spike" superimposed on this complex, likely representing safety pacing in CRT-D.

The complications and malfunctions inherent with conventional cardiac pacing are also observed with biventricular pacing. In addition, biventricular pacing has unique complications related to placement of the left ventricular pacing lead through the coronary sinus. Dislodgement of the left ventricular electrode with resultant loss of pacing occurs as an early complication in approximately 10% of patients. Patients with malfunction of a biventricular pacing system frequently report palpations or acute decompensation of chronic heart failure.

Left Ventricular Assist Devices

Mechanical ventricular assistance devices have been used as a "bridge" to transplantation since the 1960s. These implanted devices replace or support the pump function of the LV and were originally bulky and mechanically complex owing to the pulsatile nature of the pump mechanisms. This usually resulted in extended in-hospital care while the patient awaited cardiac transplantation. Newer devices, such as the Jarvik 2000 and HeartMate II, are continuous flow pumps that are portable and powered with a comparatively smaller battery pack. Implantation is associated with fewer infectious complications and lower immediate postoperative mortality, and survival for more than 1 yr is increasingly common. The greatest mortality is noted within the first 30 d after implantation and during hospitalization. Left ventricular assistance devices (LVAD) is commonly used as "destination" therapy in patients who do not qualify for cardiac transplantation.

Patients with an LVAD typically require care at cardiac transplant centers. As technology progresses, emergency physicians not based at a transplant center may encounter a patient with an LVAD. In such cases, telephone consultation with an expert at a transplant center may help avoid missteps. The more common complications with this device include infection and embolic stroke. Device failure usually results in severe heart failure. If necessary, dopamine, dobutamine, or a combination of these drugs may be given to treat CHF symptoms while the patient awaits transfer. If cardiac arrest occurs, chest compressions may dislodge the device. The hand pump should be used to provide circulation if this backup method is available and early transition to CPB should be considered (Table 7-3).

Table 7-3 Comparison of Common Ventricular Assist Devices

	THORATEC VAD	HEARTMATE Ⅱ	HEARTMATE Ⅰ OR XVE
Flow type	Pulsatile—patient will have a pulse and BP.	Axial—patient will not have a pulse or BP.Use Doppler to confirm flow.	Pulsatile—patient will have a pulse and BP.
Backup method	Hand pump	No external method	Hand pump
Battery life	Up to 3 hr	Up to 10 hr	Up to 10 hr
Defibrillation or cardioversion	No precautions	No precautions	Use hand pump during procedure
Cardiac arrest	Use hand pump	No external method	Use hand pump

(CHEN Yuguo)

Chapter 8

Blood and Blood Components

KEY CONCEPTS

Massive transfusion has no formal definition. Administration of at least 10 units of RBC in 24 hr is a commonly used cutoff.

Patients receiving massive transfusion are prone to coagulopathy and thrombocytopenia.

In considering the use of blood component therapy, the patient's age, severity of symptoms, cause of the deficit, underlying medical condition, ability to compensate for decreased oxygen-carrying capacity, and tissue oxygen requirements are all important.

TRALI is now considered the leading cause of transfusion-related mortality.

Chronically anemic, normovolemic elderly patients are at greatest risk for developing CHF with the rapid infusion of blood.

During or after the transfusion, the patient with bacterial contamination may develop rigors, vomiting, abdominal cramps, fever, shock, AKI, and DIC.

PERSPECTIVE

The modern blood transfusion era began with discovery of the ABO red cell antigen system in the early 1900s. It was soon found that adding citrate enabled the storage of anticoagulated blood. Energetic pioneers, such as John Lundy of the Mayo Clinic, gained a wealth of clinical experience, prompting dissemination of expertbased advice, such as Lundy's recommendation that blood transfusion was appropriate when a patient's hemoglobin (Hgb) was less than 10 g/dL or when a patient lost more than 15% of circulating blood volume.Rapid expansion of blood banking occurred after World War Ⅱ, and in subsequent decades, research focused on such critical issues as prolonging the storage life of blood products, component therapy, and reducing the risk of transfusion reactions and transfusion-related infections.

PATHOPHYSIOLOGIC PRINCIPLES

Blood Banking

RBC storage methods aim to ensure viability of at least 75% of the cells 24 hr after infusion. Blood collection bags contain an anticoagulant preservative of citrate, phosphate, dextrose, and adenine (CPDA-1), ensuring a shelf life of 35 d and hematocrit (HCT) of 70% to 80% for PRBC. Additive solutions (Adsol, Nutricel, Optisol) provide additional nutrients, extending maximum storage to 42 d and lowering viscosity, which makes infusion easier.

Storage, however, impairs red cell function. Although PRBC are maintained at 1 to 6℃, cell metabolism continues, and changes occur. These changes are collectively referred to as the "storage lesion." Documented alterations are numerous and include a decrease in both pH and the level of 2,3-diphosphoglycerate.In addition, the deformability of stored RBC changes over time. After infusion, however, many of these changes are readily reversed. The decrease in 2,3- diphosphoglycerate, for example, results in a left shift in the Hgb-oxygen dissociation curve, but 2,3-diphosphoglycerate levels begin to recover within minutes and are fully restored within 24 hr.

Additional well-established changes in stored blood include cell leakage of potassium, although the amount (approximately 6 mEq/U) is readily tolerated by most otherwise healthy patients. PRBC contain essentially no functional platelets or granulocytes.

Blood Typing

A blood specimen from the patient is then sent for the following tests: ABO grouping, Rh typing, and an antibody screen for unexpected antibodies (non-ABO/Rh antibodies). Completion of these steps speeds the delivery of crossmatched blood if it is subsequently required.

Identified RBC antigens include the ABO and related carbohydrate antigens (H, P, I, and Lewis), the 48 Rh system antigens, and more than 200 non-ABO/Rh antigens.ABO incompatibility results in acute hemolysis, the most serious transfusion reaction.

ABO grouping requires that the recipient's red cells be tested with anti-A and anti-B serum and that his or her serum be tested with A and B red cells. Patients with type O have antibodies against both. The major clinically significant Rh antigen is the D antigen. Rh typing is usually done by adding a commercial reagent (anti-D) to recipient RBC.

The antibody screen identifies unexpected antibodies in the patient's serum.When transfusion is delayed by a positive antibody screen in a critically ill patient, clinicians should communicate directly with the blood bank to determine the best course of action.Administering blood that is not completely crossmatched is therefore an option if the need is emergent.

The type and screen allows for quicker selection of appropriate banked blood for complete crossmatch if a transfusion is later ordered.

When a unit of blood is ordered for transfusion, a crossmatch is done.Patients with blood group AB (who lack anti-A and anti-B antigens), for example, are "universal recipients"—they can receive blood from any of the ABO groups. Type O blood (lacking the A and B antigens), also known as "universal donor" blood, conversely, can be given to anyone. Rh sensitization can occur in Rh-negative patients exposed to Rh-positive blood, and this sensitization in turn can result in hemolytic disease of the newborn with subsequent pregnancies.

If the antibody screen is negative, an "immediate spin crossmatch" at room temperature serves as a final check for ABO incompatibility. A "complete crossmatch" is generally done before transfusion if the antibody screen is positive. This requires incubation to 37℃ and the addition of antihuman globulin (Coombs' reagent) to promote agglutination.

Special Clinical Circumstances

To select the most appropriate blood products in the emergency setting, clinicians should consider the patient's hemodynamic stability, the likelihood of ongoing hemorrhage, and the amount of time available to intervene. When time is short, waiting for fully crossmatched blood may result in a dangerous delay, and alternatives should be considered. When the clinician anticipates large and ongoing blood losses,complications resulting from massive transfusion are a concern as well.

Administering Blood before Completion of Compatibility Testing

An antibody screen and immediate spin crossmatch at a minimum take approximately 45 to 60 min. If the antibody screen is positive, the antibody is identified via more elaborate procedures, and a complete crossmatch is required. This process can take up to several hours (or even days).

Universal (group O) blood is used when RBC are needed in hemorrhaging, unstable patients before any testing can be done. Type-specific blood (with ABO and Rh testing) can generally be made available within 15 min of receiving a sample of the patient's blood.

Massive Transfusion

Massive transfusion has no formal definition. Administration of at least 10 u of RBC in 24 hr is a commonly used cutoff. Patients receiving any amount of blood are susceptible to a variety of complications ,for example,infectious, physiologic, and immunologic insults. Hypothermia is common in these patients, and can reduce clotting factor activity. Warmed intravenous fluids, blood warmers, and warming lights and blankets are often needed. Acidosis is a common finding with massive hemorrhage but can also be caused by hypoperfusion, and the contribution of transfused blood to acidosis is felt to be variable.Citrate from banked blood, for example, is metabolized in the liver to bicarbonate, which can sometimes result in metabolic alkalosis. A rational response to metabolic acidosis is to optimize DO_2 and ventilation. Administering sodium bicarbonate may be considered in severe cases.

Patients receiving massive transfusion are also prone to coagulopathy and thrombocytopenia.

Coagulopathy often occurs in massive trauma. Commonly recommended goals in this setting would be to consider maintaining an INR below 1.5, a fibrinogen level greater than 1 to 2 g/L, and platelet count above 50,000 to 100,000/μL.

Administration

Legal Aspects

Before a blood product can be infused, two qualified personnel check it at the bedside to prevent a potentially fatal clerical error. This check includes recipient and unit identification, as well as confirmation of compatibility, and the expiration date.

If typed and crossmatched blood arrives with the patient from a transferring facility, it is important that the temperature be maintained between 1 and 10℃ during transport. If the blood is not used right away and the blood bank is asked to hold the blood for the patient, it is processed and crossmatched as for other issued blood and quarantined for 24 hr. It can be sent back to the blood bank to have this done only if (1) it has been constantly maintained at a temperature between 1 and 10℃, (2) all container seals are intact, and (3) tubing segments have remained attached to the blood container.

Infusion Adjuncts

Urgent transfusion situations require flow rates faster than gravity can provide. An administration set with an in-line pump is the simplest method to speed infusion.With high-pressure infusion, large-bore needles are recommended.

If only a small-gauge needle is available, the transfusion may be diluted with normal saline.In elective transfusions, no significant hemolysis occurs when small-gauge needles are used if the maximum rate of infusion is less than 100 mL/hr.

MANAGEMENT

Decision-Making

In considering the use of blood component therapy, the patient's age, severity of symptoms, and underlying medical condition are all important. Clinical evaluation, including appearance (pallor, diaphoresis), mentation (alert, confused), HR, BP, and the nature of the bleeding (active, controlled, uncontrolled), can be supplemented by laboratory evaluation.

Whole Blood

The use of fresh whole blood in civilian practice is generally unavailable and rarely used.

Packed Red Blood Cells

PRBC are indicated only to improve DO_2 to tissues at the microvascular level and thus improve intracellular oxygen consumption (VO_2).For decades, transfusion of RBC was guided by the so-called "10/30 rule": transfusion wasindicated for an Hgb of less than 10 g/dL or a HCT of less than 30%. In the critical care setting, a transfusion threshold of 7 g/dL was as safe as a threshold of 10 g/dL. A higher trigger was more appropriate in patients with CAD.

The recommendations of the American Society of Anesthesiologists seem reasonable: transfusion is rarely needed with an Hgb concentration greater than 10 g/dL and is usually needed when the Hgb is less than 6 g/dL. Patients with an Hgb of 6 to 10 mg/dL require careful clinical judgment.

Fresh Frozen Plasma

Transfused trauma patients receiving fewer than 10 units of blood found that administration of FFP was associated with no survival benefit, yet with a higher risk of complications, including ARDS, pneumonia, sepsis, and multiple organ dysfunction. The following indications seem reasonable based on current evidence: coagulopathy of trauma, hemorrhaging patients with coagulopathy resulting from hepatic dysfunction or DIC, plasma exchange for TTP, and emergency reversal of a vitamin K antagonist in the presence of clinically significant hemorrhage. Because of the volume of FFP needed to reverse coagulopathy caused by vitamin K antagonism (at least 10 mL/kg, and perhaps as much as 30 mL/kg),however, some guidelines call for the use of prothrombin complex concentrate or recombinant factor VIIa instead.FFP is not indicated for volume expansion, nonurgent reversal of a vitamin K antagonist.Thromboelastography may prove useful in guiding coagulation therapy.This test provides information on function of both platelets and coagulation factors (including fibrinogen).

If a specific factor deficiency is identified (e.g., hemophilia), targeted replacement of that factor, if available, is usually more practical.

Platelets

Platelet transfusion is indicated prophylactically when the count is less than 10,000/μL,as it appears that hemostasis is well maintained even at counts of 5000/μL. Platelets are often given to adults in a dose of 6 units of platelet concentrate , which typically raises the platelet count about 40,000 to 60,000/μL.Retrospective data support the safety of performing LP with platelet counts as low as 10,000/μL.A platelet count of 20,000 to 30,000/μL is generally considered adequate, and for major surgery, a count of 50,000/μL is generally acceptable, although higher cutoffs (70,000-100,000/μL) are often used for neurosurgical and retinal procedures.Patients with anemia appear more prone to bleeding.Lastly, when thrombocytopenia results from immune-mediated platelet destruction caused by ITP or TTP, transfusion is generally ineffective.

Autotransfusion

Autotransfusion may be used in the emergency setting in the event of severe chest trauma. This strategy has numerous advantages: immediate availability, blood compatibility, elimination of donor-to-patient disease transmission, avoidance of the storage lesion, lower risk of circulatory overload, and fewer direct complications (e.g., hyperkalemia, hypothermia, hypocalcemia, and metabolic acidosis).

Therapeutic Modalities

Packed Red Blood Cells

In acute hemorrhage, PRBC are used to supplement initial crystalloid replacement. In an average adult, 1 unit (450 mL) of PRBC increases the Hgb by about 1 g/dL or the HCT by about 3%. Lactated Ringer's solution can lead to clotting secondary to the added calcium, and hemolysis may result with a hypotonic solution. Most transfusions are given over 60 to 90 min (never longer than 4 hr). Unused blood should be returned promptly to the blood bank. Any units unrefrigerated for more than 30 min are discarded.

Fresh Frozen Plasma

A unit of FFP contains all clotting factors and typically has a volume of 200 to 250 mL. It must be ABO compatible and is given through blood tubing. FFP can be used to replace the most labile components (factors Ⅴ and Ⅷ), but it is given within 24 hr of thawing.One unit of activity for any coagulation factor is equal to the clotting activity found in 1 mL of FFP.In massive transfusion, many centers now use FFP in a 1 : 1 ratio with red cells.

Platelets

Crossmatching is generally unnecessary,but Rh-negative patients are treated with Rh-negative platelets because there may be enough red cells in the platelet concentrate to cause Rh sensitization.In adults the traditional dose has been 4 to 6 units (a "six-pack" of platelets),use of smaller, more frequent transfusions is considered in patients who are being admitted. Once sensitization has occurred and patients have developed immune-mediated platelet refractoriness.

OUTCOMES

Adverse effects of RBC transfusion can be divided into immune-mediated and non–immune-mediated categories, as well as acute, delayed, and chronic effects.

Immune–Mediated Adverse Effects

Acute

Intravascular Hemolytic Transfusion Reaction. Intravascular hemolytic transfusion reaction is the most serious transfusion reaction.The onset of symptoms is immediate and may include any of the following symptoms: fever, chills, headache, nausea,vomiting,a sensation of chest restriction,severe joint or low back pain,and a burning sensation at the site of the infusion.Clinical effects can include hypotension, DIC, and ATN.Treatment includes stopping the transfusion immediately, and initiating vigorous crystalloid fluid therapy. Diuretic therapy can also be used to maintain urine output at 1 to 2 mL/kg/hr.Some patients may require pressors.Blood and urine specimens are sent to the laboratory, as well as the remainder of the transfusion and the blood tubing.Detection of free Hgb (blood and urine) and a positive result of Coombs'test on post-transfusion,but not pretransfusion,specimens confirms the diagnosis.

Febrile Transfusion Reaction. It is defined as a 1°C or greater temperature elevation that occurs with transfusion and for which no other medical explanation is found. Reactions are believed to result from antileukocyte antibodies, most commonly as a result of prior transfusion. Treatment is symptomatic with analgesics, antipyretics, and antihistamines.

The use of leukoreduced RBC can help decrease, but not eliminate, the risk of this reaction. If a febrile reaction occurs in a first-time transfusion, it should be treated in the same way as an extravascular hemolytic reaction until proven otherwise.

Allergic Reactions (Urticaria to Anaphylaxis). Urticaria, or hives, may occur during a transfusion without other signs or symptoms and with no serious sequelae. The transfusion does not need to be stopped, and treatment with an antihistamine is usually sufficient. Consider prophylactic antihistamines in patients with a history of this reaction. The patient is likely to have a genetic IgA deficiency. Presentation is similar to anaphylactic reactions from other causes. Treatment is with epinephrine and corticosteroids. Use of washed RBC, and plasma products from IgA-deficient individuals can be used to avoid recurrence with subsequent transfusions.

Transfusion-Related ALI. Transfusion-related ALI (TRALI) is now considered the leading cause of transfusion-related mortality. It has been defined as new ALI resulting in bilateral pulmonary edema and hypoxemia (ratio of arterial oxygen concentration to fraction of F_iO_2 $[P_aO_2/F_iO_2] \leqslant 300$, or oxygen saturation as measured by Pox <90% on room air) and occurring during or within 6 hr after a transfusion without temporal relationship to an alternative explanation for ALI.If an alternative explanation is also present, the diagnosis of possible TRALI is appropriate.Implicated blood components include PRBC, FFP, platelets, and cryoprecipitate. The initial clinical presentation is that of a noncardiogenic pulmonary edema, with dyspnea,hypoxemia, and bilateral infiltrates on chest radiograph. Fever, hypotension, and transient leukopenia may also be seen.It is safe to continue transfusion of blood products from a different donor, if necessary. Complete resolution is usually seen within 48 to 96 hr. Overall prognosis is better than would be expected with many other causes of ALI.

Delayed

Extravascular Hemolytic Transfusion Reaction. Extravascular hemolytic transfusion reactions result from a non–ABO-mediated immune reaction, most often caused by an anamnestic response in a patient previously sensitized to red cell antigens by transfusion, pregnancy, or transplant. After repeat exposure from transfusion, however, antibody levels rise, and extravascular hemolysis occurs days to weeks later. The patient may have fever, anemia, and jaundice. Symptoms are not usually severe, but rare cases of oliguria or DIC do occur.

Transfusion-Associated Graft-versus-Host Disease. A rare but life-threatening complication, transfusion-associated graft-versus-host disease results when transfused lymphocytes proliferate and attack the recipient. Mortality is greater than 90%. Cell-mediated immunodeficiency puts patients at risk, as does having an HLA type that is identical between donor and recipient. Symptoms, which begin 3 to 30 d after transfusion, include fever, erythematous skin rash, diarrhea, elevated liver enzymes,and pancytopenia. The only effective treatment is bone marrow transplant, and most deaths result from coagulopathy or infection. Efforts are therefore directed at prevention by using gamma irradiation of all cellular components. The use of leukocyte-poor components is also advocated. This condition should be kept in mind when transfusion is being considered for anemic leukemia or lymphoma patients, especially those who have recently received chemotherapy.

Non-Immune-Mediated Adverse Effects

Acute

Circulatory Overload. Chronically anemic, normovolemic elderly patients are at greatest risk for developing CHF with the rapid infusion of blood. Transfusing more slowly (over a period of 4 hr) and administering diuretics are useful in preventing this complication.

Bacterial Contamination. The risk of bacterial contamination is greater, however, with platelets, which are stored at a higher temperature. During or after the transfusion, the patient may develop rigors,vomiting, abdominal cramps, fever, shock, AKI, and DIC. If contamination is suspected, the transfusion should be stopped, blood cultures obtained from both the bag and the patient, and broad-spectrum antibiotics and hemodynamic support initiated.

Chronic

Risk of Transfusion-Transmitted Viruses.It is common for acquiring hepatitis C and HIV infection from transfusion. Cytomegalovirus can be transmitted by blood transfusion as well.

(Shou Songtao YU Muming)

SECTION 2

Medical Emergencies

Cardiac Emergencies

Chapter 9

Chest Pain

KEY CONSEPTS

Chest pain is a symptom caused by several life-threatening diseases and has a broad differential diagnosis. It is complicated by a frequent disassociation between intensity of symptoms and signs and seriousness of underlying pathology.

All patients undergo electrocardiography as soon as possible after reporting their pain. Patients with positive ECG findings and those considered at high risk are triaged directly to the treatment area and monitored.

The two most commonly performed studies in patients with chest pain are the chest radiograph and 12-lead ECG

A serum D-dimer assay may help discriminate patients with PE from those with a possible gastrointestinal cause.

Patients with suspected thoracic aortic dissection may be evaluated by CT angiography, transesophageal echocardiography, or MRI.

CK-MB, an isoform of CK, is more specific for cardiac ischemia but largely has been supplanted by troponin testing.

Any patient with almost any type of chest pain may be having coronary ischemia, PE, or aortic dissection.

PERSPECTIVE

Chest pain has a broad differential diagnosis. ACS, aortic dissection, PE, pneumothorax, pericarditis with tamponade, and esophageal rupture are potentially catastrophic causes of chest pain.

It is complicated by a frequent disassociation between intensity of symptoms and signs and seriousness of underlying pathology.

DIAGNOSTIC APPROACH

Differential Considerations

The differential diagnosis of chest pain includes many of the most critical diagnoses and nonemergent conditions in medicine (Table 9-1).

Table 9-1 Differential Diagnosis of Chest Pain

ORGAN SYSTEM	CRITICAL DIAGNOSES	EMERGENT DIAGNOSES	NONEMERGENT DIAGNOSES
Cardiovascular	AMI Acute coronary ischemia Aortic dissection Cardiac tamponade	UA Coronary spasm Prinzmetal's angina Cocaine-induced pericarditis or myocarditis	Valvular heart disease Aortic stenosis Mitral valve prolapse Hypertrophic cardiomyopathy
Pulmonary	Pulmonary embolus Tension pneumothorax	Pneumothorax Mediastinitis	Pneumonia Pleuritis Tumor Pneumomediastinum

Continued

ORGAN SYSTEM	CRITICAL DIAGNOSES	EMERGENT DIAGNOSES	NONEMERGENT DIAGNOSES
Gastrointestinal	Esophageal rupture (Boerhaave's syndrome)	Esophageal tear (Mallory-Weiss) Cholecystitis Pancreatitis	Esophageal spasm Esophageal reflux Peptic ulcer Biliary colic
Musculoskeletal			Muscle strain Rib fracture Arthritis Tumor Costochondritis Nonspecific chest wall pain
Neurologic			Spinal root compression Thoracic outlet Herpes zoster Postherpetic neuralgia
Other			Psychological Hyperventilation

Rapid Stabilization and Assessment

The patient's appearance, ECG and vital signs should be assessed as soon as he/she arrives at ED. All patients, except those with obvious benign causes of chest pain, undergo electrocardiography as soon as possible after reporting their pain. The ECG should be read for AMI by the emergency physician as soon as it is completed. Patients with positive ECG findings and those considered at high risk are triaged directly to the treatment area and monitored. Most patients also require a chest radiograph to evaluate the chest pain.

If vital signs are stable, a focused history and physical examination are performed. But patients with severe derangements in vital signs require stabilizing treatment during a search for the precipitating cause. If a patient has unilateral chest pain, respiratory distress, shock, and unilateral reduction or absence of breath sounds, immediate intervention with needle or tube thoracostomy is required. (Fig. 9-1).

If myocardial ischemia is suspected, aspirin and nitroglycerin may be appropriate. Patients with pain and findings suggestive of aortic dissection and with significant hypertension are candidates for immediate reduction of blood pressure. Patients with low voltage on the ECG, diffuse ST segment elevation, elevated jugular venous pressure on examination, and signs of shock should undergo prompt bedside cardiac ultrasound.

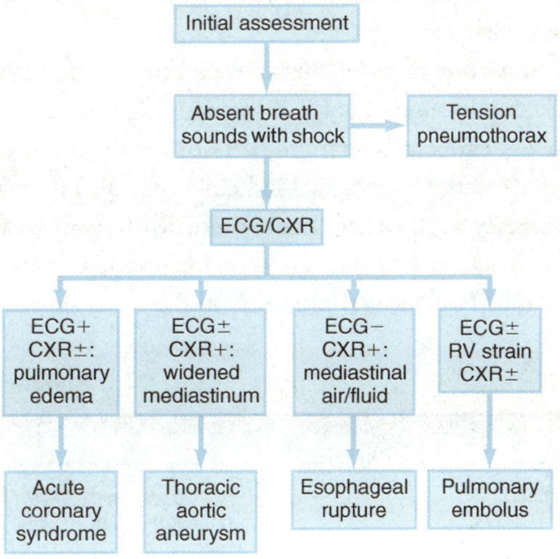

Fig. 9-1 Initial assessment of critical diagnoses.

Pivotal Findings

The history and physical examination are key to diagnosis.

History

Characteristic of chest pain. "Squeezing," "crushing," or "pressure" pain leads the emergency physician to suspect a cardiac ischemic syndrome, although cardiac ischemia can also be characterized by nonspecific discomfort, such as "bloating" or "indigestion." "Tearing" pain that may migrate from the front to back or back to front is the classic description in aortic dissection. "Sharp" or "stabbing" pain is seen more in pulmonary and musculoskeletal diagnoses. Patients reporting a "burning" or "indigestion" type of pain may initially be thought to have a gastrointestinal condition, but owing to the visceral nature of chest pain, patients with all causes of pain may use any of the preceding descriptions.

Patient's activity at the onset. Pain occurring during exertion suggests an ischemic coronary syndrome, whereas progressive onset of pain at rest suggests AMI. Pain of sudden onset is more typical with aortic dissection, PE, or pneumothorax. Pain after meals is more indicative of a gastrointestinal cause.

Severity of pain. Alterations in pain severity are documented at times of onset, peak, present, and after intervention.

Location of the pain. Pain that is localized to a small area is more likely to be somatic versus visceral in origin. Pain localized at the periphery of the chest is more likely to have a pulmonary rather than a cardiac cause. Lower chest or upper abdominal pain may be of cardiac or gastrointestinal origin.

Radiation of pain. Transthoracic pain through to the back should suggest aortic dissection or gastrointestinal causes, especially pancreatitis or posterior ulcer. Inferoposterior myocardial ischemia may also manifest primarily as thoracic back pain. Radiation to the arms, neck, or jaw increases the likelihood of cardiac ischemia. Pain located primarily in the back, especially interscapular back pain that migrates to the base of the neck, suggests aortic dissection.

Duration of pain. Pain that lasts a few seconds or minutes is rarely of cardiac origin. Pain that is exertional but abates with a few minutes of rest may be a manifestation of cardiac ischemia. Pain that is maximal at onset may be caused by aortic dissection.

Aggravating or alleviating factors. Pain that worsens with exertion and improves with rest is more likely related to coronary ischemia. Pain related to meals is more suggestive of a gastrointestinal cause. Pain that worsens with respiration is seen more often with pulmonary, pericardial, and musculoskeletal causes.

Other associated symptoms. This may suggest the visceral nature of the pain (Table 9-2). Diaphoresis should lead to an increased clinical suspicion for a serious or visceral cause. Hemoptysis, a classic PE sign, is rarely seen. Near-syncope and syncope lead to higher likelihood of a cardiovascular cause or PE. Dyspnea is seen in cardiovascular and pulmonary disease. Nausea and vomiting may be seen in cardiovascular and gastrointestinal complaints.

Prior presumptive diagnoses. A prior history of cardiac testing, such as stress testing, echocardiography, or angiography, may be useful in determining if the current episode is suggestive of cardiac disease. Similarly, patients with previous spontaneous pneumothorax or PE are at increased risk of recurrence.

Table 9-2 Significant Symptoms of Chest Pain

SYMPTOM	FINDING	DIAGNOSIS
Pain	Severe, crushing, pressure, substernal, exertional, radiation to jaw, neck, shoulder, arm	AMI Coronary ischemia UA Coronary spasm
	Tearing, severe, radiating to or located in back, maximum at onset, may migrate to upper back or neck	Aortic dissection
	Pleuritic	Esophageal rupture Pneumothorax Cholecystitis Pericarditis Myocarditis
	Indigestion or burning	AMI Coronary ischemia Esophageal rupture UA Coronary spasm Esophageal tear Cholecystitis

Continued

SYMPTOM	FINDING	DIAGNOSIS
Associated syncope or near-syncope		Aortic dissection PE AMI Pericarditis Myocarditis
Associated dyspnea (SOB, DOE, PND, orthopnea)		AMI Coronary ischemia PE Tension pneumothorax Pneumothorax UA Pericarditis
Associated hemoptysis		PE
Associated nausea, vomiting		Esophageal rupture AMI Coronary ischemia UA Coronary spasm Esophageal tear Cholecystitis

Presence of risk factors. The presence of risk factors for a particular disease is primarily of value as an epidemiologic marker for large population studies (Box 9-1).

Box 9-1 Risk Factors Associated with Potentially Catastrophic Causes of Chest Pain

- ACS
  - Past or family history of CAD
  - Age
    - Men older than 33 yr
    - Women older than 40 yr
  - DM
  - Hypertension
  - Cigarette use or possible passive exposure
  - Elevated cholesterol (low-density lipoprotein) or triglycerides
  - Sedentary lifestyle
  - Obesity
  - Postmenopausal
  - LVH
  - Cocaine abuse
- Pulmonary embolism
  - Prolonged immobilization
  - Surgery longer than 30 min in last 3 mo
  - Prior deep vein thrombosis or pulmonary embolus
  - Pregnancy or recent pregnancy
  - Pelvic or lower extremity trauma
  - Oral contraceptives with cigarette smoking
  - CHF
  - COPD
  - Obesity
  - Past medical or family history of hypercoagulability
- Aortic dissection
  - Hypertension
  - Congenital disease of the aorta or aortic valve
  - Inflammatory aortic disease
  - Connective tissue disease
  - Pregnancy
  - Arteriosclerosis
  - Cigarette use
- Pericarditis or myocarditis
  - Infection
  - Autoimmune disease (e.g., systemic lupus erythematosus)
  - Acute rheumatic fever
  - Recent myocardial infarction or cardiac surgery
  - Malignancy
  - Radiation therapy to mediastinum
  - Uremia
  - Drugs
  - Prior pericarditis
- Pneumothorax

Prior pneumothorax
Valsalva's maneuver
Chronic lung disease
Cigarette use

Physical Examination

Specific findings may be found in a variety of causes (Table 9-3).

Table 9-3 Pivotal Findings in Physical Examination

SIGN	FINDING	DIAGNOSES
Appearance	Acute respiratory distress	PE Tension pneumothorax AMI Pneumothorax
	Diaphoresis	AMI Aortic dissection Coronary ischemia PE Esophageal rupture UA Cholecystitis Perforated peptic ulcer
Vital signs	Hypotension	Tension pneumothorax PE AMI Aortic dissection (late) Coronary ischemia Esophageal rupture Pericarditis Myocarditis
	Tachycardia	AMI PE Aortic dissection Coronary ischemia Tension pneumothorax Esophageal rupture Coronary spasm Pericarditis Myocarditis Mediastinitis Cholecystitis Esophageal tear (Mallory-Weiss)
	Bradycardia	AMI Coronary ischemia UA
	Hypertension	AMI Coronary ischemia Aortic dissection (early)
	Fever	PE Esophageal rupture Pericarditis Myocarditis Mediastinitis Cholecystitis
	Hypoxemia	PE Tension pneumothorax Pneumothorax

Continued

SIGN	FINDING	DIAGNOSES
Cardiovascular examination	Significant difference in upper extremity blood pressures	Aortic dissection
	Narrow pulse pressure	Pericarditis (with effusion)
	New murmur	AMI Aortic dissection Coronary ischemia
	S_3/S_4 gallop	AMI Coronary ischemia
	Pericardial rub	Pericarditis
	Audible systolic "crunch" on cardiac auscultation (Hamman's sign)	Esophageal rupture Mediastiniti
	JVD	AMI Coronary ischemia Tension pneumothorax PE Pericarditis
Pulmonary examination	Unilateral diminished or absent breath sounds	Tension pneumothorax Pneumothorax
	Pleural rub	PE
	Subcutaneous emphysema	Tension pneumothorax Esophageal rupture Pneumothorax Mediastinitis
	Rales	AMI Coronary ischemia UA
Abdominal examination	Epigastric tenderness	Esophageal rupture Esophageal tear Cholecystitis Pancreatitis
	Left upper quadrant tenderness	Pancreatitis
	Right upper quadrant tenderness	Cholecystitis
Extremity examination	Unilateral leg swelling, warmth, pain, tenderness, or erythema	PE
Neurologic examination	Focal findings	Aortic dissection
	Stroke	AMI Coronary ischemia Aortic dissection Coronary spasm

Ancillary Studies

ECG. The two most commonly performed studies in patients with chest pain are the chest radiograph and 12-lead ECG (Table 9-4). An ECG should be performed within 10 min of arrival in all patients with chest pain in whom myocardial ischemia is a possibility. Rapid acquisition of the ECG facilitates the diagnosis of AMI and expedites "door to treatment" times from arrival to PCI or thrombolytic therapy in AMI. Patients with a new injury pattern on ECG (Table 9-5) or new ischemic ECG changes should have appropriate therapy instituted at this point (Fig. 9-2). An ECG showing right ventricular strain pattern, in the appropriate setting, should raise the clinical suspicion for PE. Diffuse ST segment elevation helps make the diagnosis of pericarditis.

Imaging study. Chest radiography is performed for patients with a possibly serious cause of chest pain. Pneumothorax, pneumonia, empyema, and pleural effusion are definitively diagnosed at this point. A wide mediastinum or ill-defined aortic knob increases the clinical suspicion for acute aortic dissection. Pleural effusion, subcutaneous air, or mediastinal air-fluid level may be seen in esophageal rupture. Increased cardiac silhouette may indicate pericarditis or cardiomyopathy.

Table 9-4 Ancillary Testing of Patients with Chest Pain

TEST	FINDING	DIAGNOSIS
ECG	New injury	AMI, Aortic dissection
	New ischemia	Coronary ischemia, Coronary spasm
	RV strain	PE
	Diffuse ST segment elevation	Pericarditis
CXR	Pneumothorax with mediastinal shift	Tension pneumothorax
	Wide mediastinum	Aortic dissection
	Pneumothorax	Esophageal rupture Pneumothorax
	Effusion	Esophageal rupture
	Increased cardiac silhouette	Pericarditis
	Pneumomediastinum	Esophageal rupture Mediastinitis
ABG	Hypoxemia, A-a gradient	PE
$\dot{V}/\dot{Q}$ scan or Spiral CT	High probability or any positive in patient with high clinical suspicion	PE

Table 9-5 Electrocardiogram Findings in Ischemic Chest Pain

Classic MI	ST segment elevation (>1 mm) in contiguous leads; new LBBB Q waves >0.04 sec duration
Subendocardial infarction	T wave inversion or ST segment depression in concordant leads
UA	Most often normal or nonspecific changes; may see T wave inversion
Pericarditis	Diffuse ST segment elevation; PR segment depression

Patients with suspected thoracic aortic dissection may be evaluated by CTA, TEE, or MRI. Patients at high pretest probability for PE should undergo MDCT or pulmonary angiography or a ventilation-perfusion lung scan.

CT with a 64 or higher detector scanner has the potential to rule out all of the life-threatening causes of chest pain. Although ACS, PE, and thoracic dissection (the "triple rule out") are the causes most commonly discussed, pneumothorax, mediastinitis, and pericardial effusions are also diagnosed with CT.

Bedside ultrasound in ED plays an important role in distinguishing chest pain of cardiogenic from other originals. Regional wall motion abnormality suggests myocardial ischemia, and acute dilation of right heart accompanied by pulmonary artery hypertension is the strong evidence of pulmonary embolus. The absence of "slide sign" may indicate pneumothorax. For patients suspect of cardiac tamponade, ultrasound may be the best option.

Laboratory testing. CK is associated with multiple false-positive results and has no use in the evaluation of unstable angina. CK-MB, an isoform of CK, is more specific for cardiac ischemia but largely has been supplanted by troponin testing. CK-MB produces fewer false-positive results than CK, and peak sensitivity approaches 98%. CK-MB isoforms improve sensitivity at 4 hr to 80%, approaching 93% at 6 hr. The current universal definition of AMI places CK and CK-MB in a secondary role to troponins.

Troponins (I and T), when elevated, identify patients with ACS who have the highest risk for an adverse outcome. Sensitivity for AMI at 4 hr is 60%, rising to nearly 100% by 12 hr. Elevated troponin in the correct clinical setting is synonymous with AMI and is embedded in the universal definition of MI.

A serum D-dimer assay may help discriminate patients with PE from those with a possible gastrointestinal cause. A low serum D-dimer in a patient without a high pretest probability of PE effectively excludes the diagnosis.

DIAGNOSTIC TABLE

After the patient is stabilized and assessment is completed, the findings are matched to the classic

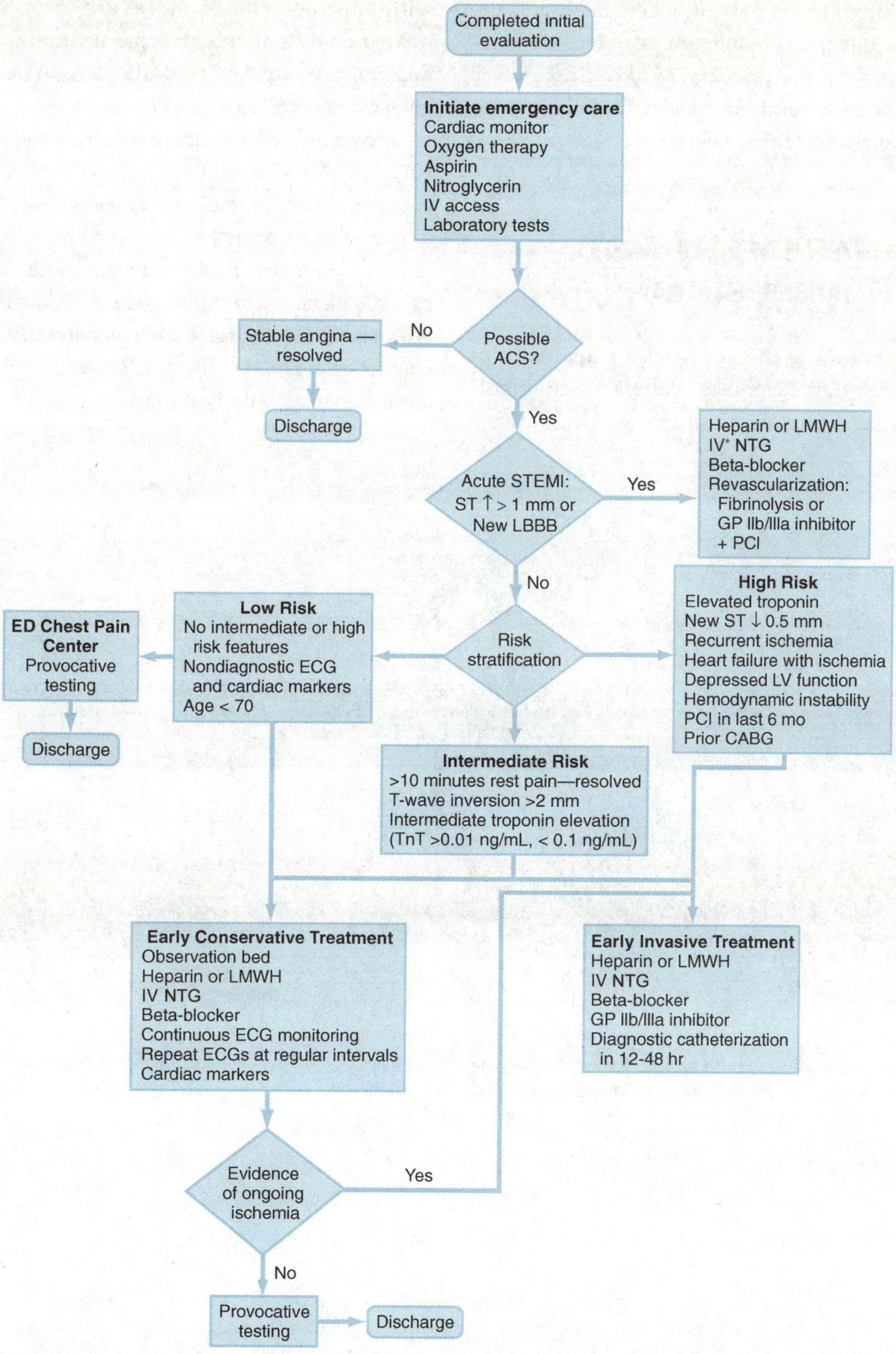

Fig. 9-2 Clinical guidelines for emergency department management of chest pain of myocardial ischemic origin.
∗ IV: intravenous injection.

and atypical patterns of the seven potentially critical diseases causing chest pain. This matching process is continual while the patient is evaluated and the response to therapy is monitored. Any inconsistency in findings with the primary working diagnoses requires a rapid review of the pivotal findings and the potential diagnoses (Table 9-6).

MANAGEMENT AND DISPOSITION

Fig. 9-3 outlines the approach to treatment of critical noncardiac diagnoses. Patients with critical diagnoses generally are admitted to ICU. Patients with emergent diagnoses typically are admitted to the hospital, most often on telemetry units. Patients with nonemergent diagnoses are most frequently treated as outpatients. Hospitalization is required in certain circumstances, particularly when patients have other comorbid conditions.

Frequently, no definitive diagnosis is established. Any patient with almost any type of chest pain may be having coronary ischemia, PE, or aortic dissection. When a clear pattern does not emerge to allow the emergency physician to make an alternative diagnosis confidently, or if the pattern of symptoms clearly is not compatible with a serious disorder, such as coronary ischemia, continued evaluation, hospitalization, or observation admission may be the best course.

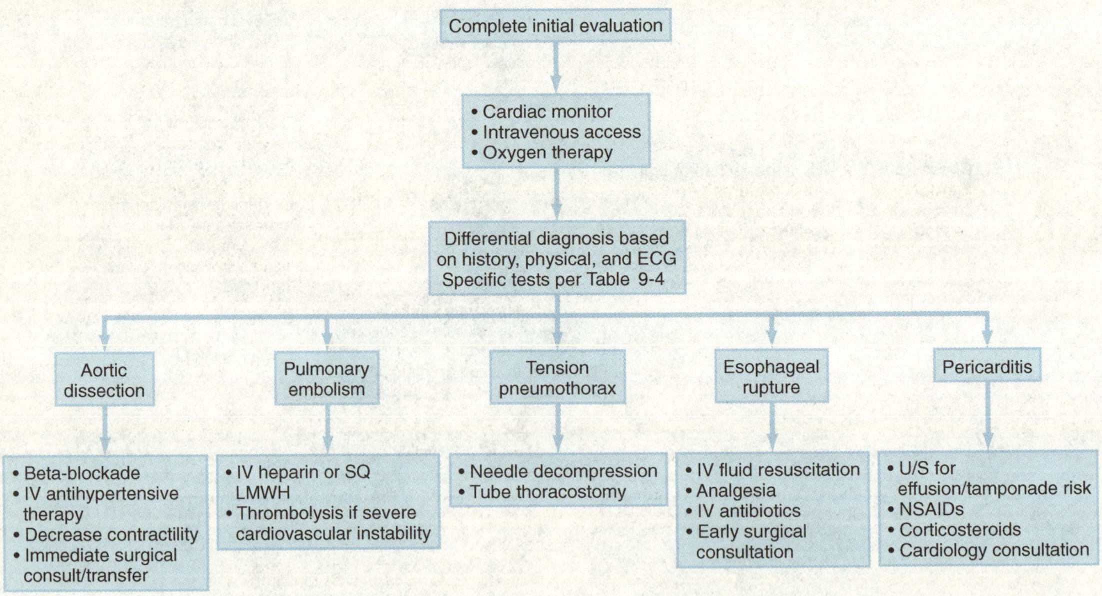

Fig. 9-3 Clinical guidelines for ED management of chest pain from potentially catastrophic nonmyocardial origins.

Table 9-6 Causes and Differentiation of Potentially Catastrophic Illness Presenting with Central Chest Pain or Discomfort

	PAIN HISTORY	ASSOCIATED SYMPTOMS	SUPPORTING HISTORY	PREVALENCE IN EMERGENCY DEPARTMENT	PHYSICAL EXAMINATION	USEFUL TESTS	ATYPICAL OR ADDITIONAL ASPECTS
MI	Discomfort is usually moderately severe to severe and rapid in onset. May be more "pressure" than pain. Usually retrosternal, may radiate to neck, jaw, both arms, upper back, epigastrium, and sides of chest (left more than right). Lasts more than 15-30 min and is unrelieved by NTG	Diaphoresis, nausea,vomiting, dyspnea	May be precipitated by emotional stress or exertion. Often comes on at rest. May come on in early awakening period. Prodromal pain pattern often elicited. Previous history of MI or angina. Age >40 yr, positive risk factors, and male sex increase possibility	Common	Patients are anxious and uncomfortable. Blood pressure usually is elevated, but normotension and hypotension are seen. The heart rate is usually mildly increased, but bradycardia can be seen. Patients may be diaphoretic and show peripheral poor perfusion. There are no diagnostic examination findings for MI, although $S_3$and S_4 heart sounds and new murmur are supportive	ECG changes (new Q waves or ST segment–T wave changes) occur in 80% of patients. CK-MB and troponins are helpful if elevated, but may be normal	Pain may be reported as "indigestion" or "unable to describe." Other atypical presentations include altered mental status, stroke, angina pattern without extended pain, severe fatigue, syncope. Elderly may have weakness, CHF, or chest tightness. 25% of nonfatal MIs are unrecognized by patient. The pain may have resolved by the time of evaluation
Unstable angina	Changes in pattern of preexisting angina with more severe, prolonged, or frequent pain (crescendo angina). Pain usually lasts >10 min. Angina at rest lasting 15-20 min or newonset angina (duration <2 mo) with minimal exertion. Pattern of pain change important in gauging risk for AMI. Unpredictable responses to NTG and rest	Often minimal. May have mild diaphoresis, nausea, dyspnea with pain. Increasing pattern of dyspnea on exertion	Not clearly related to precipitating factors. May be a decrease in amount of physical activity that initiates pain. Previous history of MIor angina. Older than 40 yr, presence of risk factors, and male sex increase probability	Common	Nonspecific findings of a transient nature, may have similar cardiac findings as in MI, especially intermittent diaphoresis	Often no ECG or enzyme changes. Variant angina (Prinzmetal's) has episodic pain, at rest, often severe, with prominent ST segment elevation	May be pain-free at presentation. Full history is essential. Fewer than 15% of patients hospitalized for unstable angina go on to AMI. May respond to NTG. May manifest similarly to non–Q wave infarction

Continued

	PAIN HISTORY	ASSOCIATED SYMPTOMS	SUPPORTING HISTORY	PREVALENCE IN EMERGENCY DEPARTMENT	PHYSICAL EXAMINATION	USEFUL TESTS	ATYPICAL OR ADDITIONAL ASPECTS
Aortic dissection	90% of patients have rapid-onset severe chest pain that is maximal at beginning. Radiates anteriorly in chest to the back interscapular area or into abdomen. Pain often has a"tearing" sensation and may migrate.	Neurologic complications of stroke, peripheral neuropathy, paresis or paraplegia, abdominal and extremity ischemia possible	Median age 59 yr. History of hypertension in 70%-90% of patients. 3:1 ratio males to females. Marfan syndrome and congenital bicuspid aortic valves have increased incidence.	Rare	Often poorly perfused peripherally but with elevated BP. In 50%-60% of cases, there is asymmetrical decrease or absence of peripheral pulses. 50% of proximal dissections cause aortic insufficiency. Other vascular occlusions: coronary (1%-2%), mesentery, renal, spinal cord. New-onset pericardial friction rub or aortic insufficiency murmur supportive of diagnosis	ECG usually shows left ventricular hypertrophy, nonspecific changes. Chest film shows abnormal aortic silhouette (90%). Aortic angiography has diagnostic accuracy of 95%-99%. TEE, CT, MRI most useful in screening.	Rare for patient to be painfree. May have neurologic complications. Physical examination findings may be minimal. Dissection into coronary arteries can mimic MI Ascending aortic aneurysms are more often approached surgically. Descending are generally managed medically.
Pulmonary embolism	Pain is more often lateralpleuritic. Central pain is more consistent with massive embolus. Abrupt in onset and maximal at beginning. May be episodic or intermittent	Dyspnea and apprehension play a prominent role, often more than pain. Cough accompanies about half the cases. Hemoptysis occurs in <20%. Anginalike pain may occur in 5%	Often some period of immobilization has occurred, e.g., postoperative. Pregnancy, oral contraceptives, heart disease, and cancer are all risk factors. Previous DVT or PE is the greatest risk factor.	Uncommon in ambulatory patients but common in departments with high volumes of elderly or medically complex patients	Patients are anxious and often have arespiratory rate >16 breaths/min. Tachycardia, inspiratory rales, and an increased pulmonic second sound are common. Fever, phlebitis, and diaphoresis are seen in 30%-40% of patients. Wheezes and peripheral cyanosis are less common.	ABG show PO_2<80 mm Hg in 90%. Widened A-a gradient is helpful. Chest film is usually normal, although 40% show some volume loss, oligemia, or signs of consolidation caused by pulmonary infarction. Lung perfusion scan rules out, if truly negative	Patients may have dyspnea with or without bronchospasm. Acute mortality rate is 10%. Emboli usually from lower extremities above knee, prostate or pelvis venous plexus, right side of heart. May be subtle cause of COPD exacerbation

Continued

	PAIN HISTORY	ASSOCIATED SYMPTOMS	SUPPORTING HISTORY	PREVALENCE IN EMERGENCY DEPARTMENT	PHYSICAL EXAMINATION	USEFUL TESTS	ATYPICAL OR ADDITIONAL ASPECTS
Pneumothorax	Pain is usually acute and maximal at onset. Most often lateralpleuritic, but central pain can occur in large pneumothorax	Dyspnea has a prominent role. Hypotension and altered mental states occur in tension pneumothorax	Chest trauma, previous episode, or asthenic body type	Infrequent	Decreased breath sounds, increased resonance on percussion. Elevated pressure in neck veins occurs in tension pneumothorax	Chest film definitive. Inspiratory and expiratory films may enhance contrast between air and lung parenchyma. Tension pneumothorax should be diagnosed on physical examination	May be subtle in COPD, asthma, cystic fibrosis. Can be complicated by pneumomediastinum
Esophageal rupture	Pain usually is preceded by vomiting and is abrupt in onset. Pain is persistent and unrelieved, localized along the esophagus, and increased by swallowing and neck flexion	Diaphoresis, dyspnea (late), shock	Older individual with known gastrointestinal problems. History of violent emesis, foreign body, caustic ingestion, blunt trauma, alcoholism, esophageal disease	Rare	Signs of lung consolidation, subcutaneous emphysema may be present	Chest film usually has mediastinal air, a leftsided pleural effusion, pneumothorax, or a widened mediastinum. pH of pleural effusion is <6.0. Diagnosis supported by watersoluble contrast esophagram or esophagoscopy	Patient may be in shock state. This entity often considered late in differential diagnostic process
Pericarditis	Dull, aching recurrent pain unrelated to exercises or meals, or it may be a sharp, stabbing, pleuritic-type pain that does not change with chest wall motion. May be severe. Not relieved by NTG	Dyspnea, diaphoresis	Pain is often worse when supine but improves sitting up. Often preceded by viral illness or underlying disease (SLE or uremia)	Rare Tamponade even more rare complication	Friction rub may be heard, often fleeting, position dependent (50% of patients)	ECG pattern typical for ST segment elevation across the precordial leads. Erythrocyte sedimentation rate may be elevated.	More common in 20- to 50-year-olds. May have associated tachycardias, ventricular dysrhythmias. Idiopathic most common (80%). Treated with aspirin, NSAID.

(CHEN Yuguo)

Chapter 10

Acute Coronary Syndrome

KEY CONSCEPTS

ACS includes the "acute" subtypes of CAD, including UA, AMI, and SCD.

Usually the reduction of coronary blood flow does not cause ischemic symptoms at rest until the vessel stenosis exceeds 95%.

RVMI rarely occur in isolation and are usually associated with IWMIor inferoposterior MI.

Several other conditions, particularly LBBB and LVH, also feature ST segment elevation that mimics AMI.

Particularly in individuals with nondiagnostic ECG, the presence of regional systolic wall motion abnormalities in a patient without known CAD is a moderately accurate indicator of AMI.

The AHA recommends that all patients with STEMI receive fibrinolytic therapy within 30 min of arrival or undergo primary PCI no later than 90 min after arrival.

Emergency revascularization with PCI or CABG is preferred in patients with STEMI complicated by cardiogenic shock irrespective of the delay to treatment.

Empirical therapy of beta-adrenergic blocking agents in the ED should be reconsidered and reserved for only those patients who have adverse effects from significantly elevated BP despite application of NTG, or significant tachydysrhythmia.

PERSPECTIVE

ACS includes a spectrum of clinical presentations ranging from UA to non-ST segment elevation myocardial infarction (NSTEMI) and STEMI. ACS and in particular AMI remain the leading causes of death in much of the developed world.

EPIDEMIOLOGY

CAD continue to be the leading causes of death among adults in many developed countries. The incidence of cardiovascular disease is expected to continue to increase owing to lifestyle and behavioral changes that promote heart disease.

Reduction in cigarette smoking, management of lipids, and improved management of HTN and DM undoubtedly play a role, along with significant advances in medical treatment.

SPECTRUM OF DISEASE

CAD includes the spectrum from asymptomatic CAD and stable angina to UA, AMI, and SCD. ACS includes the "acute" subtypes of CAD, including UA, AMI, and SCD.

Stable Angina

Stable angina pectoris is transient, episodic chest discomfort resulting from myocardial ischemia. Physical or psychological stress may provoke an attack of angina that resolves spontaneously over a constant, predictable period of time with rest or NTG.

Unstable Angina

UA is broadly defined as angina occurring with minimal exertion or at rest, new-onset angina, or a worsening change in a previously stable anginal syndrome in terms of frequency or duration of attacks, resistance to previously effective medications, or provocation with decreasing levels of exertion or stress. Rest angina is defined as angina occurring at rest, lasting longer than 20 min, and occurring within 1 w of presentation. New-onset angina is angina of at least class Ⅱ severity with onset within the previous 2 mo. Increasing or progressive angina is diagnosed when a previously known angina becomes more frequent, longer in duration, or increased by one class within the previous 2 mo of at least class Ⅲ severity. Symptoms that last longer than 20 min despite cessation of activity are consistent with angina at rest and reflect UA.

UA is often referred to as preinfarction angina, accelerating or crescendo angina, intermediate coronary syndrome, and preocclusive syndrome. UA should be considered a possible harbinger of AMI.

Plaque rupture accompanied by thrombus formation and vasospasm illustrate the intracoronary events of UA.

Variant angina—also known as Prinzmetal's angina—is caused by coronary artery vasospasm at rest with minimal fixed coronary artery lesions; it may be relieved by exercise or NTG. The ECG reveals ST segment elevation that is impossible to discern from AMI electrocardiographically.

Acute Myocardial Infarction

AMI is defined as myocardial cell death and necrosis of the myocardium.

AMI is further classified by findings on the ECG at presentation, as either STEMI or NSTEMI.

PATHOPHYSIOLOGY

The underlying pathophysiology of ACS is myocardial ischemia. Inadequate perfusion most commonly results from coronary arterial vessel stenosis as a result of atherosclerotic CAD. Usually the reduction of coronary blood flow does not cause ischemic symptoms at rest until the vessel stenosis exceeds 95%. Myocardial ischemia, however, may occur with exercise and increased myocardial oxygen consumption with as little as 60% vessel stenosis.

CAD is characterized by thickening and obstruction of the coronary vessel arterial lumen by atherosclerotic plaques.

Thrombus formation is considered an integral factor in ACS, including all subtypes ranging from UA to NSTEMI and STEMI. The most important factors in the infarction are the acute events of plaque rupture, platelet activation, and thrombus formation.

Another important aspect of ACS is vasospasm. Approximately 10% of MI occur as a result of coronary artery spasm and subsequent thrombus formation without significant underlying CAD.

CLINICAL FEATURES

Diabetic patients frequently exhibit nontraditional symptoms of AMI, such as dyspnea. The elderly commonly note only weakness, confusion, or other nonclassic symptoms as the primary manifestation of ACS.

Preadmission Evaluation

Chest pain is a poor predictor of the diagnosis. Preadmission 12-lead ECG offers high specificity and positive predictive value for AMI in patients with atraumatic chest pain.

Emergency Department Evaluation

The History

The character of the chest discomfort as well as the onset, location, radiation, duration, prior presence, and any exacerbating or alleviating factors should be sought. Associated symptoms, especially of a cardiac, pulmonary, gastrointestinal, and neurologic nature, should be elicited.

The Classic History

The term angina refers to "tightening," not pain. Classically, it is substernal or precordial in location and may radiate to the neck, jaw, shoulders, or arms.

Furthermore, classic features of angina pectoris include exacerbation with exertion, a heavy meal, stress, or cold, and alleviation with rest. Anginal discomfort characteristically lasts from 2 to 5 min up to 20 min (Table 10-1).

Table 10-1 Clinical Characteristics of Classic Anginal Chest Discomfort

CHARACTERISTIC	MORE LIKELY TO BE ANGINA	LESS LIKELY TO BE ANGINA
Type of pain	Dull, pressure	Sharp, stabbing
Duration	2-5 min, often 15-20 min	Seconds or hours
Onset	Gradual	Rapid
Location	Substernal	Lateral chest wall, back
Reproducible	With exertion	With inspiration
Associated symptoms	Present	Absent
Palpation of chest wall	Not painful	Painful

The Atypical History

In patients with AMI or UA, atypical presenting complaints include dyspnea, nausea, diaphoresis, syncope, or pain in the arms, epigastrium, shoulder, or neck.

Before age 85, chest pain is found in the majority of patients with AMI. In those older than 85 yr, however, atypical symptoms are more common than chest pain.

Patients with DM are at heightened risk for ACS as well as an atypical presentation.

Physical Examination

The physical examination focuses on the cardiac, pulmonary, abdominal, and neurologic examinations, looking for signs of complications of ACS (Table 10-2).

Table 10-2 Key Entities in the Differential Diagnosis of Chest Pain

AMI	UA
Stable angina	Prinzmetal' s angina
Pericarditis	Myocardial or pulmonary contusion
Pneumonia	PE
Pneumothorax	Pulmonary hypertension
Pleurisy	Aortic dissection
Boerhaave's syndrome	Gastroesophageal reflux
Peptic ulcer disease	Gastritis or esophagitis
Esophageal spasm	Mallory-Weiss syndrome
Cholecystitis or biliary colic	Pancreatitis
Herpes zoster	Musculoskeletal pain

Outcomes in Atypical Presentations

Atypical presentation of patients with ACS is associated with a delay in diagnosis and poorer outcomes.Patients with MI without chest pain were significantly more likely to die .Patients with atypical symptomatology seek medical care later and are less likely to receive standard therapies.

Early Complications of AMI

Bradydysrhythmia and AVB occur in 25% to 30% of patients with AMI. Patients with AVB in the setting of anterior AMI have a poor prognosis.

Tachydysrhythmias are quite common in the setting of AMI.

Cardiogenic shock is hypotension with end-organ hypoperfusion. Other causes of shock with similar presentations should be considered, such as aortic dissection, PE, pericardial tamponade, and ventricular free wall rupture accompanying AMI.

Pericarditis, when associated with AMI, can occur early or in a delayed fashion; the former is termed infarct pericarditis, and the latter is known as post-MI syndrome or Dressler's syndrome. Infarct pericarditis is associated with transmural insult. This pain is characteristically pleuritic and worse in the supine position.

Stroke may also complicate AMI, most commonly ischemic or thromboembolic.

Hyperglycemia in the setting of AMI may be viewed as a complication in AMI. Hyperglycemia is present in up to one half of all patients with STEMI.

DIAGNOSTIC INVESTIGATIONS

Electrocardiography

In the patient with chest discomfort or other symptoms suggestive of ACS, the 12-lead ECG helps establish the diagnosis.

Other 12-lead ECG determinations include cardiac rhythm, evolution of the ACS event, response to therapy, and clinical information suggesting an alternative diagnosis, such as PE or acute myopericarditis.

In ACS, morphologic changes may occur in the T wave, the ST segment, the QRS complex, and even the PR segment (e.g.ST segment depression in atrial infarction or infarct-related pericarditis).

Various rhythm disturbances also occur.

Electrocardiographic Abnormalities in ACS

The earliest electrocardiographic finding in AMI is the hyperacute T wave, but becomes tall and peaked within minutes of the interruption of blood flow. The hyperacute T wave progresses to ST segment elevation in classic MI. The differential diagnosis of the tall T wave includes hyperacute T waves of ischemia, hyperkalemia, benign early repolarization (BER), LVH, LBBB, and pericarditis (Fig. 10-1).

As the AMI progresses, ST segment elevation may become evident. The concave morphology, if noted in all elevated ST segments, is atypical for AMI and more commonly seen with other ST segment elevation syndromes (Table 10-3 and Fig. 10-2).

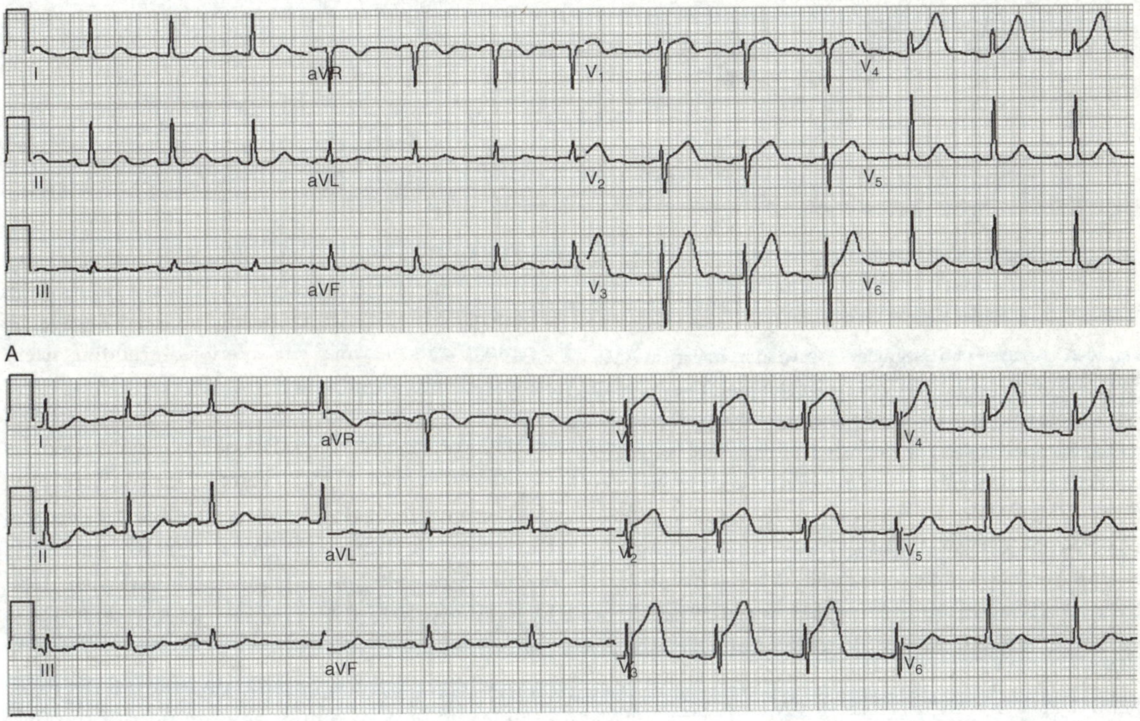

Fig. 10-1 Hyperacute T wave of AMI. A, Note the broad, tall T waves in leads V_3 and V_4 in this patient with chest pain and diaphoresis. These are the hyperacute T waves of early STEMI. The ST segment is just beginning to rise in leads V_3 and V_4; leads V_1 and V_2 are also suspicious. B, This tracing is from the same patient, roughly 30 min after the ECG in A. Note the prominent ST segment elevation in leads V_1 to V_4.

Table 10-3 Differential Diagnosis of ST Segment Elevation on the ECG

AMI	Acute pericarditis
LVH	Left ventricular aneurysm
Ventricular paced rhythm	BER
Normal variant	Osborn wave of hypothermia
Hyperkalemia	Brugada's syndrome
PE	Acute cerebral hemorrhage
Prinzmetal's angina	Postelectrical cardioversion

ST segment depression generally represents subendocardial or noninfarction ischemia. The differential diagnosis of ST segment depression includes myocardial ischemia or AMI, repolarization abnormality of ventricular hypertrophy (the "strain" pattern), bundle branch block, ventricular paced rhythm (VPR), digoxin effect, hyperkalemia, hypokalemia, PE, intracranial hemorrhage, myocarditis, rate-related ST segment depression, postcardioversion of tachydysrhythmias, and pneumothorax (Fig. 10-3).

T wave inversions should suggest possible myocardial ischemia. The T wave inversions of ACS are classically narrow and symmetrically inverted. T wave inversions are best evaluated in

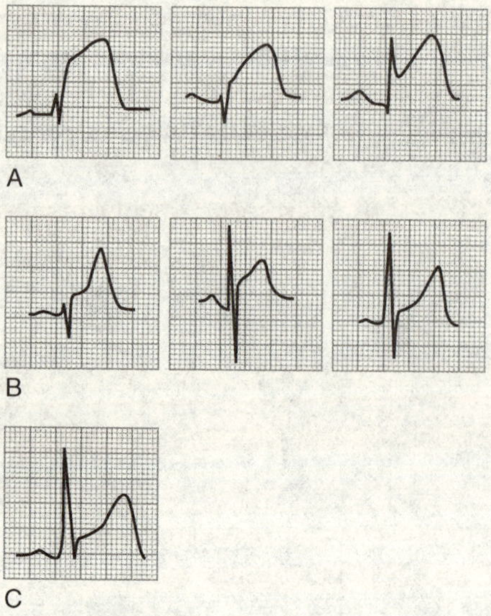

Fig. 10-2 Analysis of ST segment–T wave morphology in AMI, BER, and acute pericarditis. An analysis of the ST segment–T wave morphology (from the beginning at the J point to the end at the apex of the T wave) may be particularly helpful in distinguishing among the various causes of ST segment elevation (STE) and identifying the AMI case. A, The initial upsloping portion of the ST segment is usually either flat (horizontally or obliquely) or convex in the patient with AMI. This morphologic observation, however, should be used only as a guideline; it is not infallible. B, Non-AMI causes of STE are seen here with concavity of the ST segment–T wave (left BER, middle pericarditis, right BER). C, Patients with STE related to AMI may demonstrate concavity of this portion of the waveform.

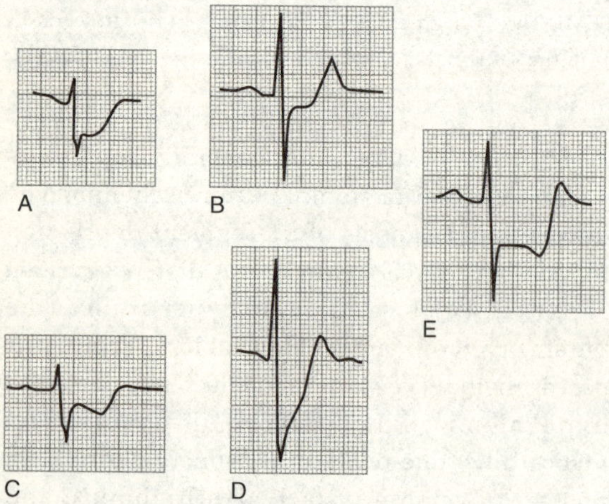

Fig. 10-3 ST segment depression (STD) in ACS. A, Horizontal STD unstable angina pectoris.(USAP). B, Horizontal STD (NSTEMI). C, Downsloping STD (USAP). D, Upsloping STD (USAP). E, Horizontal STD as seen in lead III in a patient with anterior wall AMI, an example of reciprocal STD, also known as reciprocal change.

comparison with the most recent prior ECG, given the multitude of normal variations (Fig. 10-4.)

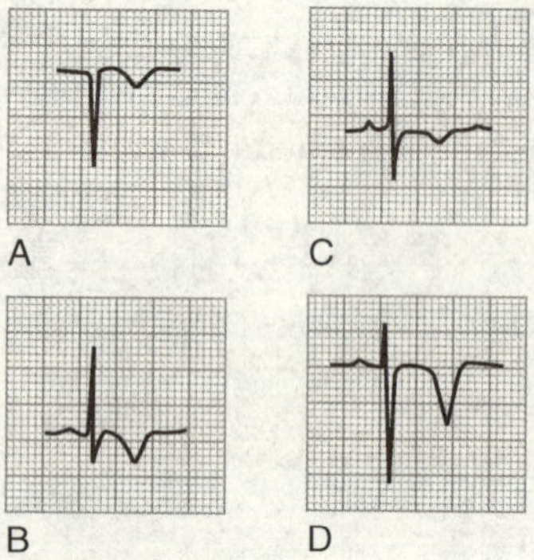

Fig. 10-4 T wave inversions of ACS. A and B, T wave inversions in patients with ACS. C, T wave inversion in a patient with NSTEMI. D, Deeply inverted T waves in a patient with proximal left anterior descending artery stenosis, Wellens syndrome.

The differential diagnosis of T wave inversion is broad and includes ACS, ventricular hypertrophy, bundle branch block, VPR, myocarditis, pericarditis, PE, pneumothorax, WPWS, cerebrovascular accident, hypokalemia, gastrointestinal disorders, hyperventilation, persistent juvenile T wave pattern, and normal variants. Q waves are generally representative of irreversible myocardial necrosis. Pathologic Q waves may emerge within the first hour of infarction but most commonly develop 8 to 12 hr into the infarction. Q waves may persist after MI as enduring markers of previous MI on the ECG.

Anatomic Location of Acute Myocardial Infarction

The regional distribution of AMI can be derived from noting the pattern of the various morphologic changes that are described (Table 10-4). *Anterior wall myocardial infraction(AWMI)* are primarily evidenced by changes in the precordial leads V_1 to V_4 (Fig. 10-5). Septal involvement is reflected by changes in V_1 and V_2. Extension to the lateralwall is evident if the pathologic changes extend beyond leads V_1 to V_4 to include leads V_5, V_6, Ⅰ, and aVL. In anterior ST segment elevation AMI, reciprocal ST segment depression may occur in leads Ⅲ and aVF. The anterior wall is served by the left anterior descending artery. The first diagonal branch of the left anterior descending artery is likely to be involved when the ST segment elevation extends to

Table 10-4 Regional ST Segment Changes in AMI

LOCATION	LEADS	ST SEGMENT
AWMI	V_1 through V_4	Elevation
LWMI	Ⅰ, aVL, V_5, and V_6	Elevation
IWMI	Ⅰ, Ⅱ, and aVF	Elevation
RVWMI	V_{4R}	Elevation
PWMI	V_8 and V_9	Elevation
	V_1 through V_3	Depression

leads I and aVL. Isolated occlusion of the diagonal branch of the left anterior descending artery displays similar findings, but of smaller amplitude, to those seen with left anterior descending artery occlusion (ST segment elevation in leads V_2 and V_3, and possibly leads V_1 and V_4, or both, along with ST segment depression in lead Ⅱ and either Ⅲ, aVF, or both).

*Lateral wall MI(LWMI)*are frequently seen in concert with AWMI (anterolateral), inferior wall MI (IWMI)(inferolateral), or IWMI with posterior extension (inferoposterolateral).Lateral involvement is manifested by changes in some or all of the lateral leads Ⅰ, aVL, V_5, and V_6. So-called "high lateral MI" are restricted to leads I and aVL (Fig. 10-6) and are suggestive of occlusion of the left circumflex coronary artery; ST segment elevation in these leads may be accompanied by reciprocal ST segment depression in leads Ⅲ, aVF, and V_1. Based on cardiac MRI localization of some of these lesions, new Q waves appearing in leads I and aVL (but not V_6) indicate a "mid-anterior wall MI," previously referred to as a "high lateral MI."

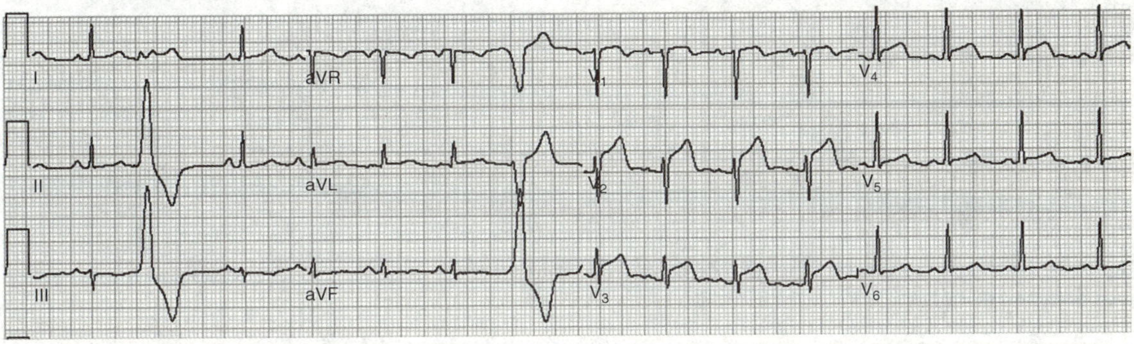

Fig. 10-5 AWMI. STE is evident in leads V_1 to V_4.

IWMI are characterized by morphologic changes in limb leads Ⅱ, Ⅲ, and aVF. The inferior wall of the heart and the AV node are served by the right coronary artery in roughly 90% of cases (right dominant); in the remainder, the left circumflex artery serves that function (left dominant). An inferior STEMI is present if two or more contiguous inferior leads (Ⅲ, aVF, Ⅱ)

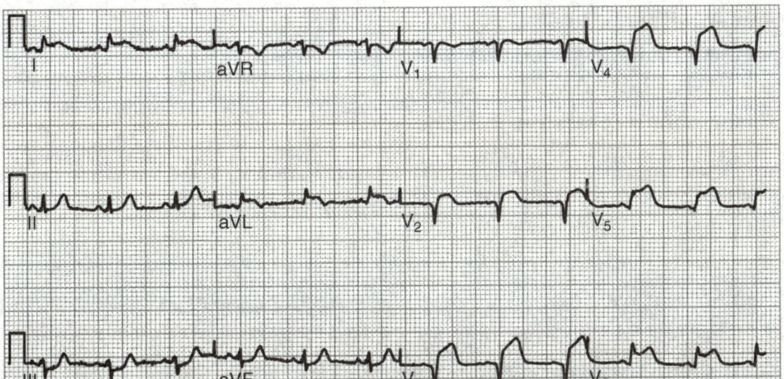

Fig. 10-6 Anterolateral AMI. STE is seen in leads Ⅰ, aVL, V_5, and V_6. A proximal left anterior descending artery lesion with thrombus was noted at emergent percutaneous coronary intervention.

are involved; reciprocal ST segment depression is frequently seen in lead aVL, lead I, or both (Fig. 10-7): V_1 less than V_2 and V_3. ST segment depression in leads V_1 to V_3 in the presence of inferior MI can be caused by reciprocal change, posterior extension, or simultaneous anterior ischemia during IWMI. ST segment elevation inferiorly that is greater in lead Ⅲ than in lead Ⅱ, accompanied by ST segment depression in lead aVL, Ⅰ, or both, is 90% sensitive and 71% specific for right coronary artery occlusion. ST segment elevation in lead V_1 in the presence of an ST segment elevation inferior MI (with elevation greater in lead Ⅲ than in lead Ⅱ) suggests concomitant right MI. Occlusion of the left circumflex artery may be occult on the 12-lead ECG.

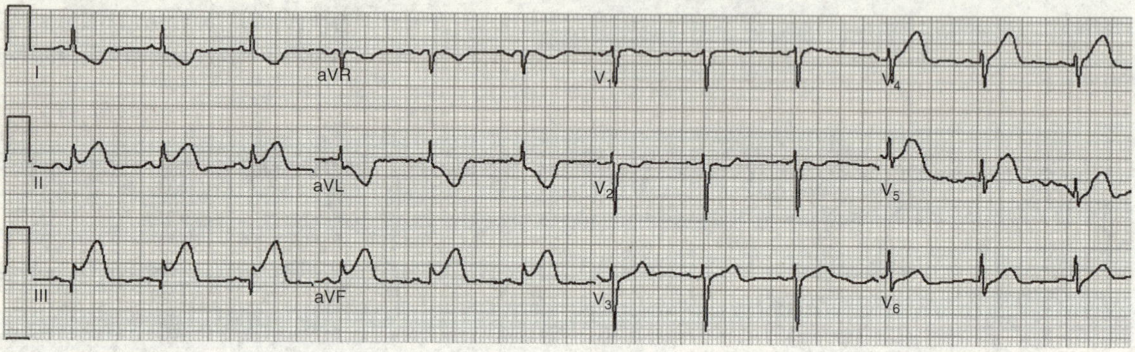

Fig. 10-7 IWMI with reciprocal changes. Marked STE is seen IWMI (leads Ⅱ, Ⅲ, and aVF).Classic reciprocal STD is evident in leads I and aVL.

PWMI are usually seen along with inferior or inferolateral MI. The culprit lesion may be in the right coronary artery, its posterior descending branch, or the left circumflex artery. Findings include (1) horizontal ST segment depression; (2) a tall, upright T wave; (3) a tall, wide R wave; and (4) an R wave amplitude/S wave amplitude ratio greater than 1 (Fig. 10-8). The combination of horizontal ST segment depression with an upright T wave increases the diagnostic accuracy of the 12-lead ECG for PWMI. In that the tall R wave in the right precordial leads is actually the mirror image of a posterior Q wave, its emergence may be delayed in PWMI. Additional leads (posterior leads V_8 and V_9) increase the sensitivity for detection of acute PWMI. Patients with IWMI who have either ST segment depression in leads V_1 to V_3 or ST segment elevation in the posterior leads V_8 and V_9 generally have larger infarction zones. Cardiac MRI suggests that these "PWMI" producing tall R waves in leads V_1 and V_2 are actually lateral left ventricular wall MI.

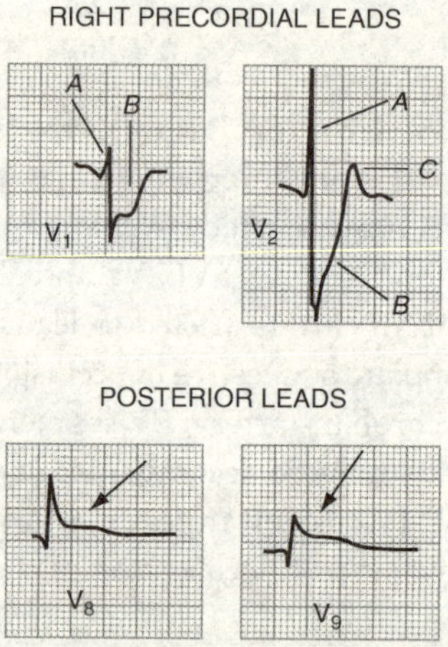

Fig. 10-8 Isolated PWMI; complexes from right precordial leads and posterior leads. The right precordial leads V_1 and V_2 reveal typical findings of PWMI with prominent R wave (A), STD (B), and upright T wave (C). The posterior leads V_8 and V_9 in the same case demonstrate STE (arrows), confirming isolated PMI.

RVMI rarely occur in isolation and are usually associated with IWMI or inferoposterior MI. At times, AWMI involves some (but less than half) of the right ventricular wall. Clinically, RVMI features include elevated jugular venous pressure and hypotension in the setting of IWMI.

ST segment elevation in lead V_1 in the setting of IWMI is suggestive of RVMI. ST segment elevation is usually greater in lead Ⅲ than in lead Ⅱ when RVMI coexists with inferior AMI. Application of "right-sided" precordial leads is the best means to diagnose RVMI with the ECG. These leads, as a mirror image of the left precordial leads, demonstrate ST segment elevation with RVMI in leads V_{3R} to V_{6R}, with V_{4R}

having the highest sensitivity. ECG changes in the right-sided precordial leads with RVMI may be subtle (Fig. 10-9). Patients with IWMI with concomitant RVMI have larger MI.

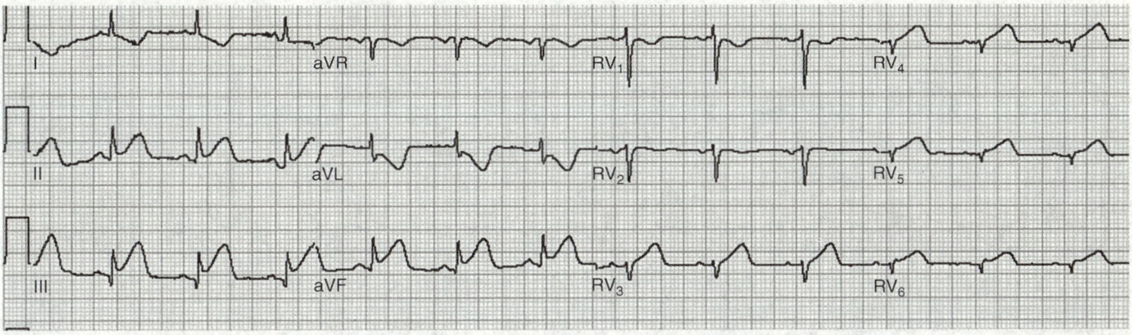

Fig. 10-9 RVMI demonstrated with right-sided precordial leads (RV_1 to RV_6). This tracing is taken from the same patient as in Figure 10-7. The STE of IWMI is still present, as is the reciprocal STD in leads I and aVL. The precordial leads are right-sided chest leads, as might be inferred from the relatively low voltage. STE is noted in leads RV_3 to RV_6 (V_{3R} to V_{6R}), consistent with RVMI.

Left Main Coronary Artery Occlusion. In a patient with symptoms of ACS, ST segment elevation in lead aVR should prompt consideration of occlusion of the left main coronary artery.

ECG Differential Diagnosis of ST Segment Elevation

Several other conditions, particularly LBBB and LVH, also feature ST segment elevation that mimics MI(Table 10-3).

BER includes the following ECG characteristics: (1) ST segment elevation; (2) upward concavity of the initial portion of the ST segment; (3) notching of the terminal portion of the QRS complex at the J point ; (4) symmetrical, concordant T waves of large amplitude; (5) diffuse ST segment elevation on the ECG; and (6) relative temporal stability over the short term. J point elevation is usually less than 3.5 mm, and the concave ST segment is usually elevated less than 2 mm (although it may be elevated as much as 5 mm in some cases) in the precordial leads and 0.5 mm in the limb leads. Maximal ST segment elevation in BER is typically seen in leads V_2 to V_5. Isolated BER in the limb leads is quite rare and should prompt reconsideration of AMI (Fig. 10-10A and Fig. 10-11).

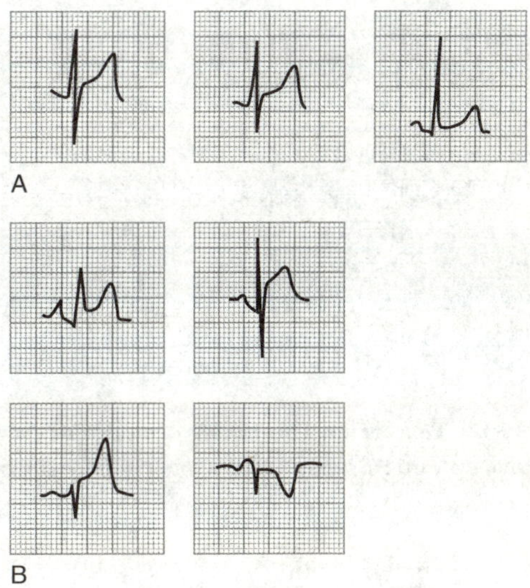

Fig. 10-10 Noninfarctional STE. A, BER with concave STE. B, Acute pericarditis with concave STE and PR segment depression (upper two examples); concave STE without PR segment abnormalities (lower left example); and "reciprocal" STD and PR segment elevation in lead aVR (lower right example).

Pericarditis, in the acute phase, features diffuse ST segment elevation as well. The ST segment elevation is usually seen in all leads with the exception of aVR; V_1 is variable.(Fig.10-12, Fig.10-10B).

LVA, wherein a focal area of myocardium paradoxically bulges outward during systole, has characteristic ECG changes that can be difficult to differentiate from those of AMI. Anatomically, LVA is most commonly found anteriorly, and changes are most often seen in leads V_1 to V_6 as well as leads I and aVL. ST segment elevation may be of any morphology (e.g., convex or concave), and Q waves may be present(Fig. 10-13). The calculation of the ratio of the amplitude of the T wave to the QRS

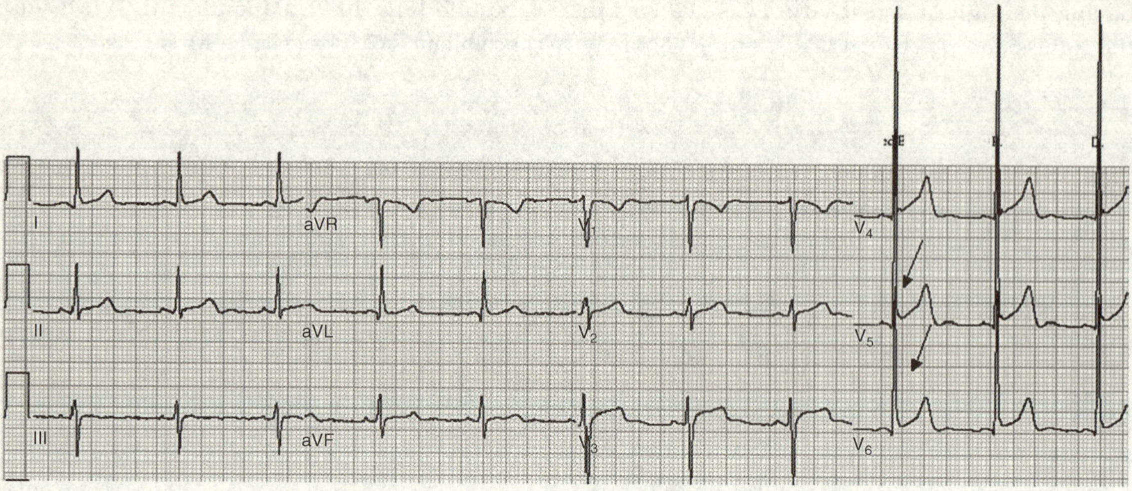

Fig. 10-11 BER. Note the upwardly concave STE, best seen in leads V_4 to V_6. The T waves are relatively large in the same leads. Subtle notching is also seen at the J point in leads V_4 and V_5 . Prior ECGs of this patient were unchanged.

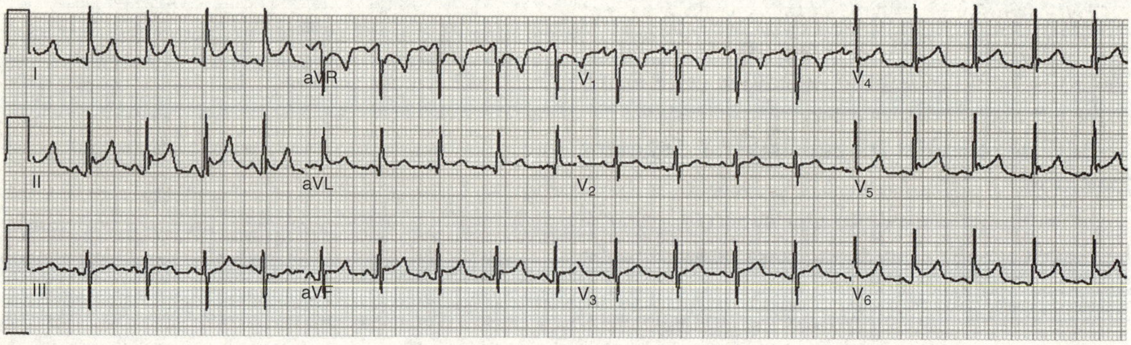

Fig. 10-12 Pericarditis. This tracing demonstrates several classic signs of pericarditis: (1) sinus tachycardia; (2) diffuse, concave upward ST segment elevation; (3) PR segment depression, best seen in lead Ⅱ; and (4) PR segment elevation in lead aVR.

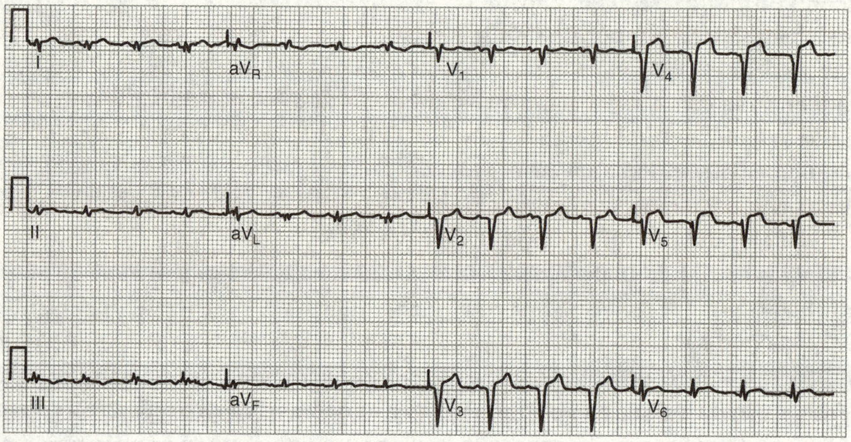

Fig. 10-13 LVA: representative example of 12-lead ECG from patient with anterior LVA. Note well-developed, completed Q waves in leads V_2 through V_5 and absence of reciprocal changes in contralateral leads.

complex may help distinguish acute AWMI from LVA. If the ratio of the amplitude of the T wave to the QRS complex exceeds 0.36 in any single lead, the ECG probably reflects AMI. If the ratio is less than 0.36 in all leads, however, the findings are probably a result of LVA.

A new, or presumably new, *LBBB* is strongly suggestive of ACS when noted in the appropriate clinical presentation. In the right precordial leads (leads V_1 to V_3), ST segment elevation and tall, vaulted, upright T waves mimic those seen in acute AWMI. The QS pattern of LBBB in these leads resembles the Q waves seen in MI. Depressed ST segments with T wave inversions are seen in some or all of the lateral leads (leads V_5, V_6 , I, and aVL) in LBBB; both of these resemble ischemic changes seen in ACS. Because LBBB is a frequent finding on the ECG of a patient at risk for CAD, the normal findings in LBBB (Fig. 10-14) and the presentation of ST segment AMI in a patient with LBBB must be distinguished.

Three independent ECG predictors of MI in the presence of LBBB were identified: (1) ST segment elevation of at least 1 mm that is concordant with the QRS complex; (2) ST segment depression of at least 1 mm in lead V_1, V_2, or V_3 ; and (3) ST segment elevation of at least 5 mm that is discordant with the QRS complex. For accuracy in diagnosis, a specificity of 90% requires a score of at least 3. Thus if an ECG features only discordant ST segment elevation of 5 mm or more but neither of the other two criteria, further testing is recommended before one can conclude that the ECG is indicative of AMI (Fig. 10-15).

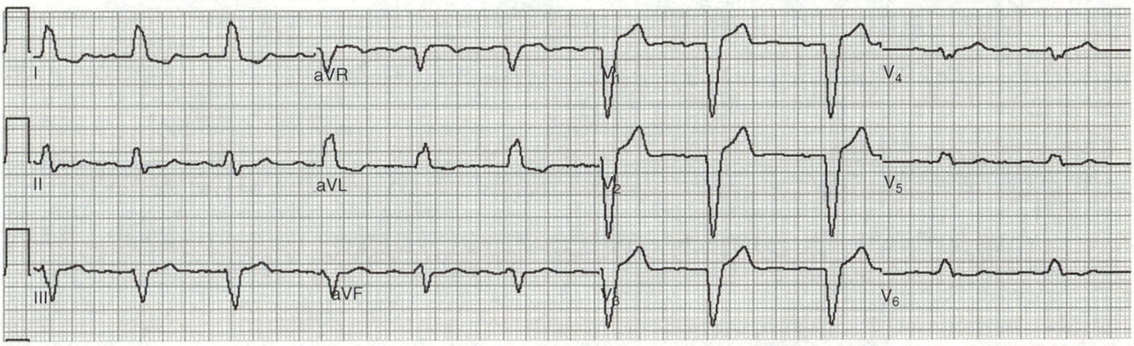

Fig. 10-14 LBBB (normal). This tracing demonstrates the classic findings of LBBB: (1) QRS complex width greater than 0.12 second; (2) absence of Q wave in lead V_6; (3) broad monophasic R wave in leads V_5, V_6, I , and aVL; (4) discordant ST segment–T wave changes in leads V_1 to V_3 (simulating acute MI), I , and aVL. A first-degree AVBis also apparent.

VPR can mimic and mask the manifestations of AMI. VPR originating in the right ventricular apex create a wide QRS complex, with a pseudo-LBBB pattern. As with LBBB, the right precordial leads in VPR typically feature predominantly negative QRS complexes with discordant ST segments and T waves that are elevated and tall or vaulted, respectively. Unlike LBBB, however, VPR originating in the right ventricular apex often yields a predominantly negative QRS complex in leads V_5 and V_6 as well. As with the LBBB scenario, the VPR pattern represents a significant confounding variable in the evaluation of the patient with chest pain suspected of having ACS. Sgarbossa and associates advanced criteria essentially the same as the LBBB criteria: (1) ST segment elevation of at least 5 mm that is discordant with the QRS complex; (2) ST segment elevation of at least 1 mm that is concordant with the QRS complex; and(3) ST segment depression of at least 1 mm in lead V_1, V_2, or V_3 (Fig. 10-16).

LVH may mimic or obscure ACS on the ECG. LVH that may feature prominent left-sided forces, manifesting as large rS or QS complexes in the right precordial leads. The initial portion of the elevated ST segment in LVH is generally concave, as opposed to the obliquely straight or convex pattern that usually (but not always) is seen with ST segment elevation in AMI. In LVH, the left precordial leads (and at times leads I and aVL) may show evidence of repolarization abnormality(or strain pattern), with ST segment depression and asymmetrically inverted T waves. The changes in LVH should be static over time (Fig. 10-17).

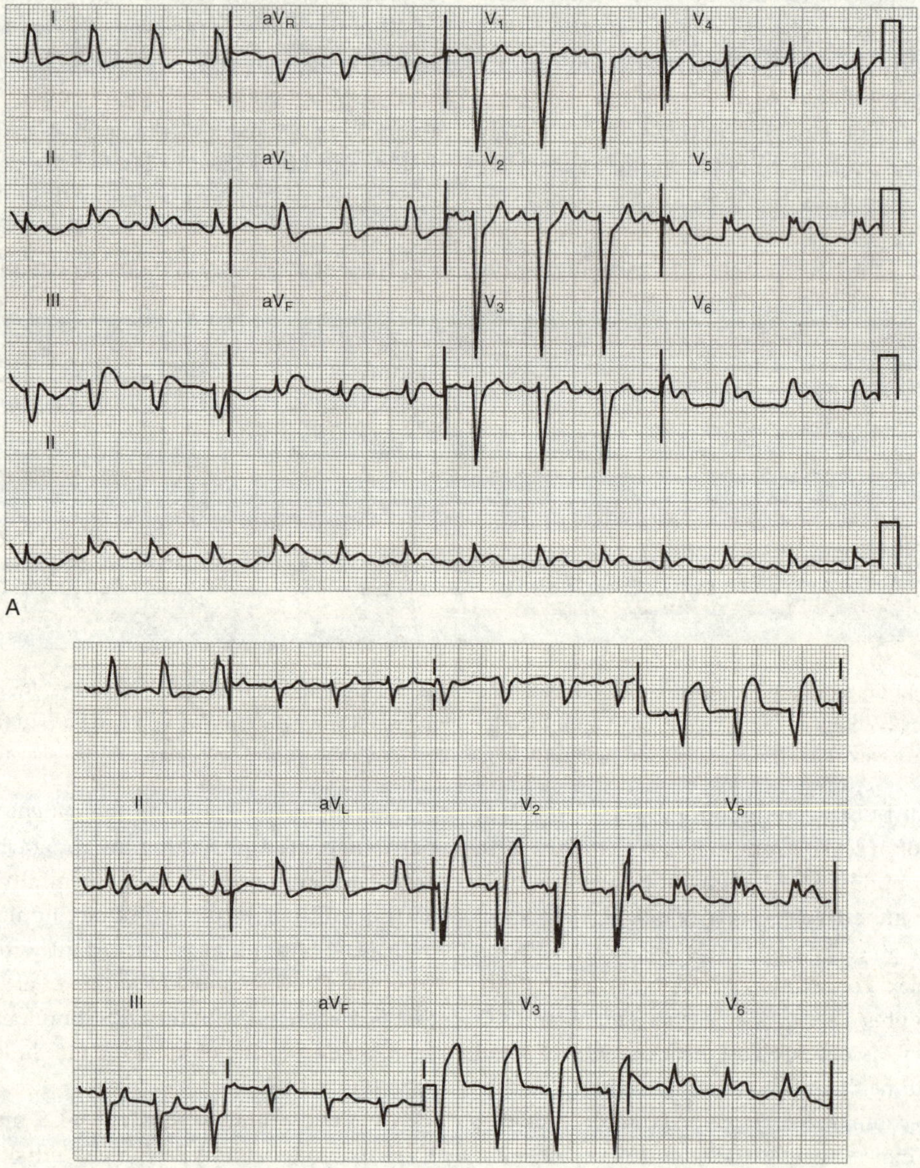

Fig. 10-15 AMI in LBBB. A, Using the Sgarbossa criteria, there is strong evidence of AMI because of the concordant ST segment elevation greater than 1 mm in leads Ⅱ, V_5, and V_6; also suggestive is the ST segment depression seen in V_2. B, Again, applying the Sgarbossa criteria to this tracing with underlying LBBB, AMI is strongly suggested. There is concordant ST segment elevation in leads V_5 and V_6 that appears to exceed 1 mm; furthermore, there is excessively discordant ST segment elevation in leads V_2 and V_3, probably greater than 5 mm.

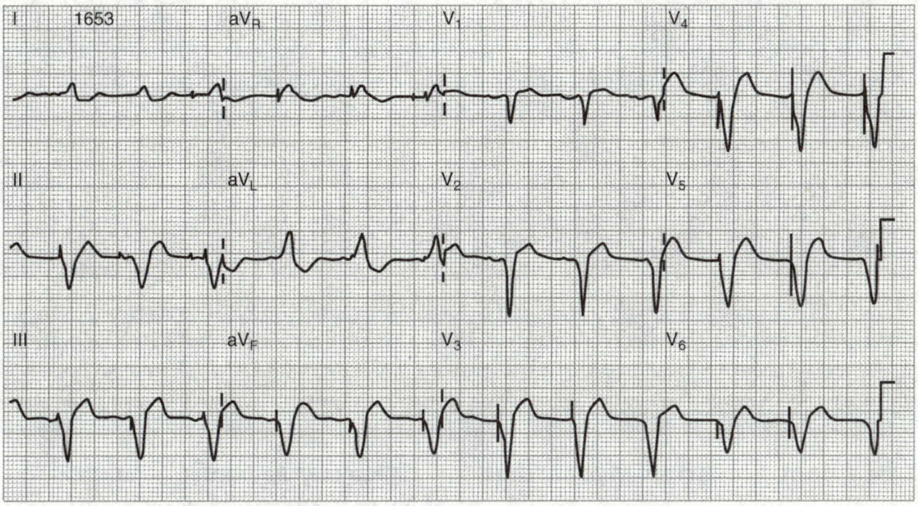

A

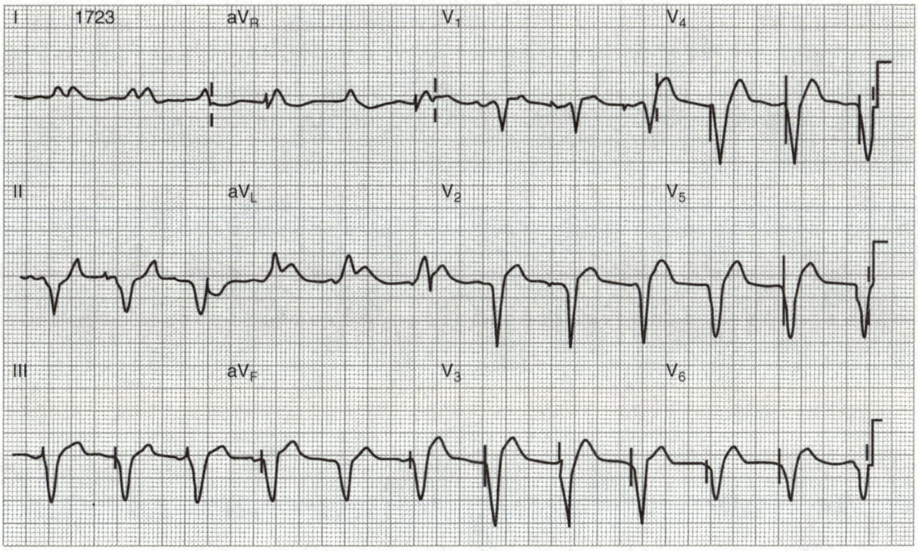

B

Fig. 10-16 Permanent right ventricular paced pattern with AMI; ventricular paced rhythm. A. Appropriate ST segment–T wave findings in the patient with a paced rhythm. B. Serial ECG from the patient in A, revealing evolution of changes worrisome for AMI, including concordant ST segment elevation in leads I and aVL consistent with LWMI.

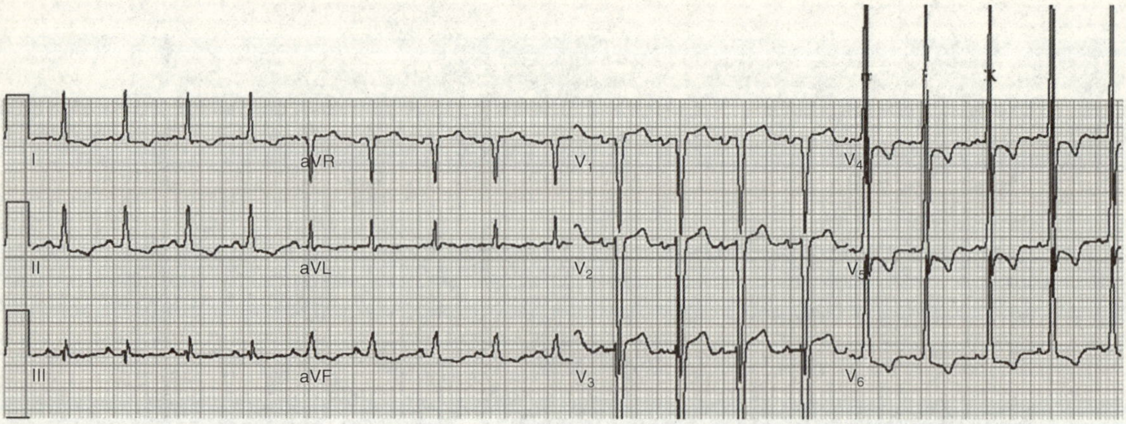

Fig. 10-17 LVH with repolarization abnormality. This tracing demonstrates classic repolarization abnormality, with STD in the left-sided precordial leads following large-amplitude R waves. The T waves in these leads are asymmetrically inverted. The right precordial leads (V_1 and V_2) show a mirror image of the changes seen in V_3 to V_6, with slight STE (contour initially concave) and asymmetric tall T waves. See Fig10-20B for evidence of evolving AMI in a patient with LVH and repolarization abnormality.

Non-ST Segment Elevation Myocardial Infarction

NSTEMI supplants non–Q wave MI, previously termed subendocardial MI.

ECG manifestations of NSTEMI include ST segment depression and T wave inversion, which may be deep and symmetrical.

Electrocardiographic Adjuncts in the Diagnosis of Acute Coronary Syndrome

Most commonly, additional lead ECG use posterior(leads V_8 and V_9) and right ventricular (V_{4R}) electrodes, thus constituting the 15-lead ECG (Fig. 10-18). Posterior leads V_8 and V_9 are placed under the tip of the left scapula and at the left

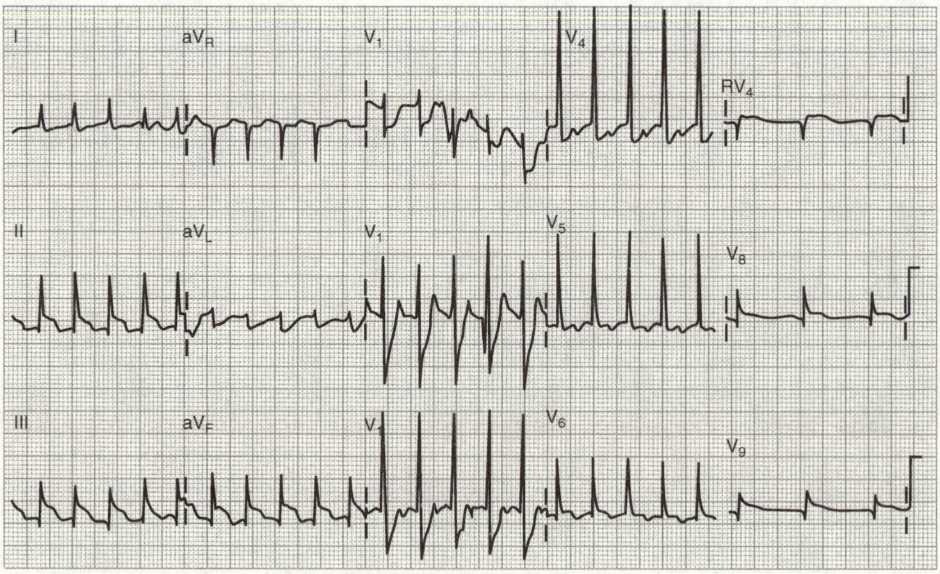

Fig. 10-18 Fifteen-lead ECG with inferior, lateral, posterior, and RVMI. The standard 12-lead ECG reveals the typical STE in the inferior and lateral leads as well as STD with prominent R wave in the right precordial leads. PWMI is indicated by both the right precordial STD with prominent R wave and the STE in posterior leads V_8 and V_9. Note that the degree of STE is less pronounced than that seen in the inferior leads because of a relatively longer distance from the posterior epicardium to surface leads. The RVMI is noted in this case, using the simplified approach with only RV_4, which demonstrates STE of relatively small magnitude.

paraspinal area, at the same level as leads V_4 to V_6.

ECG imaging of the right ventricle is enhanced with the use of the right-sided chest leads V_1R to V_6R .Of the right precordial leads, V_4R has the highest sensitivity for RVMI and is the lead of choice to include in the 15-lead tracing.

Possible applications for additional lead ECG include the following: (1) ST segment changes (depression or elevation) in leads V_1 to V_3, either in an isolated lead or in more than one; (2) equivocal ST segment elevation in the inferior (Ⅱ, Ⅲ, aVF) or lateral (Ⅰ, aVL) limb leads or both; (3) all inferior STEMI; and (4) hypotension in the setting of ACS. Additional lead applications can be used, including the 18- and 24-lead ECG.

Examination of ST segment trends (measured every 20 s for at least the first hour) and automated serial ECG (at least every 20 min) in ED patients with chest pain can significantly increase the sensitivity and specificity for detection of AMI (16%) and ACS compared with the initial ECG (Fig. 10-19).

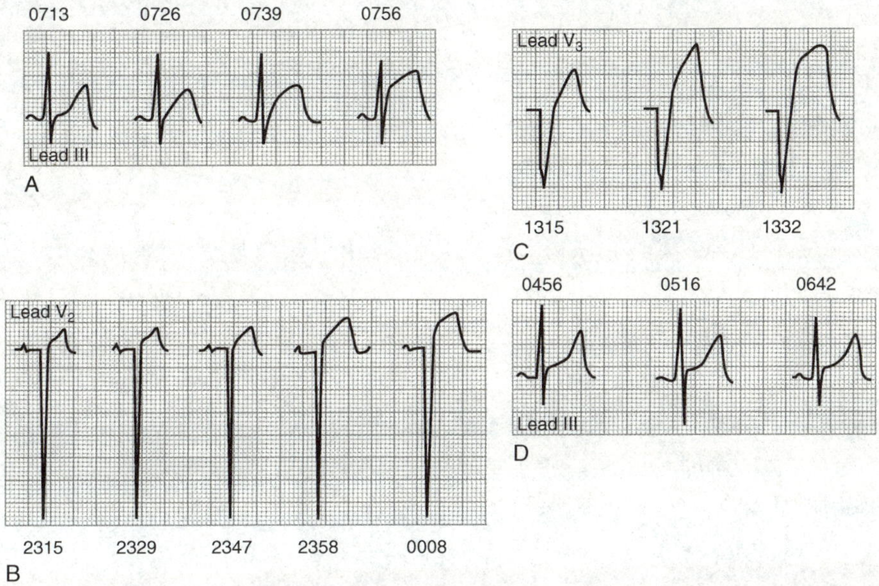

Fig. 10-19 Serial electrocardiography. A, Representative example of lead III in a patient with chest pain and an initially nondiagnostic ECG depicting the evolution of STE AMI. B, Representative example of lead V_2 in a patient with the left ventricular hypertrophy pattern. Serial sampling of this patient with ongoing chest pain and a confounding ECG pattern reveals the progression to STE AMI. C, Representative example of lead V_3 in a patient with LBBB and evolving AMI. D, Representative examples of lead III in a patient with chest pain and noninfarctional STE; note the lack of change (degree of elevation as well as morphology of elevation) over time in this patient with BER.

Limitations of Electrocardiography in Acute Coronary Syndrome

The sensitivity and specificity of a single ECG for AMI are approximately 60% and 90%, respectively. Serial ECG in the setting of continued or recurrent pain increase the diagnostic utility. The initial ECG is nondiagnostic in approximately half of the patients in the ED who are ultimately diagnosed with AMI. In patients being evaluated for ACS, only serial electrocardiography, combined with serial cardiac marker determinations, can exclude AMI.

Chest Radiography

Patients with AMI complicated by pulmonary edema who have a normal heart size most often have no past history of CHF. In fact, AMI is the most frequent cause of pulmonary edema with a normal cardiac size.

Serum Markers

Biochemical markers play a pivotal role in

the diagnosis, risk stratification, and guidance of treatment.

For patients with a nondiagnostic ECG, early elevation of serum markers of myocardial necrosis confirms a presumptive diagnosis of NSTEMI. This single test is too insensitive to be used to support a decision that the patient can be discharged or to determine that no acute coronary event has occurred. The patient's history remains the most vital portion of the diagnostic evaluation of potential ACS. Serial testing substantially improves the sensitivity of these tests (Table 10-5 and Fig.10-20, see color illustration).

Table 10-5 Summary of Test Performance Studies of Diagnostic Technologies for ACS in the ED

TECHNOLOGY	DISEASE STUDIED	NO. OF STUDIES (SUBJECTS)	PREVALENCE RANGE OF STUDIES, %	DISEASE SENSITIVITY, % (95% CI)	DISEASE SPECIFICITY, % (95% CI)
CK (single)	AMI	12 (3195)	7-41	37 (31-44)	87(80-91)
CK(serial)	AMI	2 (786)	26-43	69-99	68-84
CK-MB(presentation)	ACS	1 (1042)	20	23	96
	AMI	19 (6425)	6-42	42 (36-48)	97 (95-98)
CK-MB (serial)	ACS	1 (1042)	20	31	95
	AMI	14 (11,625)	1-43	79 (71-86)	96 (95-97)
Myoglobin (presentation)	AMI	18 (4172)	6-62	49 (43-55)	91 (87-94)
Myoglobin (serial)	AMI	10 (1277)	11-41	89 (80-94)	87 (80-92)
TNI(presentation)	AMI	4 (1149)	6-39	39 (10-78)	93 (88-97)
TNI(serial)	AMI	2 (1393)	6-9	90-100	83-96
TNT(presentation)	AMI	6 (1348)	6-78	39 (26-53)	93 (90-96)
TNT(serial)	AMI	3 (904)	5-78	93 (85-97)	85 (76-91)
CK-MB and myoglobin combination (presentation)	AMI	3 (2283)	9-28	83 (51-96)	82 (68-90)
CK-MB and myoglobin combination (serial)	AMI	2 (291)	11-20	100	75-91
Exercise stress ECG	ACS	2 (312)	6-10	70-100	82-93
Rest echocardiography	ACS	2 (228)	3-30	70 (43-88)	87 (72-94)
	AMI	3 (397)	3-30	93 (81-91)	66 (43-83)
Stress echocardiography	AMI	1 (139)	4	90	89
Sestamibi (rest)	ACS	3 (702)	9-17	81 (74-87)	73 (56-85)
	AMI	3 (702)	92 (78-98)	67 (52-79)	

Troponins

Because of their superior sensitivity and specificity compared with other biochemical markers, cardiac troponins are the best markers for myocardial cell injury. Two myocardium-specific proteins, myocardial TnI and TnT, precede the release of CK-MB into the serum.

After injury a biphasic rise in serum troponins corresponds to early release of the free cytoplasmic proteins, followed by a slower and greatly prolonged rise with breakdown of the actual muscle fiber. Serum troponin concentrations begin to rise measurably in the serum at about the same time as CK-MB elevations become detectable, as early as 3 hr after onset, but troponin levels remain elevated for 7 d or more.

The cardiac-specific troponins, determined serially, are highly sensitive for the early detection

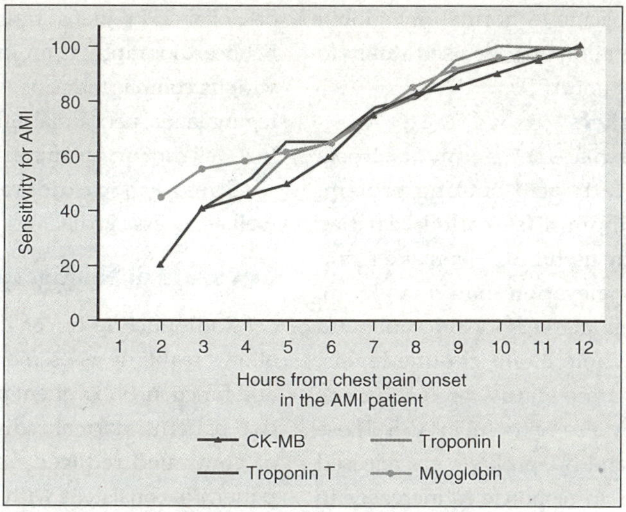

Fig. 10-20 Serum marker sensitivity relative to the time of onset of chest pain in the patient with AMI.

of myocardial injury. A positive test result is associated with significant risk, and serial negative results predict low risk. Serial measurements, particularly when performed at least 6 hr after symptom onset, markedly improve the sensitivity of the cardiac troponins for AMI. The sensitivity of TnT approaches 50% within 3 to 4 hr of the event. The test result is positive in about 75% of patients at 6 hr after onset of symptoms; at 12 hr, the test is almost 100% sensitive.

Cardiac conditions that can result in significant increased troponin levels in patients without evidence of ACS include myocarditis, pericarditis, CHF, LVH, and nonpenetrating cardiac trauma.

Troponin elevations can also be seen in noncardiac conditions, including PE, sepsis, and renal insufficiency. Elevated troponin levels are commonly seen in asymptomatic patients with end-stage renal disease.

Creatinine Phosphokinase

CK is found in large quantities not only in cardiac muscle but also in skeletal muscle, brain, kidney, lung, and the gastrointestinal tract. Myocardial cells are by far the most abundant potential sources of CK-MB; thus the appearance of CK-MB in the serum is highly suggestive of MI. In the setting of AMI, CK-MB is released and is detectable in the serum as early as 3 hr after onset of the necrosis. CK-MB characteristically peaks at 20 to 24 hr and becomes normal within 2 to 3 d after injury. Elevated CK-MB values identify a patient at considerable risk for a poor outcome but do not correlate well with infarct size. Abnormal CK-MB elevations may be seen in patients with trauma, muscular dystrophies, myositis, and rhabdomyolysis and after extremely vigorous exercise.

CK-MB determinations obtained beyond this 3hr time period have increasing sensitivities for the diagnosis of AMI, particularly when obtained 12 to 16 hr after onset. Serial sampling, even over relatively short time periods (12 hr), increases sensitivity considerably, particularly when considered with serial ECG and repeated assessments of the patient.

Myoglobin

Myoglobin is rapidly released into the circulation after myocardial cellular injury. In cases of myocardial injury, myoglobin rises in the initial 1 to 2 hr, peaks at 5 to 7 hr, and returns to baseline by 24 hr. Myoglobin is attractive as an early indicator of myocardial injury. Thus myoglobin is elevated in any clinical situation involving the skeletal muscle, such as trauma, exercise, and significant systemic illness. In addition, myoglobin increases are seen in patients with renal failure because of reduced clearance.

A doubling of the level as soon as 1 to 2 hr after the initial measurement greatly increases the sensitivity for the diagnosis of AMI, but this approach is very nonspecific. A normal myoglobin value 2 hr after presentation may be used safely to rule out active AMI but not ACS.

Other Cardiac Markers

One such new cardiac-specific myonecrosis marker is heart-type fatty acid-binding protein. Ischemic-modified albumin (so-called "cardiac albumin") is a potentially useful ACS biomarker, and may have even earlier elevation than myoglobin. Other potential ischemia markers include unbound free fatty acids and whole blood choline levels. Markers of hemodynamic status, including the natriuretic peptides, may also be useful in ACS. These markers, such as BNP and NT-proBNP, are released from cardiac myocytes in response to increases in ventricular wall stress. BNP is most commonly used as a marker for CHF. The natriuretic peptides are excellent predictors of both short and long-term mortality in patients with UA, NSTEMI, and STEMI.

The inflammatory markers CRP and hsCRP have long-term prognostic value for cardiac events in healthy individuals as well as potential short-term prognostic value when combined with other markers for ACS.

Multiple Marker Strategies

Diagnostic, risk stratification, and prognostic accuracy might be enhanced by the use of multiple markers for AMI and ACS. The combination of CK-MB and myoglobin measurement has a sensitivity of 62% to 100% and specificity of 72% to 89% for AMI on presentation. A three-marker approach (CK-MB, TnI, and myoglobin) in an accelerated critical pathway was reported to have 100% sensitivity and 100% negative predictive power for AMI. In ED chest pain patients with an initial nondiagnostic ECG, a 2 hr delta CK-MB combined with a 2 hr delta TnI had a sensitivity of 93% and specificity of 94% for AMI.

Echocardiography

Two-dimensional echocardiography detects regional wall motion abnormality associated with ACS. After AMI, paradoxical wall motion and decreased EF observed during systole indicates the subsequent loss of muscle tone from necrosis.

Particularly in individuals with nondiagnostic ECG, the presence of regional systolic wall motion abnormalities in a patient without known CAD is a moderately accurate indicator of AMI.

Resting echocardiography provides an assessment of global and regional function in patients with ACS. Echocardiography is an important tool to assess for various complications of AMI, including acute mitral regurgitation, pericardial effusion, ventricular septal and free wall rupture, and intracardiac thrombus formation.

Stress echocardiography can detect CAD as well as assess cardiac function early after an AMI.

Myocardial Scintigraphy

Radionuclide tracer injection and scintigraphy allows real-time assessment of myocardial perfusion and function. Subsequent imaging then reveals one of two patterns: normal redistribution (normal uptake) or continued reduced uptake. The redistribution pattern is consistent with active coronary ischemia, and the continued reduced uptake is found in patients with MI, either remote or recent.

The probability of a cardiac event is tenfold higher in patients with abnormal scans than in patients with a normal scan.

Computed Tomography

Ectron beam computed tomography (EBCT) was introduced nearly two decades ago to screen for coronary calcium as a marker of underlying atherosclerotic heart disease and risk of ACS. Whereas calcium scoring systems exist to assess cardiovascular disease risk, few studies have examined the role of EBCT in the assessment of patients with acute chest pain.

Technical advances in imaging include MDCT with multislice 16-, 64-, and 256-slice CT scanning, as well as ECG-gated MDCT.

Cardiac CT provides excellent detection of calcified and noncalcified coronary artery plaque and stenosis, indicative of atherosclerosis and risk of ACS.

The triple rule-out or global assessment protocol refers to the use of CT to assess for three life-threatening causes of chest pain, including PE and aortic dissection as well as ACS.

EMERGENCY DEPARTMENT BASED CHEST PAIN CENTERS

The goal of the chest pain center (CPC) is to

provide an integrated approach to patients with chest pain or potential ACS that includes rapid triage, early identification, and treatment of low-risk ACS patients.

A CPC protocol should rapidly direct patients with possible ACS into a high-level treatment area where an ECG and clinical examination can be performed within the first 10 min.

The CPC can have assigned nursing personnel who rapidly evaluate the patient with chest pain with a 12-lead ECG, as well as screening vital signs and cardiac monitoring, and deliver the ECG directly to a clinician capable of making a decision about activation of the catheterization laboratory or administration of fibrinolytic therapy.

Many CPC now use further ACS evaluation with stress testing, echocardiography, or myocardial scintigraphy before disposition.

MANAGEMENT OF ACUTE CORONARY SYNDROME

Relationship of Time to Treatment with Outcome

Timely treatment within the first hour after symptom onset may result in substantial, if not complete, myocardial salvage. Delivered later, from 2 to 12 hr after AMI onset, treatment may result in a more modest, but significant benefit.

Overall, the average time to fibrinolysis ranges from 45 to 90 min. The AHA recommends that all patients with STEMI receive fibrinolytic therapy within 30 min of arrival or undergo primary PCI no later than 90 min after arrival.

STEMI patients who receive hospital-based reperfusion therapies (fibrinolytic agent or PCI) progress through a sequence of steps that can define process time points (Fig. 10-21).

Fibrinolytic agents should be stored and administered in the ED. In a system in which fibrinolysis is the sole reperfusion therapy, the decision to administer that therapy rests solely with the emergency physician.

Pharmacologic Intervention

Nitroglycerin

Patients with possible ACS and SBP greater than 90 mm Hg should receive a sublingual NTG tablet on presentation. If symptoms and pain are not fully relieved with three sublingual tablets, intravenous NTG should be considered. With bradycardia, hypotension, IWMI, and RVMI, a sudden decrease in preload associated with NTG can result in profound hypotension.

Morphine

If a patient with possible ACS is unresponsive to

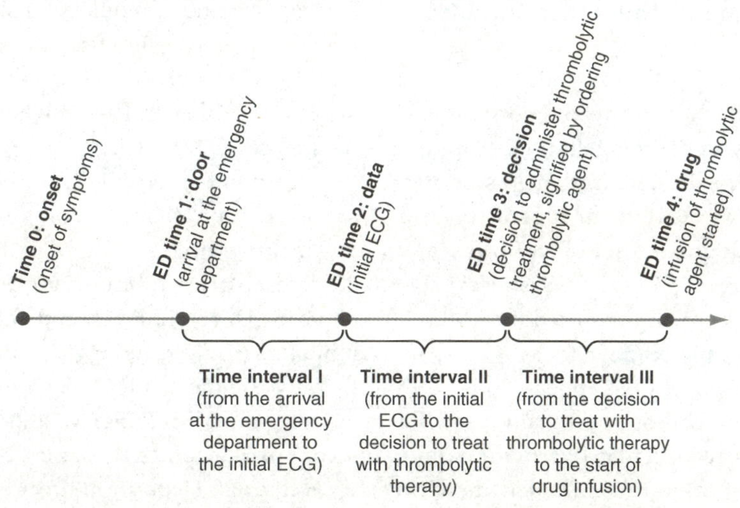

Fig. 10-21 The four Ds of ED-based diagnosis and management of the patient with AMI. Shown are the process time points and intervals through which the patient with AMI passes until treatment in ED.

NTG or has recurrent symptoms despite maximal anti-ischemic therapy, administration of morphine sulfate is reasonable. Standard doses of morphine sulfate are 2 to 5 mg delivered intravenously, repeated every 5 to 30 min as necessary.

Beta-Adrenergic Blockers

The early intravenous use of beta-adrenergic blocking agents, when coupled with contemporary therapy, does not appear to offer significant benefit and is associated with an increased rate of adverse events. Oral administration to patients without contraindication during the first day of management is an appropriate approach to the ACS patient. Empirical therapy in the ED should be reconsidered and reserved for only those patients who have adverse effects from significantly elevated blood pressure despite application of NTG, or significant tachydysrhythmia.

Angiotensin-Converting Enzyme Inhibitors

ACEI may also reduce morbidity and mortality after AMI. These benefits increase when ACEI are used in conjunction with other agents, such as aspirin and fibrinolytics.

Captopril, enalapril, lisinopril, or ramipril may be used in this setting. Therapy should be initiated within the first 24 hr. In patients with asymptomatic left ventricular dysfunction, therapy should continue for a minimum of 2 to 4 mo. Contraindications to ACEI therapy include hypotension, volume depletion, and borderline perfusion. Renal function must be monitored closely.

HMG-Coenzyme A Reductase Inhibitors (Statins)

Initiation of *Statins* therapy should occur within the first 24 hr or should continue if patients are already undergoing statin therapy, as discontinuation during hospitalization is associated with an increase in near-term mortality and adverse events. Administration of statin therapy before elective or urgent PCI for ACS is reasonable to decrease the incidence of periprocedure AMI.

Calcium Channel Blockade

The primary benefit of CCB appears to be with symptom resolution. Unless specifically used for rate control of supraventricular dysrhythmia in a patient who cannot tolerate beta-blockade, CCB agents are not recommended for ACS.

Antiplatelet Therapy

Aspirin. Aspirin independently reduces the mortality of patients with AMI without fibrinolytic therapy. The usual dose is 324 mg of non-enteric-coated aspirin, chewed and swallowed, unless significant allergy, hemorrhage, or other issue, such as a potential aortic dissection, contraindicates its use.

Glycoprotein Ⅱb/Ⅲa Receptor Inhibitors. The glycoprotein Ⅱb/Ⅲa inhibitors (GPI) are potent antiplatelet agents and include abciximab, eptifibatide, and tirofiban. Therefore the primary indication regarding GPI administration is planned mechanical coronary intervention.

GPI therapy, in the invasively managed patient, continues to offer improved outcome.

PSY_{12} Receptor Inhibitor Agents. The thienopyridines—ticlopidine, clopidogrel, and prasugrel—are more potent platelet inhibitors than aspirin. They irreversibly inhibit platelet aggregation for the duration of the life of the platelet. Ticlopidine has nonlinear kinetics and, with repeated administration, reaches a maximal effect after 8 to 11 d of use. Clopidogrel, a ticlopidine analogue, and prasugrel have the advantage of a rapid onset of action.

Clopidogrel and prasugrel are the preferred agents in this class because of their more rapid onset of action and improved safety profile. Prasugrel incurs a higher bleeding risk than clopidogrel, however, in patients older than 75 yr, those who weigh more than 60 kg, those who have had a previous TIA or stroke, and those at high risk for bleeding. Ticlopidine is associated with a risk of neutropenia and agranulocytosis. With clopidogrel, maximal platelet inhibition occurs after 3 to 5 d of clopidogrel therapy with 75 mg daily; an earlier onset of platelet inhibition is seen when a higher loading dose is used (300 to 600 mg).

Ticagrelor is rapidly absorbed reaching peak serum concentration at 2.5 hr.

Antithrombins

The antithrombins include unfractionated heparin (UFH), LMWH, and the direct thrombin inhibitors (hirudin and bivalirudin). Antithrombotic therapy is indicated in ACS patients with recurrent anginal pain, AMI (NSTEMI and STEMI), a positive serum marker, and a dynamic 12-lead ECG.

Heparins. Heparin indirect effect on thrombin inhibits clot propagation.

UFH should be administered early in patients with the following ACS features: recurrent or persistent chest pain, AMI, positive serum marker, and dynamic ECG. Therefore the weight adjusted regimen recommended is an initial bolus of 60 U/kg (maximum 4000 U) and an initial infusion of 12 U/kg/hr with an activated partial thromboplastin time goal of 1.5 to 2.5 times the control value.

The combination of aspirin, beta-blocker, and LMWH (dalteparin) significantly decreases the rate of nonfatal AMI or death at 1 w of therapy, with a less pronounced effect at 40 to 150 d.

Enoxaparin is administered in a twice-daily regimen subcutaneously at a dose of 1 mg/kg for all ACS patients. Contraindications to heparin therapy include known allergy, active ongoing hemorrhage.

The vast majority of patients with AMI require therapy with heparin.

Other Antithrombins (Hirudin, Bivalirudin, and Fondaparinux). The direct thrombin inhibitors hirudin and bivalirudin (formerly known as Hirulog) are potent antithrombin anticoagulants providing significant theoretical advantages compared with heparin. Hirudin can inhibit thrombin-induced platelet aggregation. Hirudin offers little value in the ACS patient.

Bivalirudin, however, is more effective than heparin in reducing death or reinfarction in patients with ACS, particularly those patients undergoing very early PCI.

Fondaparinux is the first widely used selective factor Xa inhibitor. The increased risk of catheter-associated thrombi during PCI prevents its use without additional UFH administration.

Reperfusion Therapies

Pharmacologic and mechanical methods of reperfusion are both effective under specific clinical conditions.

Fibrinolytic therapy unequivocally improves survival in patients with STEMI .Patients with absolute contraindications to fibrinolytic therapy, certain relative contraindications, cardiogenic shock, and UA may not be eligible.

Fibrinolytic Therapy

Fibrinolytic Agent Selection. TNK has several potential benefits: (1) its longer half-life allows it to be administered as a single bolus; (2) it is 14 times more fibrin specific than t-PA and even more so than r-PA; and (3) it is 80 times more resistant to plasminogen activator inhibitor type 1 than t-PA. At the present time it appears that TNK is marginally more effective, minimally safer, and easier to administer than t-PA and thus is recommended.

Eligibility Criteria for Fibrinolytic Agent Therapy

The 12-Lead ECG. Combined with the patient's history and physical examination, the 12-lead ECG is the key determinant of eligibility for fibrinolysis. The ECG findings include two basic issues: (1) ST segment elevation of 1 mm or more in two or more anatomically contiguous standard limb leads or elevation of 2 mm or more in two or more contiguous precordial leads, and (2) new or presumed new LBBB.

Patients with new LBBB and AMI are at an increased risk for a poor outcome and need rapid reperfusion therapy. Patients with AMI in anterior, inferior, or lateral anatomic locations benefit from fibrinolytic therapy.

Patient's Age. Patients older than 75 yr do have a higher incidence of hemorrhagic stroke than younger patients.

Time from Symptom Onset. The generally accepted therapeutic time window for administration of a fibrinolytic agent after the onset of ST segment elevation AMI is 12 hr. Patients treated within the first 6 hr of AMI have the best outcome. Later administrations, from 6 to 12 hr after AMI onset, also confer benefit.

Blood Pressure Extremes. Patients with a history of chronic hypertension should not be excluded from fibrinolytic therapy if their blood pressure is under control at the time of presentation or can be lowered to acceptable levels with standard therapy for ischemic chest pain. The admission blood pressure is also an important indicator of risk of intracerebral hemorrhage.

Retinopathy. Active diabetic hemorrhagic retinopathy is a strong relative contraindication to fibrinolytic therapy.

Cardiopulmonary Resuscitation. CPR is not a contraindication to fibrinolytic therapy unless CPR is prolonged—more than 10 min—or extensive chest trauma from manual compression is evident.

Previous Stroke or Transient Ischemic Attack. A history of previous ischemic stroke should remain a strong relative contraindication to fibrinolytic therapy, and previous hemorrhagic stroke an absolute contraindication.

Previous MI or Past Coronary Artery Bypass Graft. In the setting of AMI, a previous MI should not preclude consideration for treatment with fibrinolytic agents.

Recent Surgery or Trauma. Recent surgery or trauma is considered a relative contraindication to fibrinolytic therapy. Patients were excluded if they had had surgery or trauma within the previous 10 d.

Menstruation. Because natural estrogen is partially cardioprotective, there is little experience with fibrinolysis among premenopausal women.

Contraindications. A list of absolute and relative contraindications is shown in Box 10-1.

Box 10-1 Fibrinolysis in AMI: Absolute and Relative Contraindications

- Recent (within 10 d) major surgery (e.g., coronary artery bypass graft, obstetric delivery, organ biopsy, previous puncture of noncompressible vessels)
- Cerebrovascular disease
- Recent gastrointestinal or genitourinary bleeding (within 10 d)
- Recent trauma (within 10 d)
- Hypertension: systolic BP 180 mm Hg or diastolic BP 110 mm Hg
- High likelihood of left heart thrombus (e.g., mitral stenosis with atrial fibrillation)
- Acute pericarditis
- Subacute bacterial endocarditis
- Hemostatic defects, including those secondary to severe hepatic or renal disease
- Significant liver dysfunction
- Diabetic hemorrhagic retinopathy or other hemorrhagic ophthalmic condition
- Septic thrombophlebitis or occluded AV cannula at seriously infected site
- Advanced age (older than 75 yr)
- Patients currently receiving oral anticoagulants (e.g., warfarin sodium)
- Any other condition in which bleeding constitutes a significant hazard or would be particularly difficult to manage because of its location

Percutaneous Coronary Intervention

Patients with absolute contraindications to fibrinolytic therapy, certain relative contraindications, cardiogenic shock, and UA may be ineligible to receive fibrinolytic therapy.

Thus PCI with stenting appears to be superior to standard angioplasty.

Rescue Percutaneous Coronary Intervention. Historically, rescue PCI has been considered advantageous in patients whose infarct related arteries fail to reperfuse after fibrinolytic therapy. These patients are profoundly ill, with a markedly worse outcome.

Facilitated Percutaneous Coronary Intervention. Facilitated percutaneous coronary intervention refers to combination therapy involving fibrinolysis coupled with emergent PCI. This concept originally was developed to maximize therapy in STEMI patients;

Choice of Reperfusion Therapy

The principal choices for reperfusion therapy in the STEMI patient include fibrinolysis and PCI. The systems goal should be a first medical contact–to-[therapy] time within 90 min. The system goal for fibrinolytic therapy is to deliver the drug within 30 min of patient presentation.

PCI is the preferred reperfusion strategy in the STEMI patient. PCI provides improved outcome over fibrinolysis in the STEMI patient. Patients who are not able to rapidly reach the PCI suite should receive fibrinolysis.

Reperfusion Therapy in Cardiogenic Shock

Patients with AMI with cardiogenic shock demand special consideration because of a mortality rate approaching 80%. Fibrinolysis is not effective in these patients owing to a significantly lower coronary perfusion pressure. In shock, the occlusive thrombus is not exposed to the fibrinolytic agent, resulting in clinical failure of the drug. Thus, emergency revascularization with PCI or CABG is preferred in patients with STEMI complicated by cardiogenic shock irrespective of the delay to treatment . Fibrinolytic therapy should be given to eligible patients who are otherwise unsuitable candidates for PCI or CABG.

Resuscitated Cardiac Arrest with ST Segment Elevation Myocardial Infarction

The management of the STEMI patient resuscitated from cardiac arrest includes: (1) rapid revascularization with PCI, (2) strict hemodynamic monitoring, (3) serum glucose control, (4) oxygen and volume-limiting ventilation, and (5) immediate application of therapeutic hypothermia for those patients whose cardiac arrest was caused by ventricular fibrillation or pulseless ventricular tachycardia. A clinical presentation of coma after cardiac arrest should not be considered a contraindication to reperfusion therapy, as such findings are commonly present.

Therapeutic hypothermia, when combined with PCI, in resuscitated cardiac arrest STEMI patients demonstrates an impressive rate of survival with good neurologic outcome.

Transfer of a Patient with Acute Coronary Syndrome

There are several indications for the transfer of a patient with ACS to a facility with PCI capability. These include rapid access to PCI (catheter across the lesion within 90 min of arrival to the initial hospital), persistent hemodynamic instability or ventricular dysrhythmias, and postinfarction or postreperfusion ischemia. Hospital transfer for PCI is also suggested for patients with fibrinolytic contraindications who may benefit from PCI or CABG.

Potential Pharmacologic Management Approach

The patient with stable chest pain with a normal to minimally abnormal ECG and a negative serum marker is best managed initially with NTG sublingually or topically in combination with aspirin. Continued or recurrent pain in the ED may be treated with parenteral morphine sulfate. Continued pain may ultimately require intravenous NTG and heparinization with UFH or LMWH, with additional antiplatelet therapy with either a thienopyridine or GPI.

The ACS patient with an abnormal ECG, particularly ST segment and T wave abnormalities, or elevated serum markers may warrant numerous therapies, including ASA, heparin, and other antiplatelet agents. NTG may be administered by the topical or intravenous route. Heparin therapy is generally indicated in this instance.

The AMI patient without ST segment elevation requires aspirin, NTG, heparin, and morphine sulfate. The patient with ST segment elevation AMI is treated with the preceding medications and is considered for urgent revascularization, achieved by fibrinolytic agents, PCI, or, in the rare case, CABG.

(CHAI Yanfen)

Chapter 11

Aortic Dissection

KEY CONCEPTS

Aortic dissection is a longitudinal cleavage of the aortic media created by a dissecting column of blood.

Most patients with aortic dissection have chest pain, typically of sudden onset, sharp, and migratory. Chest pain associated with neurologic symptoms or syncope increases the likelihood of aortic disease.

Imaging(CT aortography or TEE) is essential to establish or exclude the diagnosis of aortic dissection.

Medical therapy including pain relief and BP control is recommended. A target SBP of 100 to 120 mmHg and HR below 60 beats/min are recommended.

PERSPECTIVE

Aortic dissection is a longitudinal cleavage of the aortic media created by a dissecting column of blood. The term "dissecting aortic aneurysm" has been inaccurately applied to this entity since 1819, when Laënnec first used the term *aneurysme dissequant*. The term *aortic dissection* is preferred to dissecting aortic aneurysm because the affected aorta is only rarely aneurysmal. In 1955, DeBakey outlined the principles that remain the basis for the surgical treatment of this entity. Medical treatment of aortic dissection was first advocated in the 1960s and is indicated for certain types of dissections. The in-hospital mortality rate for patients treated for aortic dissection is 27%.

Epidemiology

The incidence of aortic dissection is estimated at 6 per 100,000 population per year, and the mortality is 1 to 5 per 100,000 population per year. Aortic dissection occurs more often in men and increases with age.HTN is the most common risk factor associated with aortic dissection and is seen in 65%-75% of patients.A history of cardiac surgery is present in 18% and a bicuspid aortic valve in 14% of all patients with aortic dissections but more often in proximal dissections. Atherosclerosis is rarely involved at the site of dissection. Patients with aortic dissection may have a positive family history.

Aortic dissection is uncommon before age 40 except in association with congenital heart disease, Ehlers-Danlos or Marfan's syndrome, or giant-cell arteritis. As many as 44% of patients with Marfan's syndrome develop aortic dissection and account for about 5% of cases.Women with Marfan's syndrome are at particular risk during pregnancy.In patients without connective tissue disease and with an aortic root size of less than 40 mm, pregnancy does not appear to be an independent risk factor. Acute aortic dissection also occurs with stimulant use, exertion, cardiac surgery, or intraaortic balloon pump insertion.

PRINCIPLES OF DISEASE

Anatomy and Physiology

With each contraction the heart swings from side to side, resulting in flexion of both the ascending aorta and the descending aorta. The descending aorta flexes just distal to the left subclavian artery, where the mobile aorta is tethered. At an average of 70 heartbeats per minute, this sequence occurs about 37 million times a year, causing repetitive stress on the aorta.

The aortic wall has three distinct layers: the intima, the media, and the adventitia. The media is composed of elastic tissue and smooth muscle.

Dissection occurs through a degeneration of the media characterized by loss of smooth muscle cells and elastic tissue, accompanied by scarring, fibrosis, and hyalin-like changes. Pathologic studies show that this process is neither cystic nor necrotic; therefore the old term cystic medial necrosis is no longer used.

Pathophysiology

Medial degeneration is now considered to be part of normal aging, although it is augmented by HTN and with aortic dissection. The anatomic differences between the "normal" aorta and a dissection are quantitative rather than qualitative. More recent evidence suggests that medial degeneration results from inflammatory cell infiltration.

The repetitive hydrodynamic forces produced by the ejection of blood into the aorta with each cardiac cycle contribute to weakening of the aortic intima and to medial degeneration. These hydrodynamic forces primarily affect the ascending aorta. Sustained HTN intensifies these forces and results in an increase in medial degeneration. A bicuspid valve, present in 1% to 2% of the population, is the most common congenital abnormality affecting the aortic valve and proximal aorta. A bicuspid aortic valve may disrupt laminar flow and reorient the flow of blood toward the aortic wall, producing local injury. In Marfan and Ehlers-Danlos syndromes, normal hydrodynamic forces act on an aortic media that is already weakened.

As a result of medial degeneration and repeated flexion of the aorta, hydrodynamic stress tears the aortic intima and a column of blood gains access into the aortic media. An alternative theory suggests that these forces damage the vasa vasorum of the aorta, which rupture and hemorrhage into the aortic media, which may explain the absence of an intimal tear in some cases of dissection. Regardless of which of these theories is correct, the depth of penetration into the media and the distance and direction of dissection are at least partially determined by the degree of medial degeneration.

Once a dissecting hematoma is established in the media, migration of the hematoma occurs in an antegrade or retrograde fashion, or both, forming a "false lumen". The false lumen forms in the outer half of the media and propagates until it ruptures back into the "true lumen" of the aorta, resulting in a rare "spontaneous cure" or through the adventitia into the pericardial sac or pleural cavity. Because the outer wall of the aorta that contains the hematoma is thin, rupture is much more likely to occur to the outside. The most important factors favoring continued dissection of the aorta are (1) the degree of elevation of BP and (2) the steepness (slope) of the pulse wave (upstroke pattern on apex cardiogram, dP/dt). Both of these hemodynamic factors must be controlled to halt migration of the hematoma.

Classification

Anatomic classification is important for diagnosis and therapy. The *Stanford classification* is based on the involvement of the ascending aorta. Type A dissections involve the ascending aorta; type B dissections do not (Fig. 11-1). Dissections that involve the ascending aorta are more often lethal than those limited to the distal aorta and call for a different therapeutic approach. In the International Registry of Acute Aortic Dissection (IRAD), 62% of dissections are type A and 38% are type B.Patients with distal dissections tend to be older, heavy smokers with chronic lung disease and more often have generalized atherosclerosis and HTN compared with patients who have proximal aortic dissectons.

Two other aortic conditions are closely related to aortic dissection: intramural hemorrhage and penetrating aortic ulcer. Both groups of patients have clinical symptoms and management recommendations similar to those for patients with aortic dissection. An intramural hemorrhage is a contained hematoma within the aortic wall and occurs in about 10% of aortic dissections.Rupture of the vasa vasorum is believed to be the initial event. Penetrating atherosclerotic ulcers of the aorta occur in older hypertensive patients with evidence of CAD. CT shows a focal ulceration without dissection, most commonly in the distal descending aorta. The progression of penetrating ulcers results in progressive aortic enlargement with saccular and fusiform aneurysm formation. Patients can have both an intramural hematoma and a penetrating atherosclerotic ulcer.

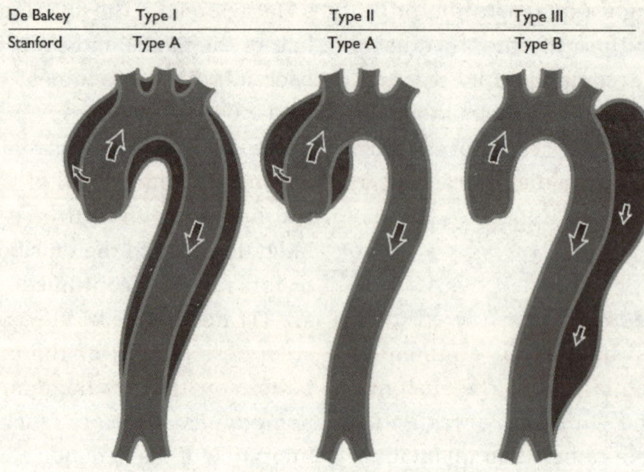

Fig. 11-1 Classification of aortic dissection localization.

A dissection is acute if it is of less than 2 w duration and chronic if has been present for more than 2 w.

CLINICAL FEATURES

History

Pain is by far the most common presenting complaint, affecting more than 90% of patients. The pain is usually excruciating, occurs abruptly, is most severe at onset, and is typically described as "sharp", "tearing", "ripping" and "knife-like". Most cases of painless aortic dissection are chronic in nature.

The location of the pain may help localize the dissection. Anterior chest pain is associated with the ascending aorta, neck and jaw pain with the aortic arch, pain in the interscapular area with the descending thoracic aorta, and pain in the lumbar area or abdomen with involvement below the diaphragm. Migration of the pain consistent with propagation of the dissection suggests aortic dissection but occurs in only 17% of cases.The onset of aortic dissection is often accompanied by visceral pain symptoms, such as diaphoresis, nausea, vomiting, lightheadedness, and severe apprehension.

Syncope occurs early in aortic dissection in approximately 9% of cases and may be the sole presentation in some patients. It most often heralds dissection into the pericardium, causing pericardial tamponade, but may occur from transient interruption of blood flow to the cerebral vasculature. Other causes of syncope secondary to aortic dissection are hypovolemia, excessive vagal tone, and cardiac conduction abnormalities. Patients with aortic dissection and syncope have a higher mortality. Neurologic symptoms such as focal weakness or change in mental status occur in up to 17% of cases.

Physical Examination

The presentation varies greatly, depending on the patient and the location and extent of the dissection (Table 11-1). Generally, the patient appears apprehensive. Most of the patients have a history of chronic HTN that may be exacerbated by a catecholamine release related to the acute event. Severe HTN refractory to medical therapy may occur if the dissection involves the renal arteries with subsequent renin release. If hypotension is present, either the dissection has progressed back into the pericardium with resulting pericardial tamponade or hypovolemia has occurred from rupture through the adventitia. *Pseudohypotension*, a condition in which the BP in the arms is low or unobtainable and the central arterial pressure is normal or high, may be present. This results from the interruption of blood flow to the subclavian arteries.

Table 11-1 Main clinical presentations and complications of patients with acute aortic dissection

	Type A (%)	Type B (%)
Chest pain	80	70
Back pain	40	70
Abrupt onset of pain	85	85
Migrating pain	<15	20
Aortic regurgitation	40-75	N/A
Cardiac tamponade	<20	N/A
Myocardial ischaemia or infarction	10-15	10
Heart failure	<10	<5
Pleural effusion	15	20
Syncope	15	<5
Major neurological deficit (coma/stroke)	<10	<5
Spinal cord injury	<1	NR
Mesenteric ischaemia	<5	NR
ARF	<20	10
Lower limb ischaemia	<10	<10

Aortic regurgitation occurs in up to 32% of patients and is more common with type A dissections. The murmur of aortic insufficiency may have a musical, vibrating quality with variable intensity, and CHF may develop. The patient with presumed aortic dissection should be examined carefully for findings that suggest hemorrhage into the pericardium or tamponade, such as jugular venous distention, muffled heart sounds, tachycardia, and hypotension.

When the integrity of one of the branches of the aorta is compromised, the expected ischemic findings occur. Pulse deficits and discrepancies in BP between limbs can be helpful if present but have a sensitivity of only around 30%.Usually these are present in the upper extremities and result from involvement of one or both of the subclavian arteries.Obstruction of one or both common iliac or superficial femoral arteries may produce pulse deficits in the lower extremities. Arterial obstruction may occur by either of two mechanisms. An intimal flap produced by the dissection may cover the true lumen of a branch vessel, or the dissecting hematoma may compress an adjacent true lumen. Frequent reexamination may detect transient pulse deficits.

Neurologic findings are related to the site of blood flow interruption. Proximal dissections are a more frequent cause of strokes or coma. Stroke treatment with a fibrinolytic agent in the patient with aortic dissection can be fatal. Distal dissections occluding the anterior spinal artery commonly cause ischemic paraparesis or ischemic peripheral neuropathy.

In up to 3% of cases, a proximal dissection can dissect into the ostium of a coronary artery, most frequently the right coronary artery, and cause an AMI, usually inferior to posterior.Failure to identify the inciting aortic dissection with incorrect administration of a fibrinolytic agent occurs in about 0.1% to 0.2% of MI.Distal extension of aortic dissections into the abdomen can cause mesenteric ischemia, renal failure, femoral pulse deficits, and lower extremity ischemia.

DIAGNOSTIC STRATEGIES

Routine laboratory tests are of little value in the diagnosis of aortic dissection but are useful for differential diagnoses. The hemoglobin usually is normal or unchanged from the patient's baseline. The leukocyte count is commonly mildly elevated. Recently, there has been increasing interest in the biochemical diagnosis of acute aortic dissection, including CRP, myosin heavy chain, soluble elastin, and D-dimer levels.

Choice of Diagnostic Test

Although aortic dissection can be suspected on the basis of history and physical examination, diagnostic imaging is necessary for the diagnosis to be established. Frequently, more than one test is required to make the diagnosis and to assess associated complications.

The clinical strategy should consider (1) the technology available at the institution, (2) the institution-specific sensitivities and specificities for the diagnostic tests, (3) the benefits of diagnosing nondissection causes of chest pain, and (4) the ease of performing each test, especially "after hours". A recent meta-analysis suggested that TEE, helical CT, and MRI are of similar diagnostic value in ruling aortic dissection in or out.

Unless institutional circumstances do not permit,

contrast CT aortography is recommended as the test of first choice. In patients with renal failure or contrast allergy, or for those considered too unstable to undergo CT scan, TEE is recommended. If the patient has a diagnostic (i.e., positive) transthoracic echocardiography(TTE), the diagnosis is established, but an additional confirmatory study may or may not be required, depending on the preference of the physician who will be assuming care of the patient. A negative TTE does not exclude dissection, and further imaging is indicated in such cases.

Electrocardiography

The ECG is often useful in excluding myocardial infarction; however, 15% of patients with aortic dissection may have ECG abnormalities suggesting ischemia.Proximal dissections that involve the right coronary artery may show an inferior wall myocardial infarction, and the constellation of symptoms and signs (pain, diaphoresis, hypotension) may be difficult to distinguish from those associated with primary AMI. The ECG typically shows LVH in 26%, reflecting long-standing HTN. Other findings include nonspecific ST-T wave changes and prior Q wave infarction. No abnormalities are noted on the ECG in 31% of cases (Table 11-2).

Chest Radiography

Routine chest radiographic studies are abnormal in 80% to 90% of patients, but the abnormalities are nonspecific and rarely diagnostic.Mediastinal widening occurs in the majority of cases and may be difficult to differentiate from the aortic tortuosity that is associated with chronic HTN. Up to 12% of patients with aortic dissection have a normal chest radiograph (Table 11-2).

Table 11-2 Characteristics of Aortic Dissection from the International Registry of Acute Aortic Dissection

	NORMAL CXR (%)	WIDENED MEDIASTINUM ON CXR (%)	NORMAL ECG (%)	ISCHEMIA (%)	LEFT VENTRICULAR HYPERTROPHY (%)
All(*n*=464)	12	62	31	15	26
Type A (*n*=289)	11	63	31	17	25
Type B (*n*= 175)	16	56	32	13	32

Echocardiography

TTE is an insensitive tool for detecting aortic dissection, because it does not visualize the aortic arch or much of the descending aorta, and imaging quality may not be optimal because of the patient's body habitus. However, TTE can provide valuable information about pericardial effusion or aortic regurgitation and can help determine whether cardiac tamponade is the cause of hypotension in a patient with aortic dissection.

TEE is highly sensitive (Table 11-3) for the diagnosis of aortic dissection,and is the procedure of choice in unstable patients.TEE can be quickly performed at the patient's bedside with sedation or light anesthesia and requires no radiation or contrast agent injection. Visualization of the distal ascending aorta and proximal arch used to be difficult because of the interposition of the air-filled trachea and left mainstem bronchus, but evaluation of this "blind spot" has been aided by biplane and multiplane probes.

Table 11-3 Sensitivities and Specificities of Imaging Modalities for Diagnosing Aortic Dissection

TEST	TEE	HELICAL CT	MRI
Sensitivity (%)	98	100	98
Specificity (%)	95	98	98

Computed Tomography

CT aortography is a reliable test for diagnosing aortic dissection (see Table 11-3) and is the diagnostic test of choice in most institutions.Findings suggestive of aortic dissection include dilation of the aorta, identification of an intimal flap, and the clear demonstration of both the false and true lumina

(Fig. 11-2). Dynamic scanning, in which rapid scans are obtained at multiple levels immediately after a bolus injection of an intravenous contrast agent, improves the accuracy of the CT scan in the diagnosis of aortic dissection by allowing detection of differential filling rates in the true and false lumina . Dynamic scanning performed with helical CT improves sensitivity and specificity. Sixty-four-slice MDCT may soon alter the approach to chest pain in the ED. MDCT may reliably evaluate for coronary artery disease, pulmonary embolus, and aortic dissection as a "triple" scan.

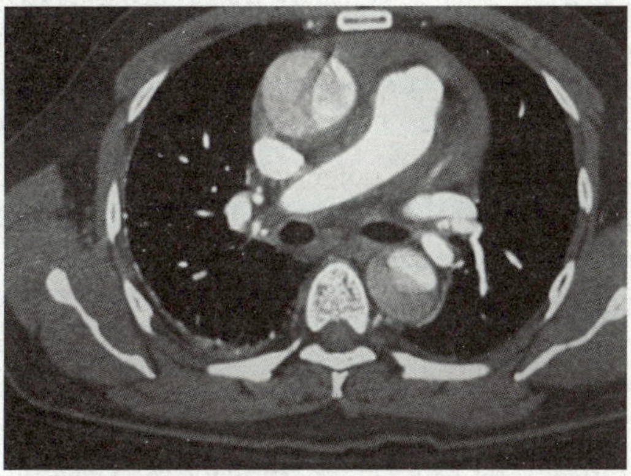

Fig. 11-2 CT scan demonstrating the true lumen and false lumen.

Magnetic Resonance Imaging

MRI is an appealing option in the detection of low-grade aortic dissection in stable patients whom the diagnosis is uncertain. Sensitivity and specificity are excellent (Table 11-3). MRI shows the site of intimal tear, type and extent of dissection, presence of aortic insufficiency, and differential flow velocities in the true and false channels and in the aortic side branches. It requires no contrast material or ionizing radiation and is noninvasive. It is particularly useful in the evaluation of chronic aortic dissection, in the follow-up of postoperative patients, and for monitoring nonoperative patients for progression of the dissection. Its availability, however, is limited, and it is difficult to perform in unstable patients.

DIFFERENTIAL CONSIDERATIONS

The differential diagnosis for the patient with symptoms suggestive of aortic dissection is extensive. Signs and symptoms associated with aortic dissection vary and depend on the extent of aortic and branch vessel involvement. Patients with the ultimate diagnosis of aortic dissection are often initially thought to have other conditions such as myocardial ischemia, CHF,or pulmonary embolus. Several clinical syndromes are particularly suggestive of aortic dissection—chest pain that is of sudden onset, migratory pain, chest pain with concomitant neurologic deficits or syncope, and chest pain with pulse deficits.

Although chest pain is the most common symptom of aortic dissection, it is also the most common presenting complaint of at least three other serious and more common clinical entities: AMI, pulmonary embolus, and pericarditis. An ECG can be helpful in excluding AMI, although aortic dissection and AMI may coexist as a result of the dissection proceeding retrograde to the ostium of a coronary artery and causing infarction. In cases in which aortic dissection is excluded, CT may reveal other abnormalities that explain a patient's presentation (e.g., pulmonary embolus). TEE is helpful in identifying causes of chest pain other than aortic dissection (e.g., cardiac ischemia).

When the initial presentation of the aortic dissection is pain or dysfunction in an extremity resulting from disruption of the blood supply, peripheral neurologic diagnoses should be included in the differential diagnosis. An aortic dissection may involve the carotid artery and may initially mimic a primary central nervous system lesion such as a stroke. The diagnosis of aortic dissection should be considered in any patient with a new diagnosis of pericardial effusion, pericardial tamponade, or aortic insufficiency.

MANAGEMENT

In all patients with aortic dissection, medical therapy including pain relief and BP control is recommended. While urgent surgery is recommended in patients with Type A aortic dissection, and medical therapy is always recommended in patients with uncomplicated Type B aortic dissection.

Emergency Department

Early therapy for aortic dissection is critical and should be initiated while diagnostic tests are being performed. Opioids should be administered in adequate doses to control pain and decrease sympathetic tone.Patients with aortic dissections are typically hypertensive. The two goals of medical management are to (1) reduce BP and (2) decrease the rate of rise of the arterial pulse (d*P*/d*t*) to diminish shearing forces. A target BP of 100 to 120 mmHg systolic and a heart rate below 60 beats/min are recommended.Beta-adrenergic blockers are the cornerstone of aortic dissection management and are effective when used as the sole agent (in addition to opioid analgesia for pain). Because vasodilators such as sodium nitroprusside or fenoldopam reflexively increase the heart rate and may also increase the d*P*/d*t*, they necessitate concomitant use of a beta-blocker and so are a more complicated form of therapy. Initial therapy with either esmolol or labetalol, as described later, and use of opioid analgesia, such as morphine or fentanyl, for pain are recommended.

Recommended Therapy

Esmolol and labetalol are titratable short-acting beta-blockers that can be used as monotherapy for hemodynamic control in aortic dissection. Esmolol is an ultra-short-acting beta-blocker that is given as an initial bolus of 500 μg/kg, followed by an infusion of 50 to 200 μg/kg/min. Labetalol has both alpha- and beta-blocking activity and is given as an initial series of 20-mg intravenous boluses every 5 to 10 min, incrementally increased to 80 mg until a target HR of 60 has been reached or a total of 300 mg has been given. A maintenance infusion of labetalol is then given at 1 to 2 mg/min. If a patient is normotensive, a beta-blocker should still be used to lower the d*P*/d*t* and maintain a HR of 60 beats/min. In patients with a history of COPD or at risk for bronchospasm, a selective beta-blocker, such as metoprolol or atenolol, should be considered.

Alternative Agents

Sodium nitroprusside was widely used before esmolol and labetalol became available and is a reasonable agent to use but necessitates concomitant use of a beta-blocker to mitigate reflex tachycardia and requires more effort to prepare and administer. The initial infusion is 0.5 to 3 μg/kg/min, and the infusion is adjusted to reach the same hemodynamic goals described earlier.

The CCB nifedipine is not recommended to treat aortic dissection. Nifedipine has minimal inotropic or chronotropic effects and may reflexively stimulate sympathetic activity and increase shear stress on the aortic wall. Intravenous NTG is often used initially in patients with hypertensive chest pain and possible or uncertain aortic dissection. NTG is a less effective arterial dilator than NTG and less desirable than nitroprusside for the treatment of patients with aortic dissection. Like nitroprusside, NTG should be accompanied by a beta-blocker. Some physicians prefer an infusion of fenoldopam over nitroprusside, but this has not been specifically studied in patients with aortic dissection.

Patients with hypotension secondary to aortic rupture or pericardial tamponade should be resuscitated with intravenous fluids and immediately transported to the operating room if they are to have a chance to survive. BP should be measured in all four limbs, if necessary, to ensure that the condition is not a pseudo hypotension caused by an intimal flap obstructing the extremity in which the BP is measured. In patients with electromechanical dissociation or marked hypotension, pericardiocentesis may raise the BP pending definitive surgery.

Surgery

Type A acute aortic dissections require prompt surgical treatment. The aortic segment containing the original intimal tear is resected when possible, with graft replacement of the ascending aorta to redirect blood into the true lumen. If aortic insufficiency is present, it can be corrected through aortic valve resuspension or replacement. Patients with type A dissections have an in-hospital mortality rate of 27% when treated surgically versus an in-hospital mortality of 56% when treated medically.

Definitive treatment of type B acute aortic dissections is less clear.These patients in general tend to be worse surgical risks. Uncomplicated distal dissections have traditionally been treated with BP control, and patients have an in-hospital mortality of 10% when treated in this manner. Surgery has been reserved for patients who have persistent pain, uncontrolled HTN, occlusion of a major arterial trunk, frank aortic leaking or rupture, or development of a localized aneurysm. These patients have an in-hospital, 30-day mortality rate of 32%. A "deadly triad" of absence of chest pain, hypotension, and branch vessel involvement is an independent predictor of in-hospital death.

Interventional Therapy

Interventional stent-graft and fenestration techniques are replacing surgery for complicated type B dissections in some centers, especially for patients with renal and mesenteric ischemia. Patients treated with interventional therapy have an in-hospital mortality rate of 6.5%.Interventional therapy for stable type B dissections is currently under study, and treatment decisions should rest with the primary treating physician.In general, interventional endovascular techniques are not applicable to type A dissections.

DISPOSITION

Patients with chronic aortic dissections have already survived their period of greatest mortality risk and are usually treated by BP control and close monitoring unless complications lead to surgery. Regardless of the type of definitive therapy, all patients who have sustained and survived an aortic dissection require careful long-term treatment. Major complications that may occur with time are redissection, the development of a localized aneurysm, and progressive aortic insufficiency.

(LI Lijun)

Chapter 12

Pericardial and Myocardial Disease

KEY CONCEPTS

Thrombolytic therapy is contraindicated in pericarditis because of the potential for hemorrhagic pericarditis or tamponade.

Cardiac tamponade is suspected on the basis of distended neck veins, hypotension, and muffled heart sounds. Diagnosis is by echocardiography or by presumptive pericardiocentesis in severe cases.

Myocarditis should be considered in any patient with the combination of viral illness symptoms and a new presentation of cardiac disease (dysrhythmia, failure.).

Cardiomyopathies are a heterogeneous group of diseases associated with mechanical or electrical dysfunction.

Patients with newly diagnosed HCM should avoid strenuous exertion until evaluated by a emergency physician. Beta-blockers are the mainstay of therapy for HCM, and nitrates are avoided.

PERICARDIAL DISEASE(PERICARDITIS)

PERSPECTIVE

Our knowledge of pericardial function and disease has increased greatly since Hippocrates described the pericardium in 460 BC as "a smooth tunic that envelops the heart and contains a small amount of fluid resembling urine."Galen provided the first description of a pericardial effusion and performed the first pericardial resection. Lancisi first described the appearance of constrictive pericarditis at autopsy in 1728.In 1935, Beck described the clinical presentation of cardiac tamponade, known as Beck's triad (hypotension,jugular venous distention, and muffled heart sounds).Despite the passage of time and the modern availability of many diagnostic tools, the diagnosis and treatment of pericardial disease still present a challenge.

ETIOLOGY

Each of the disorders listed in Box 12-1 can produce acute pericarditis,with or without pericardial effusion.In addition,most of these disorders can progress to cardiac tamponade or constrictive pericarditis.Most cases of pericarditis in developed countries are idiopathic.

EPIDEMIOLOGY

Acute pericarditis is a syndrome caused by inflammation of the pericardium. Although the exact incidence is unknown, autopsy series show an incidence of pericarditis of approximately 5%. The incidence of pericarditis in the ED is not known.

Box 12-1 Etiology of Pericarditis

Infectious

- Viral
- Bacterial
- Fungal
- Parasite
- Rickettsia

Postinjury

- Trauma

- Surgery
- MI
- Radiation

Metabolic diseases
- Uremia
- Medications

Systemic diseases
- RA
- SLE
- Sarcoidosis
- Scleroderma
- Dermatomyositis
- Amyloidosis

Tumors

Aortic dissection

PRINCIPLES OF DISEASE

Pericardial Anatomy and Physiology

The normal pericardium envelops the heart and attaches to the great vessels. It consists of parietal and visceral layers, with a narrow potential space between them.Its blood supply comes from the internal mammary artery, and its nerve supply from the phrenic nerve.

An ultrafiltrate of plasma, 15 to 35 mL of fluid, is normally contained in the pericardial space. Abnormal amounts of pericardial fluid can accumulate when the venous or lymphatic drainage of the heart is obstructed. The pericardium serves several functions: it maintains the heart's position, lubricates the heart's surface, prevents the spread of infection, prevents cardiac overdilation, augments atrial filling, and maintains the normal pressurevolume relationships of the cardiac chambers. Patients with congenital absence (or surgical removal) of the pericardium, however, show few, if any, problems.

PATHOPHYSIOLOGY

The inflammation of pericarditis is characterized by a granulocytic and lymphocytic infiltration of the pericardium. There is an increase in the number of antibodies in the pericardial fluid.

IDIOPATHIC PERICARDITIS

Clinical Features

The classic symptoms of pericarditis include chest pain, pericardial friction rub, and ECG abnormalities. A history of fever and myalgia is common. Pericarditis chest pain usually is sharp and pleuritic and varies with position. It is typically relieved by sitting forward and is worsened by lying down, deep inspiration, or swallowing. Pericarditis pain is usually retrosternal, can radiate to the trapezius muscles, and may manifest as isolated shoulder pain. Pain can also be felt in the area of the diaphragm.

The physical examination hallmark of acute pericarditis is the pericardial friction rub. It may be audible anywhere over the anterior chest wall but usually is best heard at the lower left sternal border. Friction rubs are best heard via the diaphragm of the stethoscope, with the patient leaning forward in full expiration. The rub also can be accentuated by a full inspiration, followed by a breath hold, during which auscultation is performed.

Diagnostic Strategies

There is no single test that is diagnostic for pericarditis. The ECG is the most reliable diagnostic tool. It evolves through stages that occur over time. The first stage occurs in the first hours to days of illness. It includes diffuse ST segment elevation seen in leads Ⅰ, Ⅱ, Ⅲ, aVL, aVF, and V_2 through V_6 and also reciprocal ST segment depression in aVR and V_1. Most patients with acute pericarditis have concurrent PR segment depression (Fig.12-1). In the next stages, the ST and PR segments normalize, but the T waves flatten, and then there is deep, symmetrical T wave inversion. At the last stage, the ECG reverts to normal, although the T wave inversions may become permanent

The early ECG findings of acute pericarditis may be difficult to distinguish from AMI, coronary artery spasm, or benign early repolarization.

When the ECG pattern suggests ACS and the pain is not clearly pericarditic in nature,

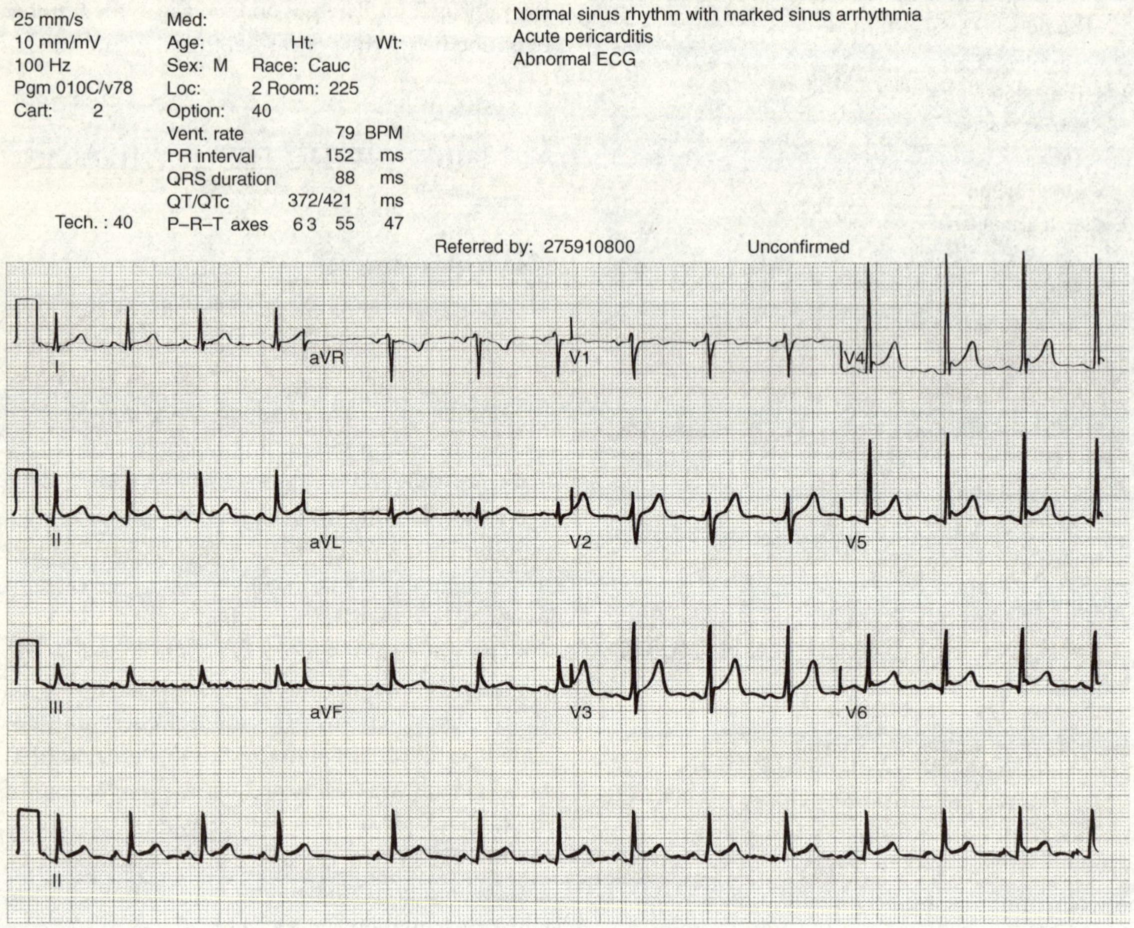

Fig. 12-1 ECG showing acute pericarditis.

often the best course is early diagnostic coronary angiography.

Echocardiography facilitates the definitive diagnosis of pericarditis with effusion,and a normal echocardiogram cannot be used to exclude pericarditis.

Some patients with acute pericarditis have elevated cardiac markers caused by myopericarditis, myocarditis, or AMI.The WBC count and ESR may be elevated or normal and are not sensitive or specific.

Management and Disposition

If a specific cause of pericarditis is found, therapy should be specific for that cause. Otherwise, therapy for acute pericarditis is symptomatic. Anti-inflammatory therapy will reduce pain, and a NSAID is the treatment of first choice.If the chosen NSAID is not effective within 1 w, a different class of NSAID should be tried,such as indomethacin. Colchicine is effective for recurrent pericarditis, and steroid therapy has shown mixed results.

Complications

Effusion, tamponade, and constriction are main complications of acute pericarditis.Patients with fever, pericardial effusion, a subacute course, or failure of initial NSAID treatment have a worse prognosis. Eighteen percent of patients can have recurrent pericarditis that may require serial echocardiography to exclude effusion or tumor.

UREMIC PERICARDIAL DISEASE

Perspective and Etiology

Pericarditis may occur secondary to renal failure

or dialysis. It occurs more frequently in hemodialysis patients than in those receiving peritoneal dialysis. ARF is also associated with pericarditis, and the cause is unknown. The evaluation of a chronic renal disease patient with pericarditis requires a diligent search for infectious causes.

Clinical Features and Diagnostic Strategies

Patients with uremic pericarditis have chest pain, unexplained fever, and possibly a coarse friction rub.They also may have significant effusions. The ECG in uremic pericarditis is often normal.In a dialysis patient, cardiac enlargement on chest radiograph in the absence of signs of volume overload or CHF should prompt consideration of pericardial effusion. An echocardiogram will provide the definitive answer.Pericardiocentesis may be needed to exclude infection.

Management and Disposition

Uremic pericarditis is initially treated with intensive dialysis. NSAID is ineffective and often is contraindicated by the patient's underlying renal impairment. Systemic steroids may require 1 or 2 w of therapy in the few patients who do not respond to dialysis.

Complications

Uremic pericardial effusions are among the most common causes of cardiac tamponade. Uremic pericardial effusions may be locular and difficult to fully drain with a catheter, and surgical options should be considered.

POST-MYOCARDIAL INFARCTION PERICARDITIS

Approximately 20% of patients with transmural MI experience a different quality of chest pain 2 to 4 d after infarction. This pain may represent early post-MI pericarditis. There is frequently low-grade fever and a transient pericardial friction rub. A large pericardial effusion is unusual. Early post-MI pericarditis is generally short-lived and disappears with 1 to 3 d with aspirin therapy.

The ECG changes of pericarditis usually are masked by the AMI changes. Patients with early post-MI pericarditis have more dysrhythmias and heart failure. Pericarditis in AMI may be an indicator of greater myocardial damage and a worse outcome.

Dressler reported a syndrome of fever, pleuritis, leukocytosis, pericardial friction rub, and chest radiograph evidence of new pericardial or pleural effusions in post-MI patients. Dressler's syndrome is a delayed complication of AMI. The cause of late post-MI pericarditis may be immunologic, but the syndrome may also occur with pulmonary embolus and after pericardiotomy. Anticoagulants should be discontinued to reduce the risk of hemorrhage. Delayed post-MI pericarditis is treated with NSAID such as ibuprofen or indomethacin.

POSTINJURY PERICARDITIS

Perspective

Postcardiac injury syndrome is defined as pericarditis after MI, cardiac surgery, or trauma. The incidence ranges from approximately 5% after MI to 30% after thoracic surgery or trauma. Pericarditis develops in 20% of patients with a penetrating cardiac injury.

Principles of Disease

Injury to the pericardium in blunt trauma may range from contusion to laceration or rupture.

Penetrating wounds to the heart usually cause laceration of the pericardium and the myocardium, with secondary pericarditis and pericardial infections. Although the exact incidence is unknown, infection, tamponade, myocarditis, and inflammatory pericarditis may occur.

An immune pathogenesis is suggested by the development of cardiac autoantibodies. Constrictive pericarditis occurs secondary to trauma. This may be caused by pericardial blood, possibly secondary to the decreased resorptive power of damaged pericardium, with secondary fibrosis and constriction.

Clinical Features

Symptoms and signs of postcardiac injury syndrome include pericardial rub, fever, and chest pain. Although the diagnosis is usually established clinically, confirmation by echocardiography is helpful. The interval between injury and the onset of pericarditis ranges from 4 to 12 d.

Management and Disposition

Most patients respond to aspirin or NSAID (ibuprofen 600 mg four times per day).The patient of uncomplicated pericarditis should be observed until other life-threatening disease processes have been excluded.

NEOPLASTIC PERICARDIAL DISEASE

Perspective

Malignant pericardial tumors typically manifest late, which complicates diagnosis and treatment. The most common causes are lung cancer , breast cancer, lymphoma and leukemia. Primary malignancies of the pericardium are rare.

Principles of Disease and Pathophysiology

The pattern of cardiac involvement by a malignant tumor is determined by the heart's lymphatic drainage system.

Malignant pericardial effusions contribute directly to the patient's death in most cases commonly from cardiac tamponade.

Clinical Features

Primary cardiac neoplasms, such as angiosarcoma and teratoma, can initially cause symptoms consistent with pericarditis. The typical course is that of an acute pericarditis that resolves and subsequently recurs. Malignant pericardial disease is difficult to diagnose. Most patients are asymptomatic or have nonspecific symptoms, such as shortness of breath, cough, palpitations, ill-defined chest pain, weakness, dizziness, hiccups, or fatigue.

Diagnostic Strategies

The diagnostic workup for malignant pericardial effusion includes an echocardiogram, CT, or MRI. When a pericardial effusion is identified, pericardial fluid cytology is recommended if the underlying malignancy is undiagnosed.

Management and Disposition

Malignant pericardial effusion treatment may include pericardiocentesis, local instillation of sclerosing or chemotherapeutic agents, systemic chemotherapy, cardiac radiation, and pericardial window.

PERICARDIAL DISEASE RELATED TO CONNECTIVE TISSUE DISORDERS

Pericarditis occurs in approximately one third of patients with RA, usually within 3 yr of the initial diagnosis. Rheumatoid pericardial disease is rarely clinically significant. Occasional patients develop effusions, constrictive pericarditis, or cardiac tamponade. Corticosteroid treatment is useful. Prednisone is the initial treatment, with close follow-up appointment.

Pericarditis is found at autopsy in more than 50% of patients with SLE. The effusion is usually thick and fibrinous. Either cardiac tamponade or constrictive pericarditis may develop. Corticosteroid therapy is indicated.

Other connective tissue diseases that may cause pericarditis include Sjögren's syndrome, giant cell arteritis, ankylosing spondylitis, Reiter's syndrome, Behçet's disease, systemic sclerosis, and polyarteritis nodosa.

MISCELLANEOUS INFECTIOUS CAUSES OF PERICARDITIS

Other causes of pericarditis include Rickettsia conorii, which causes Mediterranean spotted fever (treated with doxycycline), Mycoplasma pneumoniae (treated with a macrolide), Nocardia asteroids (treated with pericardiectomy and long-term use of antibiotics such as sulfisoxazole), Chlamydia trachomatis, Epstein-Barr virus, cytomegalovirus infection, Haemophilus actinomycetemcomitans (treated with chloramphenicol), and coccidioidomycosis. Viral and bacterial causes of pericarditis can coexist.

PERICARDIAL EFFUSION

Etiology and Clinical Features

The most common causes of pericardial effusion are viral or idiopathic pericarditis, malignancy, uremia, trauma, and radiation therapy. Drug reactions and autoimmune diseases are less common causes.

Pericardial effusion is often asymptomatic. Patients with known associated conditions with cough, fever, chest pain, or dyspnea may have an effusion.

Diagnostic Strategies

Pericardial effusion may cause an enlarged cardiac silhouette on chest radiograph, usually with normal pulmonary vasculature. A minimum of 200 to 250 mL of pericardial fluid is necessary to produce cardiomegaly on a chest radiograph.

Echocardiography is the diagnostic modality of choice (Fig. 12-2, see color illustration). It easily differentiates pericardial fluid from cardiac chamber enlargement and provides information about myocardial wall motion.

CT may be useful in diagnosing pericardial effusion when the echocardiogram is technically unsatisfactory. MRI can also be diagnostic. Nuclear scans may be useful in detecting purulent pericardial effusions.

Pericardiocentesis may be performed for either diagnostic or therapeutic purposes. Elective diagnostic pericardiocentesis is indicated in cancer patients, for failure to respond to usual treatment, or when bacterial infection is suspected. Common complications of pericardiocentesis include induction of cardiac dysrhythmias, pneumothorax, perforation of myocardium, laceration of coronary or internal mammary arteries, and liver laceration. Echocardiographic-guided pericardiocentesis is the procedure of choice.

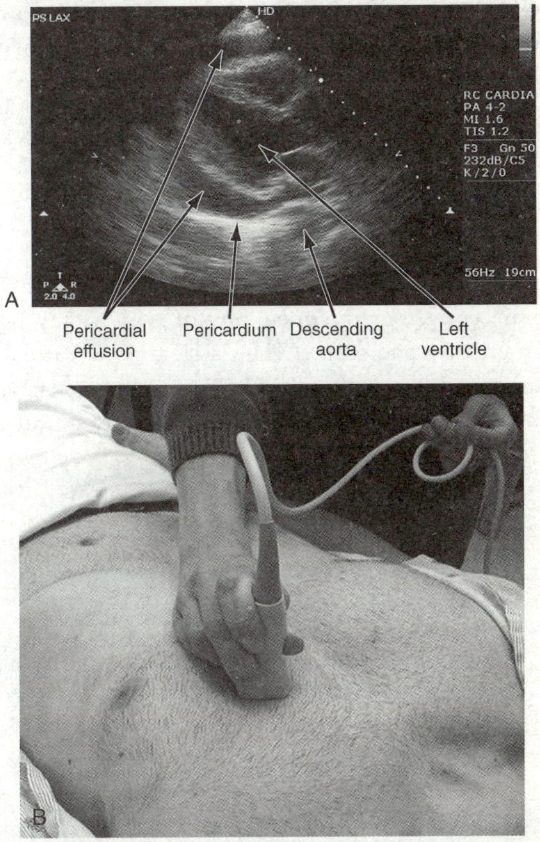

Fig. 12-2 A, Bedside ultrasound showing a pericardial effusion. The effusion is best seen superior to the left ventricle at the top of the image. B, The proper technique for ED ultrasound of pericardial effusion.

CARDIAC TAMPONADE

Etiology and Pathophysiology

Ten percent of all patients with cancer develop cardiac tamponade. Cardiac tamponade should be suspected in patients with penetrating chest wounds. It is also common in patients with uremic pericarditis.

Cardiac tamponade is the result of compression of the myocardium by the contents of the pericardium. This compression is usually caused by fluid, but it may be caused by gas, pus, blood, or a combination of factors.

Cardiac tamponade is a physiologic continuum reflecting the amount of fluid, the rate of accumulation, and the nature of the heart. The final result is increased pericardial pressure, which causes decreased ventricle compliance and decreased flow of blood into the heart. The reduction of blood inflow into the right ventricle results in decreased stroke volume that leads to decreased cardiac output.

The heart initially responds to tamponade by increasing heart rate to maintain CO.

Symptoms and Signs

Cardiac tamponade symptoms are often nonspecific, but particularly include chest pain, cough, or dyspnea, any of which may be progressive and severe. The classic triad of cardiac tamponade signs described by Beck is hypotension, distended neck veins, and muffled heart sounds. These signs may not be present if tamponade develops quickly.

Diagnostic Strategies

The chest radiograph shows cardiomegaly only if there is a large accumulation of fluid (250 mL). The ECG classically shows decreased voltage or electrical alternans (Fig. 12-3), but the latter is rare. Echocardiography confirms the diagnosis when an effusion and paradoxical systolic wall motion are seen. Thermodilution catheters can also be diagnostic, showing equalization of right and left ventricular pressure.

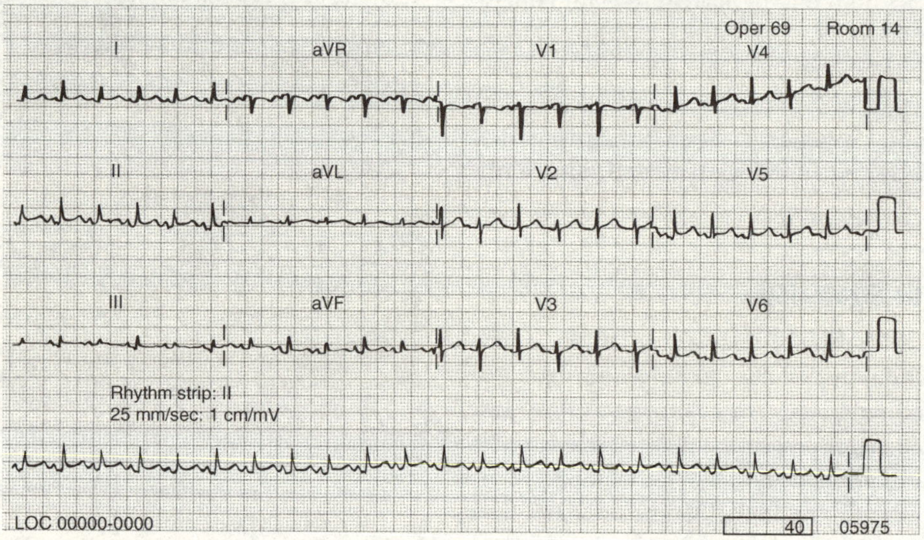

Fig. 12-3 Electrocardiogram showing electrical alternans.

Management and Prognosis

Initial treatment includes volume augmentation to the right ventricle with intravenous fluids to increase the filling pressure to overcome the pericardial constriction. Pericardiocentesis or pericardial window is the treatment of choice.Cardiac tamponade has a high mortality that depends on the severity and nature of the underlying disease, the time course of onset, and the rapidity of diagnosis and intervention.

PURULENT PERICARDITIS

Epidemiology and Etiology

Purulent pericarditis is a life-threatening process that is seen most commonly in a hospitalized patient with systemic illnesses who develops sepsis. It can occur in any age group and can be caused by any type of infectious agent, with bacteria, especially Streptococcus and Staphylococcus, being the most common.

Principles of Disease and Pathophysiology

Purulent pericarditis occurs by several mechanisms: (1) spread from an adjacent infection, such as pneumonia or empyema; (2)hematogenous spread from a distant site; (3) direct inoculation of bacteria (trauma or procedure); and (4) spread from an intracardiac source. The most common mechanism is spread from a distant site.

Clinical Features and Diagnostic Strategies

Purulent pericarditis usually manifests as a febrile illness lasting 2 or 3 d. Common presenting signs include tachycardia, dyspnea, hepatomegaly, elevated central venous pressure, chest pain, friction rub, and leukocytosis. The most common presentation is a hospitalized patient with a serious underlying disease who initially improves after treatment of the primary process but later develops fever, dyspnea, and chest pain.

The diagnosis should be suspected in any febrile patient with multisystem illness who has a pericardial effusion. Pericardiocentesis is necessary to establish the diagnosis, obtain fluid for microbiologic studies, and relieve cardiac tamponade.

Management and Disposition

Pericardiectomy is the traditional treatment of choice. Indwelling catheters, coupled with lavage, antibiotics and fibrinolytics, may avoid the need for surgery. Intravenous antibiotics or antifungals are also needed.

In addition to the initial complications related to sepsis and tamponade, long-term sequelae of purulent pericarditis include the development of constrictive pericarditis.

CONSTRICTIVE PERICARDITIS

Perspective and Etiology

Constrictive pericarditis may be a late consequence of acute pericarditis of virtually any cause. Other predisposing conditions include radiation, trauma, purulent pericarditis, actinomycosis, and postpericardiotomy adhesions. Tuberculosis is still the leading cause of constrictive pericarditis in some countries.

Principles of Disease and Pathophysiology

Constrictive pericarditis usually results from fibrous reaction of the pericardium. The key pathophysiologic feature is impaired diastolic filling from external cardiac compression caused by the thickened pericardium. In advanced cases the visceral and parietal pericardial layers may be adherent.

Because the pericardium limits volume, ventricular filling is rapid and completed within the first third of diastole, after which left ventricular volume and pressure remain unchanged. Early ventricular filling followed by a period of unchanging pressure yields a corresponding dip and plateau pattern or square root sign on the left ventricular diastolic pressure curve, which suggests the diagnosis of constrictive pericarditis.

Clinical Features

The symptoms and signs of constrictive pericarditis are identical to those of CHF. Dyspnea, fatigue, and weight gain are the most common complaints. Hepatomegaly, marked pitting lower extremity edema, and ascites can be seen on physical examination. The characteristic auscultatory finding of constrictive pericarditis is a pericardial knock in early diastole. A friction rub may also be heard.

Diagnostic Strategies

The diagnosis is considered in a patient with right-sided heart failure symptoms. Heart size on the chest radiograph is typically small but may be increased by atrial enlargement. Pericardial calcification is suggestive when present on CT or MRI. Liver function tests are consistent with passive congestion. ECG findings include low QRS voltage, nonspecific ST-T wave abnormalities, and atrial dysrhythmias.

Doppler echocardiography may help differentiate constrictive pericarditis from RCM or cardiac tamponade. Cardiac catheterization and simultaneous measurement of right ventricular and left ventricular end-diastolic pressures or endomyocardial biopsy may be necessary.

Differential Considerations and Management

Constrictive pericarditis is often confused with CHF. The diagnosis should also be considered with signs of elevated venous pressure but no history of myocardial dysfunction. Pericardiectomy is the therapy of choice.

MYOCARDIAL DISEASES (MYOCARDITIS)

PERSPECTIVE

The term myocarditis was coined initially by Sobernheim in 1837. Romberg reported the association with scarlet fever and typhus in 1891, and "isolated idiopathic interstitial myocarditis" was described by Fiedler in 1899.

EPIDEMIOLOGY AND ETIOLOGY

Some degree of myocarditis is detected in almost 10% of routine autopsies but is often not recognized clinically.In reality, any infectious agent can cause myocarditis (Box 12-2). Cytomegalovirus and Toxoplasma gondii have emerged as potential causes of myocarditis in cardiac transplant patients. Of patients who have died of AIDS, 67% have myocarditis on autopsy.The mortality rate is approximately 20% at 1 yr and 50% at 5 yr.

Box 12-2 Infectious Causes of Myocarditis

- Adenovirus
- Chagas' disease
- Coxsackie B virus
- Chlamydia
- Cytomegalovirus
- H_1N_1 virus
- Hepatitis A
- Hepatitis B
- Hepatitis C
- Human herpesvirus 6
- Influenza A
- Influenza B
- Lymphocytic choriomeningitis virus
- Mononucleosis
- Mumps
- Mycoplasma
- Parainfluenza
- Parvovirus 19
- Rabies
- Rubeola
- Rubella
- Streptococcus
- *Toxoplasma gondii*
- Varicella zoster

PRINCIPLES OF DISEASE AND PATHOPHYSIOLOGY

Myocarditis occurs by (1) necrosis from direct invasion of an offending infectious agent and its replication within or near myocytes, (2) destruction of cardiac tissue from infiltration of host cellular immune components or from cytotoxic effects of host immunity activated by the infectious agent, or (3) the toxic effect of exogenous or endogenous chemicals produced by a systemic pathogen. Three stages are proposed: acute (early after infection), with viral cytotoxicity and focal necrosis; subacute, in which there is an increase in humoral factors leading to autoimmune injury; and chronic, in which there is diffuse myocardial fibrosis and cardiac dysfunction that may lead to DCM.

Cardiac autoantibodies develop after myocarditis. Because myocarditis is linked to the development of DCM, idiopathic DCM after myocarditis may be predominantly autoimmune in origin, resulting from either shared antigens or molecular mimicry.

CLINICAL FEATURES

Flulike complaints, including fever, fatigue, myalgias, vomiting, and diarrhea, are usually the first symptoms and signs of myocarditis. The most common presentation is dyspnea, chest pain, and dysrhythmias. Altered vital signs include fever, tachycardia, tachypnea, and, uncommonly, hypotension. No symptom or sign is sensitive or specific. Cardiac examination is often unremarkable. When chest pain or CHF occurs at initial presentation, there is a worse prognosis.

DIAGNOSTIC STRATEGIES

Common ECG changes include sinus tachycardia, a widened QRS, and low electrical activity. There may be a prolonged corrected QT interval, atrioventricular block, or AMI pattern abnormalities.

Cardiac troponin may be elevated although when in the course of the disease is unknown. The prognostic significance of elevation is not known, although one can assume that a higher level correlates with more myocardial damage. The WBC count and ESR may be elevated or normal and so are not of diagnostic value. The echocardiographic features of myocarditis, although nonspecific, include reduced left ventricular ejection fraction, global hypokinesis, and regional wall motion abnormalities. Contrast-enhanced MRI may be diagnostic.Acute and convalescent viral titers are positive in less than 40% of cases.

Endocardial biopsy, the historical gold standard, has variable sensitivity and specificity owing to sampling error when the tissue taken is different from the tissue involved (Fig. 12-4, see color illustration). Because of the limitations of biopsy, MRI may become the diagnostic test of choice and the next gold standard.

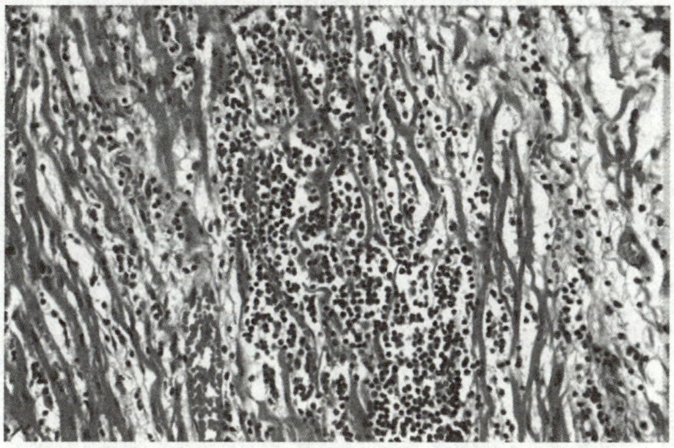

Fig. 12-4 Myocardial biopsy specimen showing myocarditis. Note the lymphocytic infiltrate.

DIFFERENTIAL DIAGNOSIS

Myocarditis can masquerade as AMI with severe chest pain, ECG changes, elevated cardiac markers, and heart failure. Patients with myocarditis are usually young and have few risk factors for CAD. ECG abnormalities may extend beyond the distribution of a single coronary artery, or there may be global, rather than segmental, wall motion abnormalities on echocardiography.

If the differentiation of myocarditis from AMI is unclear, catheterization may be necessary. Coronary angiography is usually normal in myocarditis, which should prompt consideration of endomyocardial biopsy.

MANAGEMENT

Treatment is supportive and aimed at preserving left ventricular function. The type of supportive care necessary is determined by the patient's clinical presentation and the stage and severity of disease. This may extend from simple limitation of activity to rhythm and CHF treatment, extracorporeal membrane oxygenation,ventricular assist devices,and eventual cardiac transplantation.

Therapy is stage specific. In the first phase, demonstration of replicating virus suggests that early antiviral agents, such as pleconaril or ribavirin, may be effective. Unfortunately, the diagnosis is often made after the initial viral phase.

Immunosuppressive therapy for the subacute phases of myocarditis have shown no benefit.

In the chronic stage, CHF symptoms predominate and standard pharmacologic treatment for CHF is indicated.

DISPOSITION

All patients should be monitored, and those with persistent hemodynamic instability require intensive care. Paradoxically, patients with fulminant myocarditis have the best prognosis. Complications of myocarditis include ventricular dysrhythmias, LVA, and cardiac failure.

The mortality rate is 20% at 1 yr and 50% at 5 yr.The long-term prognosis in survivors is variable.

CARDIOMYOPATHIES AND SPECIFIC HEART MUSCLE DISEASE

Cardiomyopathies are a heterogeneous group of diseases associated with mechanical or electrical dysfunction. They usually exhibit inappropriate ventricular hypertrophy or dilation and have a variety of causes. It is becoming increasingly evident that many of these diseases result from genetic mutations. The diseases included are listed in Box 12-3.

Box 12-3 The Cardiomyopathies

Arrhythmogenic right ventricular
Dilated
Hypertrophic
Ion channel disorders

Inflammatory
Mitochondrial
Peripartum
Restrictive
Takotsubo

A variety of pathologic processes may initiate myocyte injury. Neurohumoral factors, immune factors, and cytokines cause myocyte dysfunction and subsequent remodeling. At the organ level the remodeling is hypertrophy or dilation. There is also an increase in interstitial fibrosis.

DILATED CARDIOMYOPATHY

Epidemiology and Etiology

DCM is a spectrum of disorders that have in common a dilated and failing heart. The incidence of DCM is estimated to be 1 case per 2500 adults. Many cases previously thought to be of unknown cause may be secondary to infection. It is now known that 30% to 40% of DCM cases have a genetic cause.

DCM affects men more often than women, affects African Americans more often than whites, and may occur in any age group, with middle age (40-65 yr old) being the most common. Risk factors include ethanol and tobacco abuse, pregnancy, HTN, and infection.

Pathophysiology

There are both primary and secondary causes for DCM. Possible pathophysiologic causes include myocardial inflammation; direct reaction of antibodies with receptors on myocardial muscle; toxins impairing myocardial biochemical processes; and loss or dysfunction of myocardial matrix proteins. Myocardial damage initiates a vicious cycle of hypertrophic cell death that increases the burden of the remaining cells; this leads to signaling, more work, and cell death.

Clinical Features

Symptoms of DCM have an insidious onset. Left-sided heart failure occurs as the initial manifestation in 75% of adults, with dyspnea (usually with exertion or while supine) being the major symptom. Exacerbation of heart or renal disease, dietary indiscretion, and medication noncompliance are key contributors. Chest pain on exertion is the initial symptom in 10% of adults, and systemic or pulmonary emboli are the initial manifestation in 4%. Right-sided heart failure is a late and ominous sign.

Diagnostic Strategies

ECG findings are nonspecific and may include poor R wave progression, intraventricular conduction delay, or a LBBB pattern. Holter monitoring may show frequent premature ventricular contractions and occasional ventricular tachycardia. Sudden death is uncommon. The chest radiograph reveals cardiomegaly.

Echocardiography shows left ventricular dilation, reduced systolic function, and variable wall motion abnormalities. Abnormal ventricular contractility defines DCM, and an ejection fraction less than 45% is required for diagnosis. End-diastolic and systolic volumes are increased, as are pulmonary capillary wedge pressure and central venous pressure.

Endomyocardial biopsy may also be necessary. MRI may help diagnose cardiomyopathy.

Obtaining a family history and genetic counseling may be indicated.

Management and Disposition

Therapy includes supportive measures, such as adequate rest, weight control, abstinence from tobacco, moderate salt and ethanol consumption, and reduced physical activity. Medical treatment includes standard measures for CHF.

ACEI reduce morbidity and mortality. Other afterload-reducing agents, such as isosorbide dinitrate and hydralazine, also prolong survival in patients with heart failure. Spironolactone and the angiotensin receptorblocking agents also prolong survival. Implantable defibrillators improve survival and should be considered in patients with an ejection fraction less than 30% or symptoms for more than 9 mo. Short-term statin therapy may help.

Beta-blockers can reduce symptoms and improve left ventricular function, functional capacity, and survival.

Outcome

Because medical therapy usually fails, DCM is the leading indication for cardiac transplantation in adults. Mortality from DCM is 18% by 1 yr, 35% by 5 yr, and 50% by 10 yr. Patients with DCM show progressive deterioration, with 75% of patients dying within 5 yr of diagnosis.

HYPERTROPHIC CARDIOMYOPATHY

Perspective

Hypertrophic cardiomyopathy (HCM), formerly called idiopathic hypertrophic subaortic stenosis, is a complex disorder with variable clinical manifestations. The prevalence is estimated to be 1 in 500 persons in the general population. It affects all races, men and women equally, and can manifest at any age.

Principles of Disease

Anatomy

HCM is a disease involving abnormalities of heart muscle at anatomic, cellular, and genetic levels. Specifically, it is a genetic disease of sarcomere proteins. The defining anatomic feature of HCM is a hypertrophied left ventricle in the absence of another cause of left ventricular hypertrophy. The thickening is usually asymmetrical and involves the septum more than the free ventricular wall. The dimensions of the left ventricular and right ventricular cavities are small or normal. Atrial dilation is another feature.

Histologically, individual muscle cells are hypertrophied, with a disorganized, characteristic whorled pattern. Sarcomere disarray is the histologic hallmark. Abnormal fibrous tissue is often found in the left ventricle, and the scarring mimics a healed MI.

Pathophysiology

HCM is an autosomal dominant disease caused by mutations in genes that encode for sarcomere contractile proteins.

The hypertrophy in HCM may be a compensatory response to the cardiac protein abnormalities. The usual cardiac response to physiologic stress is hypertrophy, dilation, or a combination of both.

Clinically, patients with HCM have asymmetrical LVH. They have an abnormal echocardiogram or cardiac magnetic resonance image that shows hyperdynamic ventricles. There may be an outflow obstruction, although this usually occurs with exertion. The thickness of the ventricle and degree of outflow obstruction correlate with disease severity. The pathophysiology involves impaired ventricular filling during diastole.

Genetic studies of families with HCM identify specific mutations that correlate with SCD.

Clinical Features

Although HCM occurs at all ages, the average age at diagnosis is 30 to 40 yr. HCM gained notoriety after the press coverage of the sudden deaths of several young athletes.The presentation of HCM varies widely, and it may be discovered by screening relatives of patients who have HCM.

In many patients the initial event is sudden death, which usually occurs during exertion. Ninety percent of patients have shortness of breath. Other symptoms include chest pain, syncope, near-syncope, and palpitations.

Physical examination may reveal a loud S_4 gallop and a harsh crescendo-decrescendo midsystolic murmur. This murmur is accentuated by the Valsalva maneuver or changing from a standing to a squatting position. Such position interventions change preload and afterload, which accentuates the murmur. Other physical findings may include a bifid arterial pulse, paradoxical splitting of the second heart sound, and, rarely, a mitral leaflet septal contact sound. Many dysrhythmias are seen in HCM, including premature atrial and ventricular contractions, multifocal ventricular ectopy, and ventricular and supraventricular tachydysrhythmias. In the ED, the diagnosis should be suspected in anyone with a family history, characteristic murmur, and cardiopulmonary symptoms (i.e., chest pain, dyspnea, and dysrhythmia) not explained by other life-threatening conditions.

Diagnostic Strategies

Patients with suspected HCM should have an ECG, chest radiograph, and echocardiogram. The ECG is abnormal in approximately 90% of patients.

The most common abnormalities are LVH, ST segment alterations, T wave inversion, left atrial enlargement, abnormal Q waves, and diminished or absent R waves in the lateral leads. The chest radiograph may be normal or may show left ventricular or atrial enlargement.

Echocardiography is the most important clinical diagnostic strategy. Findings include asymmetrical LVH, left ventricular outflow tract narrowing, a small left ventricular cavity, and reduced septal motion. The dynamic characteristic of HCM distinguishes it from the discrete forms of obstruction to ventricular flow. Doppler techniques help assess the severity of this obstruction at rest and with provocative maneuvers.

Magnetic resonance is helpful when the echocardiogram is not. Nuclear studies can be used to assess systolic and diastolic ventricular function and ventricular scarring. Electrophysiologic studies may show dysrhythmias but are not more predictive of sudden death than clinical factors.

Differential Diagnosis

HCM mimics many disorders.ECG changes, without a history of preceding MI, may also suggest HCM. Echocardiography is often helpful, but ultimately cardiac catheterization may be necessary to confirm the diagnosis.

Management

Long-term beta-blocker therapy is the mainstay of therapy. This prolongs diastole, increases ventricular filling, and results in symptomatic improvement (primarily dyspnea and chest pain) and exercise tolerance. CCB is also useful. Verapamil reduces obstruction, decreases contractility, and improves diastolic relaxation and filling. This improves exercise capacity, and the negative effects on heart rate and BP decrease oxygen consumption and the incidence of angina. Verapamil is contraindicated when conduction blocks are present but should be considered when there is no response to beta-blockers. Another option is disopyramide.

NTG is avoided in HCM-associated chest pain because it decreases ventricular volume. Amiodarone is the drug of choice for treatment of ventricular dysrhythmias in HCM. Amiodarone may also control Af. Automatic implantable cardioverter defibrillators are indicated for patients with sudden death or a history of a sudden death risk factor.

Surgical treatment is reserved for patients with large (>50 mm Hg) systolic gradients, severe symptoms, and poor quality of life who do not respond to drug therapy. The most common procedure is septal myomectomy. Dual-chamber pacing decreases outflow gradient and improves symptoms, but it does not improve outcome.

Disposition

The natural history of HCM is variable and probably reflects the many different genetic causes. The annual mortality rate is 1%.

The onset of Af in patients with HCM may precipitate marked hemodynamic compromise and severe CHF. Cardioversion is indicated, as is rate control and anticoagulation to prevent thromboembolism.

Risk factors for sudden death include malignant genotype, unexplained syncope, sudden death in first-degree relatives, abnormal hemodynamic response to exercise, and greater than 30-mm ventricular thickening.

Patients with HCM who have angina, syncope, near-syncope, dysrhythmias, and abrupt changes in cardiopulmonary status should be hospitalized.

RESTRICTIVE CARDIOMYOPATHY

Perspective

The hallmark of restrictive cardiomyopathy (RCM) is a gradual and progressive limitation of ventricular filling secondary to myocardial infiltration. RCM is the least common type of cardiomyopathy, accounting for less than 5% of all cases.

The most common cause of RCM worldwide is tropical endomyocardial fibrosis, which is endemic to India, Africa, and Latin America. Symptoms include an initial viral-like illness followed by persistent fever, malaise, and the development of severe rightsided heart failure.

Pathophysiology

Restriction of ventricular filling results in low ventricular volumes, high end-diastolic ventricular pressures, and decreased cardiac output. Systolic function is maintained. Grossly, there is atrial enlargement with small ventricles. As the disease progresses the ventricular cavities may become obliterated by fibrous tissue, scarring, or thrombus.

Clinical Features and Diagnostic Strategies

Symptoms are those of worsening diastolic dysfunction and include exercise intolerance, elevated central venous pressure, peripheral edema, pulmonary edema, and S_3 and S_4 gallops.

Differentiation from constrictive pericarditis requires CT, MRI, or Doppler echocardiography. Pericardial calcification favors a diagnosis of constrictive pericarditis over the diagnosis of RCM. Myocardial biopsy may be necessary.

Management and Disposition

Most of the underlying causes of RCM are untreatable. The exception is hemochromatosis. Symptomatic treatment with vasodilators and diuretics may help in all patients. Patients with RCM should be maintained in sinus rhythm. Transplantation is a possibility in some patients with better survival than controls. RCM is relentless, with 90% of patients dying within 10 yr of diagnosis. Patients with hemochromatosis are treated with phlebotomy.

PERIPARTUM CARDIOMYOPATHY

Perspective

Peripartum cardiomyopathy(PPCM) is uncommon and represents less than 1% of the cardiovascular problems associated with pregnancy. PPCM is a form of DCM with symptoms and signs of heart failure that appear initially during the last 3 mo of pregnancy or the first 5 mo postpartum. The diagnosis is made if there is no previous heart disease and no other cause for the heart failure.

Etiology and Epidemiology

The cause of PPCM is unknown. Risk factors include myocarditis, excessive use of tocolytics, preeclampsia, advanced maternal age, multiparity, twins, and genetic predisposition. The incidence is estimated to be 1 case of PPCM per 13,000 to 15,000 live births.

Clinical Features and Diagnostic Strategies

PPCM is clinically identical to DCM. Patients usually have symptoms of CHF but may also have chest pain, palpitations, or thromboembolism. Physical examination often reveals tachycardia, tachypnea, pulmonary rales, an enlarged heart, and an S_3 heart sound.

The ECG may show LVH or nonspecific ST-T wave changes. On echocardiography, all four chambers are enlarged with reduction in left ventricular systolic function.

Management and Disposition

Treatment of PPCM includes limitation of physical activity, beta-blockers, alteration of preload with nitrates and diuretics, increase in ventricular contractility, and afterload reduction. ACEI are teratogenic and should be avoided, if possible, in pregnancy. Hydralazine and labetalol are effective choices.

Mortality for PPCM in the United States is approximately 2%.Half of the survivors have complete or near-complete recovery of cardiac function within the first 6 mo. Patients who do not recover completely show either continuous clinical deterioration or persistent left ventricular dysfunction. Subsequent pregnancies may be associated with a high risk of maternal mortality. In the ED, patients with signs of hemodynamic instability or failure to maintain oxygenation should be admitted for treatment and fetal monitoring.

SPECIFIC HEART MUSCLE DISEASES

Amyloidosis

Massive amyloid deposition results in an increased cardiac weight and the diastolic dysfunction of RCM. CHF occurs in most cases of cardiac amyloidosis. Treatment involves standard CHF and antidysrhythmic therapy, although the dysrhythmias in amyloid heart disease are often refractory to treatment. The prognosis is poor, with death often resulting from progressive heart failure within 1 yr of symptom onset.

Sarcoidosis

Cardiac granulomas occur in approximately 25% of cases of systemic sarcoidosis. Granulomas located in the septum cause severe conduction defects, those in the papillary muscles cause mitral regurgitation, and those in the ventricular walls produce scarring and wall motion abnormalities. Complete heart block is the most common conduction block. Ventricular dysrhythmias are often refractory to therapy. Myocardial involvement in sarcoidosis is an indication for systemic corticosteroid therapy. Refractory cardiac failure and dysrhythmias are indications for heart transplantation.

Connective Tissue Disorders and Disease of the Myocardium

Myocarditis associated with various connective tissue diseases occurs more often than is recognized clinically. Cardiac abnormalities occur in RA, juvenile RA, mixed connective tissue disease, and primary Sjögren's syndrome. SLE is the connective tissue disease most commonly associated with cardiac abnormalities. Cardiac involvement in SLE includes pericarditis, endocarditis, and myocarditis.

The clinical presentation includes CHF, angina, and dysrhythmias. Pericardial disease can also occur. Although prognosis is poor, azathioprine may be a beneficial adjunct to steroid therapy.

Sudden Death

Approximately 25% of sudden deaths in patients younger than age 21 yr can be attributed to disease of the myocardium. Cardiac causes include myocarditis, HCM, and anomalous coronary artery circulation. In patients with sudden death attributed to cardiac causes, prodromal symptoms are reported in more than half of the patients, most commonly chest pain (25%) in patients older than age 20 yr and dizziness (16%) in patients younger than age 20 yr.

CAD becomes the leading cardiac cause (58%) in sudden death in people ages 30 to 39 yr. HCM and anomalous coronary arteries are seen more often in sports-related deaths.

(CHEN Yuguo)

Chapter 13

Hypertension

KEY CONSEPTS

The definitive cause of elevated BP remains unknown in more than 90% of patients. These individuals are labeled as having *primary or essential HTN*, and the cause is considered idiopathic.

The patients for whom an identifiable cause can be ascertained. These individuals are labeled as having *secondaryecondary HTN* .

A true hypertensive emergency is defined by the presence of acute target-organ dysfunction.

Acute BP reduction is not indicated for patients with asymptomatic HTN who lack evidence of acute target-organ injury.

PERSPECTIVE

The vast majority of those with HTN will be asymptomatic, and their BP elevation often will diminish without treatment within a few hours of arrival. When patients are symptomatic, however, uncontrolled HTN may represent a true emergency.

PRINCIPLES OF DISEASE

Definition of Hypertension and Relevant Terminology

Although BP below 120/80 mm Hg is considered normal, delineation of what constitutes HTN is evolving. For decades, 140/90 mm Hg has existed as the universally established threshold that separates HTN from prehypertension . Manual BP measurements obtained by specifically trained personnel in an office using proper technique in a nonstressful setting. Automated BP measurement is more reliable than office-based manual assessment. Newer automated office BP measurement devices are so much more precise that recent guidelines have suggested lowering the cutoff for establishing a diagnosis of HTN to 135/85 mm Hg when BP is obtained via this approach.

Prior attempts to classify patients have relied on ambiguous and overlapping terms such as "hypertensive crisis", "hypertensive urgency" and "accelerated" or "malignant" HTN, causing confusion on the part of clinicians and reliance on non–evidence-based interventions. A better approach focuses on the presence (or absence) of signs or symptoms attributable to acute target-organ injury within the context of established or newly "diagnosed" severe HTN, thus distinguishing patients with active vasculopathy from those without.Moreover,such categorization helps to identify patients in whom acutely elevated BP may be transient or reactive rather than indicative of an underlying chronic disease process. Along these lines, three distinct classes of HTN are relevant to emergency medicine practice:

1. *Hypertensive emergency*: A condition distinguished by acute target-organ dysfunction, manifesting with newly developed clinical sequelae or consequential diagnostic test abnormalities.
2. *Poorly controlled chronic HTN*: A presentation in which patients with established HTN are found to have elevated BP without specific attributable symptoms or evidence of acute target-organ damage. Such presentations most often result from nonadherence to treatment regimens or inadequate medical management but also may reflect refractory disease. Concurrent use of seemingly innocuous medications,

including NSAID, steroids, decongestants, appetite suppressants, over-the-counter stimulants, oral contraceptives, and tricyclic antidepressants or rebound from short-acting antihypertensives, such as clonidine, may be contributory.

3. *Elevated BP without prior history of HTN*: Approximately 70% of those with high BP in the ED but no established history of HTN will have elevated BP on ABPM or at clinic follow-up. Patients should not be diagnosed with HTN, however, until a series of properly performed BP measurements in a nonemergency ambulatory setting confirms the diagnosis.

Pathophysiology of Chronic Hypertension

Whereas BP is known to rise with increasing age, onset of HTN in the nonelderly represents a complex interplay of multiple inciting factors including neurohormonal dysregulation, vascular modulation, sodium intake, psychosocial stress, and obesity. Alterations in cardiac and renal function are also important. The definitive cause of elevated BP remains unknown in more than 90% of patients. These individuals are labeled as having *primary or essential HTN*, and the cause is considered idiopathic. In the subset of patients for whom an identifiable cause can be ascertained, the term *secondary HTN* applies (Table 13-1).

Table 13-1 Secondary Causes of HTN

CAUSE	DIAGNOSTIC TEST	CLINICAL CLUES
Endocrine		
Cushing's syndrome and other glucocorticoid excess states	History; dexamethasone suppression test	Glucose intolerance; purple striae
Hyperaldosteronism and other mineralocorticoid excess states	24hr urinary aldosterone level or other mineralocorticoids	Unexplained hypokalemia
Oral contraceptive use	History	
Pheochromocytoma	24hr urinary metanephrine and normetanephrine	Labile or paroxysmal HTN with palpitations, pallor and perspiration
Thyroid disease	Serum TSH	Temperature intolerance, weight loss, tachycardia
Parathyroid disease	Serum PTH	Hypercalcemia
Pulmonary		
Obstructive sleep apnea	Sleep study with O_2 saturation	Obesity; narcolepsy
Renal		
Chronic pyelonephritis	History; urinalysis, urine culture	
Diabetic nephropathy and other chronic kidney disease	Estimated GFR; urine albumin/Cr ratio	
Nephritic and nephrotic syndromes	Urinalysis	
Polycystic kidney disease	Renal US	
Renovascular conditions (renal artery stenosis)	Doppler flow study; magnetic resonance angiography	HTN onset before the age of 30 yr or after 55 yr; abdominal bruit; refractory HTN control; recurrent pulmonary edema; unexplained renal failure
Toxic or Metabolic		
Chronic alcohol abuse	History; ETOH level	
Sympathomimetic drug use	History; drug screen	
Tyramine containing foods	History	Paroxysms of HTN, especially in those taking monoamine oxidase inhibitors
Vascular		
Atherosclerosis		
Coarctation of the aorta	CTA	Decreased lower extremity pulses

ETOH, ethyl alcohol. TSH, thyroid-stimulating hormone.

Neurohormonal Dysregulation

The SNS has a pivotal role in the development of HTN. Norepinephrine is a potent stimulator of vasoconstriction. The SNS also stimulates beta1-adrenergic receptors in the heart, leading to an increase in CO. Sympathoactivation exerts additional, direct effects on the kidney that promote sodium reabsorption and trigger renin release, which results in angiotensin II production and further vasoconstriction.

Independent of SNS activity, the RAAS is critical to BP dynamics. Renin is an enzyme produced by juxtaglomerular cells in the kidney. Renin cleaves angiotensin I from its plasma globulin precursor, angiotensinogen. Angiotensin I is then converted to angiotensin II by circulating and tissue-bound (especially lung) ACE. Angiotensin II exerts systemic and renal effects by binding to AT_1 receptors, which results in arterial vasoconstriction, sodium reabsorption, and modulation of GFR. Angiotensin II also serves as a potent stimulator of aldosterone release.

Vascular Modulation

Continued vascular stimulation by both the SNS and RAAS coupled with an increase in wall tension caused by HTN.

Sodium Intake

Randomized trials have consistently demonstrated a reduction in systolic BP with diminished daily sodium intake. Salt sensitivity is defined by an increase in BP with intake of a high-sodium diet. Relative hypokalemia plays a critical role, and the entire effect of salt sensitivity on BP can be abolished with high-dose (approximately 4000 mg or 100 mEq per day) potassium supplementation.

Psychosocial Stress

Life stress is an important modulator of BP and a specific contributor to disparities in HTN.

Obesity

Increased body mass index (>30 kg/m^2) is a known risk factor for HTN. Elevated BP in obese individuals correlates with high circulating aldosterone and cortisol levels, which in turn may be a related to salt sensitivity. Obesity, especially truncal, is also strongly associated with diabetes and obstructive sleep apnea, both of which contribute to poor BP control.

Pathophysiology of Target-Organ Damage

Uninterrupted by treatment, continued vasoconstriction leads to a number of deleterious consequences that culminate in target organ damage. On a macrocirculatory level, the central component of the cardiovascular system is most affected. Active contraction against this resistance also increases intraventricular wall tension, which, together with ongoing stimulation from, among other things, the SNS and RAAS, triggers cardiomyocyte hypertrophy and myocardial fibrosis. Initially, this leads to an increase in LV mass, which enhances the heart's pumping against excessive afterload. When progressive, however, this process results in LV stiffening and impaired diastolic function with a reduction in LV filling and diminished flow from the left atrium to the LV. If the increase in afterload is sudden, an abrupt decrease in stroke volume occurs, precipitating backflow of fluid into the lungs and rapid onset of "flash pulmonary edema." Over time, this contributes to LV wall thinning, chamber dilation, and eventually systolic dysfunction.

Autoregulation works to maintain relatively constant blood flow and is protective with moderate fluctuations. Small-vessel ischemic episodes are the primary cause of chronic target-organ damage, including progressive white matter (i.e., multi-infarct) disease in the brain and hypertensive nephropathy. In a hypertensive emergency, however, an abrupt rise in vascular pressure overwhelms autoregulatory mechanisms, triggering endothelial injury. Unchecked wall tension ensues, and terminal arterioles dilate and eventually rupture, leading to a proinflammatory, hypercoagulable state with fibrin deposition and diffuse ischemia .Rising pressure in the proximal capillary beds causes fluid leakage and tissue edema, which, combined with the process of fibrinoid necrosis, produces acute target-organ damage and possibly microangiopathic hemolytic anemia.

CLINICAL FEATURES

Hypertensive Emergency

Most hypertensive emergencies occur in patients with chronic HTN. Organ systems involvement is dominated by injury to the brain, heart, or kidneys (Table 13-2). Focal neurologic deficit or altered mentation therefore point to brain injury, whereas chest pain or shortness of breath is indicative of cardiac or vascular involvement.

Table 13-2 Hypertensive Emergencies by Organ System

INJURY PATTERN BY TARGET ORGAN	APPROXIMATE INCIDENCE (%)
Brain (cumulative)	37-45
Acute ischemic stroke	6-25
Hypertensive encephalopathy	8-16
Intracerebral or subarachnoid bleed	5-23
Heart (cumulative)	27-49
Acute heart failure syndromes	14-37
ACS	11-12
Kidney	
Acute renal risk	15
AKI	8
Vascular	
Aortic dissection	1-2
Other	
Eclampsia	2
Acute hypertensive retinopathy	1

Hypertensive Encephalopathy

Hypertensive encephalopathy is a manifestation of diffuse vasogenic cerebral edema. It is caused by a failure of autoregulation in the brain, with vasospasm, ischemia, increased vascular permeability, punctate hemorrhages, and interstitial edema. The patient generally has severe headache, vomiting, and altered mental status, which may progress to seizures or coma. Retinal involvement may cause blurred vision progressing to complete blindness. Papilledema is often present, along with significant hypertensive retinopathy. CT does not show acute hemorrhage or other acute pathology.

Acute Stroke, Heart Failure Syndromes, and Other Hypertension-Related Emergencies

Acute stroke is not a hypertensive emergency. Chronic HTN is the primary population attributable risk factor for development of heart failure. AKI in the setting of elevated BP may be a consequence of associated target organ damage.

Blood Pressure Elevation in the Absence of Target-Organ Dysfunction

These patients do not have target-organ injury and most often have poorly controlled chronic HTN. When symptoms are present, they generally are nonspecific (e.g., low-grade or recurrent headache, atypical chest pain, dyspnea, dizziness, generalized weakness, focal but anatomically uncorrelated weakness or numbness, vague visual disturbances) and, with the exception of dyspnea, appear to be unrelated to the degree of BP elevation. The patient should be observed in a quiet area of the ED and reassured; in many cases the BP spontaneously improves.

DIAGNOSTIC STRATEGIES

The diagnostic evaluation of hypertensive emergency is guided by symptoms and signs identified on clinical examination but will often involve a number of tests. In nearly all instances, laboratory testing may be required to look for acute or worsening renal dysfunction and microangiopathic hemolytic anemia (i.e.,CBC with manual differential and peripheral smear).Individuals with chest pain or shortness of breath may require a chest radiograph, an ECG, and cardiac biomarker (i.e., troponin and NP) measurement. Echocardiography is a reasonable consideration, routine CT of the thorax is indicated for patients with suspected aortic dissection. When focal neurologic deficits or altered mentation is present, nonenhanced brain imaging with CT is helpful, often with follow-up MRI.

Funduscopy can provide evidence of hypertensive target-organ damage. Findings of acute hypertensive retinopathy. The spectrum of retinal findings in HTN can be graded on a 5point scale (Box 13-1).

Box 13-1 Funduscopic Grading of Suspected Hypertensive Retinopathy

Grade 0—Normal

Grade 1—Minimal arterial narrowing

Grade 2—Obvious arterial narrowing with focal irregularities

Grade 3—Arterial narrowing with retinal hemorrhages and/or exudate

Grade 4—Grade 3 plus disk swelling

There is no simple, efficient test for detecting subclinical cardiac disease in the ED. Although chest x-ray examination and ECG are often used, they have poor sensitivity for target-organ damage (especially LV hypertrophy), and abnormalities, when identified, are unlikely to alter clinical management. Serum NP levels (i.e., BNP and NT-proBNP) have yielded conflicting results and are not optimal screening tests.

CONSIDERATION OF DIFFERENTIAL DIAGNOSES

For those with a suspected hypertensive emergency, the decision point centers on the potential causal relationship between patient presentation and acutely elevated BP. Clinical entities within this broader heading, such as stroke syndromes and acute heart failure, do carry their own differentials. For patients with poorly controlled chronic HTN, a consideration of etiology (i.e., primary vs. secondary) may be warranted. Related diagnostic workup (Table 13-1) can usually be pursued on an outpatient basis. For those without a previous history of HTN, definitive diagnosis will require reassessment in an outpatient setting.

MANAGEMENT

Acute Blood Pressure Control

Antihypertensive Therapy

Antihypertensive therapy is indicated in treatment of acute hypertensive encephalopathy and in the presence of specific target-organ injury. The goal of acute antihypertensive therapy is to safely and effectively lower BP.

Blood Pressure Goals

Optimal treatment of a true hypertensive emergency is best achieved when therapy is directed toward (1) the precipitant of specific target-organ dysfunction and (2) the acute consequences of elevated BP rather than the BP itself.

Chronic Antihypertensive Therapy

Initiation of oral antihypertensive therapy for new onset HTN and reinitiation or up-titration for patients with chronic HTN is appropriate from the ED if follow-up cannot be ensured.

DISPOSITION

Asymptomatic individuals without evidence of acute target-organ dysfunction can be discharged home, but hypertensive emergency patients warrant admission, most often to an EICU.

(CHAI Yanfen CUI Shuzhang)

Chapter 14

Dysrhythmias

> **KEY CONCEPTS**
>
> There are three electrophysiologic mechanisms of dysrhythmias: enhanced automaticity, triggered activity, and reentry.
>
> A regular, new-onset, symptomatic wide-complex tachycardia should be assumed to be VT until proven otherwise.
>
> Type II second-degree AVB is never a normal variant and implies a conduction block below the AV node. When the conduction ratio is 2 : 1, type II block should be assumed until proven otherwise.
>
> The possibility of an accessory pathway should be considered in any tachycardia exceeding a rate of 200 to 250, regardless of the QRS complex morphology, and nodal blocking agents should not be used without careful consideration.
>
> Treatment of torsades de pointes instable patients involves correcting any underlying metabolic or electrolyte abnormalities and increasing the heart rate to shorten ventricular repolarization.

The term dysrhythmia denotes any abnormality in cardiac rhythm.

CARDIAC CELLULAR ELECTROPHYSIOLOGY

The function of individual cells in the conductive and contractile tissues of the heart depends on an intact resting membrane potential(MP). Na^+, K^+, and Ca^{2+} ions create MP and regulate conduction and contractility. MP is the result of a differential concentration of Na^+ and K^+ on either side of the cell membrane, measuring approximately −90 mV in normal resting, nonpacemaker cells(Fig. 14-1). The resting MP is generated from the flow of K^+ down a concentration gradient toward the extracellular fluid.

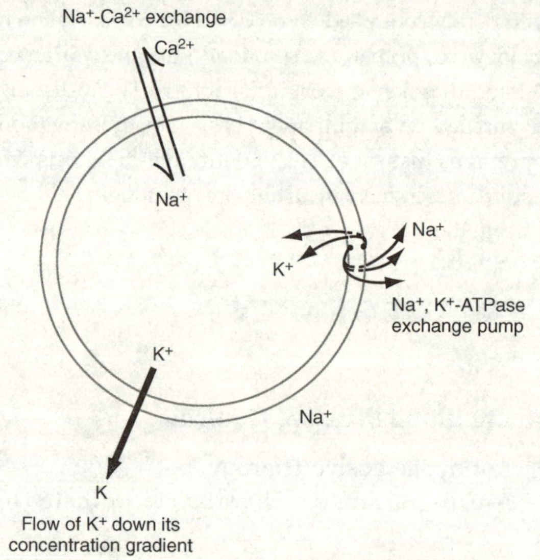

Fig. 14-1 Flow of various ions across the myocardial cell membrane. Na^+–K^+pump exchanges three Na^+ions for each two K^+ions, generating a net negative flow of 10 mV. The flow of K^+ down the concentration gradient (dark arrow) generates another 80 mV of current. The Na^+–Ca^{2+} exchange adds little to the resting MP.

In normal nonpacemaker cells, the application of an electrical stimulus causes MP to become less negative, termed depolarization. When MP reaches −70 mV, specialized Na^+ channels open, causing a rapid influx of positive charge into the cell. This "fast" channel activity further decreases MP and is augmented at 30 to 40 mV by a second "slow" channel that allows Ca^{2+} influx. When these channels close, resting MP is restored by Na^+–K^+ pump, an event known as repolarization (Fig. 14-2).

In nonpacemaker cells, additional depolarization from a second electrical stimulus is not possible when MP is more positive than

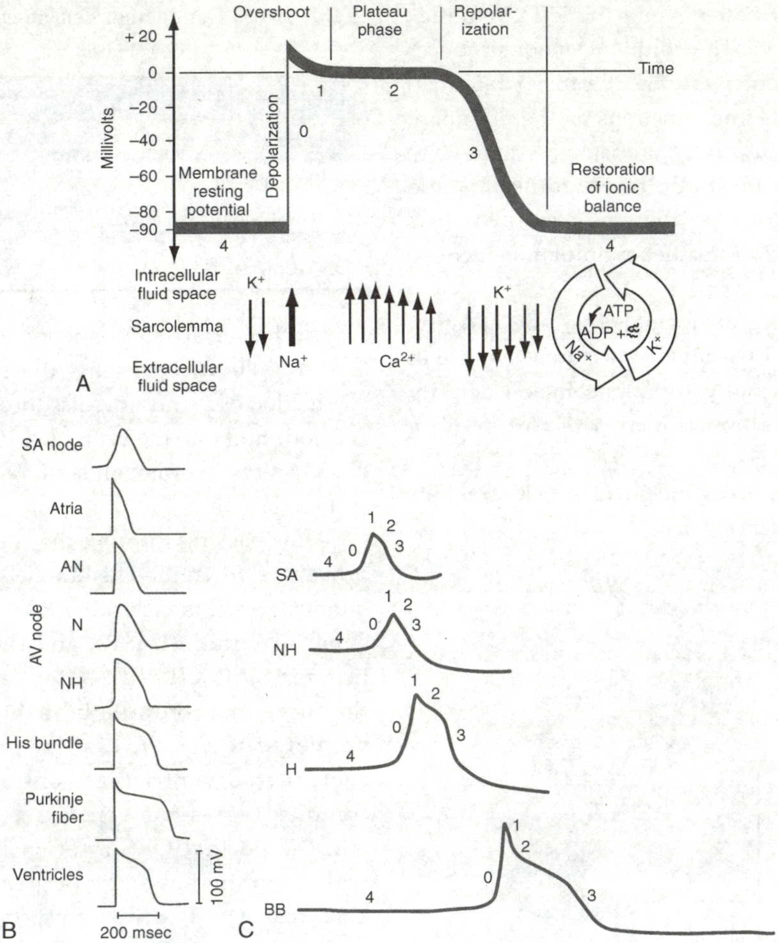

Fig. 14-2 A, Action potential of a myocardial cell and its relation to ion flow. B, Action potentials of various myocardial tissues. C, Action potentials of various pacemaker cells.

−60 mV. This period is termed the effective refractory period (Fig. 14-3). At MP of −60 to −70 mV, a strong impulse can cause a response; this response represents the relative refractory period. At MP of −70 mV or less, virtually all fast channels are ready for activity if properly stimulated (Fig. 14-3).

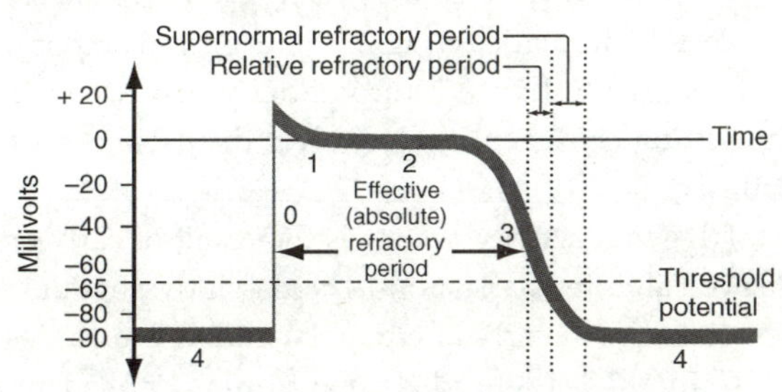

Fig. 14-3 Action potential showing various refractory periods.

Pacemaker cells differ from non–impulse-generating cells in two ways: their resting MP is less negative, and they can spontaneously depolarize via slow Na^+ influx. Nonpacemaker cells may undergo spontaneous depolarization under pathologic conditions, especially during ischemia.

ANATOMY AND CONDUCTION

The SA node is an area of specialized impulse-generating tissue located at the junction of the right atrium and the superior vena cava. Its blood supply is from the right coronary artery

(RCA) in 55% of patients and the left circumflex artery(LCA) in 45%. The normal SA node produces spontaneous depolarizations at a faster rate than other pacemakers and functions as the dominant pacemaker. The SA node maintains a rate of 60 to 90 beats/min in most adults. Hypothermia and vagal stimulation slow the sinus rate, whereas hyperthermia and sympathetic stimulation increase the rate.

In the absence of normal SA node activity, other myocardial tissues may assume the role of pacemaker. Rates of ectopic pacemaker activity vary widely depending on the underlying pathology.

Fig. 14-4 correlates the surface ECG tracings with tissue electrical events.

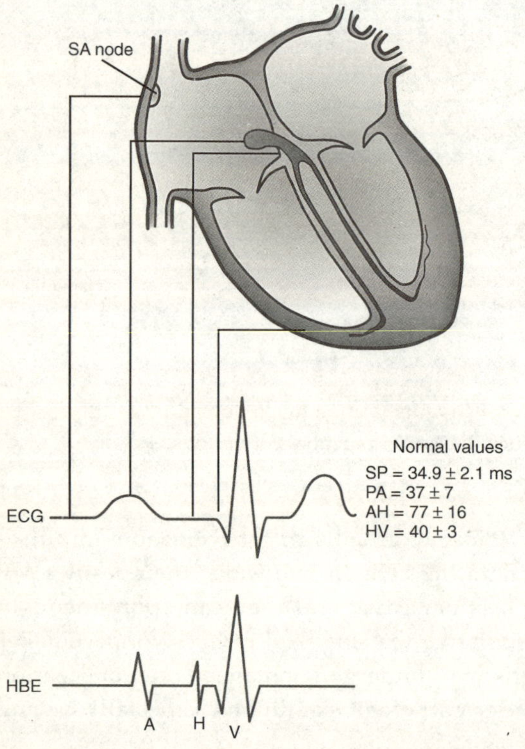

Fig. 14-4 Electrical events in the heart related to surface ECG and His bundle electrogram.

The AV node is an area of specialized tissue between the atria and the ventricles of the heart. Its blood supply is from a branch of the RCA in 90% of patients (right dominant) and from the LCA in the remaining 10% (left dominant). Transmission of impulses within the AV node is slower than in parts of the conducting system (Table 14-1).

Table 14-1 Conduction Velocities in Various Heart Tissues

TISSUE	VELOCITY (M/S)
Atrium	1000
AV node	200
His-Purkinje system	4000
Ventricles	400

On the surface ECG, the PR interval (normally 0.10 to 0.20 s) represents the time it takes for conduction of a sinus impulse through the atria and AV node and into the ventricles. PR prolongation is usually a result of nodal or supranodal conduction system disease.

After passing through the AV node, impulses propagate down the His bundle to the three main bundle branch fascicles: the RBB, the left anterior-superior bundle(LASB), and the left posterior-inferior bundle(LPIB). After conduction down the three main bundle branches, impulses are delivered to the Purkinje fibers, allowing for coordinated ventricular contraction. The QRS complex represents ventricular depolarization, and the normal QRS interval is 0.09 s or less, with a duration of 0.12 s or greater being clearly abnormal. The T wave corresponds to ventricular repolarization and varies in duration depending on the length of the cardiac cycle. The total time of ventricular depolarization and repolarization is represented by the QT interval.

MECHANISMS OF DYSRHYTHMIA FORMATION

There are three electrophysiologic mechanisms: enhanced automaticity(Fig. 14-5), triggered activity, and reentry.Enhanced automaticity can occur in the setting of ischemia, electrolyte disturbances, or drugs.

Triggered activity occurs as the result of early or delayed afterdepolarizations. The classic dysrhythmia associated with early afterdepolarization is torsades de pointes. Triggered dysrhythmias caused by delayed after depolarizations occurs with digitalis toxicity or with reperfusion therapy for AMI.

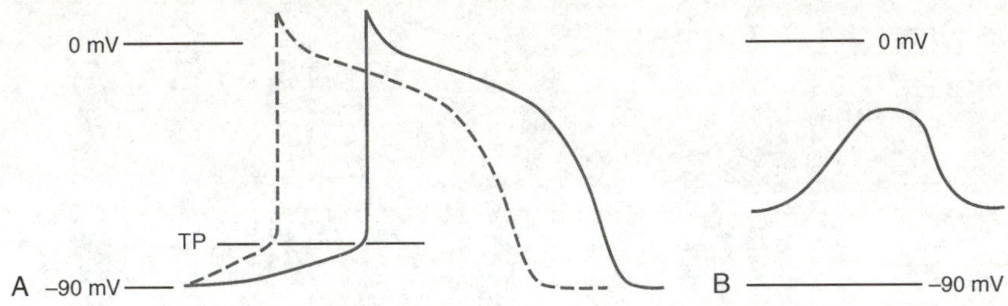

Fig. 14-5 A, Enhanced normal automaticity (dashed line). B, Abnormal automaticity. TP, threshold point.

Reentry dysrhythmias occur as a consequence of abnormal conduction (Fig. 14-6). The cycle is then repeated, creating a self-sustaining or "circus movement" tachycardia that can appear orderly or disorderly (i.e., fibrillatory).

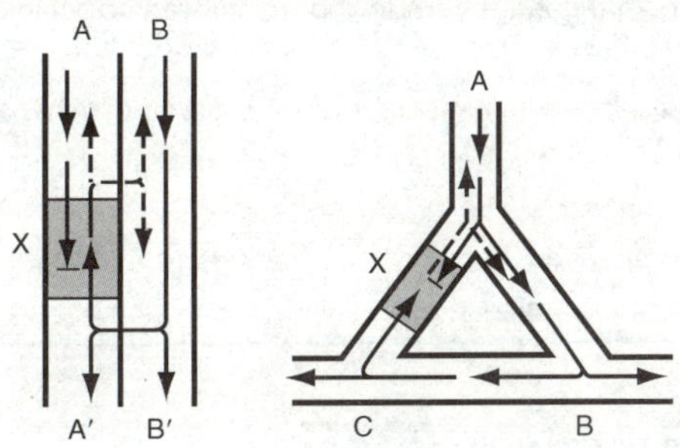

Fig. 14-6 Mechanism of reentry.

Reentry mechanisms are responsible for most narrow complex tachycardias and many VTs.

APPROACH TO DYSRHYTHMIA RECOGNITION AND MANAGEMENT

Dysrhythmias are classified according to their electrophysiologic origin, ECG appearance, and underlying ventricular rate. Although overlap exists, the following categorization is useful:

- Bradycardias
- Extrasystoles
- Narrow-complex (QRS less than 0.12 s) tachycardias (regular and irregular)
- Wide-complex (QRS 0.12 s or greater) tachycardias(regular and irregular)

Classically, the approach to any specific dysrhythmias is defined on the basis of the clinical stability.

Initial Assessment of Stable Patients

Stable patients may be asymptomatic or have mild symptoms, such as light-headedness, dyspnea on exertion, palpitations, or mild anxiety.

The approach to the patient with a stable dysrhythmia begins with gathering evidence from the history, physical examination, 12 lead ECG, and a rhythm strip. The nature of any symptoms, including the timing, velocity of onset (gradual vs. abrupt), and duration, is important. For the patient with "palpitations," questions about the rate and regularity of the heartbeat are often asked, inquiring about precipitating events and associated symptoms such as dizziness, chest pain, dyspnea, or syncope is critical to understanding the context of any dysrhythmia. The past history of rhythm disturbances or a prior history of ischemic or structural heart disease and a thorough medication history are essential. Occasionally the family history can suggest an inherited disorder such as an accessory pathway or Brugada's syndrome.

Multiple leads ECG are often required to detect such things as the presence or absence of P waves (often best seen in inferior leads or V_{1-2}; Fig. 14-7), the relationship between P waves and QRS complexes, prolongation of the QRS and QT interval, and evidence of ischemia or prior MI (Box 14-1).

Vagal maneuvers, such as carotid sinus massage and the Valsalva maneuver, transiently slow AV conduction, which may help terminate or uncover a supraventricular rhythm disturbance.

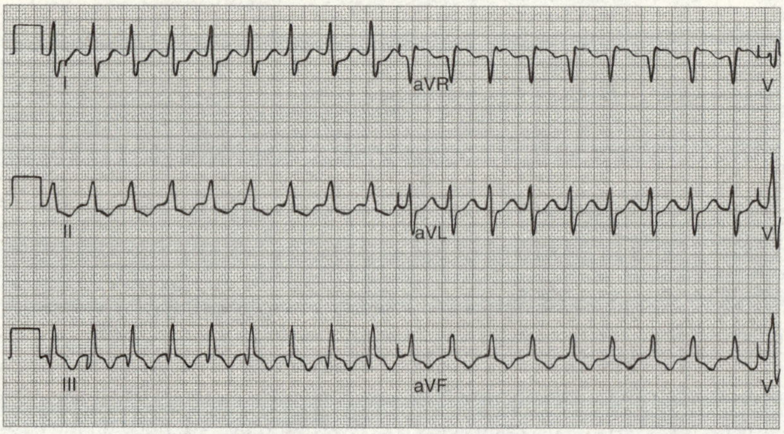

Fig. 14-7 Note the P waves before the QRS complexes in lead aVF.

Box 14-1 Basic ECG Observations during Dysrhythmia Analysis

1. Ventricular rate: Fast (>100 complexes/min), slow (<60 complexes/min), or normal (60-100 complexes/min).
2. Rhythm: Regular, completely irregular (irregularly irregular or chaotic), regular with occasional irregularity, or grouped impulses. Calipers and long strips are recommended to detect subtle irregularity.
3. QRS width: Prolonged (>0.12 s), borderline (0.09-0.12 s), or normal. If determined without ECG being physically present (e.g., prehospital radio medical command), it is helpful to ask for QRS duration in number of small boxes from printed rhythm strip (each box equals 0.04 s) to ensure accuracy.
4. P wave presence and relationship to QRS complexes: This may require mapping of P waves with calipers to detect those falling within QRS complex or T wave.
5. Rhythm changes: Examine these areas closely for clues.
6. Multiple leads, especially chest leads or esophageal lead if difficulties with P wave visualization are experienced.
7. Comparison with previous tracings (if available) is often valuable.

Pseudodysrhythmias

Loose leads, muscle contraction, shivering, tremors, and other patient movement can produce artifactual findings on a monitor, rhythm strip, or 12-lead ECG (Fig. 14-8).Such pseudodysrhythmias can mimic and are often mistaken for serious dysrhythmias.

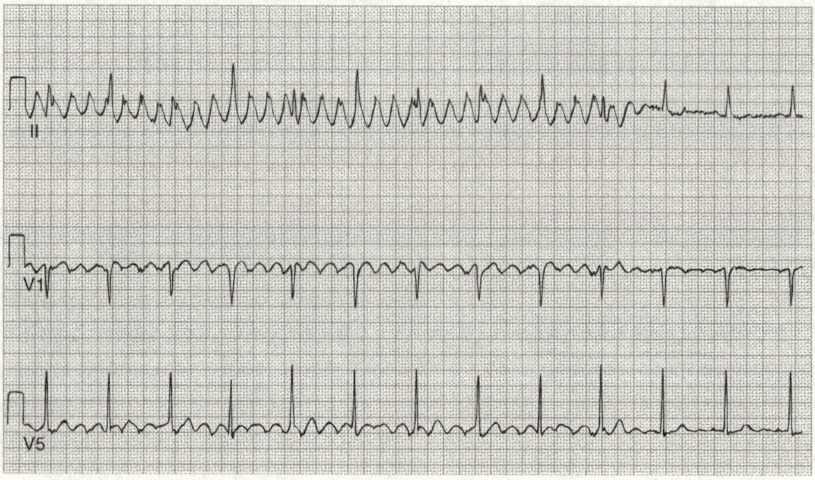

Fig. 14-8 Pseudodysrhythmia.

SPECIFIC DYSRHYTHMIAS

Sinus Bradycardia, Sinoatrial and Atrioventricular Block

Sinus Bradycardia

Bradycardia is defined as a ventricular rate of less than 60 beats/min. Sinus bradycardia is characterized by a P wave with normal morphology and a fixed P-P interval that is equal to the R-R interval, with a ventricular rate below 60 beats/min (Fig. 14-9). Sinus bradycardia is described in the early stages of an acute inferior wall MI. Other pathologic causes of sinus bradycardia include hypothermia, hypoxia, drug effects, and sick sinus syndrome(SSS).

Treatment for symptomatic sinus bradycardia is atropine. Occasionally, dopamine or epinephrine infusion may be required.

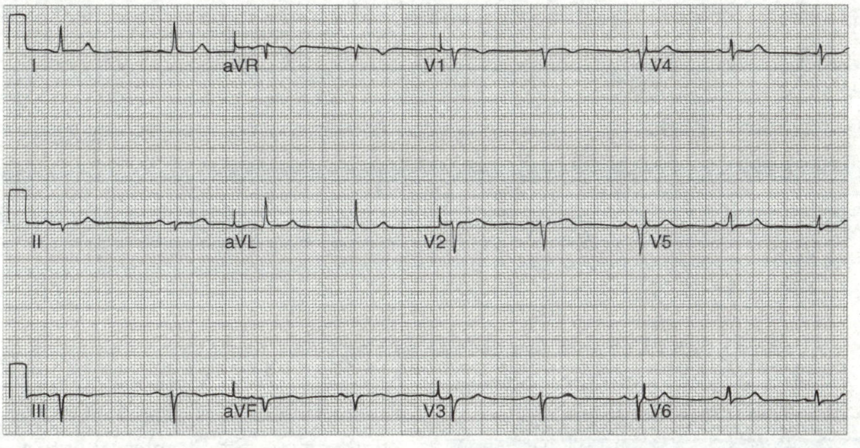

Fig. 14-9 Sinus bradycardia.

Sinus Dysrhythmia

Sinus dysrhythmia is diagnosed when a variable P-P interval is seen.

Sinus Arrest and Sinoatrial Exit Block

Disturbances in sinus rhythm are characterized by an absence of atrial depolarization, diagnosed by missing P waves on the ECG (Fig. 14-10).When the patient is symptomatic, the approach to treatment is similar to that for sinus bradycardia.

Sick Sinus Syndrome

Sick Sinus Syndrome(SSS) refers to a group of dysrhythmias from disease of the sinus node and its surrounding tissues, including sinus bradycardia, sinus arrest, and SA exit block. A variant of SSS known as bradycardia-tachycardia syndrome is characterized by one or more of these bradydysrhythmias

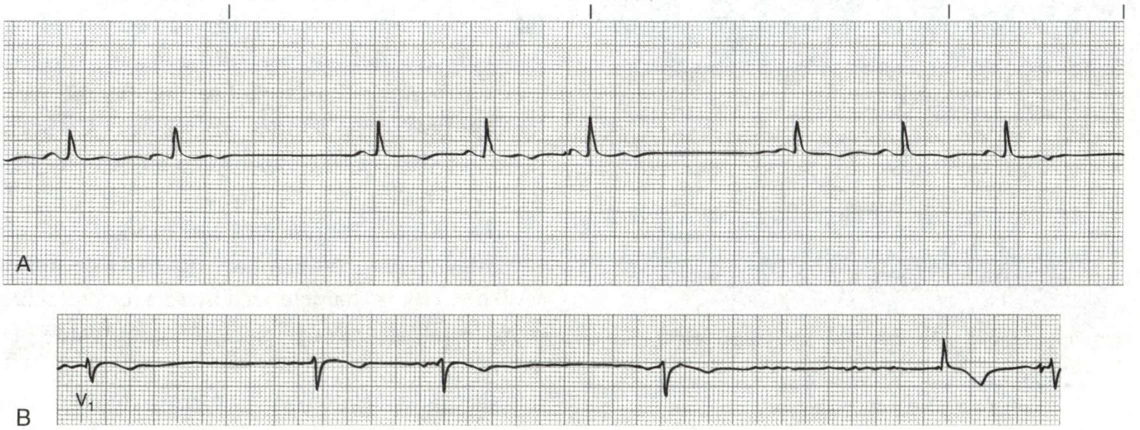

Fig. 14-10 A, Incomplete sinus block. B, sinus arrest with ventricular escape rhythm.

alternating with a tachydysrhythmia, typically Af. SSS is most common in elderly adults. It is also associated with cardiomyopathies, connective tissue diseases, and certain drugs. SSS is suspected when a patient has syncope and the ECG demonstrates sinus impulse abnormalities. Long-term management often requires permanent pacemaker placement for symptomatic bradycardia.

Atrioventricular Block

First-Degree Atrioventricular Block.

On the ECG, first-degree AVB is defined by a prolonged PR interval (>0.20 s), typically with a narrow QRS complex (Fig. 14-11).First-degree AVB requires no specific treatment.

Second-Degree Atrioventricular Block.

Second-degree AVB is characterized by one or more sinus impulses failing to reach the ventricles.

Second-degree AVB can be further classified into two types on the basis of the underlying pathophysiology and ECG appearance(Table 14-2).

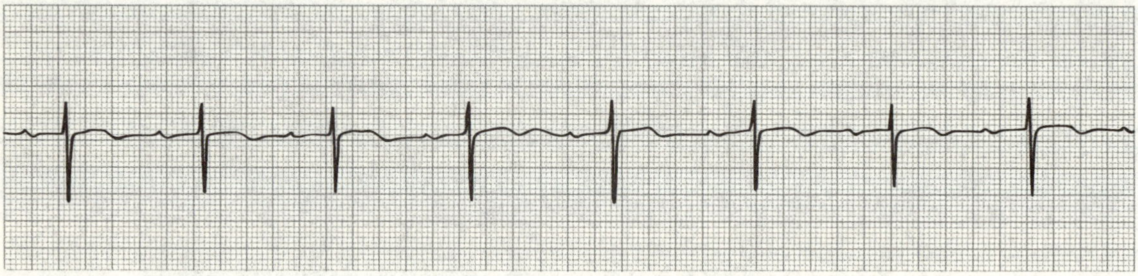

Fig. 14-11 First-degree AVB.

Table 14-2 Features of Type Ⅰ and Type Ⅱ Second-Degree Atrioventricular Block

FEATURE	TYPE Ⅰ (Wenckebach or Mobitz Ⅰ AVB)	TYPE Ⅱ (Mobitz Ⅱ block)
Clinical	Usually acute	Often chronic
	Inferior MI	Anteroseptal MI
	Rheumatic fever	Lenègre's disease Lev disease
	Digitalis or beta-blockers	Cardiomyopathy
Anatomic	Usually AV node	Infranodal
Electrophysiology	Increased relative refractory period	No relative refractory period
	Decremental conduction	All-or-none conduction
ECG features	RP/PR reciprocity	PR interval stable
	Prolonged PR interval	PR interval usually normal
	QRS duration normal	QRS duration prolonged
Response to atropine and exercise	Improves	Worsens
Response to carotid massage	Worsens	Improves*

*Primarily refers to conduction ratio.

Type Ⅰ Second-Degree AVB. Type Ⅰ second degree AVB, also called Wenckebach or Mobitz Ⅰ AVB. The surface ECG is characterized by a progressive lengthening of the PR interval until an impulse is not conducted(Fig. 14-12). By definition, the longest R-R interval (i.e.following the dropped beat) is less than twice the length of the shortest.

In the setting of an inferior AMI, this type of AVB is generally transient.

Type Ⅱ Second-Degree AVB. Type Ⅱ second-degree AVB, or Mobitz Ⅱ block, represents a conduction block just below the level of the AV node. On the surface ECG, conduction of atrial impulses is sporadic and typically periodic, but the PR interval does not widen (Fig. 14-13).

Type Ⅱ second-degree AVB generally carries a worse prognosis than type Ⅰ second-degree AVB. In AMI, type Ⅱ AVB often progresses to CHB. For patients with signs of hypoperfusion at rest, immediate temporary pacing is the treatment of choice.

Third-Degree Atrioventricular Block.

Third-degree AVB (also known as complete AVB or CHB) is characterized by absent conduction of all atrial impulses (Fig. 14-14) accompanied by a slow escape rhythm. Pacemakers above the His bundle are associated with anarrow-complex QRS at a rate of 45 to 60 beats/min, whereas pacemakers

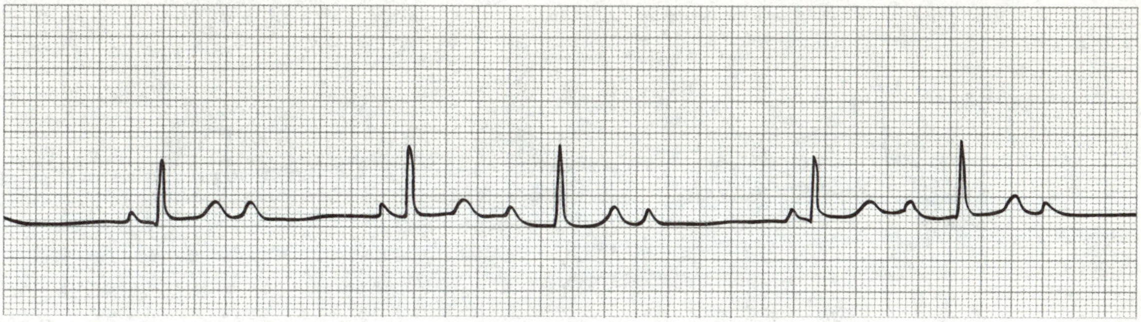

Fig. 14-12 Second-degree AVB, type Ⅰ (Wenckebach).

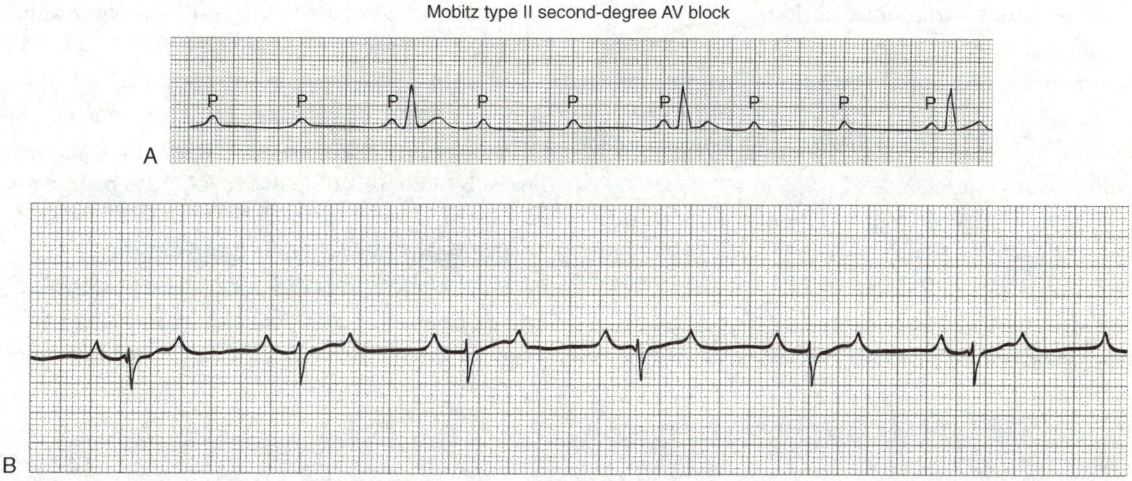

Fig. 14-13 A, Second-degree AVB, type Ⅱ. In this example, 3 : 1 conduction is shown. B, Second-degree AVB with 2 : 1 conduction.

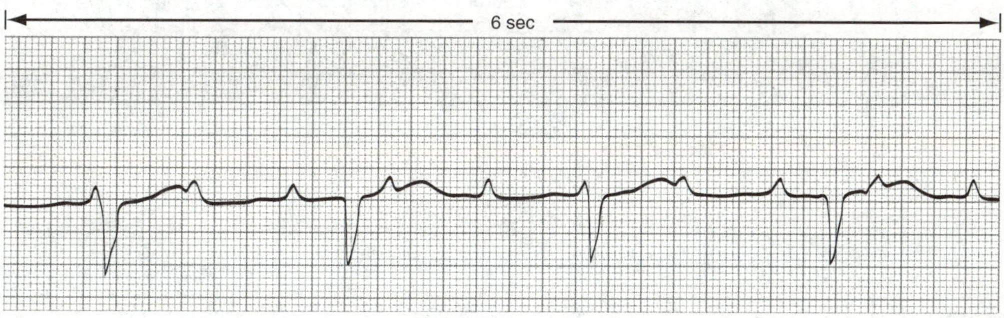

Fig. 14-14 CHB.

at or below the His bundle produce a wide-complex QRS at a rate of 30 to 45 beats/min.

The hallmark of CHB is AV dissociation, with an R-R interval that is longer than the P-P interval. Regularized Af occurs when accompanied by CHB.

CHB can be congenital, but newly symptomatic CHB is commonly acquired, which is an indication for admitting.

For patients with CHB who are markedly symptomatic, temporary pacing or a permanent pacemaker is placed.

Extrasystoles

An extrasystole is an electrical impulse originating from an ectopic atrial or ventricular focus. Bigeminy (Fig. 14-15) occurs when there is an extrasystole after every native beat; trigeminy (every third beat) and quadrigeminy (every fourth beat) are similar.

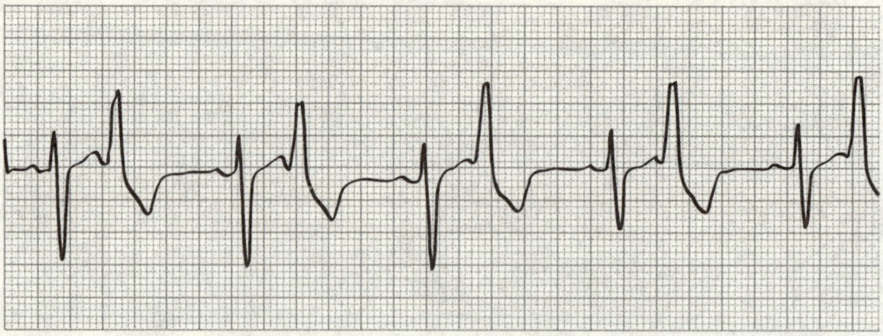

Fig. 14-15 Ventricular bigeminy.

Premature Atrial Contractions

Premature atrial contraction(PAC)(Fig. 14-16) are common. On occasion, a PAC can be the precipitant of Af, AF, or SVT. PAC can be distinguished on the ECG by the presence of an abnormal P wave early within a cardiac cycle.

Most PAC will depolarize the sinus node. Thus, the P-P interval between two sinus beats surrounding a PAC will be less than twice the intrinsic P-P cycle length (Fig. 14-16). A nonconducted (or blocked) PAC typically results in a noncompensatory pause (i.e.,R-R interval less than twice the intrinsic R-R cycle;Fig. 14-17).

If a PAC reaches the infranodal conducting system during its relative refractory period, the QRS complex may appear wide or aberrant, typically with a RBBB pattern. PAC are benign and require no specific treatment.

Premature Ventricular Contractions

PVC occurr in wide a variety of pathologic and nonpathologic states. Pathologic conditions associated with frequent PVC include AMI,

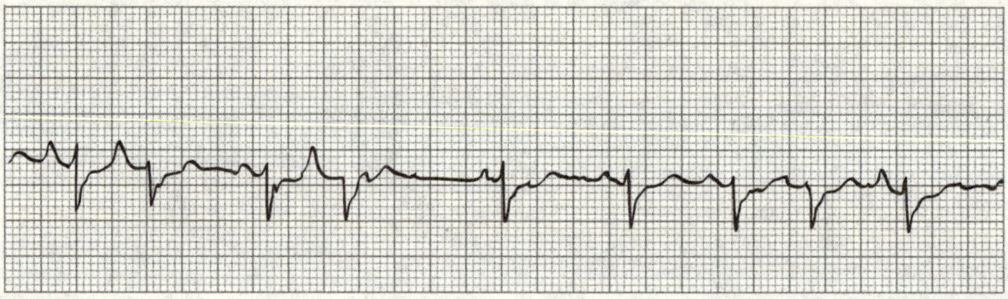

Fig. 14-16 PAC.

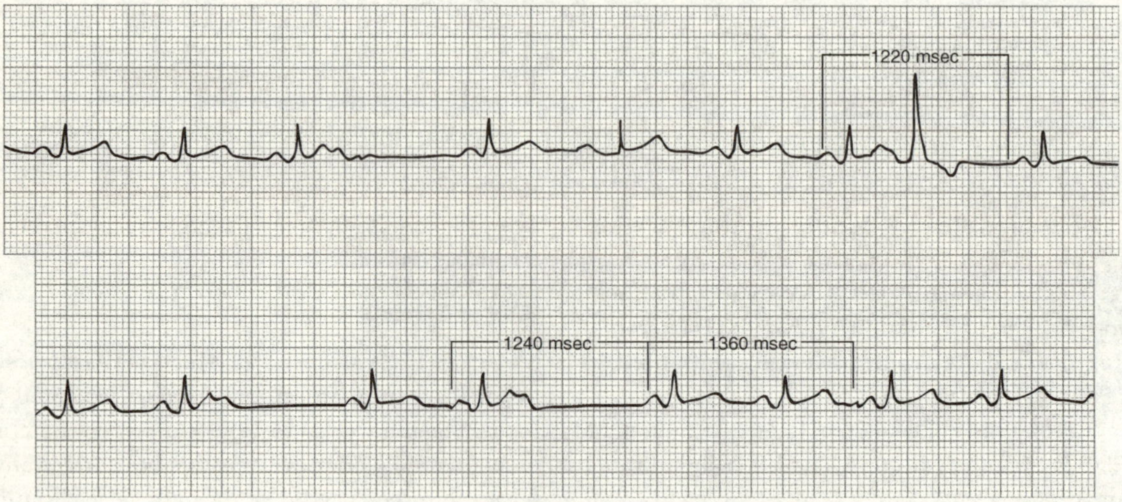

Fig. 14-17 PAC with noncompensatory pauses and one aberrantly conducted impulse (upper strip).

electrolyte disturbances, and medication toxicity.

A PVC appears as a wide-QRS complex extrasystole without a preceding P wave (Fig. 14-18). As a result, the R-R interval surrounding a PVC ends up being equal to twice the intrinsic R-R interval length (Fig. 14-18),known as a compensatory pause. Rarely, a PVC will capture the SA node, resulting in a noncompensatory pause, or will fail to capture the AV node, leaving the underlying rhythm completely unaffected (a so-called interpolated PVC; Fig. 14-19).

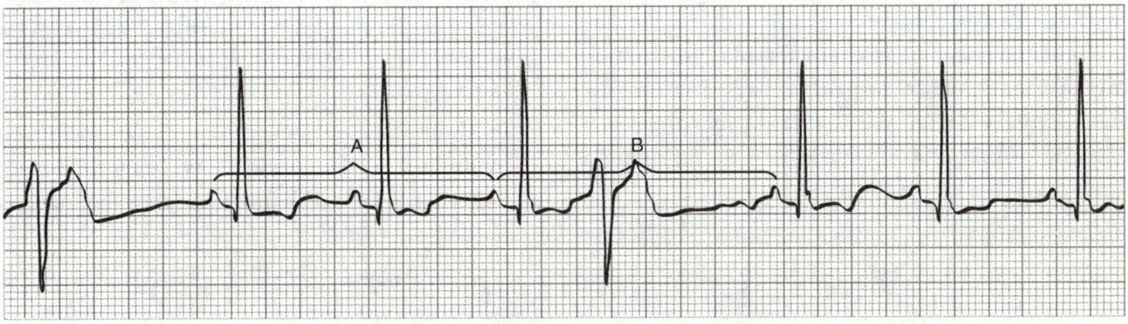

Fig. 14-18 PVC with compensatory pause. Note that a sinus P wave can be seen in the T wave of the extrasystolic beat. Also note the secondary T wave changes in beats 1 and 4 (T wave is opposite the main deflection of the QRS complex).

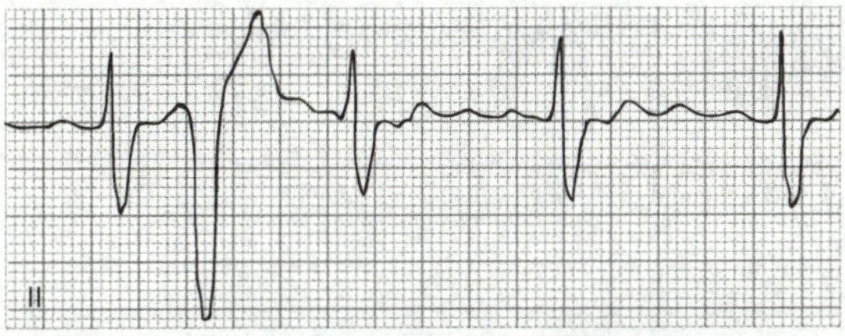

Fig. 14-19 Interpolated PVC.

The morphology of a PVC depends on the origin of the impulse. Table 14-3 notes common features of PAC and PVC.

Therapy for PVC is directed toward correcting any precipitating condition (Box 14-2), symptomatic PVC can be treated with low-dose beta-blocker. For patient with VTlidocaine is recommended .

Table 14-3 Features to Distinguish PAC with Abnormal Conduction from PVC

PAC	PVC
No compensatory pause	Fully compensatory pause (unless interpolated)
Preceding P wave (different from sinus P wave; occasionally buried in T wave)	No preceding P waves (although retrograde atrial conduction can cause inverted P wave after QRS)
Usually classic RBBB pattern (especially if long-short cycle sequence appears) identical to sinus QRS	LBBB, RBBB, or hybrid pattern
QRS axis normal or near normal	Frequently bizarre QRS axis
QRS rarely >0.14 s	QRS often >0.14 s

Box 14-2 Causes of PVC and VT

- AMI or previous MI or ischemia
- Hypokalemia
- Hypoxemia
- Ischemic heart disease
- Valvular disease
- Catecholamine excess*
- Other drug intoxications (especially cyclic antidepressants)
- Idiopathic causes
- Digitalis toxicity
- Hypomagnesemia
- Hypercapnia
- Class I antidysrhythmic agents
- Ethanol
- Myocardial contusion
- Cardiomyopathy
- Acidosis
- Alkalosis
- Methylxanthine toxicity

*Relative increase in sympathetic tone from drugs or conditions that augment catecholamine release or decrease parasympathetic tone.

Narrow-Complex Tachycardia

Narrow-complex tachycardias are defined by a QRS complex duration of 0.12 s or less on surface ECG with a ventricular rate of greater than 100 beats/min.

Sinus Tachycardia

Sinus tachycardia is characterized electrocardiographically by a regular, narrow-complex tachycardia with normal P waves preceding each QRS complex (Fig. 14-20). In adults, sinus tachycardia rarely exceeds a rate of 170 beats/min.

Sinus tachycardia is often a response to physiologic stress, as seen with hypovolemia, anemia, pain, anxiety, fever, hyperthyroidism, drugs or hypoxemia.

Atrial Tachycardia

The hallmark of atrial tachycardia (AT) is the presence morphologically abnormal P waves on the surface ECG (Fig. 14-21).

AT is often precipitated by the occurrence of a PAC. Multifocal atrial tachycardia (MAT) is a form of AT with three or more distinct P wave morphologies, and varying PR and P-P intervals from the multiple

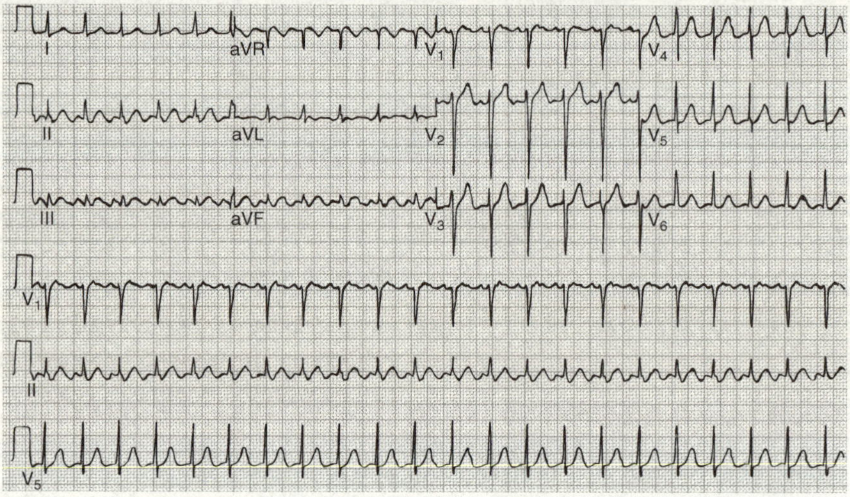

Fig. 14-20 Sinus tachycardia.

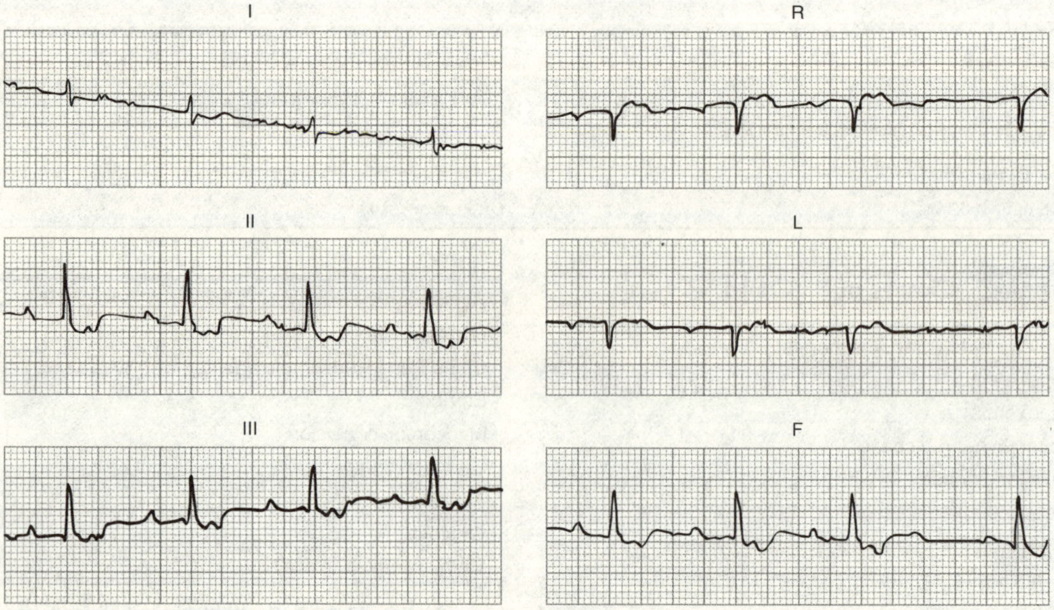

Fig. 14-21 AT(with 2 : 1 conduction) in a patient with digitalis toxicity.

ectopic atrial foci (Fig. 14-22).MAT is associated with COPD and primary cardiac pathology. The approach to patients with AT or MAT is based on identifying and treating any precipitating factors.

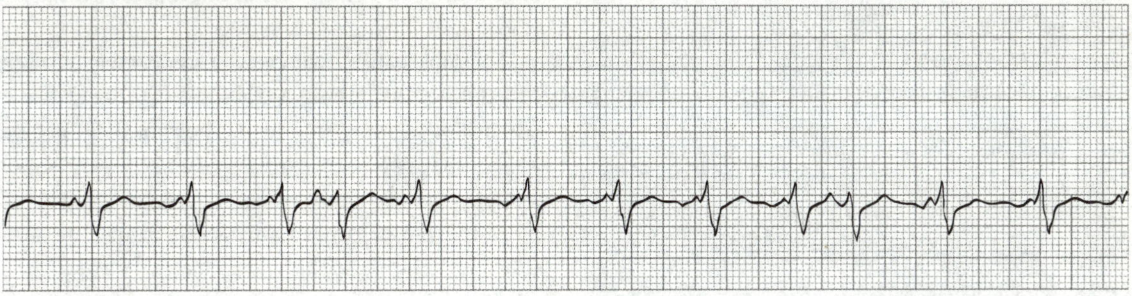

Fig. 14-22 MAT.

Atrial Fibrillation

Af may be paroxysmal, persistent, or permanent, and long-term approaches to management depend on many factors, including chronicity, symptomatology, underlying heart disease, and other comorbidities.

The ECG hallmark of Af is a"irregularly irregular" QRS pattern (Fig. 14-23). Af is the most common cause of an irregular ventricular rhythm. Af waves appear "coarse" or "fine" on the basis of their amplitude and are often best appreciated in the inferior leads or lead V_1.The ventricular rate in Af rarely exceeding 150 to 170 beats/min .Patients with Af are at risk for developing left atrial thrombi.

The Ashman phenomenon refers to aberrant ventricular conduction (Fig. 14-24). Ashman beats can be mistaken for PVC or paroxysmal VT.

Af is most commonly associated with underlying heart disease, HTN or hyperthyroidism (Box 14-3).

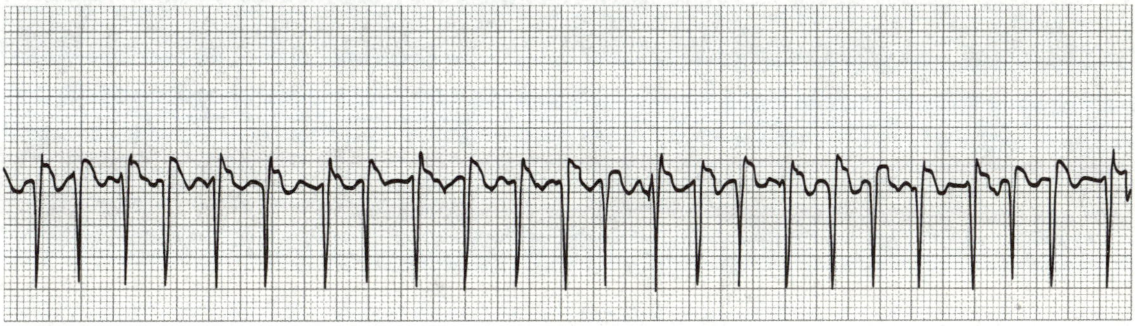

Fig. 14-23 Af with rapid ventricular response.

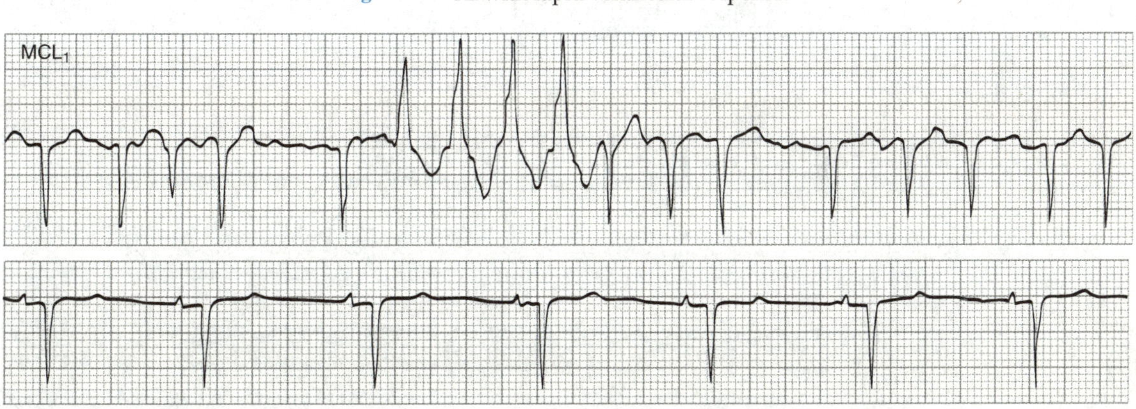

Fig. 14-24 Af with classic Ashman phenomenon series of beats. Note long-short cycle before aberrantly conducted impulses that are sustained for four beats.

Box 14-3 Causes of Atrial Fibrillation

- Hypertensive heart disease
- Cardiomyopathy
- Ischemic heart disease
- Valvular disease (especially mitral)
- CHF
- Pericarditis
- Hyperthyroidism
- SSS
- Myocardial contusion
- Acute ethanol intoxication
- Idiopathic
- Cardiac surgery
- Catecholamine excess
- PE
- Accessory pathway syndrome or(Wolff-Parkinson-White syndrome,WPWS)

For stable patients with recurrent rapid Af, administration of a nodal blocking agent. Intravenous diltiazem and verapamil or metoprolol offer the advantage of being easily titrated.

For stable patients with new-onset or newly recurrent Af—defined as having a duration of 72hr or less—ED cardioversion is an option. The choice of electrical versus pharmacologic cardioversion is dependent on institutional factors and patient preference.

Many patients with Af benefit from long-term anticoagulation as prophylaxis against stroke.

Atrial Flutter

AF is defined by atrial depolarization occurring at a regular rate of 250 to 350 beats/min caused by an atrial reentry mechanism (Fig. 14-25). So-called flutter waves are distinguished by their broad, sawtooth appearance on the surface ECG. With 2:1 conduction, the ventricular rate is approximately 150 beats/min.

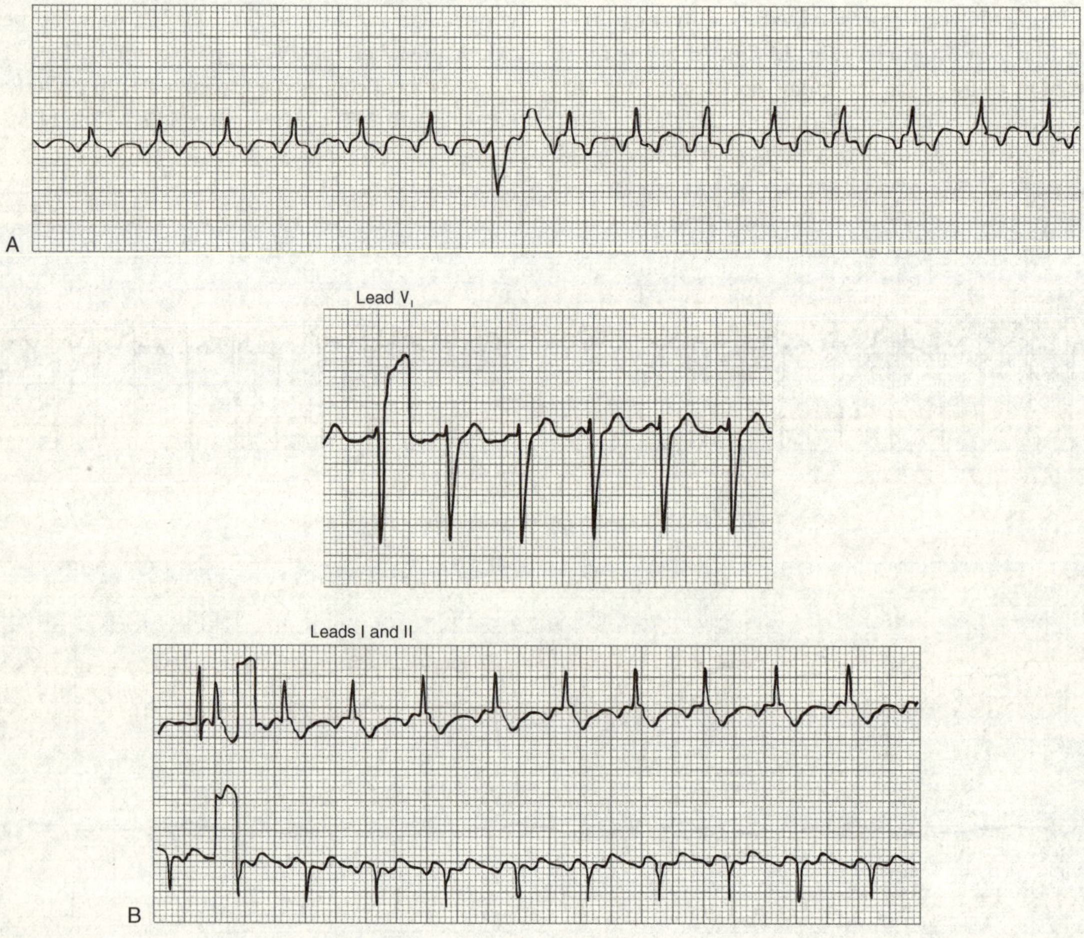

Fig. 14-25 A, AF with 2 : 1 conduction . B, AF with 2 : 1 conduction.

AF can be associated with structural heart disease, particularly valvular heart disease and cardiomyopathies.

Atrioventricular Nodal Reentrant Tachycardia

Also known by the less precise term paroxysmal supraventricular tachycardia, AV nodal reentrant tachycardia(AVNRT) is characterized by a regular narrow complex rhythm and a ventricular rate of 160 beats/min or greater (Fig. 14-26).

The onset of AVNRT is typically abrupt and frequently arises. Termination is also abrupt. Most patients with AVNRT are symptomatic. If vagal maneuvers fail to restore sinus rhythm, ED therapy for AVNRT is adenosine. In refractory cases, diltiazem, esmolol, or metoprolol may be used. Rarely, synchronized cardioversion is required.

Patients with frequent recurrences are candidates for prophylaxis (typically with a beta-blocker or calcium channel blocker) or ablation therapy.

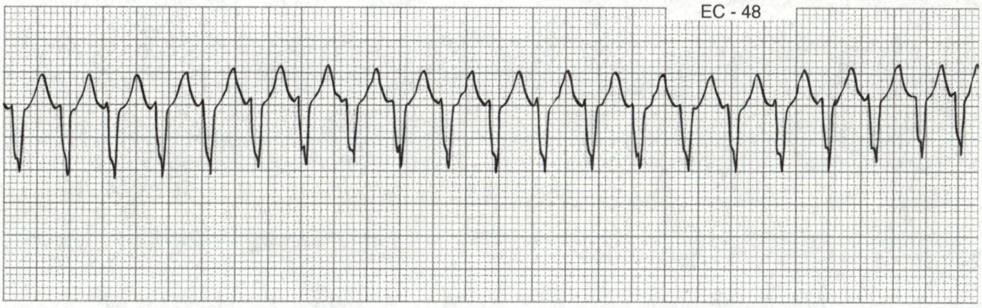

Fig. 14-26 paroxysmal supraventricular tachycardia.

Junctional Tachycardia

JT (also known as nonparoxysmal or sustained JT) showed sustained ventricular rates but rarely exceed 130 beats/min. JT is commonly associated with structural heart disease, metabolic disturbances, or drug toxicity. Treatment is aimed at addressing underlying conditions.

Preexcitation and Accessory Pathway Syndromes

Preexcitation refers to depolarization of the ventricular myocardium by circumvention of the AV node via an accessory pathway or bypass tract linking the atria to the ventricles. Accessory pathways lend themselves to reentry tachycardias and very rapid ventricular rates. WPWS characterized by paroxysmal tachycardia and the following three resting ECG features (Fig. 14-27):

- A short PR interval (<0.12 s)
- QRS duration greater than 0.10 second
- A slurred upstroke to the QRS complex, referred to as a delta wave

The majority of patients with WPWS have no underlying structural heart disease .

Orthodromic AV-reentrant tachycardia is indistinguishable clinically from AVNRT and is treated with vagal maneuvers and adenosine as first-line therapy, followed by CCB and beta-blockers as second-line agents.

In contrast, antidromic AV-reentrant tachycardia often causes a very rapid rate (200 beats/min or greater) and a wide-complex QRS. In this situation, AV nodal blocking agents are contraindicated.

Unopposed retrograde conduction through the AV node can result in Vf. Likewise, with a very rapid irregular tachycardia accompanied by a wide-complex QRS. Procainamide is recommended any time an accessory pathway with wide QRS complexes or very rapid rates exists, with amiodarone as a secondary choice.

Electrical cardioversion (100-200 J) is indicated for ventricular rates greater than 250 beats/min.

The Lown-Ganong-Levine syndrome is an uncommon accessory pathway syndrome associated with paroxysmal narrow-complex tachycardia, a short PR interval, and a normal QRS complex without a delta wave. The treatment parallels that for the WPWS.

Wide-Complex Tachycardias

Wide-complex tachycardia accompanied by a QRS duration of 0.12 s or more can derive from the ventricles themselves or can result from a tachycardia originating at or above the AV node accompanied by aberrant AV conduction (Table 14-4).

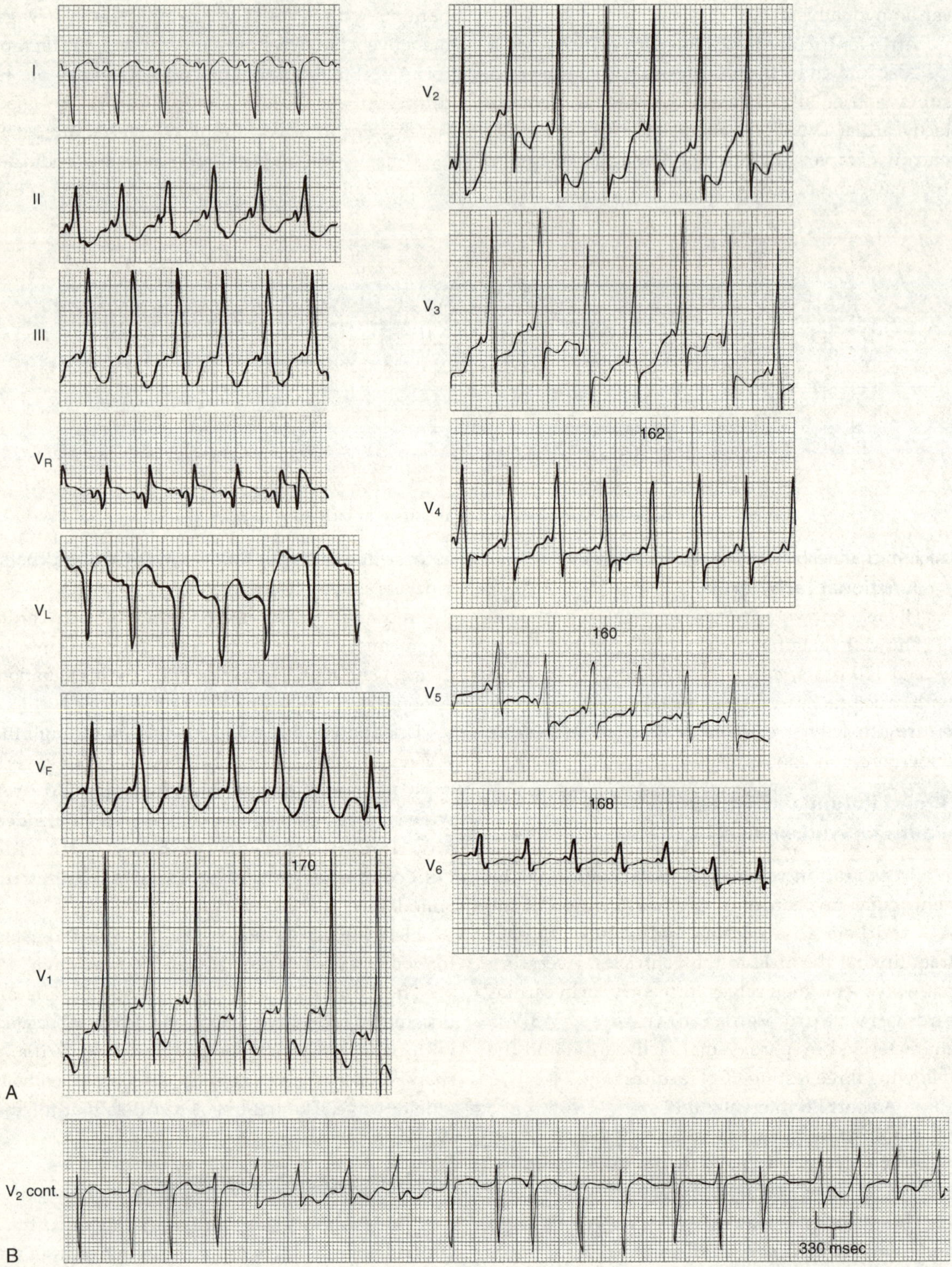

Figure. 14-27 A, WPWS. B, WPWS with Af.

Table 14-4 **Features Helpful in Distinguishing VT from SVT with Abnormal Conduction**

	VENTRICULAR TACHYCARDIA	SVT PLUS ABERRANCY
Clinical features	Age 50 or older	Age 35 or younger
	History of MI,CHF, CABG, or CAD	None
	Previous history of VT	Previous history of SVT
Physical examination	Cannon A waves	Absent
	Variation in arterial pulse	Absence of variability
	Variable first heart sound	Absence of variability
ECG	Fusion beats	None
	AV dissociation	Preceding P waves with QRS complexes
	QRS >0.14 s	QRS usually <0.14 s
	Extreme LAD artery (30 degrees)	Axis normal or near normal
	No response to vagal maneuvers	Slow or terminate with vagal maneuvers
Specific QRS patterns	V_1: R, qR, or RS	V_1: rSR′
	V_6: S, rS, or qR	V_6: qRs
	Identical to previous VT tracing*	Identical to previous SVT tracing*
	Concordance of positivity or negativity	

*If proven by electrophysiologic studies or by a preponderance of evidence.

Ventricular Tachycardia

VT originates within or below the His bundle. Nonsustained VT refers to short episodes (<30 s).Monomorphic VT is the most common form of VT at a rate of 150 to 200 beats/min (Fig. 14-28). Polymorphic VT is seen with varying QRS morphologies and suggests more severe underlying disease (Fig. 14-29, Fig. 14-30).Most patients with VT have ischemic or nonischemic cardiomyopathy.

For stable patients with VT, amiodarone or lidocaine are first-line choices in ED. Procainamide is a second-line agent. Unstable patients or those with VT refractory to drug therapy should undergo synchronized cardioversion with 100 J, with escalating doses (up to 200 J biphasic or 360 J monophasic) as needed.

Torsades de Pointes

Torsades de pointes is literally translated as "twisting of the points" and is a paroxysmal form of polymorphic VT that meets the following clinical criteria (Fig. 14-30):

1. Ventricular rate greater than 200 beats/min
2. Undulating QRS axis, with the polarity of the complexes appearing to shift about the baseline
3. Paroxysms of less than 90 s

A prolonged QT interval can be congenital or acquired. Acquired torsades de pointes is much more common than congenital and is termed "pause dependent". Acquired QT prolongation is often multifactorial (Box 14-4).Common triggers include electrolyte disturbances (hypokalemia and hypomagnesemia) and many different drugs (notably class IA and IC agents but also many others; see Box 14-4). Treatment of torsades de pointes instable patients involves correcting any underlying metabolic or electrolyte abnormalities and increasing the heart rate to shorten ventricular repolarization. For obvious reasons, classes IA and IC antidysrhythmics are contraindicated. Intravenous magnesium sulfate should be given empirically.

A baseline ventricular rate of 100 to 120 is usually enough to prevent acquired torsades de pointes and can be achieved by overdrive pacing or via beta-adrenergic infusion. Unstable patients with sustained torsades de pointes should be electrically cardioverted.

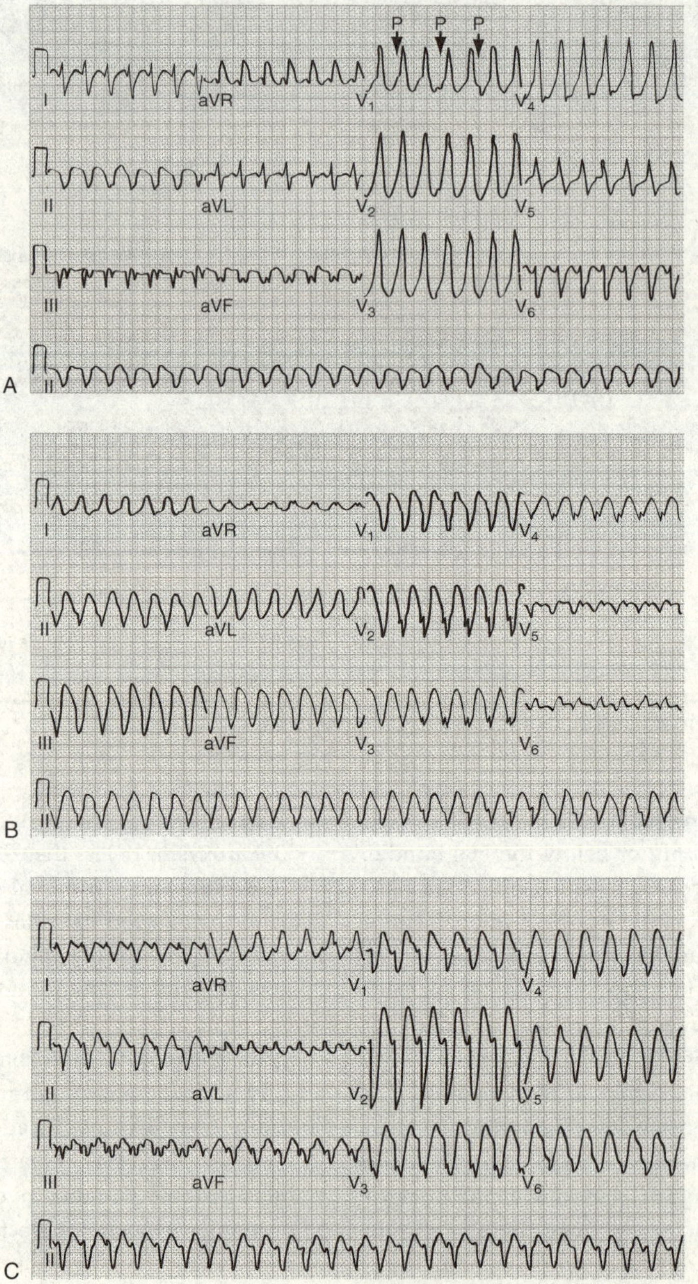

Fig. 14-28 VT. A, RS complexes are present in chest leads, but RS duration is greater than 100 ms. Although the Brugada criteria indicate that no further analysis is necessary, atrioventricular dissociation is also evident, and QRS morphology in lead V_6 is consistent with VT. B, Some RS complexes are present, RS duration is not greater than 100 ms, and atrioventricular dissociation is difficult to appreciate; morphologic criteria for VT are fulfilled because S is notched in V_1 and QR is present in V_6.C, Diagnosis is based on morphologic criteria because S is notched in V_1 and V_2 and QS is present in V_6.

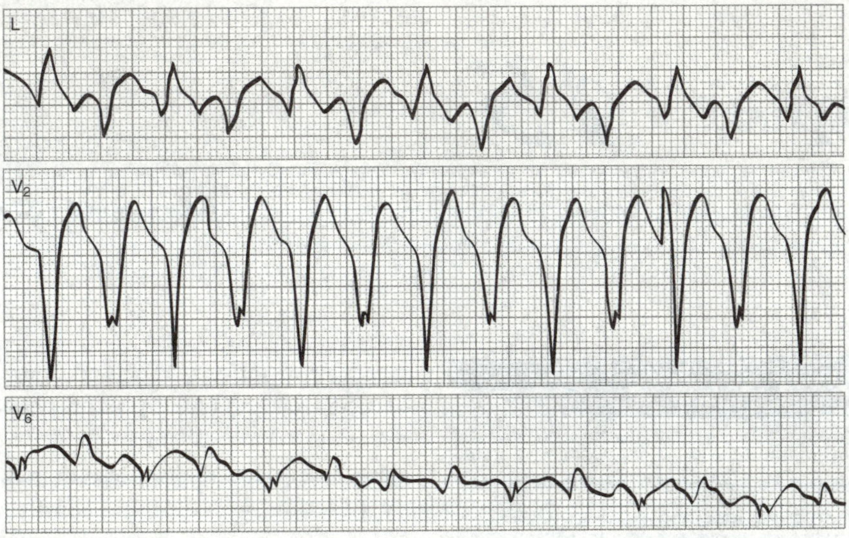

Fig. 14-29 Bidirectional VT in a patient with digitalis toxicity.

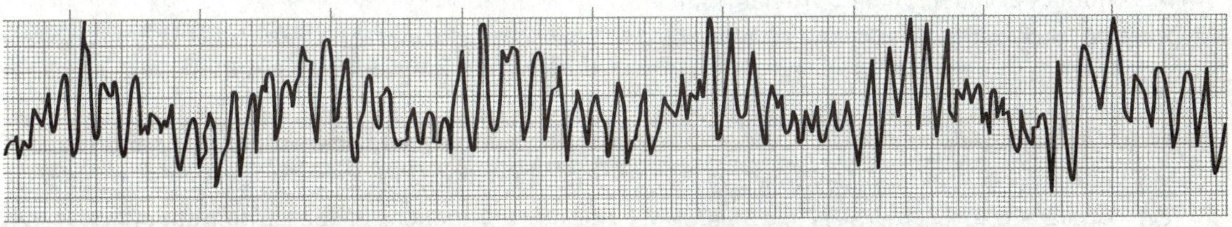

Fig. 14-30 Torsades de pointes with classic spiraling of QRS complexes around baseline.

Box 14-4 Classification and Causes of Prolonged QT Syndromes

Pause Dependent (Acquired)

Drug induced: Class IA and IC antidysrhythmics; many phenothiazines and butyrophenones (notably haloperidol and droperidol), cyclic antidepressants, antibiotics (especially macrolides), organophosphates, antihistamines, antifungals,antiseizure and antiemetic agents

Electrolyte abnormalities: hypokalemia, hypomagnesemia, hypocalcemia (rarely)

Diet related: starvation, low protein

Severe bradycardia or AVB

Hypothyroidism

Contrast injection

Cerebrovascular accident

Myocardial ischemia

Adrenergic Dependent (Tachycardia Prompted)

Congenital

Jervell and Lange-Nielsen syndrome (deafness, autosomalrecessive)

Romano-Ward syndrome (normal hearing, autosomal dominant)

Sporadic (normal hearing, no familial tendency)

Mitral valve prolapse

Acquired (Rare)

Cerebrovascular disease

Autonomic surgery: radical neck dissection, carotid endarterectomy, truncal vagotomy

Patients with congenital torsades de pointes often have syncope during exertion and a prolonged QT interval on the ECG, and it is treated with a beta-blocker.

(CHAI Yanfen)

Chapter 15

Heart Failure

KEY CONCEPTS

HF may be defined as the pathophysiologic state in which the heart is incapable of pumping a sufficient supply of blood to meet the metabolic requirements of the body or requires elevated ventricular filling pressures to accomplish this goal.

Neurohormonal mechanisms provide initial compensation for cardiac dysfunction but are ultimately deleterious in HF.

Recognition of precipitating causes in HF allows more disease-specific management.

Biomarkers such as BNP may improve recognition of HF in dyspnea of questionable cause, correlate with severity, help stratify risk, and help monitor therapeutic response.

Most acute HF can be managed with upright positioning, supplemental oxygen, vasodilators, and loop diuretics.

Patients with poor perfusion may require fluid challenge to rapidly restore preload, CO, systemic perfusion, and BP.

In hypoperfusing patients who are adequately volume repleted, norepinephrine is the pressor of choice.

In chronic HF, routine use of beta-blockers, ACEI or ARB, diuretics including spironolactone, and occasionally digoxin has resulted in sustained symptomatic improvement and reduced 5 yr mortality.

HF is a debilitating cardiac syndrome characterized by dyspnea, poor exercise tolerance, and chronic fatigue. HF may be defined as the pathophysiologic state in which the heart is incapable of pumping a sufficient supply of blood to meet the metabolic requirements of the body or requires elevated ventricular filling pressures to accomplish this goal. Conversely, low filling pressure with hypoperfusion indicates a pump-priming problem distinct from cardiac disease. The American Heart Association(AHA) and American College of Cardiology (ACC) guidelines define HF related to systolic dysfunction as a left ventricular ejection fraction (LVEF) less than 40%. Diastolic dysfunction, a pathologic condition involving failure of ventricular relaxation with consequent high filling pressures, may exist in up to half of older individuals with HF.

HF is a progressive and multifaceted disease that begins long before symptoms and signs are evident. A complex neurohormonal regulatory relationship exists between the heart and multiple organ systems(Fig. 15-1). Dysfunction of the heart or any component of the cardiopulmonary system initiates adaptive neurohormonal activation of the SNS, RAAS, NP, endothelin (ET), vasopressin, and other regulatory mechanisms. Neurohormonal activation initially compensates for circulatory system dysfunction. These mechanisms eventually lead to increased mechanical stress on the failing heart, however, causing maladaptive electrical and structural events, progressive cardiac fibrosis and apoptosis, and further impairment of systolic and diastolic function.

EPIDEMIOLOGY

HF is a common cause of poor quality of life and premature death. About 5,800,000 individuals (approximately 2% of the population) in the United States in 2009 had HF, and almost 550,000 new cases are diagnosed annually. The incidence approaches 10 per 1000 in people older than 65 yr. The ED is the main portal of entry for acute HF patients.

HF carries approximately a 50% mortality at

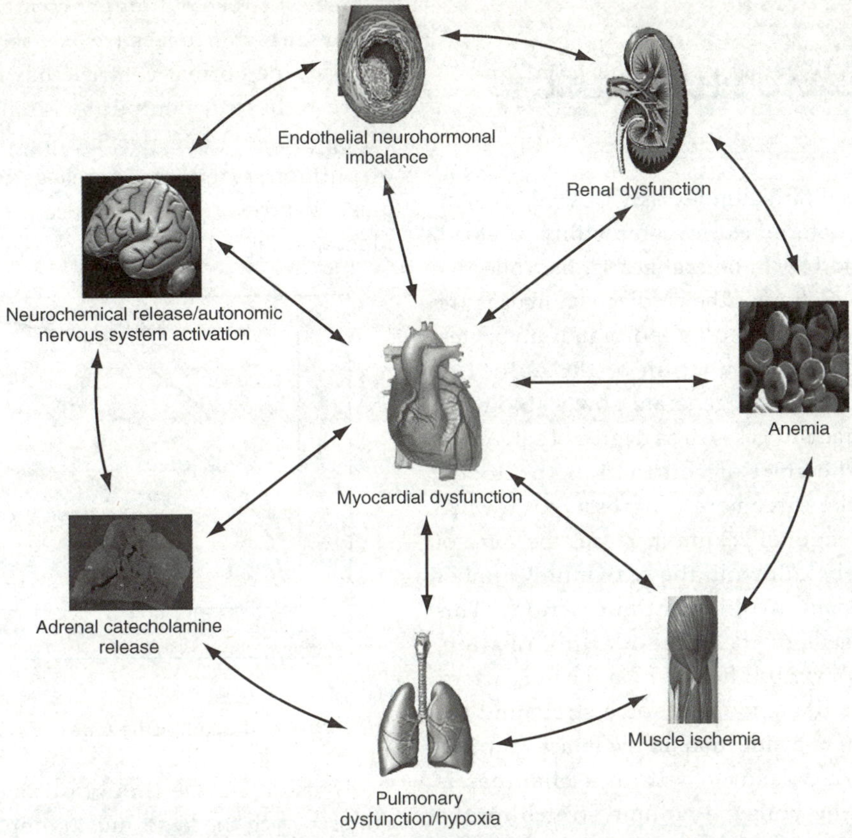

Fig. 15-1 The neurohormonal model of HF describes a complex interdependence among many organ systems in which a functional disturbance in any component causes complex compensatory changes in the others that are eventually maladaptive.

5 yr after symptom onset.

The prognosis in HF is related to a number of factors, including age, LVEF, exercise tolerance, plasma norepinephrine and BNP levels, cardiothoracic ratio on chest radiograph, resting HR, ECG evidence of LVH, Af, or presence of ventricular dysrhythmias, hemoglobin A1c level, and renal function. Renal insufficiency is one of the strongest predictors of mortality in patients with HF.

CELLULAR MECHANISMS

The heart is composed of a mass of individual striated muscle cells (myocytes) that form a branching syncytium. Each myocyte contains the sarcoplasmic reticulum, and myofibrils. Myofibrils, in turn, contain sarcomeres, which form the basic functional unit of myocardial contraction. Sarcomeres occupy approximately 50% of myocardial cell mass and are composed of contractile proteins actin and myosin along with regulatory proteins troponin and tropomyosin.

The sarcomere ranges in length from 1.6 to 2.2 μm, depending in part on the tension exerted on the muscle before contraction (preload). Sarcomere contraction occurs when thin, double-helix actin is exposed to thick myofilament myosin. Contraction as well as relaxation is controlled by calcium ion (Ca^{2+}) release from the sarcoplasmic reticulum. Intracellular ionic calcium is thus the principal mediator of the inotropic state of the heart and is mainly stored and regulated by the sarcoplasmic reticulum. Most positive inotropic agents, including digitalis and catecholamines, act by increasing availability of intracellular calcium. On the downside, increased intracellular calcium reduces diastolic relaxation.

CARDIAC PHYSIOLOGY

The normal cardiac index is 2.5 to 4.0 L/min/m^2 at rest. It is determined by contractility, preload, afterload, and HR. In normal hearts, the collective force of contraction of the cardiac chamber is the sum of forces generated by individual myocytes. Myocyte force is a function of the ability of contractile proteins to generate power (inotropic state or contractility) as well as degree of sarcomere stretch at the start of contraction (preload). Stretching the sarcomere progressively toward its optimal length of 2.2 μm increases the force of contraction by allowing the maximum number of actin-myosin myofilament interactions. This forms the basis of the Frank-Starling relation. Contractility may be affected by a host of factors.

Preload is the amount of force stretching the myofibril before contraction. In the intact ventricle, the pressure measured within a chamber is determined by both the volume stretching the chamber wall and compliance characteristics of the muscle. Changes in compliance may occur acutely with ischemia or chronically with hypertrophy and may substantially alter the relationship between chamber volume, pressure, and preload (Fig. 15-2).

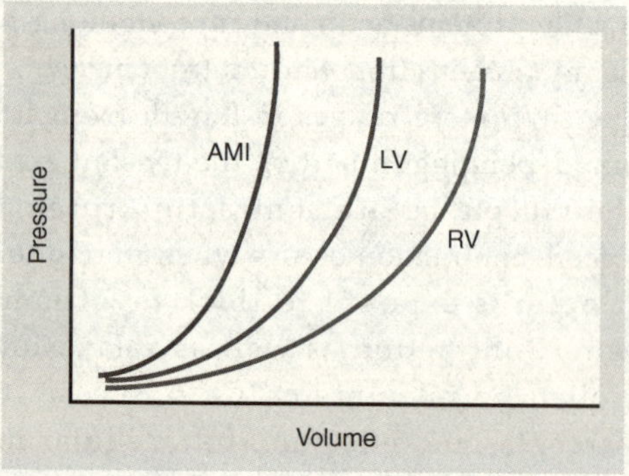

Fig. 15-2 The end-diastolic pressure of the chamber is determined by the filling volume and the compliance characteristics of the chamber. The RV is more compliant than the more muscular LV, which becomes stiffer still under conditions of ischemia or AMI.

Optimal preload is the filling pressure that stretches ventricular myofibrils maximally and leads to greatest stroke output per contraction(Fig.15-3). Accordingly, if pressure is used to estimate preload, the normal ventricle has more dramatic increases in stroke output for similar increases in filling pressure (steeper Starling curve).The risk of pulmonary edema increases when LV end-diastolic pressure rises significantly above normal ranges(6-12 mm Hg).

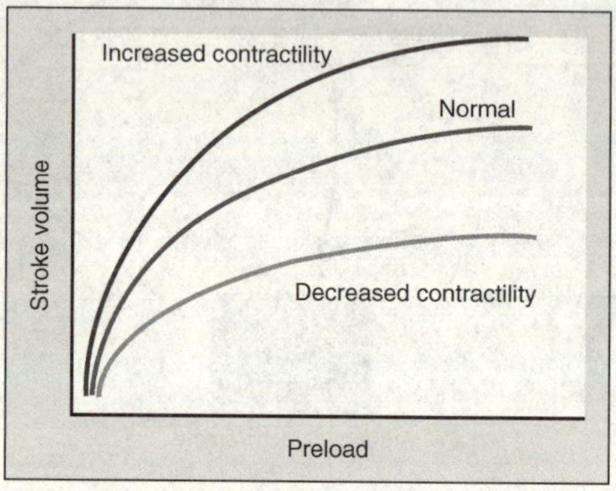

Fig. 15-3 Increased preload improves stroke volume irrespective of the contractile state of the ventricle.

Afterload can be thought of as the pressure against which the heart must pump to eject blood. BP is determined by the product of CO and systemic vascular resistance (BP = CO × SVR). HTN is a major contributor to HF in about 75% of cases. Patients with HF and low CO tend to maintain BP through peripheral vasoconstriction mediated mainly by endogenous catecholamines and the RAAS. The peripheral resistance is affected by the total cross-sectional area of the circulation, the blood viscosity, and other factors. The arterioles are the major resistance vessels in the circulation. Flow is directly proportional to the fourth power of the vessel radius (Poiseuille's law).The larger the ventricular cavity, the more mural tension and thus myocardial work is required during contraction (law of Laplace).

Failing ventricles have difficulty overcoming increases in peripheral resistance, instead dilating further, increasing end diastolic volume to maintain SV, even with decreasing ejection fraction(EF) (preload reserve).Failing hearts are therefore extremely afterload sensitive, and modest vasodilation can dramatically increase CO, particularly in those most compromised (Fig. 15-4). Afterload reduction may be beneficial because it

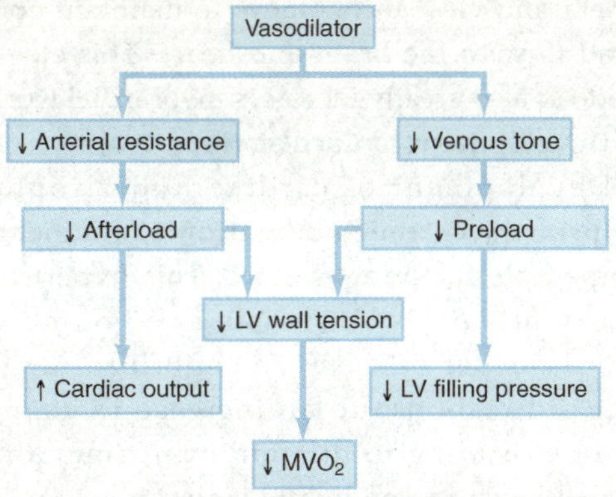

Fig. 15-4 Arterial vasodilators decrease resistance to flow and result in increased CO_2. Venodilators decrease venous return to the heart and relieve pulmonary congestion.

allows conversion of pressure work into flow work. When BP is decreased, CO increases as long as preload is maintained.

HR and rhythmic contraction are important determinants of optimal CO (CO = HR × SV).As HR increases to the range of 150 to 160 beats/min in the adult, CO increases progressively. Tachycardia above this level compromises diastolic filling time and may lead to decreased CO. Coronary perfusion, also becomes impaired by severe tachycardia.SV is maximized when atrial contraction "primes" the ventricular pumps before they contract. Therefore any derangement of intracardiac conduction or dysrhythmia can reduce SV. Loss of atrial priming (e.g., in Af) can lead to marked deterioration in CO, especially in diseased, stiffer hearts that require high filling pressures to optimize preload.

PRIMARY DISEASE PROCESSES RESULTING IN HEART FAILURE

HF can result from primary disease of coronary arteries, myocardium, cardiac valves, pericardium, peripheral vessels, or lungs. Frequently the cause is multifactorial.

Coronary Artery Disease

In developed countries, atherosclerotic CAD remains the leading cause of HF. Acute coronary thrombosis leads to focal myocardial necrosis, with resultant fibrosis and scarring. This process leads to areas of dyskinesis that result in decreased EF. Aneurysmal dilation of infarcted areas with paradoxical motion during systole may disproportionately decrease EF. When approximately 40% of the LV muscle mass is acutely infarcted, cardiogenic shock ensues. Transient loss of contractile function may result from episodes of myocardial ischemia that do not cause frank necrosis, or from an ischemic zone surrounding the infarct. This "myocardial stunning" may persist for several days.

Chronic coronary insufficiency leads to a more diffuse myocardial fibrosis termed ischemic cardiomyopathy. Revascularization of ischemic provides a survival benefit in patients with HF related to ischemic LV systolic dysfunction. Diseases affecting the coronary microcirculation, such as vaso-occlusive sickle cell anemia and diabetes mellitus, result in similar pathology. Compensatory mechanisms may occur after large AMI and progressive cardiac disease, which are collectively termed ventricular remodeling. They include cardiac dilation, reactive hypertrophy, progressive fibrosis, and changes in wall conformation. These may result from elevated chamber filling pressures as well as neurohumoral adaptive responses.

Cardiomyopathy and Myocarditis

Clinically, patients with cardiomyopathy tend to have three forms—dilated, hypertrophic, or restrictive—each associated with HF. DCM is much more common than the other two and is the second most common cause of HF.

Valvular Heart Disease

Cardiac valvular disease is the third leading cause of HF. Most acute valvular dysfunction involves either the mitral or the aortic valve, and usually results in severe regurgitation. Acutely stenotic lesions are predominantly restricted to mechanical catastrophes of prosthetic valves. These patients may be in extremis with fulminant pulmonary edema.

Pericardial Diseases

Pericardial diseases may significantly affect ventricular function, decreasing CO and increasing intracardiac pressures. In particular, cardiac tamponade may cause dyspnea and hypoperfusion not easily clinically distinguished from HF.ED use of bedside ultrasound has great usefulness in rapidly identifying this problem.

Pulmonary Disease

COPD may obscure recognition of HF. Hypoxia caused by pulmonary dysfunction leads to pulmonary arteriolar vasoconstriction, reducing lung vascular bed area and elevating pulmonary artery pressures. Chronic increases in pulmonary arterial pressure lead to RV hypertrophy and dilation. When compensatory mechanisms fail, the patient develops right-sided HF (cor pulmonale), usually with LV output preserved, at least at rest. Causes of acute cor pulmonale, such as a large pulmonary embolus, may precipitate sudden systemic hypotension and death.

Distinguishing primary pulmonary disease causing predominantly right-sided HF from LV failure with secondary right-sided dysfunction is clinically challenging. NP levels are only slightly elevated in primary pulmonary disease compared with much higher levels in LV failure.

COMPENSATORY MECHANISMS IN HEART FAILURE

Physiologic Mechanisms

Increase in Stroke Volume

Increased SV occurs in response to increase in preload (Frank-Starling mechanism).This compensatory mechanism is immediate and effective in improving CO in response to acute systemic demands. It is a limited response, however, because myofibril stretch to a sarcomere length beyond 2.2 μm does not further increase and may actually reduce stroke output. Also, this mechanism greatly increases myocardial oxygen demand, which may lead to dysfunction in the setting of significant CAD.

Increased Systemic Vascular Resistance

Increased systemic vascular resistance results in redistribution of a subnormal CO away from skin, skeletal muscles, and kidneys to maintain normal blood flow to the brain and heart. This elevated afterload also greatly increases myocardial work.

Development of Cardiac Hypertrophy

Development of cardiac hypertrophy is the primary chronic adaptation of the heart to compensate for pump failure. This hypertrophy occurs mainly by increasing the number of myofibrils per cell. New myofibrils arrange in series in response to an increase in chamber volume (leading to dilation over time) and in parallel when responding to higher pressure loads (leading to increased chamber wall thickness). In addition to myofibril hypertrophy, mitochondrial mass expands, leading to additional adenosine triphosphate(ATP) provision for the expanded myofibril mass.

Initially, hypertrophy leads to improved function of each myocardial cell but at a higher energy cost. Relative capillary blood flow is reduced, leading to progressive myocyte death with fibrosis and increased stress on the remaining myocytes. Thus the hypertrophic response eventually becomes maladaptive, accelerating myocyte death and reducing pump function. This process gradually occurs as a normal part of aging.

Neurohormonal Modulation

Neurohormonal mechanisms maintain BP and vital organ perfusion and are activated by LV dysfunction. Regrettably, these neurohormonal mechanisms also increase the hemodynamic burden and oxygen consumption of the failing ventricle and are counterproductive on a chronic basis.

Cardiac Neurohormonal Response

Increases in myocardial wall stretch activate release of cardiac natriuretic peptides, which are structurally related proteins important in volume and sodium homeostasis. They include atrial, brain (BNP), and C-type natriuretic peptide. All are elevated in patients with LV dysfunction and HF.A variety of NP receptors exist on endothelial cells, vascular smooth muscle cells, and renal epithelial cells and in the myocardium. NP promote water and sodium excretion, increase peripheral vasodilation, and inhibit the RAAS. In early HF they play a key role in compensation for LV dysfunction. Attenuation of renal response to natriuretic peptides occurs as HF progresses.

Central and Autonomic Nervous System Neurohormonal Response

Arginine vasopressin (antidiuretic hormone) is released from the pituitary gland in response to decreases in perfusion. Elevated vasopressin levels in HF increase volume overload while decreasing osmolality. This adversely affects hemodynamics and cardiac remodeling while potentiating effects of angiotensin II and norepinephrine.

HF results in a generalized stimulation of sympathetic activity and inhibition of parasympathetic tone. Increased sympathetic outflow results in release of epinephrine and norepinephrine from the adrenal glands and norepinephrine at peripheral sympathetic nerve endings, increasing cardiac contractility, HR, and vascular tone. The resulting increased vascular tone augments preload through venous contraction as well as afterload by arterial vasoconstriction. Acutely, arterial BP is improved and CO increased by catecholamines. Chronically, a decrease in the number and affinity of surface catecholamine receptors occurs in myocardial tissue, reducing responsiveness to epinephrine and norepinephrine. Elevated catecholamines adversely affect myocardial perfusion, leading to progressive apoptosis and cardiac fibrosis.

Renal Neurohormonal Response

Decreased glomerular perfusion results in reduced renal excretion of sodium. Renal arteriolar and adrenergic receptors stimulate renin release by the juxtaglomerular apparatus. Renin facilitates the conversion of angiotensinogen to angiotensin I, which is further converted to angiotensin II by ACE. Angiotensin II is a potent vasoconstrictor and an important stimulus for aldosterone release by the adrenal cortex. Aldosterone increases renal sodium retention and potassium excretion. Renal adaptation to hypoperfusion occurs mainly through production of vasodilatory hormones such as prostacyclin, along with prostaglandins PGI_2 and PGE_2. Aspirin and other NSAID interfere with prostaglandin synthesis by inhibiting cyclooxygenase.

Vascular Endothelial Neurohormonal Response

Endothelial function locally regulates vasomotor tone. This occurs in response to hemodynamic stress, hypoxia, catecholamines, angiotensin II, and many inflammatory cytokines. ET-1 is the most important ET and the most potent vasoconstrictor known. ET-1 plasma levels are elevated in HF, correlate with symptoms as well as hemodynamic stress, and are associated with adverse prognosis.

NO is produced in almost all tissues and plays a critical role in the homeostasis of cardiac function.NO-mediated endothelial dysfunction may represent the earliest stage of target organ damage, which ultimately leads to hypertensive heart disease and HF.

CLASSIFICATION OF HEART FAILURE

Many different methods of classifying HF exist, including acute versus chronic, systolic versus diastolic, right sided versus left sided, and high output versus low output. Early in HF, these may be useful clinical descriptors suggesting particular causes and treatment strategies. Late in the disease process, these distinctions blur.

Acute versus Chronic Heart Failure

The prototypical case of acute HF involves a healthy person who develops a large MI or acute valvular dysfunction. Chronic HF is best characterized by a disease state such as DCM, with gradual deterioration of cardiac function. In acute HF, early presentation may be a result of systolic dysfunction and hypoperfusion, often with acute pulmonary edema (APE)resulting from sudden reduction in chamber compliance. Chronic HF usually arises with symptoms related to fluid retention, with compensatory mechanisms adjusted so that normal perfusion exists, at least in the resting state.

Systolic versus Diastolic Dysfunction

Systolic dysfunction refers to impairment of contractility, with stroke output reduced and forward flow compromised. Systolic dysfunction is typically caused by myocyte damage such as in MI or myocarditis. Asymptomatic LV systolic dysfunction in patients 45 yr of age or older is much more common than symptomatic systolic HF. Most cases of systolic dysfunction also involve some degree of diastolic dysfunction.

Diastolic dysfunction indicates a primary problem

with ability of the ventricles to relax and fill normally. In many cases, normal or even supernormal systolic function is preserved. Asymptomatic diastolic dysfunction is much more common than asymptomatic systolic dysfunction. Diastolic dysfunction is the predominant pathophysiology in hypertrophic and restrictive cardiomyopathies, valvular aortic stenosis, and, most important, HTN.

Diastolic dysfunction occurs predominantly as a result of one of three mechanisms: impaired ventricular relaxation, increased ventricular wall thickness, or accumulation of myocardial interstitial collagen. Impaired lusitropic capacity of the myocardium leads to higher ventricular filling pressure, resulting in congestive symptoms. Myocardial relaxation is an active, energy-requiring process. Failure of myocytes to relax may be secondary to low intracellular energy stores. Patients with predominantly diastolic dysfunction have the advantage of intact myocardial contractile function. Stiffer hearts, however, have steep pressure-volume curves. Therefore small reductions in diastolic filling volume, as may occur with aggressive vasodilator or diuretic therapy, may markedly decrease ventricular filling and compromise stroke output (Fig. 15-3).

Right-Sided versus Left-Sided Heart Failure

The right and left circulations are connected and, over time, output from the two sides must be equal. Furthermore, the right and left ventricles share an interventricular septum, and dysfunction in one chamber may have an immediate impact on the other. In addition, cardiac biochemical changes such as an abnormal catecholamine response affect all chambers.

Fluid accumulation "behind" the involved ventricle is responsible for many of the clinical manifestations of HF. For example, LV failure leads primarily to pulmonary congestion with symptoms mostly of dyspnea and orthopnea. Patients with right-sided HF have symptoms of systemic venous congestion, such as pedal edema and hepatomegaly.

Patients with AMI may have APE; yet unlike patients with chronic HF, they may not have jugular venous distention or pedal edema because central venous pressure may remain within normal limits. A chest radiograph reveals evidence of pulmonary venous congestion, interstitial edema, and, in fulminant cases, alveolar edema. The cardiac shadow is often of normal size.

Acute RV infarction is an important cause of hypoperfusion with jugular venous distention and absent pulmonary congestion.

High-Output versus Low-Output Failure

High-output failure refers to a hyperdynamic state with supranormal CO and low arteriovenous oxygen difference. The hyperdynamic state may result from increased preload, decreased SVR, increased beta-sympathetic activity, or persistent tachycardia. A persistent hyperdynamic state results in myocardial damage over time. As the condition progresses, myocardial dysfunction with circulatory overload is superimposed on this background, and symptoms progress. At some point, CO becomes normal or even low, indistinguishable from classic HF.

Low-output failure is the more typical variety of HF and occurs as a result of entities such as ischemic heart disease, dilated cardiomyopathy, valvular disease, and chronic HTN. Low CO (systolic dysfunction), high filling pressures (diastolic dysfunction), and an increased systemic O_2ER (widened arteriovenous oxygen difference) characterize this more commonly encountered form of HF.

CLINICAL EVALUATION OF PATIENTS WITH SUSPECTED HEART FAILURE

Precipitating Causes of Heart Failure and Exacerbating Factors

Causes of acute cardiac decompensation are provided in Box 15-1.

Box 15-1 Common Precipitating Causes of Acute HF

- Sodium and volume excess
- Systemic HTN
- Myocardial infarction or ischemia
- Systemic infection
- Dysrhythmias
- Acute hypoxia or respiratory problems
- Anemia
- Pregnancy

- Thyroid disorders
- Acute myocarditis
- Acute valvular dysfunction
- Pulmonary embolus
- Excess exertion or trauma
- Pharmacologic complications

Iatrogenic causes of HF should also be considered, especially in patients who have recently received intravenous fluids. Patients with known renal insufficiency most often experience pulmonary edema as a consequence of salt and fluid overload. In chronic HF, the most common cause of decompensation is inappropriate decrease in intensity of treatment, including drug therapy, dietary sodium restriction, limited physical activity, or a combination of these measures.

Evaluation of Heart Failure

The NYHA classification system is a time-honored categorization for patients with chronic HF based on degree of activity causing symptoms (Box 15-2).Careful consideration of the differential diagnosis of HF is symptom based. The most common manifestation of acute HF is respiratory distress caused by pulmonary edema. Therefore the differential diagnosis includes exacerbation of COPD or asthma, pulmonary embolus, pneumonia, anaphylaxis, and other causes of acute respiratory distress. Hypoperfusion may be caused by some of these as well as by sepsis syndrome, hypovolemia, hemorrhage, cardiac tamponade, and tension pneumothorax.

Box 15-2 Classification System for Chronic HF:NYHA Functional Classes

Ⅰ. Asymptomatic on ordinary physical activity
Ⅱ. Symptomatic on ordinary physical activity
Ⅲ. Symptomatic on less than ordinary physical activity
Ⅳ. Symptomatic at rest

History

The presence and character of dyspnea, chest pain, previous heart disease, cardiac catheterization, surgery, current medications, and possible intercurrent illness should be explored.

Paroxysmal nocturnal dyspnea and Orthopnea result from pulmonary congestion precipitated by plasma volume expansion that occurs during recumbency as interstitial edema is reabsorbed into the circulation. Symptoms abate after the patient stands or props up the trunk and venous return decreases.

Physical Examination

Most HF patients are hypertensive. Clammy, vasoconstricted patients with a thready pulse and delayed capillary refill may have systemic hypoperfusion despite adequate BP.

Most patients with APE are diaphoretic because of intense sympathetic activation. Patients with pulmonary congestion secondary to HF develop interstitial and alveolar pulmonary edema, causing reduced pulmonary compliance and decreased functional residual capacity. Clinical findings include diffuse moist rales, which may be absent with decreased ventilation in more agonal patients. Peribronchial edema may cause wheezing or rhonchi, which can mimic bronchospastic disease ("cardiac asthma"). A positive response to bronchodilator therapy does not exclude HF. Jugular venous distention is present in approximately 50% of cases, and one third of patients have peripheral edema. An S_3 gallop may be present in up to 25%.

Jugular venous distention, pedal edema, and cardiomegaly may be absent in previously healthy individuals with pulmonary edema resulting from an initial episode of acute HF. Physical examination of patients with APE resulting from AMI may identify surgically correctable lesions such as acute mitral regurgitation or ventricular septal defect.

Diagnostic Testing in Heart Failure

An upright chest radiograph helps distinguish cardiogenic pulmonary edema from other causes of dyspnea. An enlarged cardiac silhouette is seen in 70% of cases. A normal heart size suggests acute cardiogenic pulmonary edema in a patient without prior HF, diastolic dysfunction, COPD, or noncardiogenic pulmonary edema. An early ECG for arrhythmia recognition and management is important, as well as for identification of ACS. Obtaining CBC to evaluate for anemia and a basic metabolic panel to determine electrolyte status as well as renal function is generally useful. Cardiac biomarkers help evaluate for ongoing myocyte injury.

When the diagnosis of HF is unclear, natriuretic peptide levels should be obtained. NT-proBNP and BNP levels help identify patients with HF. Natriuretic peptide levels correlate with ventricular function, NYHA classification, and prognosis. Plasma levels of cardiac troponins in stable HF also predict adverse outcomes.

Bedside ultrasound can be an important ED screening tool in HF, with attention to wall motion abnormalities, EF, and valvular function, as well as exclusion of cardiac tamponade. Echocardiography is similarly useful and can provide detailed measures of LV function and determine structural heart disease. MDCT coronary angiography can distinguish ischemic from other forms of cardiomyopathy but is rarely useful in acute HF. Radionuclide imaging and cardiac MRI have an expanding role in evaluating chronic HF but no utility in the acute setting.

TREATMENT OF ACUTE HEART FAILURE

The approach focuses on (1) determining underlying cardiac pathology, (2) identifying the acute precipitant, and (3) mitigating the acute decompensation. The immediate therapeutic goals are to improve respiratory gas exchange, maintain adequate arterial saturation, and decrease LV diastolic pressure while maintaining adequate cardiac and systemic perfusion.

The acute congestive state can be controlled by (1) reducing cardiac workload through decreased preload and afterload, (2) controlling excessive retention of salt and water, and (3) improving cardiac contractility. Patients may have a wide spectrum of symptoms and signs ranging from mild dyspnea on exertion to full-blown cardiogenic shock with hypotension and concomitant respiratory failure.

Acute Heart Failure

Pulmonary edema is classified clinically into cardiogenic and noncardiogenic forms. Most commonly, cardiogenic APE occurs with acute myocardial ischemia or AMI, cardiomyopathy, valvular heart disease, or hypertensive emergencies.

Patients with ACPE have substantially lower plasma volumes. Thus careful volume infusion with aliquots of normal saline is appropriate initial resuscitation for the hypoperfusing patient with ACPE.

In contrast, noncardiogenic APE generally results from an alteration in the permeability characteristics of the pulmonary capillary membrane. The alteration may have such diverse causes as septic shock, inhalation injuries, drugs or toxins, aspiration syndromes, fat emboli syndrome, neurogenic causes, and high altitude.

Acute Heart Failure with Adequate Perfusion

Many patients with acute HF demonstrate adequate systemic perfusion with elevated BP because of activation of various compensatory mechanisms. These patients should be quickly distinguished from those with APE and evidence of hypoperfusion. Hypertensive pulmonary edema is easier to manage because afterload reduction with vasodilators is extremely effective.

Therapeutic interventions should decrease both preload and afterload. Excessive preload reduction may result in an abrupt decrease in CO, however, which could cause hypotension. This occurs more readily in patients with less compliant hearts. Fluid challenge generally restores BP. Therapy for APE with adequate perfusion should begin with upright positioning, supplemental oxygen, nitrates, morphine sulfate, and loop diuretics (Fig. 15-5)

Oxygen and Ventilation

All patients with APE have hypoxemia and require high-flow oxygen by face mask if spontaneously breathing and if oxygen saturation as measured by SpO_2 is below 90%. Excessive oxygen therapy, however, may significantly increase afterload and worsen cardiac function in decompensated HF. The typical acid-base disturbance of acute HF is mixed. Patients with fulminant APE may have lactic acidosis, and many also have concomitant respiratory alkalosis resulting from the tachypnea stimulated by metabolic acidosis, hypoxemia, and decreased pulmonary compliance. In more severe cases, respiratory acidosis ensues as the patient fatigues and respirations fail. The ratio of dead space to

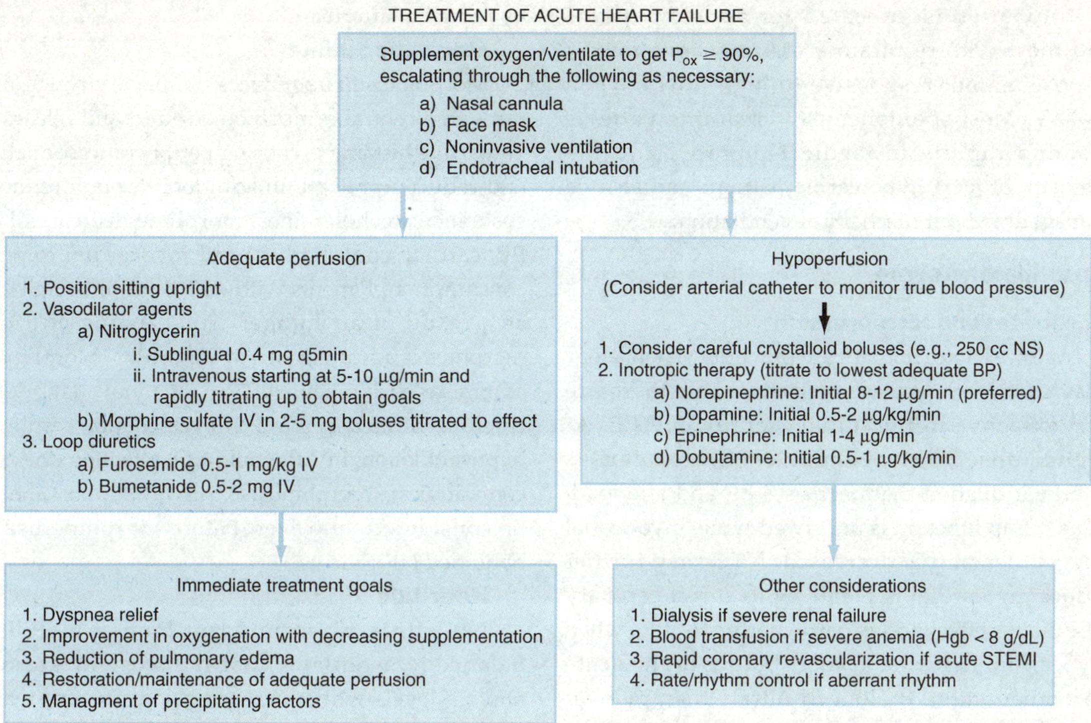

Fig. 15-5 A general therapeutic strategy for acute HF requires thoughtful application of interventions to achieve a reasonable improvement in early clinical treatment goals.

total ventilation (V_D/V_T) may be significantly increased owing to alveolar flooding. Patients with inadequate ventilation or with severe hypoxia that does not respond to supplemental oxygen require ventilatory support. Noninvasive ventilation (NIV) techniques are effective in treating severely compromised, but not agonal, APE patients. CPAP or BiPAP applied by an adjustable, snugly fitting face mask increases functional residual capacity, improves oxygenation, reduces work of breathing, and results in decreased LV preload and afterload by raising intrathoracic pressure (Fig. 15-6). These techniques result in more rapid restoration of normal vital signs and oxygenation than supplemental oxygen alone. The addition of pressure support (BiPAP) further reduces the work of breathing and more rapidly improves hypercarbia than CPAP alone. Selected patients may benefit greatly from these techniques when appropriately applied in conjunction with pharmacotherapy. These ventilatory therapies do not increase the risk of AMI in APE. NIV provides earlier improvement in respiratory distress and related metabolic abnormalities than supplemental oxygen alone in APE but does not improve short-term mortality.

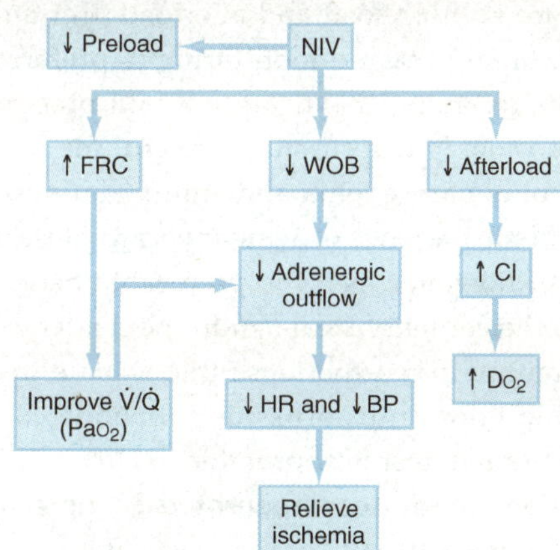

Fig. 15-6 NIV techniques recruit collapsed alveoli and increase FRC, which improves oxygenation and reduces work of breathing. NIV also acts as an afterload-reducing agent, which tends to directly improve CI, DO_2, P_aO_2, and V /Q. Preload is also reduced by NIV.

Intubation is indicated for apneic patients and those with respiratory distress, agitation, or hypoxemia not responsive to high-flow oxygen or NIV. Most spontaneously breathing patients respond rapidly to medical therapy, and the majority of alert hypercarbic patients can also be managed without mechanical ventilation.

Vasodilator Agents

Nitrates and Nitroprusside

At lower doses, nitrates are primarily venodilators. They effectively decrease preload and are therefore very effective in the initial therapy of APE. At higher doses, intravenous NTG also causes arteriolar dilation that decreases BP and afterload. Thus pump function is improved while myocardial oxygen demand is decreased. NTG may further reduce myocardial ischemia by its direct coronary vasodilator effect and is particularly effective when myocardial ischemia is contributing to the acute decompensation. Prolonged nitrate therapy over hours to days leads to tachyphylaxis secondary to depletion of intracellular sulfhydryl groups.

NTG may be initiated by the sublingual route, followed by titrated intravenous administration. Intravenous NTG has rapid onset and offset of action. Hypotension from excessive preload reduction or vagally mediated idiosyncratic reactions may occur. Sodium nitroprusside works similarly to NTG, acting as a balanced vasodilator to reduce both preload and afterload. Continuous intra-arterial pressure monitoring is preferred in patients receiving this drug to avoid precipitous hypotension. Nitroprusside is useful for patients with pulmonary edema and significant systemic HTN. In the presence of acute myocardial ischemia or AMI, however, NTG is preferable because it avoids the coronary steal syndrome. Patients with renal failure may experience thiocyanate toxicity from high-dose nitroprusside infusions. NTG is thus preferred over nitroprusside in HF.

Patients with decompensated aortic stenosis should generally not receive vasodilator agents, as flow cannot increase across a fixed obstruction. These patients may become hypotensive owing to reduced preload, with resultant decreased systemic and coronary perfusion. On the other hand, patients with mitral regurgitation benefit greatly from vasodilators, which improve antegrade flow by reducing afterload.

Morphine Sulfate

Morphine sulfate reduces pulmonary congestion through a central sympatholytic effect and release of vasoactive histamine, causing peripheral vasodilation and reduced preload. In addition, through reduced systemic catecholamines, morphine decreases HR, BP, cardiac contractility, and myocardial oxygen consumption. Patients with APE tend to be agitated as a result of air hunger. The calming effect of morphine is advantageous in this setting. Morphine is administered in repetitive 2 to 5 mg intravenous doses carefully titrated to effect. If oversedation results in hypoventilation. In APE, mild CO_2 retention does not contraindicate morphine use. Airway support should be considered, however, before morphine use in obtunded HF patients.

Nesiritide

Nesiritide, a recombinant human BNP, is a balanced vasodilator that reduces aldosterone and ET levels while increasing sodium and water excretion, without a resultant reflex tachycardia. Nesiritide, however, is not indicated in the ED treatment of episodes of acute HF.

Loop Diuretics

In patients with volume overload, this diuretic action lowers plasma volume, decreasing preload and pulmonary congestion. Although the renal effects of intravenously administered loop diuretics begin within 10 min, symptom relief in patients with APE often occurs much faster, probably the result of diuretic-induced neurohumoral changes. Furosemide acts as a vasodilator, promoting both renal PGE_2 and natriuretic peptide secretion, and as a vasoconstrictor, stimulating renin release. Loop diuretics (furosemide or bumetanide) should be administered to patients with hypertensive APE. The half-life of furosemide in patients with APE is double that in healthy volunteers, and caution is required with frequent administration. Continuous infusion of furosemide is not superior to bolus therapy.

Patients who fail to respond to loop diuretic administration may have severely compromised renal perfusion. In these situations, invasive hemodynamic monitoring may be beneficial. Diuretic therapy causes depletion of the important cations K^+ and Mg^{2+}, which may be significant in patients in whom these cations are already depleted by chronic diuretic therapy or other agents. High-dose diuretic therapy in APE is associated with deterioration in renal function and increased mortality.

Other Therapies

Most patients with APE and adequate systemic perfusion respond promptly to treatment with oxygen, nitrates, morphine, and diuretics. Hemodialysis is useful in patients with renal insufficiency. Blood transfusion candidates in acute HF have worse clinical features but derive some benefit from RBC repletion for hemoglobin levels below 8 g/dL. Therapies such as ET receptor antagonists, vasopressin receptor antagonists, betaendorphins, adenosine receptor antagonists, and other agents have undefined therapeutic potential. Urodilatin, a synthetic renal NP, has effectiveness in acutely decompensated HF. Levosimendan, a calcium-sensitizing drug that opens ATP-dependent potassium channels, provides prompt hemodynamic improvement in acute HF. In cardiogenic shock treated with PCI, levosimendan improves cardiovascular hemodynamics compared with conventional inotropic therapy. Relaxin, a vasodilating hormone produced in pregnant women, shows promise in the treatment of decompensated HF. Historical therapies (e.g., rotating tourniquets, phlebotomy, and theophylline) have no demonstrated efficacy in APE. Endotracheal intubation should be reconsidered if the patient develops severe respiratory deterioration unresponsive to NIV, significant cardiac dysrhythmias, or low CO or has ongoing chest pain.

Treatment of Acute Heart Failure in Hypotensive Patients

Patients with ACPE and apparent systemic hypotension present a therapeutic dilemma. The combination of hypotension and elevated left-sided filling pressure dramatically decreases coronary perfusion, particularly with CAD, leading to further impairment of contractility from increased ischemia. Vasopressor administration to maintain coronary perfusion pressure is necessary. Vasopressors, however, can increase afterload, decrease CO, increase myocardial oxygen demand, exacerbate ischemia, and precipitate dysrhythmias.

If the patient is truly hypoperfusing, the patient is either in true cardiogenic shock (pulmonary edema, hypotension, and decreased peripheral perfusion) or is volume depleted. Patients in true cardiogenic shock have lost as much as 40% of their ventricular muscle mass. Nearly 25% of patients with AMI and clinical evidence of systemic hypoperfusion, however, have low preload, indicating the presence of hypovolemia. Fluid challenge alone in these patients restores hemodynamic stability in half. If the patient has true cardiogenic shock, more intensive interventions, including vasopressor therapy, intra-aortic balloon pump (IABP), and endotracheal intubation with mechanical ventilation, may be needed. APE with systemic hypoperfusion in the setting of ACS represents ischemic cardiogenic shock. Emergency coronary revascularization is the treatment of choice.

Inotropic or Vasopressor Therapy

Inotropic agent use in HF increases myocardial oxygen demand, cardiac arrhythmias, and mortality. Intravenous inotropic agents with vasoactive properties should be reserved for hypoperfused patients with low CO despite a high LV filling pressure. Revascularization to reperfuse stunned or hibernating myocardium is preferable.

In hypotensive patients who are adequately volume repleted , norepinephrine is the pressor of choice. It raises BP and coronary perfusion pressure (alpha-vasoconstrictor effect) with a modest beta effect for inotropy and the least overall increase in HR and contractility. In cardiogenic shock, norepinephrine administration is a temporizing maneuver to maintain coronary perfusion pending rescue strategies, such as angioplasty, IABP, or cardiac surgery.

Dopamine has a dose-dependent effect on peripheral vascular tone and is a positive inotropic and chronotropic agent. Despite previous impressions, dopamine in HF has no clinically significant perfusion-sparing effect on the kidneys at any dose. Epinephrine is a potent alpha- and beta-agonist that maintains BP and increases CO. In cardiac surgery patients, it combats myocardial stunning after CPB. Dobutamine is a synthetic catecholamine that is mainly a beta$_2$-receptor agonist with some beta$_1$- and alpha-agonist activity. It is an inotropic vasodilator at therapeutic doses and should be used with caution in patients with borderline hypotension because it occasionally reduces BP further. Isoproterenol is a potent beta-agonist that causes profound tachycardia and vasodilation, which would be dangerous in HF.

Amrinone and milrinone are phosphodiesterase type Ⅲ inhibitors that increase cAMP in the myocardium and peripheral smooth muscle. These intravenous vasodilating inotropic agents increase CO and reduce LV pressures without producing significant changes in HR and BP. The positive inotropic effects of amrinone and dobutamine are additive, and concomitant use of both drugs appears to be better tolerated than high doses of dobutamine alone, with lower metabolic costs. Amrinone and milrinone may be useful on a short-term basis in patients awaiting heart transplantation. They should be used with caution in selected patients—in general in the context of invasive hemodynamic monitoring. These agents are prodysrhythmic, and long-term use of phosphodiesterase type Ⅲ inhibitors reduces survival in HF.

Rate and Rhythm Controllers

Compensatory tachycardia is the rule in HF, unless the patient is taking beta-blocking agents. Noncompensatory tachycardia increases myocardial oxygen consumption while reducing coronary perfusion and is a particular problem with AF or Af with rapid ventricular response. As with other causes of HF, diltiazem is a more prompt and safe alternative to digoxin in normotensive patients. Electrical cardioversion is indicated when a new-onset tachydysrhythmia is causing or exacerbating HF, especially with hypoperfusion or ongoing evidence of myocardial ischemia. Transcutaneous pacing may be necessary in severe bradycardia with hypotension.

Chronic Heart Failure

Chronic HF often involves a more gradual onset of symptoms, with a slow increase in dyspnea on exertion, progressive orthopnea, fatigue, and other symptoms. Patients with chronic HF often have complex multiorgan dysfunction and comorbidities for which polydrug medical regimens are used.

U.S. guidelines approved by the AHA and ACC reflect a new classification system for chronic HF that includes four categories: patients at risk, patients with asymptomatic LV dysfunction, patients with symptomatic HF, and those with refractory HF. Echocardiography is a very useful modality in screening for asymptomatic LV dysfunction in high-risk subgroups.

A main goal in the management of HF is to modify long-term maladaptive responses as well as achieve short-term functional improvement. Treatment should ideally be initiated in patients at risk to prevent disease progression. Atherosclerotic CAD, HTN, DM, hyperlipidemia, cocaine or ethanol abuse, smoking, and obesity are significant risk factors for HF. Paradoxically, however, overweight and obese patients have lower cardiovascular mortality in chronic HF.

The LV remodeling process is triggered by volume or pressure overload as well as loss of cardiac myocytes (e.g., MI). Therapeutic interventions in HF aim to slow remodeling. Various antihypertensive therapies allow regression of LVH and reduce the rate of SCD. Beta-blockers, ACEI, aldosterone antagonists, and ARB all inhibit or reverse remodeling.

The mainstay of treatment for chronic HF and asymptomatic LV dysfunction is vasodilator therapy, which benefits pump function by reducing both afterload and preload. The most important vasodilators for chronic HF are ACEI, angiotensin Ⅱ receptor antagonists, and nitrates.

Common Therapeutic Agents in Chronic Heart Failure

Angiotensin-Converting Enzyme Inhibitors. ACEI increase survival in all classes of chronic HF and reduce development of HF in patients with AMI and asymptomatic LV dysfunction.

The main side effects of ACEI are hypotension, deterioration of renal function, chronic cough, and upper airway angioedema.

Angiotensin Ⅱ Receptor Blockade. Both ACEI and ARB allowed reverse remodeling in HF and reduced the risk of development of Af. ARB were not superior to ACEI in reducing mortality or hospitalization for HF.ARB are most useful in patients intolerant of ACEI and have reduced side effects of cough and bradykinin accumulation.

Beta-Blocker and Combined Alpha-, Beta-Blocker Therapy. Despite the apparent paradox of use of agents that reduce myocardial contractility, beta-adrenergic blocking agents have significant efficacy in chronic HF. Beta-blockers in chronic HF significantly increase EF and decrease mortality. HR reduction with use of beta-blockers correlates with improvement in LVEF and reduced death rate in HF. AHA/ACC guidelines recommend beta-blockers for all patients with symptomatic LV systolic dysfunction.

Beta-blockers should not normally be initiated in acute HF. They are most useful in chronic HF associated with conditions having indications for beta-blocker therapy, including HTN, angina pectoris, and significant dysrhythmias. Slow upward titration of beta-blocker therapy facilitates maximal tolerability. Vasodilating beta-blockers such as carvedilol and nebivolol may have special use in chronic HF.

Diuretics. Patients with chronic HF exhibit a reduced ability to excrete a sodium and water load, with abnormal cardiac and hemodynamic adaptations to salt excess. Low-dose diuretics are one of the most effective treatments to prevent recurrence of HF. Loop diuretics are associated with significant side effects, including hypovolemia, electrolyte disturbances (low K^+, Mg^{2+}, and Na^+), hyperuricemia, worsening renal function, and metabolic alkalosis. Torasemide may block the aldosterone cascade and may be clinically a better loop diuretic in chronic HF. The addition of thiazide diuretic therapy to loop diuretics greatly increases sodium and fluid excretion but increases side effects.

The use of potassium-sparing diuretics spironolactone and eplerenone in HF is associated with a reduced risk of death.

Nitrates. Nitrate therapy improves exercise tolerance in chronic HF and offers potential hemodynamic improvement. The main problem with nitrate therapy appears to be rapid drug tolerance, which can be partially addressed by daily nitrate drug-free intervals.

Cardiac Glycosides. The cardiac glycosides inhibit the adenosine triphosphatase–dependent sodium-potassium pump in the cell membrane of the cardiac myocyte. This inhibition increases the availability of intracellular calcium to contractile proteins in myocardial cells, with modest positive inotropic effect. Digoxin is of benefit in patients with all degrees of chronic HF by reducing symptoms and improving quality of life and exercise tolerance. Digoxin should be used in low doses for most persistently symptomatic HF patients whose treatment already includes ACEI, diuretics, and beta-blocker therapy when HF is caused by systolic or diastolic dysfunction.

Admission Criteria and Predictors of Readmission in Heart Failure

In general, exacerbations of chronic HF require admission if the cause of the exacerbation cannot be readily recognized and corrected, if the disease process is unstable because of increased ischemia or new dysrhythmia, or if clinical deterioration appears likely. Precipitating events, including ACS, concomitant pneumonia, or worsening renal function increase hospital mortality and should prompt admission.

Initiation of proven therapeutic modalities at hospitalization leads to early benefits, including decreased risks of mortality and rehospitalization for HF.

SUMMARY

Evaluation and management of patients with HF remains a challenge in emergency medicine. Recognition of common precipitating events allows early understanding of appropriate management issues. Most acute decompensated HF can be managed with adequate oxygenation along with vasodilator and loop diuretic therapy. Advances in the chronic medical management of HF, including the routine use of beta-blockers, ACEI or ARB, diuretics including spironolactone, and occasionally digoxin have resulted in sustained symptomatic improvement and reduced 5 yr mortality.

(CHAI Yanfen LIU Chenyan)

Pulmonary Emergencies

Chapter 16

Dyspnea

KEY CONSEPTS

Dyspnea results from a variety of conditions, ranging from nonurgent to life-threatening.

The differential diagnosis can be divided into acute and chronic causes, of which many are pulmonary. Other causes include cardiac, metabolic, infectious, neuromuscular, traumatic, and hematologic conditions.

Bedside oxygen saturation determinations, or selective use of ABG are useful in determining the degree of hypoxia and the need for supplemental oxygen.

If dyspnea is believed to be upper airway in origin, direct or fiberoptic laryngoscopy or a soft tissue lateral radiograph of the neck may be useful.

Ultrasound may also be of benefit in rapidly distinguishing between COPD and HF.

PERSPECTIVE

Dyspnea is the term applied to the sensation of breathlessness and the patient's reaction to that sensation.Dyspnea is often ill defined by patients, who may describe the feeling as shortness of breath, chest tightness, or difficulty breathing. Neither the clinical severity nor the patient's perception correlates well with the seriousness of underlying pathology and may be affected by emotions, behavioral and cultural influences, and external stimuli.

The following terms may be used in the assessment of the dyspneic patient:

Tachypnea: A respiratory rate greater than normal. Normal rates range from 14 to 18 cycles/min in adults.

Hyperpnea: Greater than normal minute ventilation to meet metabolic requirements.

Hyperventilation: A minute ventilation (determined by respiratory rate and V_T) that exceeds metabolic demand.ABG characteristically show a normal PO_2 with an uncompensated respiratory alkalosis (low PCO_2 and elevated pH).

Dyspnea on exertion: Dyspnea provoked by physical effort or exertion. It often is quantified in simple terms, such as the number of stairs or number of blocks a patient can manage before the onset of dyspnea.

Orthopnea: Dyspnea in a recumbent position. It usually is measured in number of pillows the patient uses to lie in bed (e.g., two-pillow orthopnea).

Paroxysmal nocturnal dyspnea: Sudden onset of dyspnea occurring while reclining at night, usually related to the presence of CHF.

Epidemiology

Dyspnea is a common presenting complaint among ED patients of all ages. Causes vary widely and may include benign, self-limited conditions or significant pathology that can produce long-term morbidity and premature mortality.

Pathophysiology

The actual mechanisms responsible for dyspnea are unknown. Normal breathing is controlled both centrally by the respiratory control center in the medulla oblongata and peripherally by chemoreceptors located near the carotid bodies, and mechanoreceptors in the diaphragm and skeletal muscles. Any imbalance among these sites is perceived as dyspnea. This imbalance generally results from ventilatory demand being greater than capacity.

The perception and sensation of dyspnea are believed to occur by one or more of the following mechanisms: increased work of breathing, such as the increased lung resistance or decreased compliance that occurs with asthma or COPD, or increased respiratory drive, such as results from severe hypoxemia, acidosis, or centrally acting stimuli (toxins, central nervous system events). Pulmonary stretch receptors also play a role.

DIAGNOSTIC APPROACH

Differential Considerations

Dyspnea is subjective and has many different potential causes. The differential diagnosis can be divided into acute and chronic causes, of which many are pulmonary. Other causes include cardiac, metabolic, infectious, neuromuscular, traumatic, and hematologic conditions (Table 16-1).

Table 16-1 Differential Diagnoses for Acute Dyspnea

ORGAN SYSTEM	CRITICAL DIAGNOSES	EMERGENT DIAGNOSES	NONEMERGENT DIAGNOSES
Pulmonary	Airway obstruction Pulmonary embolus Noncardiogenic edema Anaphylaxis Ventilatory failure	Spontaneous pneumothorax Asthma Cor pulmonale Aspiration Pneumonia (CAP score >70)	Pleural effusion Neoplasm Pneumonia(CAP score ≤ 70) COPD
Cardiac	Pulmonary edema MI Cardiac tamponade	Pericarditis	Congenital heart disease Valvular heart disease Cardiomyopathy
Primarily Associated with Normal or Increased Respiratory Effort			
Abdominal		Mechanical interference Hypotension, sepsis from ruptured viscus, bowel obstruction,inflammatory or infectious process	Pregnancy Ascites Obesity
Psychogenic			Hyperventilation syndrome. Somatization disorder Panic attack
Metabolic or endocrine	Toxic ingestion DKA	Renal failure Electrolyte abnormalities Metabolic acidosis	Fever Thyroid disease
Infectious	Epiglottitis	Pneumonia (CAP score >70)	Pneumonia (CAP score ≤ 70)
Traumatic	Tension pneumothorax Cardiac tamponade Flail chest	Simple pneumothorax, hemothorax Diaphragmatic rupture	Rib fractures
Hematologic	Carbon monoxide poisoning Acute chest syndrome	Anemia	
Primarily Associated with Decreased Respiratory Effort			
Neuromuscular	CVA, intracranial insult Organophosphate poisoning	Multiple sclerosis Guillain-Barré syndrome Tick paralysis	Amyotrophic lateral sclerosis Polymyositis Porphyria

Pivotal Findings

History

Duration of Dyspnea. Chronic or progressive dyspnea usually denotes primary cardiac or pulmonary disease. Acute dyspneic spells may result from asthma exacerbation; infection; pulmonary embolus; intermittent cardiac dysfunction; psychogenic causes; or inhalation of irritants, allergens, or foreign bodies.

Onset of Dyspnea. Sudden onset of dyspnea should lead to consideration of PE or spontaneous pneumothorax. Dyspnea that builds slowly over hours or days may represent a flare of asthma or COPD; pneumonia; recurrent, small pulmonary emboli; CHF; or malignancy.

Positional Changes. Orthopnea can result from left-sided HF, COPD, or neuromuscular disorders. One of the earliest symptoms seen in patients with diaphragmatic weakness from neuromuscular disease is orthopnea. Paroxysmal nocturnal dyspnea is most common in patients with left-sided HF but also occurs in COPD. Exertional dyspnea commonly is associated with COPD but also can be seen with poor cardiac reserve and abdominal loading. Abdominal loading, caused by ascites, obesity, or pregnancy, leads to elevation of the diaphragm, resulting in less effective ventilation and dyspnea.

Trauma. Dyspnea can result from trauma, causing fractured ribs, flail chest, hemothorax, pneumothorax, diaphragmatic rupture, pericardial effusion, cardiac tamponade, or neurologic injury.

Symptoms

Patient descriptions of dyspnea vary significantly and generally correlate poorly with severity. Fever suggests an infectious cause. Anxiety or overwhelming fear, particularly if it precedes the onset of dyspnea, may point to panic attack or psychogenic dyspnea, if no organic cause can be isolated. PE or MI may cause isolated dyspnea with or without associated chest pain, particularly if the pain is constant, dull, or visceral. If the pain is sharp and worsened by deep breathing but not by movement, pleural effusion, pleurisy, or pleural irritation from pneumonia or PE are possible. Spontaneous pneumothorax also may produce sharp pain with deep breathing that is not worsened by movement.

Signs

Physical signs in dyspneic patients may be consistent with specific illnesses (Table 16-2). Physical findings found in specific diseases also can be grouped as presenting patterns (Table 16-3).

Table 16-2 Pivotal Findings in Physical Examination

SIGN	PHYSICAL FINDIN	DIAGNOSES TO CONSIDER
Vital signs	Tachypnea	Pneumonia, pneumothorax
	Hypopnea	Intracranial insult, drug or toxin ingestion
	Tachycardia	PE, traumatic chest injury
	Hypotension	Tension pneumothorax
	Fever	Pneumonia, PE
General appearance	Cachexia, weight loss	Malignancy, acquired immune disorder, mycobacterial infection
	Obesity	Hypoventilation, sleep apnea, PE
	Pregnancy	PE
	Barrel chest	COPD
	"Sniffing" position	Epiglottitis
	"Tripoding" position	COPD or asthma with severe distress
	Traumatic injury	Pneumothorax (simple, tension), rib fractures, flail chest, hemothorax, pulmonary contusion
Skin and nails	Tobacco stains or odor	COPD, malignancy, infection
	Clubbing	Chronic hypoxia, intracardiac shunts, or pulmonary vascular anomalies
	Pallid skin or conjunctivae	Anemia
	Muscle wasting	Neuromuscular disease
	Bruising	Chest wall: rib fractures, pneumothorax

Continued

SIGN	PHYSICAL FINDIN	DIAGNOSES TO CONSIDER
		Diffuse: thrombocytopenia, chronic steroid use, anticoagulation
	Subcutaneous emphysema	Rib fractures, pneumothorax, tracheobronchial disruption
	Hives, rash	Allergic reaction, infection, tick-borne illness
Neck	Stridor	Upper airway edema or infection, foreign body, traumatic injury, anaphylaxis
	JVD	Tension pneumothorax, COPD or asthma exacerbation, fluid overload or CHF, PE
Lung examination	Wheezes	CHF, anaphylaxis Bronchospasm
	Rales	CHF, pneumonia, PE
	Unilateral decrease	Pneumothorax, pleural effusion, consolidation, rib fractures or contusion,pulmonary contusion
	Hemoptysis	Malignancy, infection, bleeding disorder, CHF
	Sputum production	Infection (viral, bacterial)
	Friction rub	Pleurisy
	Abnormal respiratory pattern (e.g., Cheyne-Stokes)	Intracranial insult
Chest examination	Crepitance or pain on palpation	Rib or sternal fractures
	Subcutaneous emphysema	Pneumothorax, tracheobronchial rupture
	Thoracoabdominal desynchrony	Diaphragmatic injury with herniation; cervical spinal cord trauma
	Flail segment	Flail chest, pulmonary contusion
Cardiac examination	Murmur	PE
	S_3 or S_4 gallop	PE
	S_2 accentuation	PE
	Muffled heart sounds	Cardiac tamponade
Extremities	Calf tenderness, Homans' sign	PE
	Edema	CHF
Neurologic examination	Focal deficits (motor, sensory, cognitive)	Stroke, intracranial hemorrhage causing central abnormal respiratory drive; if long-standing, risk of aspiration pneumonia
	Symmetrical deficits	Neuromuscular disease
	Diffuse weakness	Metabolic or electrolyte abnormality (hypocalcemia, hypomagnesemia, hypophosphatemia), anemia
	Hyporeflexia	Hypermagnesemia
	Ascending weakness	Guillain-Barré syndrome

Table 16-3 Diagnostic Table: Patterns of Diseases Often Resulting in Dyspnea

DISEASE	HISTORY (DYSPNEA)	ASSOCIATED SYMPTOMS	SIGNS AND PHYSICAL FINDINGS	TESTS
PE	HPI: abrupt onset, pleuritic pain, immobility (travel, recent surgery) PMH: malignancy, DVT, PE, hypercoagulability, oral contraception, obesity	Diaphoresis, exertional dyspnea	Tachycardia, tachypnea, low-grade fever	Pulse oximetry, ABG (A-a gradient), D-dimer ECG (dysrhythmia, right-sided heart strain) CXR (Westermark sign, Hampton's hump), spiral CT, Magnetic resonance venography, Pulmonary angiogram, Ultrasound positive for DVT
Pneumonia	Fever, productive cough, chest pain	Anorexia, chills, nausea, vomiting, exertional dyspnea, cough	Fever, tachycardia, tachypnea, rales or decreased breath sounds	CXR, CBC, sputum and blood cultures
Bacterial	SH: tobacco use			Pulse oximetry Waveform capnography if altered mental status, ABG if capnography unavailable and acid-base derangement or hypercarbia suspected
Viral	Exposure (e.g., influenza, varicella)			
Opportunistic	Immune disorder, chemotherapy			
Fungal or parasitic	Exposure (e.g., birds), indolent onset	Episodic fever, nonproductive cough		
Pneumothorax	Abrupt onset: trauma, chest pain, thin males more likely to have spontaneous pneumothorax	Localized chest pain	Decreased breath sounds, subcutaneous emphysema, chest wall wounds or instability	CXR: pneumothorax, rib fractures, hemothorax Ultrasound: pneumothorax, pleural effusion
Simple				Ultrasound positive for pneumothorax
Tension	Decompensation of simple pneumothorax	Diaphoresis	JVD, tracheal deviation, muffled heart sounds, cardiovascular collapse	Clinical diagnosis: requires immediate decompression. May verify via bedside ultrasound
COPD or asthma	Tobacco use, medication noncompliance, upper respiratory infection symptoms, sudden weather change PMH:environmental allergies FH: asthma	Air hunger, diaphoresis	Retractions, accessory muscle use, tripoding, cyanosis "Shark fin" capnograph	CXR: rule out infiltrate, pneumothorax, atelectasis(mucus plug) Ultrasound: distinguish from HF Waveform capnography
Malignancy	Weight loss, tobacco, or other occupational exposure	Dysphagia	Hemoptysis	CXR, chest CT: mass, hilar adenopathy, focal atelectasis

Continued

DISEASE	HISTORY (DYSPNEA)	ASSOCIATED SYMPTOMS	SIGNS AND PHYSICAL FINDINGS	TESTS
Fluid overload	Gradual onset, dietary indiscretion or medication noncompliance, chest pain PMH:recent MI, DM, CHF	Worsening orthopnea, paroxysmal nocturnal dyspnea	JVD, peripheral edema,S_3 or S_4 gallop, new cardiac dysrhythmia,hepatojugular reflux	CXR and/or ultrasound: pleural effusion, interstitial edema, Kerley B lines, cardiomegaly ECG:ischemia, dysrhythmia NT-proBNP
Anaphylaxis	Abrupt onset, exposure to allergen	Dysphagia	Oral swelling, stridor, wheezing, hives	

FH, family history; HPI, history of present illness; PMH, past medical history; SH, social history

Ancillary Studies

Specific findings obtained from the history and physical examination should be used to determine which ancillary studies are needed (Table 16-4).Bedside SO_2 determinations, or selective use of ABG, are useful in determining the degree of hypoxia and the need for supplemental oxygen or assisted ventilation. An additional resource for quickly assessing ventilatory status is noninvasive waveform capnography. $ETco_2$ values together with the shape of the capnogram can be helpful in assessing the adequacy of ventilations as well as underlying causes of the dyspnea. An electrocardiogram may be useful if history or physical examination findings suggest HF, ischemic cardiac disease, dysrhythmia, or pulmonary hypertension. Bedside ultrasound is useful to rapidly diagnose pulmonary edema, pneumothorax, and COPD, as well as deep venous thrombosis.

Table 16-4 Ancillary Testing in the Dyspneic Patient

CATEGORY	TEST	FINDINGS AND POTENTIAL DIAGNOSES
Laborator	Pulse oximetry, selective ABG use	Hypoxia, hyperventilation (muscular weakness, intracranial event)
	Waveform capnography	CO_2 retention (COPD, sleep apnea), obstructive or restrictive pulmonary pattern Metabolic versus respiratory acidosis (DKA, ingestions) A-a gradient (PE) Elevated carboxyhemoglobin (inhalation injury or CO poisoning)
	Complete blood count	WBC Increase: infection, stress demargination, hematologic malignancy Decrease: neutropenia, sepsis Hgb, Hct: anemia, polycythemia Smear: abnormal Hgb (i.e., sickling), inclusions Platelets: thrombocytopenia (marrow toxicity)
	Chemistry	BUN, Cr: acute or chronic renal failure K, Mg, Phos: low levels resulting in muscular weakness Glucose: DKA D-dimer: abnormal clotting activity NT-proBNP: HF, PE Troponin: cardiac ischemia or infarct
Cardiac	ECG Echocardiogram	Ischemia, dysrhythmia, $S_1Q_3T_3$ (PE), right-sided heart strain Pulmonary hypertension, valvular disorders Wall motion abnormalities related to ischemia, intracardiac shunts

Continued

CATEGORY	TEST	FINDINGS AND POTENTIAL DIAGNOSES
Radiologic	Chest radiograph	Bony structures: fractures, lytic lesions, pectus, kyphoscoliosis Mass: malignancy, cavitary lesion, infiltrate, foreign body Diaphragm: eventration, elevation of hemidiaphragm, bowel herniation Mediastinum: adenopathy (infection, sarcoid), air Cardiac silhouette: enlarged (cardiomyopathy, fluid overload) Soft tissue: subcutaneous air Lung parenchyma: blebs, pneumothorax, effusions (blood, infectious), interstitial edema, local consolidation, air bronchograms, Hampton's hump, Westermark's sign
	$\dot{V}/\dot{Q}$ scan	PE
	Pulmonary angiogram	PE, intervention (thrombolysis)
	CT	Mass lesion, adenopathy, trauma, PE
	MRI	PE, bony and soft tissue lesions, vascular abnormality
	Soft tissue neck radiograph	Epiglottitis, foreign body
	Ultrasound	Pneumothorax, pleural effusion, impaired cardiac function or pericardial effusion
Fiberoptic	Bronchoscopy	Mass lesion, foreign body Intervention (stenting, biopsy)
	Laryngoscopy	Mass lesion, edema, epiglottitis, foreign body

Serum electrolytes may confirm metabolic acidosis or a less common cause, such as hypokalemia, hypophosphatemia, or hypocalcemia. A complete blood count may identify severe anemia or thrombocytopenia associated with sepsis. The WBC is not sufficiently sensitive or specific to be of discriminatory value.

Expanded availability of specific blood biomarkers relevant to emergent evaluation of dyspnea provides improved immediate decision support and allows for short- and long-term prognostication. These include cardiac markers and D-dimer assay, which are useful in pursuing causes such as cardiac ischemia or venous thromboembolic disease. NT-proBNP analysis adds both diagnostic and prognostic value for several causes of dyspnea, including HF, PE, and ischemic cardiac disease.

If venous thromboembolism is suspected, D-dimer testing, with or without chest CTA, duplex venous ultrasonography, or, rarely, ventilation-perfusion scanning, is performed. If dyspnea is believed to be upper airway in origin, direct or fiberoptic laryngoscopy or a soft tissue lateral radiograph of the neck may be useful.

DIFFERENTIAL DIAGNOSIS

The range and diversity of pathophysiologic conditions that produce dyspnea render a simple algorithmic approach difficult. The primary branch point is the determination of whether the dyspnea primarily is cardiopulmonary or toxic-metabolic in origin. After initial stabilization and assessment, findings from the history, physical examination, and ancillary testing are collated to match patterns of disease that produce dyspnea. This process is updated periodically as new information becomes available. Table 16-3 presents recognizable patterns of disease for common dyspnea-producing conditions, along with specific associated symptoms.

Critical Diagnoses

Several critical diagnoses should be promptly considered to determine the best treatment options to stabilize the patient. Tension pneumothorax is such a critical diagnosis and is diagnosed by history and physical examination. If a dyspneic patient has diminished breath sounds on one side, ipsilateral hyper-resonance, severe respiratory distress, hypotension, and oxygen desaturation, prompt decompression of presumptive tension pneumothorax is indicated. Bedside ultrasonography can confirm pneumothorax in less obvious cases. If dyspnea and stridor indicate upper airway obstruction, early, definitive assessment and intervention occur in the ED or operating room. Complete obstruction by a foreign body warrants the Heimlich maneuver until the obstruction is relieved or the patient is unconscious, followed rapidly by direct laryngoscopy for foreign body removal. HF and pulmonary edema can produce dyspnea and respiratory failure and require prompt intervention if severe. Significant dyspnea and wheezing in anaphylaxis require immediate use of parenteral epinephrine in addition to supportive measures. Severe bronchospastic exacerbations of asthma at any age may lead rapidly to respiratory failure and arrest and should receive vigorous attention, including continuous or frequent administration of a beta-agonist aerosol and steroid therapy. Ultrasound may also be of benefit in rapidly distinguishing between COPD and HF. As mentioned earlier, waveform capnography is a valuable adjunct for assessing the severity and determining the cause of respiratory distress.

Emergent Diagnoses

Asthma and COPD exacerbations can result in marked dyspnea with bronchospasm and decreased ventilatory volumes. Sudden onset of dyspnea with a decreased oxygen saturation on room air accompanied by sharp chest pain may represent PE. Dyspnea accompanied by decreased breath sounds and tympany on percussion on one side is seen with spontaneous pneumothorax. Dyspnea associated with decreased respiratory effort may represent a neuromuscular process, such as multiple sclerosis, Guillain-Barré syndrome, or myasthenia gravis. Unilateral rales, cough, fever, and dyspnea usually indicate pneumonia.

Fig. 16-1 provides an algorithm for assessment and stabilization of a dyspneic patient. The initial division is based on the degree of breathing effort associated with the symptoms. The most critical diagnoses are considered first, and appropriate intervention undertaken.

All patients experiencing dyspnea, regardless of possible cause, should be promptly evaluated in the treatment area. Bedside pulse oximetry readings should be obtained, and the patient should be placed on a cardiac monitor. If the pulse oximetry result is less than 95% on room air, the patient should be placed on supplemental oxygen .If necessary, breathing should be assisted with manual or mechanical ventilation.

When the airway has been secured, rapid assessment of the patient's appearance and vital signs can help determine the need for further stabilization. Decreased mental alertness, inability to speak in more than one-syllable words, or certain types of body positioning signal the presence of significant respiratory distress and the need for rapid intervention. After airway stabilization, the cause of the dyspnea can be further investigated.

Empirical Management and Disposition

The management algorithm for dyspnea (Fig. 16-2) outlines the approach to treatment for most identifiable diseases. Unstable patients or patients with critical diagnoses must be stabilized and may require admission to an intensive care unit. Emergent patients who have improved with ED management may be admitted to an intermediate care unit. Patients diagnosed with urgent conditions in danger of deterioration without proper treatment or patients with severe comorbidities, such as diabetes, immunosuppression, or cancer, may also require admission for observation and treatment.

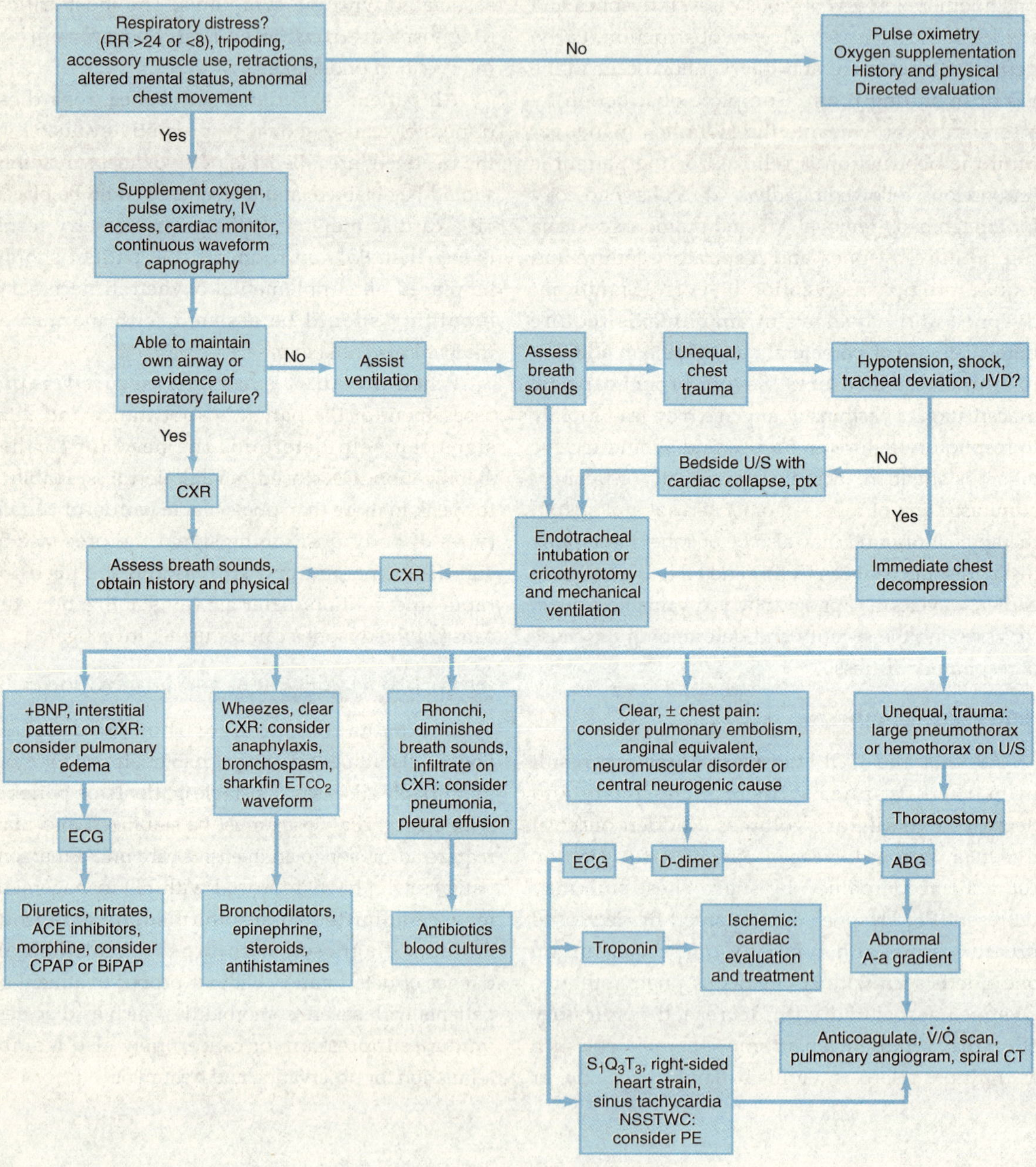

Fig. 16-1 Rapid assessment and stabilization of a dyspneic atient. NSSTWC, nonspecific ST wave changes (on ECG); ptx, pneumothorax.

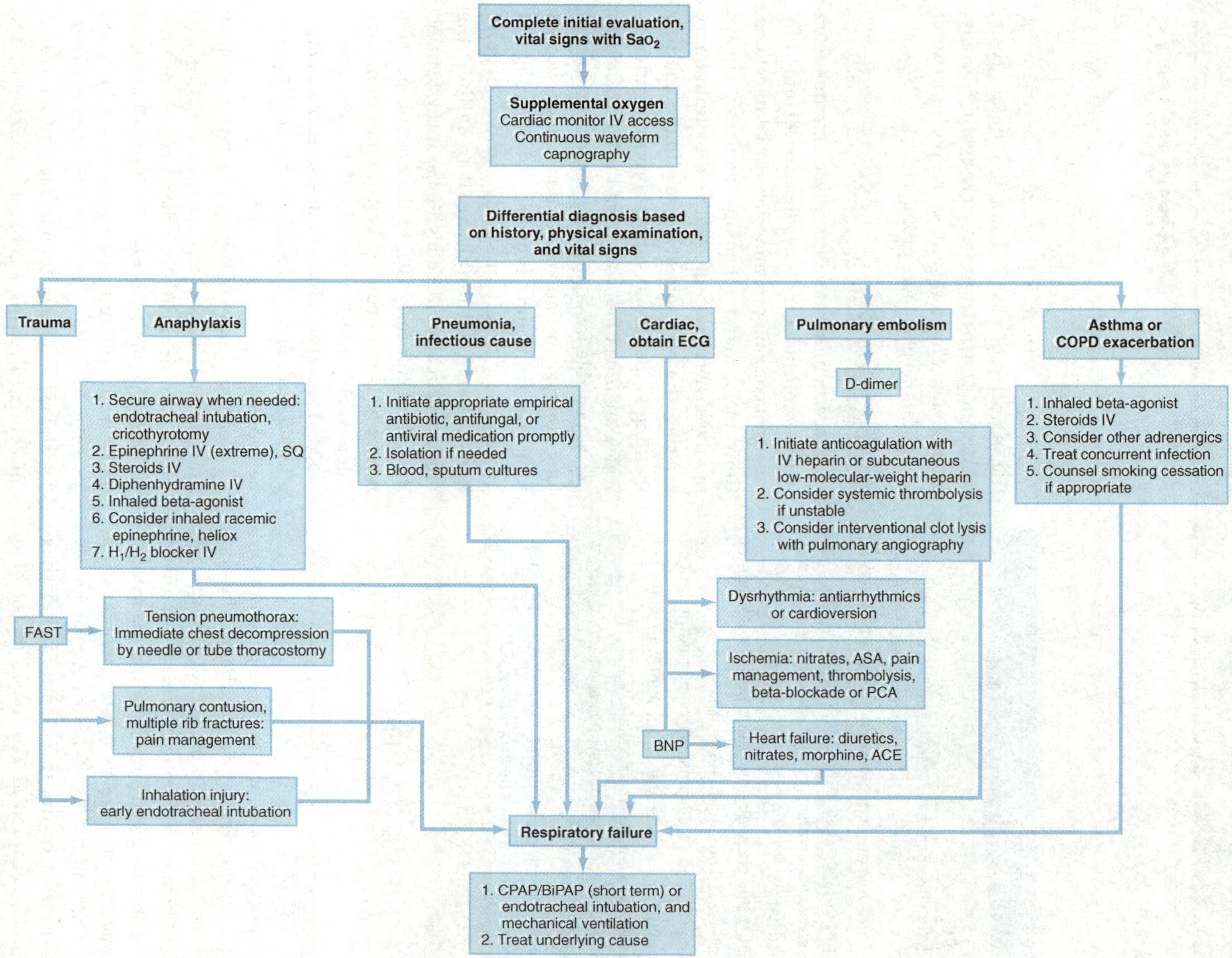

Fig. 16-2 Clinical guidelines for ED management of dyspnea.

(HUANG Liang)

Chapter 17

Hemoptysis

KEY CONSEPTS

Hemoptysis is defined as the expectoration of blood from the respiratory tract below the vocal cords.

Patients with massive or life-threatening Hemop tysis have hemorrhage generally accepted as 100 to 600 mL of blood loss in any 24 hr period, and have hemodynamic instability, shock, or impaired alveolar gas exchange.

Early bronchoscopy facilitates both localization of bleeding and therapeutic intervention.

Chest CT is as diagnostically accurate as bronch oscopy in locating bleeding peripheral vessels not accessible by a flexible bronchoscope.

Bronchial arterial embolization is an effective first-line therapy for massive hemoptysis and is the procedure of choice for patients either unable to tolerate surgery or in whom bronchoscopy has been unsuccessful.

PERSPECTIVE

Epidemiology

Hemoptysis is defined as the expectoration of blood from the respiratory tract below the vocal cords. Most cases seen in the ED are mild episodes of small-volume hemoptysis, typically consisting of either blood-tinged sputum or minute amounts of frank blood and are most commonly caused by bronchitis.Only 1% to 5% of hemoptysis patients have massive or life-threatening hemorrhage (generally accepted as 100 to 600 mL of blood loss in any 24hr period), which can result in hemodynamic instability, shock, or impaired alveolar gas exchange and has a mortality rate approaching 80%.

TB and bronchiectasis are responsible for the majority of cases of massive hemoptysis. In developed nations, cancer, cystic fibrosis, arteriovenous malformations, and postprocedural complications play more prominent roles.

Pathophysiology

Trace hemoptysis typically originates from tracheobronchial capillaries that are disrupted by vigorous coughing or minor bronchial infections. Conversely, massive hemoptysis nearly always involves disruption of bronchial or pulmonary arteries, the two sets of vessels that constitute the lung's dual blood supply. Bronchial arteries, which are direct branches from the thoracic aorta, are responsible for supplying oxygenated blood to lung parenchyma, and disruption of these vessels from arteritis, trauma, bronchiectasis or malignant erosion can result in sudden and profound hemorrhage. Although small in caliber, the bronchial circulation is a high-pressure system and the culprit in nearly 90% of the cases of massive hemoptysis requiring embolization. Pulmonary arteries, although transmitting large volumes of blood, do so at much lower pressures and, unless affected centrally, are less likely to cause massive hemoptysis.

Nearly all causes of hemoptysis have a common mechanism—vascular disruption within the trachea, bronchi, small-caliber airways, or lung parenchyma. Modes of vessel injury include acute and chronic inflammation (from bronchitis and arteritis), local infection (especially lung abscesses, TB, and aspergillosis), trauma, malignant invasion, infarction following a pulmonary embolus, and fistula formation (specifically aortobronchial fistulae).

Bronchiectasis, a chronic necrotizing infection resulting in bronchial wall inflammation and dilation, is one of the most common causes of massive hemoptysis. As tissue destruction and remodeling occur, rupture of nearby bronchial vessels can result in bleeding. Bronchiectasis can complicate chronic airway obstruction, necrotizing pneumonia, TB, or cystic fibrosis. Broncholithiasis, the formation of calcified endobronchial lesions following a wide array of granulomatous infections, is an uncommon problem with a similar propensity to erode nearby vessels. Hemorrhage control often requires surgical intervention.

Iatrogenic hemoptysis complicates 2% to 10% of all endobronchial procedures, especially percutaneous lung biopsies. Diffuse alveolar hemorrhage can be seen with autoimmune vasculitides such as Wegener's granulomatosis, systemic lupus erythematosus, and Goodpasture's syndrome. An uncommon cause of hemoptysis occurs when ectopic endometrial tissue within the lung results in monthly catamenial episodes of bleeding. Less common causes include pulmonary hereditary telangiectasias and hydatidiform infections. Any episode of hemoptysis can be exacerbated by coagulopathy and thrombocytopenia.

DIAGNOSTIC APPROACH

Differential Considerations

For a patient with apparent hemoptysis, two other potential sources of bleeding should be investigated. Nasal, oral, or hypopharyngeal bleeding sometimes contaminates the tracheobronchial tree, mimicking true hemoptysis. The clinician should closely inspect the nasopharynx and oral cavity to exclude this possibility. Gastric or proximal duodenal bleeding can similarly mimic hemoptysis, and differentiating a gastrointestinal source of bleeding is especially important because further evaluation and management of these two pathologies follow divergent pathways. Usually differentiation can be done by the patient and physician working together to differentiate coughing from vomiting.

Rapid Assessment and Stabilization

Although hemodynamic instability can occur as a result of hemorrhage, the most lethal sequela of massive hemoptysis is hypoxia, which results from the ventilation-perfusion mismatch that follows submersion of the small airways and alveoli with blood.

As a mitigating maneuver in patients with a known lateralizing source of bleeding, the "lung-down" position can be employed. For this position the patient is turned such that the bleeding lung is more dependent, promoting continued protection and ventilation of the unaffected lung and improved oxygenation. If intubation is required, a large diameter (8.0) ETT should be used to facilitate emergent fiberoptic bronchoscopy.

Pivotal Findings

History

An estimate of the rate, volume, and appearance of expectorated blood should be obtained. Additional pertinent history includes prior episodes of hemoptysis or parenchymal pulmonary disorders, including bronchiectasis, recurrent pneumonia, COPD, bronchitis, TB, and fungal infection. Inflammatory disorders that secondarily involve the lungs or pulmonary vasculature include Wegener's granulomatosis, Goodpasture's syndrome, and systemic lupus erythematosus, and a history of these should be elicited. Any risk factors for platelet dysfunction, thrombocytopenia, and coagulopathy should be noted, as should, conversely, any hypercoagulable states that might contribute to venous thromboembolic disease.

Primary or metastatic cancer can cause hemoptysis by erosion into pulmonary and bronchial vessels. Recent percutaneous or transbronchial procedures can cause immediate or delayed postprocedural bleeding, and any recent history of trauma should also be noted.

Physical Examination

After a primary survey and stabilization, a targeted examination may suggest the location and cause of bleeding but does so in less than 50% of cases. Focal adventitious breath sounds may indicate pneumonia or pulmonary abscess. A new heart murmur, especially in a febrile patient, may reflect endocarditis causing septic pulmonary emboli. Symptoms and signs of deep venous thrombosis should suggest PE. Ecchymoses and petechiae can indicate coagulopathy and thrombocytopenia, respectively.

Ancillary Testing

Initial laboratory studies include a CBC, coagulation tests, and a type and screen or crossmatch. Renal function tests should be performed if vasculitis is suggested or contrast CT is planned. Plain chest radiography screens for causes of hemoptysis (including infection and malignancy), although its sensitivity is poor.

In patients with massive hemoptysis, plain films may localize the site of hemorrhage in as many as 80% of patients; however, high-resolution MDCT of the chest is the principle diagnostic test for investigating both bronchial and nonbronchial causes of massive hemoptysis. A chest CT scan should be obtained in the high-risk patient (smokers, oncology patients) or in any patient with moderate to severe bleeding even if the initial chest radiograph is normal. CT localization of hemorrhage can expedite bronchoscopic evaluation and guide subsequent interventional procedures.

CT is diagnostically comparable to conventional angiography but less invasive and more rapidly available. Angiography is the first-line study when the cause of the hemoptysis is known (e.g., malignancy) and angiography-assisted embolization therapy is contemplated.

DIAGNOSTIC ALGORITHM

Differential Diagnosis

Potential causes of hemoptysis vary and include systemic illnesses as well as pulmonary parenchymal diseases. Box 17-1 includes the most common causes.

Box 17-1 Differential Diagnosis: Hemoptysis

Airway Disease
- Bronchitis (acute or chronic)
- Bronchiectasis
- Neoplasm (primary and metastatic)
- Trauma
- Foreign body

Parenchymal Disease
- Tuberculosis
- Pneumonia, lung abscess
- Fungal infection
- Neoplasm

Vascular Disease
- PE
- Arteriovenous malformation
- Aortic aneurysm
- Pulmonary hypertension
- Vasculitis (Wegener's granulomatosis, SLE, Goodpasture's syndrome)

Hematologic Disease
- Coagulopathy (cirrhosis or warfarin therapy)
- DIC
- Platelet dysfunction
- Thrombocytopenia

Cardiac Disease
- Congenital heart disease (especially in children)
- Valvular heart disease
- Endocarditis

Miscellaneous
- Cocaine
- Postprocedural injury
- Tracheal-arterial fistula
- SLE

Management

Since the advent of high-resolution CT, radiologic evaluation has had an integral role in the evaluation and treatment of patients with hemoptysis. The challenge to the emergency physician is to rapidly assess the need for airway control before radiographic evaluation and hemodynamic stabilization. Unless the initial chest radiograph is diagnostic or the patient is hemodynamically unstable, a chest CT should be obtained. Further management decisions should be guided by the CT results and made in conjunction with pulmonary and thoracic surgery consultants (Fig. 17-1).

Bronchoscopy

Early bronchoscopy facilitates both localization of bleeding and therapeutic intervention. Balloon and topical hemostatic tamponade, thermocoagulation, and injection of vasoactive agents can all effectively control arterial bleeding.

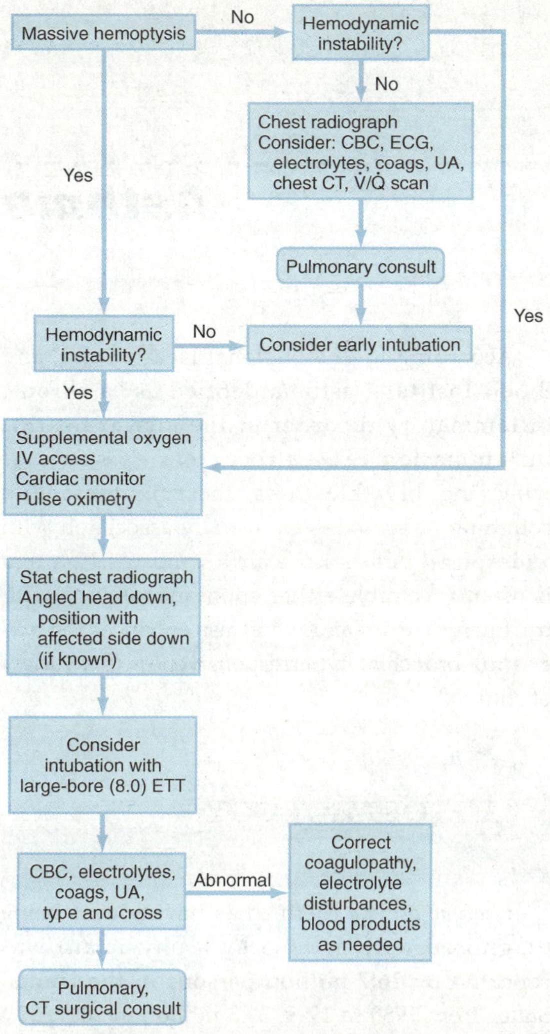

Fig. 17-1 ED management of hemoptysis.

Optimal timing for bronchoscopy remains conjectural; although stable patients with mild to moderate bleeding may benefit from early bronchoscopy, in unstable patients or those with brisk hemorrhage, bronchoscopy may facilitate airway management but is less likely to control bleeding.

Chest CT is as diagnostically accurate as bronchoscopy in locating bleeding peripheral vessels not accessible by a flexible bronchoscope. Chest CT can be used to identify the site of bleeding to determine whether angiography is indicated.

Interventional Angiography

Bronchial arterial embolization is an effective first-line therapy for massive hemoptysis and is the procedure of choice for patients either unable to tolerate surgery or in whom bronchoscopy has been unsuccessful.To guide therapy, initial localization of bleeding by bronchoscopy or CT is preferred. Rare complications include arterial perforation and dissection.

Surgery

Emergency thoracotomy, in the operating room, is reserved for life-threatening hemoptysis or for persistent, rapid bleeding that is uncontrolled by bronchoscopy and percutaneous embolization. Pulmonary arterial hemorrhage from tumor necrosis represents a surgical emergency.

DISPOSITION

Healthy patients with blood-streaked sputum or intermittent small-volume hemoptysis that has resolved and who have normal vital signs do not require imaging beyond plain chest radiography and can be discharged. Follow-up should be arranged for a few days to a week later if symptoms persist, or sooner (including return to the ED) if symptoms are worsening. High-risk patients with minor hemoptysis and all patients with moderate or large amounts of hemoptysis should undergo emergent chest CT scan.Brief hospitalization or admission to an observation unit for bronchoscopy should be considered. All patients with massive hemoptysis require admission to an ICU and expedited multidisciplinary treatment involving the emergency physician, pulmonologist, and thoracic surgeon.

(HUANG Liang)

Chapter 18

Asthma

KEY CONCEPTS

Asthma defined as a chronic inflammatory disorder of the airways and associated with widespread but variable airflow obstruction.

Hyper-responsiveness of the airways is characteristic of asthma and correlates with the severity of the disease and the need for treatment.

Serial measurements of airflow obstruction (FEV_1 or PEFR) are key components of disease assessment and response to therapy.

Guidelines for chronic use of inhaled $beta_2$-agonists, however, recommend limited daily use in a rescue-only mode. When inhaled therapy is not feasible, it is recommend that use of IV beta-agonists for severe nonresponsive acute asthma.

Inhaled and systemic steroid medications are effective in controlling airway inflammation and have important roles in management of asthma exacerbations.

Status asthmaticus refers to severe bronchospasm that does not respond to aggressive therapies within 30 to 60 min. Hypercapnia in rapid-onset near-fatal asthma normally need shorter durations of mechanical ventilation.

PERSPECTIVE

The word asthma was used initially as a synonym for "breathlessness." Since 1698, Floyer had differentiated asthma more clearly from other pulmonary disorders, subsequent definitions of asthma highlight concepts of airway hyper-responsiveness, bronchospasm, and reversible airway obstruction but fail to encompass the many facets of this disease.

According to The National Heart, Lung, and Blood Institute, asthma defined as "a chronic inflammatory disorder of the airways... this inflammation causes recurrent episodes of wheezing, breathlessness, chest tightness, and coughing ... episodes are usually associated with widespread but variable airflow obstruction that is often reversible either spontaneously or with treatment. The inflammation also enhances the pre-existing bronchial hyperresponsiveness to a variety of stimuli".

EPIDEMIOLOGY

Lifetime asthma (defined as having ever being diagnosed with asthma by a physician) was reported by 26.7 million persons in the United States from 1980 to 1999, 31.3 million in 2001, 32.6 million in 2005, and 34.1 million in 2006. The *current prevalence of asthma* in 2006 was 22.5 million (15.7 million adults), and the *asthma attack prevalence* was 12.4 million representing 54% of persons currently having asthma. Females have a 40% higher prevalence rate than males.

Asthma was responsible for more than 1.8 million ED visits in the United States in 2004 and a similar number in 2005.The asthma hospitalization rate was 35% greater in females than males.

Factors that contribute to asthma morbidity and mortality include inadequate patient and physician assessment of an acute episode resulting in undertreatment, overuse of prescribed or over-the-counter medications leading to delays in seeking treatment, failure of physicians to consider previous hospitalizations or life-threatening episodes of asthma, and failure to initiate corticosteroid therapy early in the course of an exacerbation. Socioeconomic factors, environmental influences, and over-reliance on emergency facilities for all asthma care are also contributing factors. Initiatives to educate physicians and patients about asthma pathophysiology, monitoring, and therapy may be in part responsible for the moderation of asthma mortality rates.

PRINCIPLES OF DISEASE

Pathophysiology

A variety of airway alterations occur in asthma, but airway inflammation is the final common pathway limiting airflow. Bronchoconstriction occurs due to allergic or nonallergic stimuli. Allergens induce bronchoconstriction via release of mediators and metabolic products from inflammatory cells, but nonallergic mechanisms also trigger airway inflammation in exercise, aspirin-induced, and menstrual-related asthma. Hyper-responsiveness of the airways is characteristic of asthma and correlates with the severity of the disease and the need for treatment. Edema, inflammation, mucus production, and airway smooth muscle hypertrophy contribute to bronchoconstriction and hyper-reactivity and further airway obstruction and airflow limitation. Airway remodeling may contribute to increased airway obstruction and hyper-responsiveness and decrease the response to therapy.

Evidence that inflammation is a component of asthma physiology was initially derived from autopsy findings in patients with fatal asthma. The airways revealed infiltration by neutrophils, eosinophils, and mast cells and the presence of sub-basement membrane thickening, loss of epithelial cell integrity, goblet cell hyperplasia, and mucous plugs.Inflammatory and chemotactic cytokines produced by both resident airway and recruited inflammatory cells are identified in bronchoalveolar lavage washings and pulmonary secretions.

IgE is associated with the severity of asthma and the initial and sustained responses of the airways to allergens.

Mast cells reside in the mucosa and submucosa of the airways,which may contribute to both the acute and chronic inflammatory reactions occurring in the airways.

Release of preformed histamine from mast cell granules constricts bronchial smooth muscle and causes airway edema, resulting in wheezing and airflow obstruction. This reaction usually resolves within an hour and is referred to as the *early asthmatic response*. Similar clinical manifestations occur 4 to 6 hr later as a result of cytokines generated and released by mast cells and other local and recruited inflammatory cells. The airflow obstruction and bronchospasm may be prolonged and together are referred to as the *late asthmatic response*.

Eosinophils are major effector cells in asthma. They contain granules that release inflammatory mediators including major basic protein, cationic protein, and leukotriene (LT). Major basic protein causes constriction of airway smooth muscle and desquamation of the airway epithelium. This effect exposes nerve endings, provides submucosal access for inflammatory cells and mediators, and negates epithelial cell regulation of the inflammatory process. Eosinophil cationic protein increases airway mucous production and can cause histamine release from mast cells. LTs are potent bronchoconstrictors produced by eosinophils that are more potent than methacholine. LTs also promote the secretion of thick viscid mucus, leading to airway plugging, and enhance airway vascular permeability, leading to airway edema.

It is noteworthy that preformed mediator and cytokine release from other airway inflammatory cells following the triggering stimulus also contributes to bronchial smooth muscle spasm, edema, and mucus production. The end result of persistent and self-reinforcing inflammation is airway smooth muscle stimulation and structural alterations evidenced by wheezing and airflow obstruction.

Airway epithelial cells are involved in asthma physiology. Inflammatory cells, mediators, and airway viruses can stimulate airway epithelium to produce inflammatory mediators or directly damage the epithelial barrier itself. NO is produced by airway epithelial cells. It is a potent vasodilator and may reflect the presence of inflammation in asthma.

Airway remodeling is distinctive in chronic asthma and is likely due to the presence of repetitive or chronic airway inflammation. It consists of airway wall thickening, subepithelial fibrosis, mucous gland metaplasia, increases in airway smooth muscle, myofibroblast hyperplasia, and epithelial hypertrophy. Airway remodeling may explain the resistance to therapy observed in patients with prolonged asthma histories and the decline in pulmonary function noted with age. Finally, if asthma is improperly treated, airway remodeling induced by chronic inflammation may lead to the development of chronic irreversible airflow limitation and a shortened life expectancy.

The clinical implications of the immune and inflammatory nature of the early and late asthmatic responses are crucial because therapy may be directed differently toward each phase. Mast cell stabilizers (e.g., beta$_2$-agonists) are more effective in the early asthmatic response but are of less use later in the course of an exacerbation. Anti-inflammatory therapy (e.g., corticosteroids, LT antagonists) is more effective in the late asthmatic response. Interference or inhibition of cytokine activities, suppression of chronic inflammation, and modulation of airway remodeling are potential therapeutic targets.

Miscellaneous Situations

Prevalence of aspirin-exacerbated respiratory disease (*AERD*) is 21% in adult asthmatics. It occurs more often in women. NSAID also precipitate AERD. AERD is a common life-threatening asthma.

Clinically, most patients with AERD develop symptoms in the third decade, frequently after a viral respiratory illness. Over several months, chronic nasal congestion, rhinorrhea, nasal polyps, and anosmia develop often followed by chronic pansinusitis. Bronchial asthma and sensitivity to aspirin then result. After ingestion of aspirin or a nonsteroidal drug, acute asthma symptoms occur within 3hr, usually accompanied by profuse rhinorrhea, conjunctival injection, periorbital edema, and occasionally a scarlet flushing of the head and neck. Definitive diagnosis is made by provocation challenges.

The pathogenesis of AERD is detailed in Fig. 18-1. Acetylsalicylic acid inhibits cyclooxygenase(COX), of which two isoforms are identified. COX-1 produces prostaglandin (PG) that are involved in normal physiologic maintenance of renal function, gastric mucosal integrity and hemostasis, and inflammatory states. COX-2 is not expressed in normal physiologic circumstances but produces PGs only in response to inflammatory stimuli. AERD occurs as a result of acetylsalicylic acid inhibition of COX that decreases the production of PGE$_2$. The end result is inflammatory mediator release from mast cells and eosinophils, and an increase in LT production; some of which substances are potent bronchoconstrictors. COX-2 inhibitors provide a potentially safe alternative for treatment of inflammatory conditions in patients with AERD.

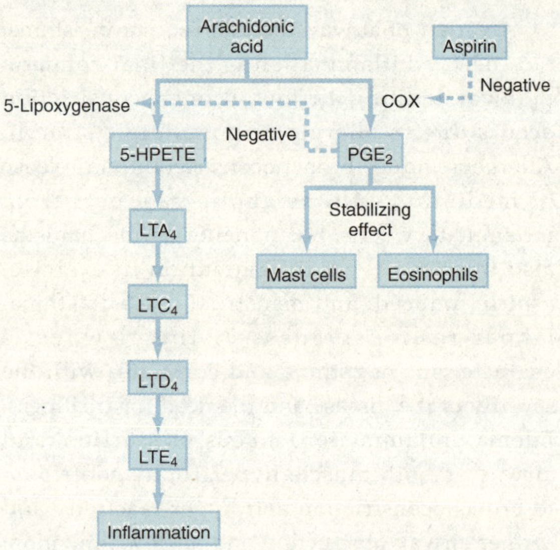

Fig. 18-1 Mechanism of AERD. Inhibition of COX decreases production of PGE$_2$. PGE$_2$ has an inhibitory effect on LT synthesis.

Exercise-induced asthma (EIA) occurs in 5% to 20% of the general population, 30% to 70% of elite winter and summer endurance athletes, and in up to 90% of patients with persistent asthma. EIA may be another reflection of chronic airway inflammation. Clinically, EIA is usually preceded by 3 to 8 min of exercise. Peak symptoms usually occur 8 to 15 min after exercise is complete and then begin to remit spontaneously; recovery occurs within 60 min.

The etiology of EIA remains unclear.

Menstruation-associated asthma affects up to 40%. The ratio of female-to-male asthma prevalence increases dramatically after puberty, and health care for asthma increases in the premenstrual phase. Fluctuations in estrogen and progesterone levels are postulated as causal factors.

Psychological factors may precipitate bronchospasm.The mechanisms of bronchospasm associated with psychological factors may be related to autonomic nervous system activation or hyperventilation. Compliance may be adversely affected by psychological factors. Relaxation as a therapy for asthma has inconsistent effects; hypnosis may be beneficial.

Genetics and Asthma

Asthma is actually a syndrome with various phenotypes. Clinicians have long recognized various asthma phenotypes (e.g., environmental, occupational, severe asthma), and researchers suspect that different pathophysiologic mechanisms may be responsible for the various manifestations of this disease.

Pathology

Airway secretions evaluated by bronchoalveolar lavage and sputum analysis in patients with mild to moderate asthma reveal increased numbers of mast cells, eosinophils, lymphocytes, and airway epithelial cells. Endobronchial biopsies may be normal, show only mild histologic changes between attacks, or reveal chronic alterations. Microscopy demonstrates submucosal infiltration with eosinophils and other inflammatory cells along with viscous mucous plugs in the bronchi and bronchioles, increased numbers of goblet cells, and mucous gland hyperplasia. Airway epithelial cells may be damaged or denuded. Immunohistochemistry demonstrates disruption of the tight junctions in the columnar cells. Airway remodeling is evidenced by squamous metaplasia, thickening of the basement membrane due to collagen and fibronectin deposition, and smooth muscle thickening. Neutrophils are the dominant cell type in the airways of some asthmatics.

In contrast to mild to moderate asthma, the acute severe asthma have inflammatory cells in the airways that consist of more neutrophils than eosinophils and elevated levels of IL-8 responsible for neutrophil activation.

Necropsies of patients with status asthmaticus reveal grossly inflated lungs that may fail to collapse on opening of the pleural cavities.

CLINICAL FEATURES

Symptoms

Most patients with acute asthma have a constellation of symptoms consisting of cough, dyspnea, and wheezing. Cough often begins early in the attack, may be the sole manifestation of the disease in cough-variant asthma and elder patients, can be associated with sputum production, and is probably the result of subepithelial vagal stimulation. Nocturnal worsening is common. Nighttime mortality is higher than in the general population.

Up to 40% of asthmatic women suffer from premenstrual worsening of symptoms, which peak 2 to 3 d before menses and are associated with more severe disease.

There are interindividual differences in the dyspnea perceived by asthmatic subjects for the same level of airway narrowing.Wheezing that develops reflects air movement velocity and turbulence, and its intensity varies according to the radius of the bronchi. With severe airway obstruction, it decreases or vanishes because air movement velocity is insufficient to produce sound.

Many asthmatics report symptoms of gastroesophageal reflux that may cause airway narrowing through a vagally mediated pathway or microaspiration. Approximately 80% of patients with asthma have symptoms of rhinitis. Approximately 5% to 15% of patients with perennial rhinitis have asthma. Overweight (BMI=25 kg/m^2) asthmatics have higher admission rates and risk of complications.

Historical Components

Slow-onset asthma with progressive deterioration over a period of at least 6 hr (usually days) occurs in over 80% of cases. This type has a female predominance, is triggered by upper respiratory tract infections, and has an airflow inflammation mechanism that results in a slower response to treatment. Sudden-onset asthma with rapid deterioration in under 6 hr occurs in less than 20%.

This type has a male predominance, is triggered by respiratory allergens, exercise and psychosocial stress, and has a bronchospastic etiology resulting in more severe airway obstruction with a faster response to therapy.

Risk factors for death from asthma are important to determine and are listed in Box 18-1.

Box 18-1 Risk Factors for Death from Asthma

Asthma History

- Previous severe exacerbation (intubation or ICU admission for asthma)
- Two or more hospitalizations for asthma in the past year
- Three or more ED visits for asthma in the past year
- Hospitalization or an ED visit for asthma in the past month
- Use of more than two MDI short-acting beta2-agonist canisters per month
- Current use of or recent withdrawal from systemic corticosteroids
- Difficulty perceiving asthma symptoms or severity of exacerbations

Social History

- Low socioeconomic status or inner-city residence
- Serious psychosocial problems
- Illicit drug use, especially inhaled cocaine and heroin

Comorbidities

- Cardiovascular disease
- Other chronic lung disease
- Chronic psychiatric disease

The brief history pertinent to the current exacerbation should include onset and possible triggers, severity of symptoms especially as compared with previous exacerbations, and other comorbidities (especially those that may be worsened by systemic corticosteroids such as diabetes, peptic ulcer, hypertension, and psychosis). In addition, all current asthma medications should be noted, including times and amounts recently used, and any potential asthma exacerbators such as aspirin or NSAID, beta-blocker (including topical agent used for glaucoma), and ACEI.

Physical Assessment

Those who suffer from mild acute asthma usually speak in sentences, moderate in phrases, and severe in words. Although alterations in mentation or consciousness indicate severe asthma, restlessness and agitation do not reliably indicate hypoxia or hypercapnia. Patients who sit upright have severe airway obstruction; cyanosis is uncommon because of the left shift of the oxyhemoglobin dissociation curve produced by respiratory alkalosis. Diaphoresis can be seen secondary to the work of breathing, but if profound it is usually accompanied by a decreasing level of agitation and interaction with caregivers and may be preterminal.

Tachypnea and tachycardia greater than 120 beats/min are associated with severe obstruction, but a lower rate does not rule out severe asthma. If tachypnea more than 40 breaths/min indicates severe airway obstruction.

A pulsus paradoxus or inspiratory fall in SBP greater than 10 mm Hg usually signifies severe disease, but its absence does not exclude it. Similarly, use of accessory muscles of respiration (sternocleidomastoid and scalenus muscles) is not prognostic.

Wheezing does not designate the presence, severity, or duration of asthma. It correlates poorly with the degree of functional derangement and may be absent when maximal effort produces minimal airflow. Physical examination may help to identify such complications of asthma as pneumonia, pneumothorax, or pneumomediastinum that may arise atypically as subcutaneus emphysema or simulate upper airway obstruction.

DIAGNOSTIC STRATEGIES

Pulmonary Function Studies

Routine pulmonary function testing (PFT) should be part of ED assessment and monitoring. The FEV_1 or the PEFR in liters per second starting with fully inflated lungs and sustained for at least 10 ms may be used. Both measurements require the patient's cooperation for maximal effort and are effort-dependent. Whenever possible, the best of three consecutive values should be recorded. Any patient not able to perform a pulmonary function study should be considered to have severe airway obstruction.

Most asthmatic assessments in the ED use single-patient-use portable peak flow meters because PEFR is easier to measure. However, the FEV_1 and PEFR measurements do not appear to be interchangeable in assessing acute airway obstruction.

Although absolute PFT measurements can be used, percentage of predicted performance (% predicted) values are preferable because they account for the individual's age (now to age 85), sex, and height. Ideally, the percentage of the patient's personal best effort individualizes the assessment and treatment.

Arterial Blood Gas Analysis

With initial onset of an asthma attack, stimulated hyperventilation leads to a modest fall in the P_aCO_2. As airway obstruction increases, the P_aCO_2 normalizes (PFT 15%–25% predicted) and then increases (PFT<15% predicted) with worsening hypoxemia.

ABG sampling should be limited to a subset of patients with predicted PFT of less than 30%, whose clinical course is perplexing and for whom capnography is not available. The assessment of ventilation may be simplified since there is a high concordance between $ETco_2$ measured by capnography and the P_aCO_2 obtained with ABG measurements.

Other Blood Testing

Leukocytosis is common in patients with acute asthma exacerbation, but is not of discriminatory value in determining whether patients have acute superimposed pulmonary infection. It's worth onting that, corticosteroid, epinephrine therapy and patients on chronic steroid therapy may have normal or significantly elevated WBC counts.

Serum electrolytes are not primarily altered unless the patient is on corticosteroids or diuretics or has cardiovascular disease and is receiving aggressive $beta_2$-agonist therapy. Frequent albuterol treatments can cause transient hypokalemia, hypomagnesemia, and hypophosphatemia.

In the older asthmatic with cardiovascular comorbidities who presents with wheezing, measure the BNP level to determine the contribution of unrecognized CHF to the clinical picture.

Radiology Studies

A chest radiograph is of little value in most acute asthma exacerbations, and its use should be restricted to patients thought to have a complicating cardiopulmonary process such as pneumonia, pneumothorax, pneumomediastinum, or CHF.

Electrocardiogram and Cardiac Monitoring

The ECG need not be routinely obtained, except in patients ⩾40 yr, with a separate complaint (e.g., chest pain), or with a history of significant cardiovascular disease. In patients with severe asthma, the ECG may show a right ventricular strain pattern that reverses with improvement in airflow. Older patients, especially those with coexistent heart disease or with severe exacerbation, may require continuous cardiac monitoring to detect arrhythmia early. All patients with severe hypoxemia, and those for whom intubation is contemplated, should have continuous cardiac monitoring.

Future Monitoring Strategies

Noninvasive monitoring of bronchial inflammation may customize the ED assessment of acute asthma. This may include measurement of biologic biomarkers such as cytokine profiles in the blood, evaluation of LTE_4 in the urine, and the monitoring of exhaled pentane, hydrogen peroxide,NO, or carbon monoxide levels.

Assessment Summary

The severity of airflow obstruction cannot be accurately judged by patients' symptoms, physical examination, and laboratory tests. Serial measurements of airflow obstruction (FEV_1 or PEFR) are key components of disease assessment and response to therapy. A more detailed analysis between commonly measured variables and patients with severe asthma (FEV_1<1 L) is shown in Table 18-1.

Table 18-1 **Objective Findings in Asthma Assessment**

FACTOR	SEVERE ASTHMA (FEV1 <1.0 L)
Pulse rate (beats/min)	≥120 but may be less with equally severe asthma
Respiratory rate (breaths/min)	≥40 but most are >20, therefore nondiscriminating
Pulsus paradoxus (mm Hg)	≥10 but may be absent with equally severe asthma in 50% of cases
Pulse rate ≥120, respiratory rate ≥20, pulsus paradoxus ≥10	If all three abnormal, 90% with severe asthma, but only 40% with FEV_1 <1.0 L have all three abnormal
Use of accessory muscles of respiration	If present, may indicate severe asthma;if absent, may have equally severe asthma in 50% of cases
ABG analysis (mm Hg)	P_aO_2 ≤60 or P_aCO_2 ≥42 indicates severe asthma; all other values difficult to interpret unless PEFR or FEV_1 known
Pulmonary function studies	PEFR and FEV_1 measure directly the degree of airflow obstruction; most useful in assessing severity and guiding treatment decisions

DIFFERENTIAL CONSIDERATIONS (BOX 18-2)

Box 18-2 The Differential Diagnosis of Asthma

- Cardiac conditions
  - Valvular heart disease
  - CHF
- COPD exacerbation
  - Pulmonary infection
  - Pneumonia
  - Allergic bronchopulmonary aspergillosis
  - Loffler's syndrome
  - Chronic eosinophilic pneumonia
- Upper airway obstruction
  - Laryngeal edema
  - Laryngeal neoplasm
  - Foreign body
  - Vocal cord dysfunction
- Endobronchial disease
  - Neoplasm
  - Foreign body
  - Bronchial stenosis
- Pulmonary embolus
- Carcinoid tumor
- Allergic or anaphylactic reaction
- Miscellaneous conditions
  - gastroesophageal reflux disease
  - Noncardiogenic pulmonary edema
  - Addison's disease
  - Invasive worm infection

MANAGEMENT OF ACUTE EXACERBATIONS

Management of Acute Asthma in the Emergency Department

The goal in the ED is to reverse the acute airflow obstruction safely, and the rapidity of this reversal is directly predictive of the outcome of the attack. As outlined in Table 18-2, the severity of attack as measured by PFT determines the aggressiveness of the therapy.

Adrenergic Medication

Controversies in Use

There is an association between death and near death from asthma and the use of inhaled beta$_2$-agonists. For this reason, guidelines for chronic use of inhaled beta$_2$-agonists, however, recommend limited daily use in a rescue-only mode.

Short-Acting Inhaled Beta2-Agonist Choice and Dosing Schedule

Racemic albuterol has been the main beta$_2$-agonist used in the ED for over 30 yr. It is more beta$_2$-selective, longer acting, and has fewer side effects than other previously available drugs such as metaproterenol or isoetharine.

Levalbuterol, the R isomer of racemic albuterol, is commercially available as a preservative-free nebulizer solution (unit doses of 0.31, 0.63, or 1.25 mg) for prevention and treatment of bronchospasm. In chronic asthma, levalbuterol provides a better therapeutic index than the standard dose of racemic albuterol.

Table 18-2 Initial Severity Assessments and Therapies in the ED

	MILD TO MODERATE	SEVERE
FEV_1 or PEFR (% predicted/personal best)	⩾40%	Unable or <40%
Oxygen therapy	Maintain SaO_2 ⩾90%	Maintain SaO_2 ⩾90%
Nebulized albuterol solution		
Levalbuterol (optimal)	1.25 mg q20min for up to three doses	1.25 mg q20min for three doses Continuous for 1 hr if severe
Racemic albuterol	2.5 mg q20min for up to three doses	5.0 mg q20min for three doses Continuous for 1 hr if severe
Albuterol MDI with VHC		
Levalbuterol (45 μg/puff) (optimal)	6-12 puffs q20min for up to three doses WS	Same for three doses (if able to do), WS
Racemic albuterol (90 μg/puff)	6-12 puffs q20min for up to three doses WS	Same for three doses (if able to do), WS
Ipratropium therapy		
Nebulized solution	If previous response (same dose as for severe)	0.5 mg q20min for three doses (may mix with albuterol solution)
MDI (18 μg/puff) with VHC	If previous response (same dose as for severe)	8 puffs q20min for three doses
Systemic corticosteroids		
Oral (preferred)	40-80 mg of prednisone or prednisolone per day if no immediate response to albuterol	40-80 mg of prednisone or prednisolone per day
Intravenous (unable to take orally or absorb)	40-80 mg of methylprednisolone per day	40-80 mg of methylprednisolone per day
Intravenous magnesium sulfate	Not indicated	2-3 g over 20 min (or at rates of up to 1 g/min) if FEV_1 ⩽ 25% predicted

WS, with supervision VHC,valved holding chamber

The amount and frequency of delivery of levalbuterol and racemic albuterol depend on the initial severity and response to therapy, as shown in Table 18-2 and Table 18-3. Patients with more severe obstruction with a poor response to initial therapy should receive higher dosing schedules and possible continuous administration. When patients are stable but require ICU admission, it may be possible to dose nebulized levalbuterol at 1.25 mg every 8 hr as opposed to racemic albuterol at 2.5 mg every 4 to 6 hr.

Nebulizer versus Metered-Dose Inhaler and Valved Holding Chamber

A metered-dose inhaler (MDI) plus a valved holding chamber, used often and frequently (see Table 18-2), provides similar bronchodilation and side effects, even in severe asthma, when compared with wet nebulization.

Intravenous Use of Adrenergic Agonists

When inhaled therapy is not feasible, it is recommend that use of intravenous beta-agonists for severe nonresponsive acute asthma. Intravenous albuterol (not available in the United States) is given as a loading dose of 4 μg/kg for 2 to 5 min followed by an infusion of 0.1 to 0.2 μg/kg/min, with close cardiopulmonary monitoring.

Howevwer, Epinephrine is used cautiously in patients older than 40 yr of age or those with

Table 18-3 Response after 1 Hour of Initial Treatment

	MODERATE EXACERBATION	SEVERE EXACERBATION
FEV_1 or PEFR(% predicted)	40%-69%	<40%
Oxygen therapy	Unnecessary	Maintain SaO_2 ⩾90%
Albuterol therapy		
Levalbuterol(optimal)	Reassess as may need less than with racemic dosing	Reassess as may need less than with racemic dosing
Racemic albuterol	q1-3h, admit decision in <4 hr	q1h or continuous
Ipratropium therapy	Unnecessary	q1h or continuous
Corticosteroids	Every 6-8 hr	Every 6-8 hr

suspected cardiovascular disease, because it might provoke myocardial ischemia. Epinephrine intravenous titrated to effect (average 1.5 μg/min with a range of 0.5-13.3 μg/min) is associated with a low rate of major (3.6% of cases) and moderate or minor adverse events.

Subcutaneous Adrenergic Agents

Subcutaneous use of adrenergic agents does not have an advantage over aerosol delivery. They may be considered in patients who cannot adequately inhale albuterol or who experience severe bronchospasm.

Given the potential for increased side effects, it can be given subcutaneously (1:1000 solution 0.2 to 0.5 mL every 20 to 30 min as needed for three doses).

Terbutaline is a longer-acting $beta_2$-agonist with bronchodilating properties equivalent to those of epinephrine in acute asthma. It can cause skeletal muscle tremor and tachycardia. A 0.25-mg dose can be given subcutaneously every 20 min for three doses.

Long-Acting $Beta_2$-Agonists and Acute Disease

Salmeterol is a long-acting (12 hr) $beta_2$-agonist that is an effective additional medication for management of daytime and nocturnal symptoms that are not adequately controlled by regular and adequate doses of effective controller medications such as inhaled steroids. It has an onset of action of 20 min and thus is not indicated for the treatment of acute attacks. Regular use of this drug without concomitant use of inhaled steroids results in greater asthma-related deaths.

Racemic formoterol dry powder and solution and single-isomer arformoterol are other long-acting $beta_2$-agonists that have an onset of action within minutes (similar to albuterol) and maximal effect within 2 hr. These drugs could evolve as acute rescue medications with extended length of action (12 hr) and similar safety profiles.

Corticosteroids

Systemic Corticosteroids in the Emergency Department

These medications should be given promptly to all patients with moderate to severe attacks or those experiencing an incomplete response to initial beta-agonist therapy. In addition, early systemic corticosteroids should be considered for patients who are taking oral or inhaled corticosteroids, have relapsed after a recent exacerbation, or have prolonged symptoms. Steroid effects begin within hours (not minutes) in acute asthma and increase to peak over 24 hr. The PEFR may improve within 2 hr of steroid therapy in those not responding to initial albuterol inhalation.

Oral corticosteroids are as beneficial as intravenous corticosteroids in the ED management of an acute asthma exacerbation. Initial oral dosing is usually 60 mg of prednisone. If intravenous methylprednisolone is used, the dose is 40 to 80 mg/d in one or two divided doses until the patient can be switched to oral therapy, or PEFR reaches 70% of predicted or personal best.

Continuing therapy with oral prednisone or prednisolone is given in an adult dose of 40 to 80 mg/d, usually as a single dose.

Side effects of short-term (hours or days) steroid use include reversible increases in glucose (important in diabetics) and decreases in potassium, fluid retention with weight gain, mood alterations including rare psychosis, hypertension, peptic ulcers, aseptic necrosis of the femur, and rare allergic reactions.

Inhaled Corticosteroids in the Emergency Department

Using inhaled corticosteroid, either alone or in addition to systemic steroids, to treat acute asthma has the potential benefits of reducing systemic side effects, directly delivering medication to the airway, and reducing airway reactivity and edema more effectively. Patients treated with these agents have early improvement in outcomes (<3 hr) because of their topical effects. High doses of inhaled corticosteroid given over hours may be necessary for them to be effective.

Corticosteroids and Discharged Patients

Discharged patients who have received systemic corticosteroids in the ED should continue oral outpatient "burst" therapy to control disease and prevent relapse. Any need for additional steroids should be determined at the patient's follow-up outpatient visit. An acceptable regimen is 40 to 60 mg of prednisone (or equivalent) in single daily dose for a total of 5 to 10 d. Dose tapering to prevent asthma rebound or out of concern for adrenal suppression is unnecessary unless the patient was already receiving systemic steroids or a prolonged course of therapy (more than 2 w) is deemed necessary. An alternative approach, if compliance may be an issue, is to give an equally efficacious single depot dose of triamcinolone diacetate (40 mg) or methylprednisolone (160 mg) before ED discharge.

Corticosteroid-Resistant Asthma

Chronic asthma is considered a steroid-responsive disease.The mechanism of this steroid resistance may be related to abnormalities in the glucocorticoid receptor number or binding properties. These patients are usually receiving alternative therapies such as cyclosporine, methotrexate, troleandomycin, hydroxychloroquine, azathioprine, gold, intravenous immune globulin, or (if with severe allergic asthma) maintenance anti-IgE recombinant humanized monoclonal antibody (omalizumab).

Anticholinergic Agents

The anticholinergic drugs available for inhalation therapy include atropine sulfate, atropine methylnitrate, glycopyrrolate, and ipratropium bromide. They are all bronchodilators.

The maximum effect with inhaled ipratropium is in 30 to 120 min, with the effect lasting for up to 6 hr. Its bronchodilating potency is lower and onset of action slower than those of the beta$_2$-agonists; hence, it should not be used alone in patients with acute asthma.

Treatment recommendations (Table 18-2) include adding ipratropium (0.5 mg) with the first three albuterol treatments in severe acute asthma (<40% predicted). The equivalent MDI dose is approximately eight puffs (18 μg/puff) every 20 min three times. Data suggest that less ipratropium might be needed in patients treated with levalbuterol nebulizations. There is evidence that ipratropium may be more effective in patients older than 40 yr, should be used in reversing bronchospasm secondary to beta-blocking agents, and might help those in whom psychological factors contribute to their disease.

Magnesium Sulfate

Magnesium relaxes bronchial smooth muscle and dilates asthmatic airways.It is reasonable to administer 2 to 3 g of intravenous magnesium sulfate over 20 min or at rates of up to 1 g/min to patients with severe refractory asthma while continuing aggressive inhalation therapy.

Inhalation magnesium in acute asthma may also have a role as an isotonic vehicle for nebulized bronchodilator therapy in improving the PFT response or even be nebulized alone for bronchodilation.

Leukotriene Modifiers

Zafirlukast (20 mg twice a day) and montelukast (10 mg daily) are rapid-acting, safe, asthma controller drugs, taken orally.

Oral zafirlukast, when given as adjunctive therapy (20 or 160 mg) for acute asthma in the ED. The acute non-beta-mediated bronchodilating effects of these relatively safe medications could be very useful in managing acute disease.

Other or Future Therapies

In patients without signs of dehydration or hypovolemia, there is no evidence that vigorous administration of fluids aids in clearing airway secretions. Mucolytics may worsen cough or airflow obstruction, and chest physical therapy is not beneficial. Sedatives are contraindicated in acute disease because of their respiratory depressant effect.

Bacterial, chlamydial, and mycoplasmal respiratory tract infections infrequently contribute to acute asthma. The decision to administer antibiotics should generally be reserved for patients with fever, purulent sputum, pneumonia, or evidence of bacterial sinusitis.

Future asthma therapies may include the second-generation antihistamines, even though earlier compounds were considered contraindicated in the disease. Neurokinin antagonists, inhaled loop diuretics (furosemide in acute attacks), and lidocaine may inhibit neurogenic inflammation, and heparin may have a role in the inhibition of mast cell products. Infused BNP can cause significant bronchodilation in patients with asthma. Lastly, specific cytokine antagonists, agonists, inhibitors of T-cell function, selective inducible nitric oxide synthetase inhibitors, and possibly gene-directed therapies may become novel treatments.

Pregnancy and Acute Asthma

The maternal and fetal risks of uncontrolled asthma are high, and acute disease should be maximally treated with the prevention of maternal and fetal hypoxia as the principal goal. Maternal asthma is not associated with preterm birth or birth defects. Many complications of pregnancy (e.g., hypertensive disorders, antepartum hemorrhage, low birth weight, need for cesarean section), however, are reported. Pregnant asthmatics receive corticosteroid therapy in the ED less often than nonpregnant women, resulting in continued exacerbation at 2w follow-up after discharge. Inhaled beta-agonists and corticosteroids should be continued during pregnancy. As the risk to mother and fetus far outweighs the potential complications, that use of systemic corticosteroids during pregnancy is suggested in severe uncontrolled exacerbations. Continuous electronic fetal monitoring should be considered at delivery. Recommendations for managing asthma during lactation are the same as those for managing the disease during pregnancy.

Severe, Near-Fatal, and Fatal Asthma

The American Thoracic Society has developed a consensus definition for identifying severe and refractory asthma that is unresponsive to conventional therapies (Fig. 18-2). Termed *severe asthma*, patients with these symptoms represent only about 10% of all asthmatics yet account for 30% of asthma-related health care costs and have the highest morbidity and mortality rates associated with this disease. To satisfy the definition of severe asthma, medical conditions that mimic asthma must be excluded, exacerbating factors (e.g., allergens) identified and treated, and patients must be generally compliant with therapies.

Clinical features of severe asthma include a lesser prevalence of atopy, a history of aspirin sensitivity, and a higher incidence of sinusitis and use of nasal corticosteroids (suggesting involvement of the upper as well as lower respiratory tract). Exacerbations are also associated with menses.

Major characteristics
- Treatment with continuous or near-continuous (≥50% of year) oral corticosteroids
- Requirement for treatment with high-dose intravenous corticosteroids

Minor characteristics
- Requirement for additional daily treatment with a controller medication (e.g., long-acting beta-agonist, theophylline, or leukotriene antagonist)
- Asthma symptoms requiring short-acting beta-agonist use on a daily or near-daily basis
- Persistent airway obstruction (FEV_1 <80% predicted, diurnal peak expiratory flow variability >20%)
- One or more urgent care visits for asthma per year
- Three or more oral steroid bursts per year
- Prompt deterioration with ≤25% reduction in oral or intravenous corticosteroid dose
- Near-fatal asthma event in the past

Fig. 18-2 American Thoracic Society workshop consensus for definition of severe/refractory asthma (requires one or both major and two minor criteria and that other conditions have been excluded, exacerbating factors have been treated, and patient is generally compliant).

Status asthmaticus refers to severe bronchospasm that does not respond to aggressive therapies within 30 to 60 min. *Near-fatal asthma* is identified by respiratory arrest or evidence of respiratory failure (P_aCO_2 > 50 mm Hg).

Two types of near-fatal asthma are recognized. Slow-onset near-fatal asthma typically reflects a gradual deterioration of asthma symptoms over several days. Rapid-onset near-fatal asthma is characterized by symptom onset and progression to life-threatening status in 3 hr or less. Clinically, rapid-onset near-fatal asthma is characterized by greater hypercapnia than occurs in the slow-onset type. Hypercapnia in rapid-onset near-fatal asthma normally need shorter durations of mechanical ventilation. Deaths associated with the slow-onset mechanism are thought to be preventable in many cases because the gradual progression of symptoms allows patients to seek medical evaluation before succumbing.

Risk factors for death from asthma are identified (Box 18-2).

Clinical Approach to the Critically Ill Asthmatic

The critically ill asthmatic appears agitated (hypoxemic), assumes an upright position, and appears to be in severe respiratory distress. Tachypnea, diaphoresis, and accessory muscle use are evident. Speech is fragmented into single or short bursts of syllables or words. Absence of wheezing indicates severe expiratory obstruction and minimal air movement. Peak expiratory testing is difficult for the patient to perform but, when possible, indicates severe expiratory obstruction. Alterations in consciousness and bradypnea indicate hypercarbia and impending respiratory arrest.

No laboratory markers identify patients with near-fatal asthma. In critically ill patients, elevated lactic acid levels reflect tissue hypoxemia and anaerobic metabolism; persistent elevations of arterial lactate levels are often associated with a poor prognosis.

Noninvasive Strategies

Therapy must be initiated immediately (Table 18-2). Attempts of termination of the attack should include high-dose frequent or continuously nebulized beta$_2$- and anticholinergic agents. If parenteral adrenergic therapy is optimal, terbutaline is preferred because of its beta$_2$ selectivity.Intravenous use of magnesium sulfate or beta$_2$-agonists (where available) may be of benefit. Oral prednisone, 60 mg, or intravenous methylprednisolone, 125 mg, should be administered early. Use of a helium/oxygen delivery system (heliox) is controversial. Heliox reduces the resistance associated with gas flow through airways with nonlaminar flow and reduces respiratory muscle work; it also increases the diffusion of carbon dioxide and may improve alveolar ventilation. Although heliox is not intrinsically therapeutic, it may decrease the work of breathing long enough to abort intubation by allowing bronchodilators and anti-inflammatory agents to achieve their effects. Close monitoring of oxygen saturation and continuous capnography are advisable. Noninvasive positive-pressure ventilation(NPPV) may benefit carefully selected patients. CPAP improves oxygenation and reduces respiratory muscle fatigue by increasing functional residual capacity and lung compliance and supplying some of the inflating pressure required during inspiration. BiPAP provides continuous positive airway pressure but delivers higher pressure during inspiration than expiration. BiPAP is well tolerated by children with status asthmaticus and may decrease the need for intubation and mechanical ventilation. BiPAP may also decrease the need for intubation and ICU care in adults with status asthmaticus.

BiPAP is not a substitute for endotracheal intubation and mechanical ventilation. Patient considerations for BiPAP include an alert mental status and intact airway reflexes.Frequent ABG monitoring after institution of this therapy identifies nonresponders. Endotracheal intubation should be performed immediately if respiratory distress persists or if clinical or laboratory signs of deterioration are observed.

Intubation and Ventilator Strategy

Endotracheal intubation is required in 2% of all asthma exacerbations and 10% to 30% requiring ICU admission. With the exception of apnea or coma, there are no absolute indications for intubation in the asthmatic patient, but intubation should occur in the failing patient before the patient develops profound acidemia or hypoxemia. Exhaustion, hypoxemia, and depression of mental status strongly mandate prompt intubation.

Orotracheal rapid sequence intubation utilizing induction agents and muscle paralysis is preferred. Ketamine (1–2 mg/kg) is the preferred agent for induction in rapid sequence intubation of the asthmatic patient. Succinylcholine (1.5 mg/kg) or a competitive NMBA, such as rocuronium (1 mg/kg) can be used for intubation paralysis. Pretreatment with lidocaine (1.5 mg/kg), given 3 min before the succinylcholine and ketamine, may mitigate the exacerbation of bronchospasm by the upper airway instrumentation and the ETT. After intubation, additional ketamine may be given as a small number of intermittent boluses of 0.5 to 1.0 mg/kg, and a benzodiazepine should be administered to keep the patient sedated and to prevent a ketamine emergence reaction. Alternatively, propofol (1.5–2 mg/kg) offers rapid-onset deep sedation and also possesses bronchodilating properties. Continued deep sedation with propofol or an equivalent agent (e.g., long-acting benzodiazepine) usually avoids the need for muscle paralysis. After intubation, an opioid that does not release histamine, such as fentanyl, can be used to improve the patient's comfort with the ventilator.

A ventilator strategy providing adequate oxygenation and ventilation while minimizing high airway pressure, barotrauma, and systemic hypotension must be instituted. The technique of *permissive hypercapnia* (also known as controlled hypoventilation) is common. Oxygenation is maintained by using a high F_iO_2; hypercarbia and respiratory acidosis (pH maintained at 7.15–7.2 using sodium bicarbonate) are tolerated. Airway pressure is kept low by providing low tidal volumes (6–8 mL/kg), thus preventing excessive increases of iPEEP, stacking of ventilations, and barotrauma. Low ventilation rates (<10 breaths/min) and high inspiratory flow rates provide prolonged time for expiration. Adjunctive therapies (in-line beta$_2$-agonists and anticholinergics, intravenous corticosteroids, intravenous ketamine, and possibly magnesium) to decrease airway pressure and airway obstruction are delivered simultaneously.

Continuous capnography is advisable.

Moderate levels of hypercapnia are well tolerated and have few deleterious effects. But, P_aCO_2 levels above 100 mm Hg should be avoided. Moreover, Hypercapnia can decrease cardiac contractility and produce cardiovascular collapse.

Neuromuscular blockade, once widely used for ventilation of asthmatic patients, is now used only in cases where deep sedation with adequate analgesia fails to provide sufficient patient relaxation for successful mechanical ventilation. Intubation and mechanical ventilation may be lifesaving in near-fatal asthma attacks. Although hazards of mechanical ventilation (nosocomial infection, barotrauma) may occur, the treatment of critically ill asthmatics with mechanical ventilation is associated with low or zero mortality and few complications. Most asthmatics requiring mechanical ventilation improve rapidly and require short ICU stays.

Complications of mechanical ventilation in the asthmatic patient include hypotension and barotrauma.

Treatment of the Refractory Critically Ill Asthmatic

If the intensively treated, intubated critically ill asthmatic continues to have elevated airway pressures, persistent hypoxemia, and continued bronchospasm, general anesthesia should be considered in the operating room. Isoflurane, a bronchodilator, has lower arrhythmogenic and hypotensive properties than halothane.

External lateral chest compression may be of assistance when patients cannot exhale. Chest compression is delivered by bilateral squeezing of the lower chest walls immediately after end inspiration occurs. Compression delivered too early (i.e., during inspiration) may increase airway pressure and result in barotrauma.

Cardiopulmonary arrest may result from unrecognized barotrauma. Empirical bilateral tube thoracostomy should be performed if unexplained cardiac arrest occurs, especially in the context of dramatic increases in peak inspiratory pressure. Intravinas Intravenous epinephrine is a logical agent to use in the setting of cardiopulmonary arrest because it has both cardiostimulatory and bronchodilatory properties. CPB and extracorporeal lung assist are also used in the treatment of near-fatal asthma.

DISPOSITION

Inpatient versus Observation or Clinical Decision Unit

Patients requiring extended care who are without life-threatening exacerbations, pregnancy, or complications of asthma can generally be treated in a clinical decision unit (CDU) for 12 hr with 8 w outcomes equal to those of patients treated in a hospital ward but with significant cost savings. The ability to predict discharge from the CDU can be assessed by the ED PEFR response to the third beta$_2$-agonist treatment (PEFR > 40% predicted is often associated with successful CDU discharge).

Table 18-4 summarizes disposition guidelines for asthmatics on the basis of their response to therapies in the ED.

Patients receiving systemic corticosteroids in the ED must continue these orally for 5

Table 18-4 ED Disposition Decision-Making Guidelines

	GOOD RESPONSE	INCOMPLETE RESPONSE	POOR RESPONSE
FEV_1 or PEFR (% predicted/ personal best)	≥70%	≥40% but <69%	<40%
Disposition site			
Home	Yes	Individualized decision (see text)	No, continue therapy
Clinical decision unit	No	Yes, if available	Yes, if available and appropriate
Hospital ward	No	Yes, if no CDU	Yes, if appropriate and available
Critical care unit	No	No	Yes, if with respiratory insufficiency/ failure

to 10 d. If the patient is not using controller medications and experiences persistent disease, moderate-dose inhaled steroids or a combination inhaled steroid and long-acting beta-agonist (e.g., salmeterol xinafoate-fluticasone propionate) should be started.

Patients should be encouraged to contact their physician or a respiratory specialist nurse for asthma-related problems within the next 3 to 5 d and to make a follow-up medical appointment within 1 to 4 w.

The asthma patient can be provided medication adjustment if the condition is not improving, and a peak flow meter for daily measurements, especially for those who have difficulty perceiving airflow obstruction or who have symptoms of worsening asthma. Lastly, all asthma patients should quit smoking.

(ZHANG Hong)

Chapter 19

Pneumonia

KEY CONCEPTS

Empirical antimicrobial therapy should be started in the ED for patients admitted with pneumonia. Empirical therapy should treat the most likely pathogens, including *S. pneumoniae, H. influenzae, M. pneumoniae,* and *C. pneumoniae.*

HIV or other immunosuppressive conditions should be considered in all patients in whom pneumonia is suspected.

Communicable diseases should be considered and isolation initiated when appropriate, including suspected TB, SARS, or influenza.

It is important to recognize the distinction between the acute aspiration of gastric contents or other liquids and bacterial pneumonia that may develop later as a complication of aspiration.

Patients with severe pneumonia, who present with severe sepsis or septic shock, require aggressive fluid resuscitation and may benefit from more intensive management with vasopressors, transfusion, and inotropic agents as part of early goal-directed therapy.

PERSPECTIVE

Pneumonia is one of the most common life-threatening infections. Most cases of community-acquired pneumonia (CAP) are managed in the outpatient setting, but pneumonia requiring hospitalization is associated with a much higher mortality rate (approximately 15%). Most deaths occur in elderly or immunosuppressed patients.

The epidemiology of CAP is changing. As the percentage of the population older than age 65 yr continues to increase, the incidence of pneumonia is expected to increase. An increasing number of patients are taking immunosuppressive drugs related to treatment of malignancy, transplantation, or autoimmune disease, resulting in more cases of pneumonia due to other opportunistic pathogens. Patients with AIDS are at increased risk of infection with *Streptococcus pneumoniae, Mycobacterium tuberculosis*, or *Pneumocystis jirovecii* (previously known as *Pneumocystis carinii*). Antibiotic resistance is more common among *S. pneumoniae* and other pathogens.

Identification of a specific etiology of pneumonia is extremely difficult within the time frame of an ED visit.

PRINCIPLES OF DISEASE

Despite the constant presence of potential pathogens in the respiratory tract, the lungs are remarkably resistant to infection.

The development of clinical pneumonia requires a defect in host defenses, the presence of a particularly virulent organism, or the introduction of a large inoculum of organisms. If the challenge of invading organisms overwhelms host defenses, microbial proliferation leads to inflammation, an immune response, and clinical pneumonia. If host defenses are weak, a minimal challenge may lead to the development of pneumonia.

Host defenses can be impaired in many ways. An altered level of consciousness (e.g., intoxication, stroke, seizures, and anesthesia) can suppress protective airway reflexes and lead to aspiration of oropharyngeal contents into the lower respiratory tract. Interventions that bypass the usual defenses of the upper airways, such as endotracheal intubation, nasogastric intubation, and respiratory therapy devices, predispose to infection. Cigarette smoking damages mucociliary function and macrophage activity. Viral infections of the respiratory tract may destroy respiratory epithelium and predispose it to bacterial infection. Increased risk of bacterial pneumonia after influenza or other viral respiratory infections is well described. The elderly are at increased risk of pneumonia related to decline of mucociliary clearance, elastic recoil of the lungs, and humoral and cellular immunity. HIV infection impairs humoral and cellular immunity.

If an infectious organism reaches the alveoli and begins replicating, a series of host immune responses occurs that ultimately may lead to the development of clinical pneumonia.As fluids and inflammatory cells enter the alveolar spaces to combat the infection, the patient develops the clinical and radiographic signs of pneumonia.

Etiologic Agents

In CAP, a microbial etiology cannot be determined in one third to one half of cases.Empiric therapy must be chosen with activity against the spectrum of likely pathogens based on the overall clinical picture.

In hospitalized adults with CAP, pathogens such as *S. pneumoniae* and *Haemophilus influenzae*, referred to as "typical" pathogens, account for approximately one fourth of cases. *Legionella*, *Mycoplasma*, and *Chlamydophila* spp. (previously known as *Chlamydia*), referred to as "atypical" pathogens, are also common. Testing for common viral agents reveals a viral etiology in approximately 18% of cases, with influenza and parainfluenza viruses most common.Atypical organisms such as *Mycoplasma* sp. or viruses account for a relatively higher proportion of pneumonia in patients who have milder illness that is amenable to outpatient therapy.Co-infection, such as with *Chlamydophila pneumoniae* and *S. pneumoniae*, is also well recognized.

"Typical" pathogens

Streptococcus pneumoniae

Streptococcus pneumoniae is the most common etiology of CAP among adults. Although this organism can cause pneumonia in healthy people, patients with a history of diabetes, cardiovascular disease, alcoholism, sickle cell disease, splenectomy, and malignancy or other immunosuppressive illness are at increased risk.It is recommended for people at increased risk because of underlying illness or age older than 65 yr.

Haemophilus influenzae

The second most frequently isolated organism in CAP among adults, is a pleomorphic gram-negative rod. It is a common pathogen in adults with COPD, alcoholism, malnutrition, malignancy, or DM.

Staphylococcus aureus

The community-associated strains of methicillin-resistant S. aureus (CA-MRSA) are emerging as a cause of severe pneumonia in previously healthy adults and children. This is often associated with influenza. Staphylococcal pneumonias are often necrotizing.

Moraxella catarrhalis

A gram-negative diplococcus that can be associated with lower respiratory tract infections in patients with COPD.

Klebsiella pneumoniae

Klebsiella pneumoniae is a gram-negative rod that rarely causes disease in a normal host and accounts for a small percentage of CAP. It may cause severe pneumonia in debilitated patients with alcoholism, DM, or other chronic illness. There is a high incidence of antibiotic resistance since the organism is often hospital acquired.

Mycobacterium tuberculosis

Mycobacterium tuberculosis is a slow-growing bacterium transmitted between people by droplet nuclei produced from coughing and sneezing. *Mycobacterium tuberculosis* survives within macrophages and may remain dormant in the body for many years.Reactivation is more likely to occur in patients with diabetes, renal failure, immunosuppressive therapy, malnutrition, or AIDS. Multidrug-resistant strains of *M. tuberculosis* are found in increasing numbers.

"Atypical" pathogens

Legionella

Another type of bacterial pneumonia caused by legionella species occurs in certain geographic locations and tends to follow specific exposures.

Mycoplasma pneumoniae and Chlamydophila pneumonia

Mycoplasma pneumoniae is one of the most common causes of CAP in previously healthy patients younger than age 40 yr. *Chlamydophila pneumoniae* is a relatively common etiology of CAP, especially in older adults.

Lower respiratory infections due to anaerobic organisms generally result from the aspiration of oropharyngeal contents with large amounts of bacteria. These infections are typically polymicrobial, including

Peptostreptococcus, *Bacteroides*, *Fusobacterium*, and *Prevotella* spp. Presentation is often subacute or chronic and may be difficult to distinguish clinically from other etiologies of pneumonia. Clinical factors that suggest an anaerobic infection include risk factors for aspiration, such as central nervous system depression or swallowing dysfunction; severe periodontal disease; fetid sputum; and the presence of a pulmonary abscess or empyema.

Viruses

Viral pneumonias are recognized as an important cause of pneumonia in adults.Influenza viruses are the most common cause of viral pneumonia in adults. Metapneumovirus is a paramyxovirus that seems to be an important cause of viral pneumonia in adults. Cytomegalovirus (CMV) primarily causes pneumonia in immunosuppressed patients, such as transplant recipients. Varicella-zoster virus causes pneumonia that seems to be more common and more severe in adults. Predisposing factors include smoking or pregnancy. Severe acute respiratory syndrome(SARS) is a respiratory illness due to a coronavirus identified in Southeast Asia.

Fungal species

Fungal infections due to organisms such as *Histoplasma capsulatum*, *Blastomyces dermatitides*, and *Coccidioides immitis* commonly present as pulmonary disease. These organisms are present in the soil in various geographic areas of the United States: *H. capsulatum* in the Mississippi and Ohio River valleys, *C. immitis* in desert areas of the Southwest, and *B. dermatitides* in a poorly defined area extending beyond that of *H. capsulatum*. These infections should be considered in people in appropriate geographic areas, especially in those who are near activities that disturb the soil, such as construction or dirt bike riding. Clinical presentation varies from an acute or chronic pneumonia to asymptomatic granulomas and hilar adenopathy.

Pneumocystis pneumonia (PCP) occurs in compromised hosts, principally people with AIDS or malignancy. PCP is one of the most common presentations leading to a diagnosis of HIV infection and AIDS.PCP typically presents subacutely with fatigue, exertional dyspnea, nonproductive cough, pleuritic chest pain, and fever.

Unusual Causes of Pneumonia

Hantaviruses are endemic in several areas of the United States and can cause a syndrome of severe respiratory distress and shock.

Plague, caused by *Yersinia pestis*, is endemic in many areas of the world, including the southwestern United States. It is an agent that could be used for biologic terrorism, but it also occurs naturally in people bitten by fleas from infected rodents or carnivores. Hematogenous spread may lead to pneumonia that is highly contagious and has a high mortality.

A number of zoonotic organisms cause pneumonia. Tularemia, caused by the bacterium *Francisella tularensis*, is spread by contact with body fluids of an infected mammal (especially rabbits) or the bite of an infected arthropod.Psittacosis can spread to humans from birds infected with *Chlamydophila psittaci*. Q fever is caused by the rickettsial organism *Coxiella burnetii*. Other zoonotic pulmonary infections include *Rhodococcus equi* associated with exposure to horses and *Bordetella bronchiseptica* associated with exposure to ill dogs ("kennel cough").

CLINICAL FEATURES

The ED evaluation should focus on establishing the diagnosis of pneumonia and determining the presence of epidemiologic and clinical features that would influence decisions regarding hospitalization and antibiotics. Key history includes the character and pattern of symptoms, the setting in which the pneumonia is acquired, geographic or animal exposures, and host factors that predispose to certain types of infections and are associated with outcome.

Pneumonia generally presents as a cough productive of purulent sputum, shortness of breath, and fever. In most healthy adults, the diagnosis can be reasonably excluded on the basis of history and physical examination, with suspected cases confirmed by chest radiography. The absence of any abnormalities in vital signs or chest auscultation substantially reduces the likelihood of pneumonia. However, no single isolated clinical finding is highly reliable in establishing or excluding a diagnosis of pneumonia.

Elder or debilitated patients with pneumonia often present with nonspecific complaints but not the classic symptoms. Pneumonia commonly presents in the elderly as acute confusion or a deterioration of baseline function. Elder patients are more likely to have advanced illness at the time of presentation and may present with sepsis in the absence of a previous syndrome suggestive of pneumonia. Rarely, patients with lower lobe pneumonia present with a complaint of abdominal or back pain.

Cough may be minimal or absent.

Pneumonia can be divided based on clinical patterns into typical pneumonia caused by pyogenic bacteria, such as *S. pneumoniae* or *H. influenzae*, and atypical pneumonia caused by organisms such as *Mycoplasma* and *Chlamydophila* spp. Factors studied prospectively and found *not* to be more frequent with atypical pneumonias than with pyogenic bacterial etiologies include gradual onset, viral prodrome, absence of rigors, nonproductive cough, lower degree of fever, absence of pleurisy or consolidation, low leukocyte count, and an ill-defined infiltrate on a chest radiograph. Although it is impossible to determine with a high degree of certainty the specific etiology of pneumonia without results of microbiologic or serologic tests, certain clinical factors suggest that a specific pathogen should be considered.

"Typical" pneumonia

The classic presentation of pneumococcal pneumonia is the abrupt onset of a single shaking chill followed by fever, cough productive of rust-colored sputum, and pleuritic chest pain. Many patients do not exhibit the classic pattern. Patients often have a preceding upper respiratory illness, and the onset of pneumonia may be insidious, especially in the elderly or with underlying lung disease. Patients with a history of asplenia, sickle cell disease, AIDS, multiple myeloma, or agammaglobulinemia are at increased risk of pneumococcal bacteremia and sepsis with high mortality rates. Extrapulmonary complications (e.g., meningitis, endocarditis, or arthritis) may rarely be present. Adults with chronic lung disease who develop pneumonia typically present with an insidious worsening of baseline cough and sputum production. *Klebsiella pneumoniae* may cause severe pneumonia in elderly or debilitated patients. Sputum is often described as "currant jelly" because of the necrotizing, hemorrhagic nature of the infection. Abscess formation, empyema, and bacteremia are common with this organism, and mortality is high.

"Atypical" pneumonia

Atypical pneumonia is caused by organisms such as *M. pneumoniae*, *C. pneumoniae*, viruses, *Legionella* sp., or rickettsiae such as *C. burnetii*. Mycoplasmal infection usually begins as a flulike illness with headache, malaise, and fever. Cough is usually nonproductive but may sometimes produce clear or purulent sputum. Skin lesions, including maculopapular, vesicular, urticarial, or erythema multiforme-type rashes, are common. Common physical findings include pharyngeal erythema, cervical adenopathy, and scattered rales and rhonchi. Rare extrapulmonary manifestations include pericarditis, glomerulonephritis, aseptic meningitis, and Guillain-Barré syndrome. Patients generally do not appear toxic, and most can be treated as outpatients. Although mucopurulent sputum generally indicates the presence of pyogenic bacterial pneumonia or bronchitis, it may also be present with mycoplasmal or viral pneumonia. Viral pneumonia in adults is often preceded by symptoms of upper respiratory infection, such as rhinitis or sore throat. Cough is usually nonproductive, and pleuritic chest pain is less common than with bacterial pneumonia.

Most *C. pneumoniae* infections in young adults cause a minor, self-limited upper respiratory illness that is subacute in onset. This organism is also associated with bronchitis, wheezing, sinusitis, pharyngitis, and atherosclerosis. Development of radiographically evident pneumonia is more common in the elderly.

Some patients with *Legionella* infection have a mild, self-limited atypical pneumonia presentation. Older patients, smokers, and those with chronic disease or immunosuppression are more prone to develop the more acute and severe systemic illness of legionnaires' disease. Gastrointestinal symptoms, such as diarrhea and abdominal cramping, are sometimes prominent.

Comorbidity

In addition to age, the presence of underlying illness, and presenting symptoms, the setting of acquisition of pneumonia may provide clues to likely etiologies.

Patients with immunosuppression due to hematologic malignancy, patients receiving chemotherapy for malignancy, and transplant recipients are prone to pulmonary infections with a wide variety of organisms.

Other risk factors for infection with multidrug-resistant pathogens include (1) hospitalization for 2 or more days in an acute care facility within 90 d of infection; (2) patients who attended a hemodialysis clinic; and (3) patients who received intravenous antibiotic therapy, chemotherapy, or wound care within 30 d of infection. Any patient with pneumonia that fulfills any one of these historical features, including patients from a nursing home or long-term care facility, is designated as having health care–associated pneumonia.

DIAGNOSTIC STRATEGIES

Chest radiographs and Computed tomography

A routine chest radiograph for all patients who present with cough is not necessary; chest radiography may be reserved for patients who have other suggestive findings (e.g., fever, tachycardia, oxygen desaturation, or an abnormal lung examination).Patients with serious underlying disease, patients with severe sepsis or shock, and patients in whom hospitalization is considered should have chest radiography performed.

CT of the chest is more sensitive than plain radiography for detecting the presence of pulmonary consolidation.

In pyogenic bacterial pneumonias, radiographs usually show an area of segmental or subsegmental infiltration and air bronchograms (Fig. 19-1). Pneumonia resulting from spread of infection along the intralobular airway results in fluffy or patchy infiltrates in the involved areas of the lung. A wide variety of bacteria and agents such as *Chlamydophila* sp. *Mycoplasma* sp., *Legionella* sp., viruses, and fungi may cause this pattern.

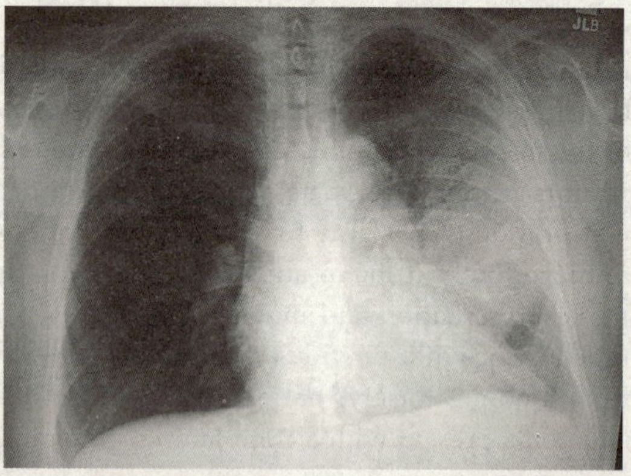

Fig. 19-1 Posteroanterior chest radiograph reveals a left upper lobe pneumonia. A variety of organisms can produce this pattern, most commonly *S. pneumoniae*, *H. influenzae*, or gram-negative bacilli, but also *C. pneumoniae*, *Mycoplasma*, or *Legionella* sp.

An interstitial pattern on a chest radiograph (Fig. 19-2) typically is caused by *Mycoplasma* sp., viruses, or *P. jirovecii*. Tiny nodules disseminated throughout both lungs represent a miliary pattern typical of granulomatous pneumonias, such as TB or fungal disease. The location of infiltrates may also give a clue to the etiology. Aspiration pneumonia occurs in dependent areas of the lung, most commonly the superior segments of the lower lobes or posterior segments of the upper lobes. Pneumonias produced by hematogenous spread (e.g., *S. aureus*) tend to be peripheral. Apical infiltrates suggest TB.

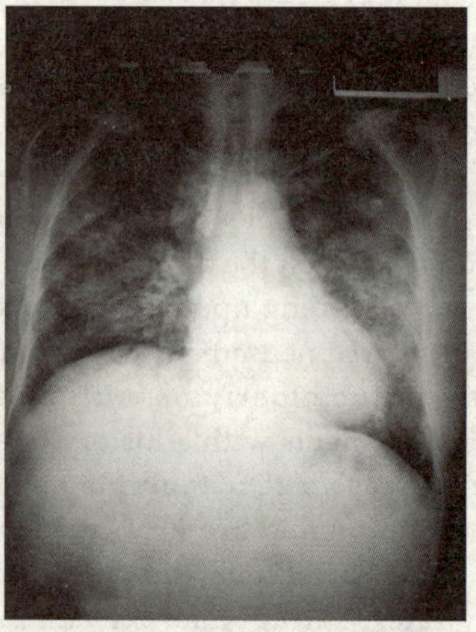

Fig. 19-2 Posteroanterior chest radiograph reveals patchy interstitial infiltrates. Viruses and *Mycoplasma* are the most likely etiologies in an otherwise healthy patient, but many bacterial organisms may also produce this pattern.

The presence of additional radiographic features in association with infiltrates may suggest a specific etiology. An infiltrate associated with hilar or mediastinal adenopathy suggests the presence of TB or fungal disease or may indicate pneumonia associated with a neoplasm. Bacteria most likely associated with cavitation (Fig. 19-3) are anaerobes, aerobic gram-negative bacilli, and *S. aureus*. Cavitation also may be present in fungal disease or TB and with noninfectious processes (e.g., malignancy and pulmonary vascular disease). Pneumatoceles or spontaneous pneumothorax may be seen in AIDS patients with PCP. Pleural effusions occur with a wide variety of organisms, including many types of pyogenic bacterial pneumonias, *Chlamydophila* sp., *Legionella* sp., and TB. Anaerobic infections associated with an effusion are especially prone to development of empyema. The diagnosis and aspiration of pleural effusions can be aided by use of ED bedside ultrasonography.

However, radiographic findings are nonspecific for predicting a particular infectious etiology. *Mycoplasma* pneumonia may present as a dense infiltrate, or pneumococcal pneumonia may present as a diffuse interstitial infiltrate. Immunocompromised patients are particularly prone to having atypical radiographic appearances. Rarely, patients with a clinical picture strongly suggestive of pneumonia have a normal chest radiograph, and some are found to have an infiltrate within the next 24 to 48 hr. The absence of findings on a chest radiograph should not preclude the use of antimicrobial therapy in appropriate patients with a clinical diagnosis of pneumonia.

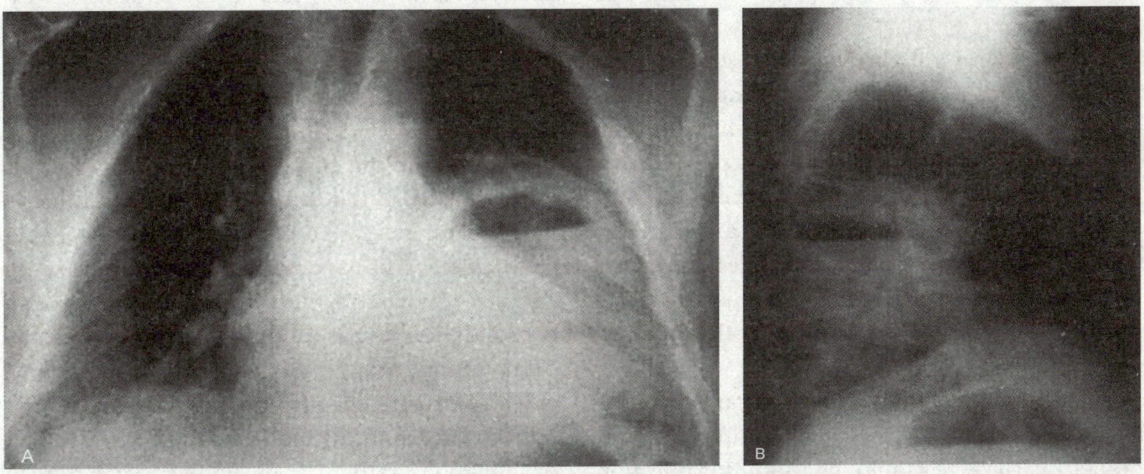

Fig. 19-3 Posteroanterior (A) and lateral (B) chest radiographs reveal a lung abscess in the left lower lobe with a distinct air-fluid level.

Laboratory

Laboratory studies also are nonspecific for identifying the etiology of pneumonia. Although the finding of a WBC greater than 15,000/mm^3 increases the probability of the patient having a pyogenic bacterial etiology rather than a viral or atypical etiology, the predictive value of this finding depends on the stage of the illness and likely prevalences of various etiologies. This is neither sensitive nor specific enough to aid decisions regarding therapy in an individual patient. A WBC may be helpful if it yields evidence of immunosuppression, such as neutropenia, or if it reveals lymphopenia that may indicate immunosuppression from AIDS. Basic metabolic panels may help identify patients with renal or hepatic dysfunction or metabolic acidosis associated with sepsis.

The assessment of respiratory function with pulse oximetry is important in the evaluation of patients with pneumonia.

Sputum Gram's stain rarely results in a change in therapy or outcome, and should not be relied on to rule out a gram-negative etiology. Empirical antimicrobial agents are usually highly clinically effective if chosen based on clinical information without sputum analysis.

Routine blood cultures are of essentially no value in nonimmunocompromised adults with pneumonia, in whom there is a very low prevalence of noncontaminant bacteremia, and management is rarely changed based on the results.Blood cultures should be obtained from immunocompromised patients, those with severe sepsis or shock, or those with risk factors for endovascular infection (e.g., prosthetic valves, intravenous drug use, or cavitary infiltrates). When cultures are drawn, they should be obtained prior to the initiation of antibiotics (although antibiotics should not be delayed for this reason).

Patients with a pleural effusion greater than 5cm on lateral upright posterior-anterior chest radiograph should have a diagnostic thoracentesis performed, with fluid sent for cell count, differential, pH (pH < 7.2 predicts the need for a thoracostomy tube), Gram's stain, and culture. Patients in significant respiratory distress, however, or with evidence of tension and mediastinal shift require emergent diagnostic and therapeutic thoracentesis.

Rapid diagnostic tests for viral antigens are available for several viruses, including RSV and influenza. These tests may be useful for infection control decisions in hospitalized patients, and they may provide an indication for influenza therapy and family prophylaxis. In the future, rapid testing using technology such as polymerase chain reaction may provide emergency physicians with a reliable method to determine the specific etiology of pneumonia.

Pneumonia Associated with Human Immunodeficiency Virus Infection

Respiratory infections are the most common type of opportunistic infection in AIDS patients. In addition to *P. jirovecii*, there is also an increased incidence of pneumonia due to *M. tuberculosis* and common bacterial pathogens such as *S. pneumoniae* and *H. influenzae*. The incidence of pneumococcal pneumonia is 7 to 10 times higher in HIV-infected people and the incidence of *H. influenzae* pneumonia is approximately 100 times higher than in non-HIV-infected individuals.

The potential for opportunistic pulmonary infection can be predicted by a recent absolute CD4 lymphocyte count less than 200/mm^3. This count is often known by patients with recognized HIV infection or may be surmised by a peripheral total lymphocyte count less than 1000/mm^3. In patients who do not know their HIV status, the presence of findings such as weight loss, hairy leukoplakia, and oral candidiasis strongly suggests immunosuppression.

Although patients with PCP may present with typical features of subacute onset of nonproductive cough, fever, shortness of breath, diffuse interstitial infiltrates on chest radiography, and arterial hypoxemia, 10% to 20% of patients subsequently proven to have PCP lack these findings. PCP usually has a subacute presentation characterized by nonproductive cough, exertional dyspnea, and weight loss. Tachypnea and tachycardia are usually present.

The classic radiographic findings in PCP are bilateral interstitial infiltrates that begin in the perihilar region. Radiographic manifestations of PCP can vary considerably, however, ranging from a normal appearance to dense consolidation. Lobar infiltrates, pleural effusions, hilar adenopathy, parenchymal nodules, and cavitary disease are also described. Hypoxemia, hypocapnia, and an increased arterial-alveolar oxygenation gradient are usually present. Serum lactate dehydrogenase is significantly elevated in AIDS patients with PCP. Confirmation of the diagnosis of PCP requires sputum induction and staining and, in some cases, further invasive procedures, such as bronchoscopy with bronchoalveolar lavage or biopsy.

There is a broad differential diagnosis for pulmonary infiltrates in AIDS patients (Fig. 19-4). The bacterial pathogens most commonly responsible for pneumonia in these patients are the same pathogens most frequently encountered in immunocompetent individuals with CAP, but they may have an atypical appearance on chest X-ray. Because AIDS patients with pulmonary TB cannot be distinguished reliably from AIDS patients with other pulmonary infections at presentation, consider TB in all HIV-infected patients with respiratory complaints and initiate respiratory isolation.AIDS patients are also at increased risk for pneumonia due to *Cryptococcus neoformans* or other fungi associated with geographic exposure. Kaposi's sarcoma may also present with pulmonary infiltrates.

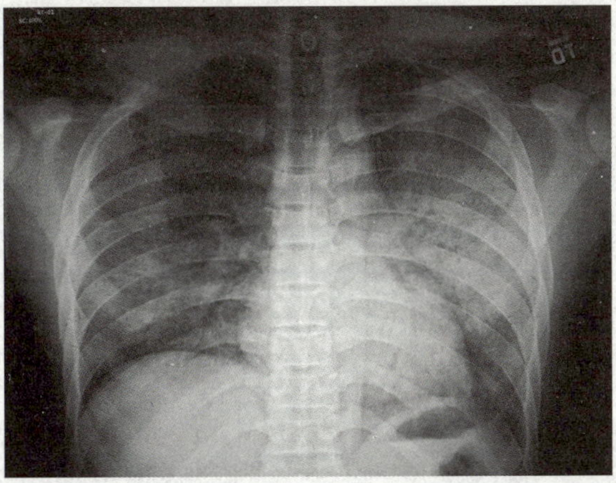

Fig. 19-4 Posteroanterior chest radiograph of an HIV-infected patient reveals interstitial disease mixed with patchy alveolar infiltrates. *Pneumocystis jirovecii* is the most common etiology, but bacterial pathogens and tuberculosis must also be considered.

DIFFERENTIAL DIAGNOSIS CONSIDERATIONS

The differentiation between upper and lower respiratory tract infections may be difficult. A chest radiograph helps differentiate between upper respiratory tract infection or bronchitis and pneumonia, but it is probably not necessary for all patients with cough and sputum production unless other factors are present that suggest the possibility of pneumonia or obscure its clinical diagnosis (e.g., toxic appearance, extremes of age, underlying illness, and abnormal chest examination).

Many noninfectious etiologies may result in inflammatory lung processes, including exposure to mineral dusts (e.g., silicosis), chemical fumes (e.g., chlorine and ammonia), toxic drugs (e.g., bleomycin), radiation, thermal injury, or oxygen toxicity. Immunologic diseases (e.g., sarcoidosis, Goodpasture's syndrome, and collagen vascular disease) or hypersensitivity to environmental agents (e.g., farmer's lung disease) may also result in pneumonia. Tumors may be confused with pneumonia radiographically or may present initially as a postobstructive infection or adenopathy with peripheral infiltrates. Lymphangitic spread of lung malignancy may resemble interstitial pneumonia.

Aspiration

It is important to recognize the distinction between the acute aspiration of gastric contents or other liquids and bacterial pneumonia that may develop later as a complication of aspiration. Aspiration of liquids into the lung disrupts surfactant and causes an inflammatory response that may lead to hypoxia and respiratory failure. Aspiration of acidic gastric contents is particularly damaging to lungs and is common in patients who are unconscious from intoxication or anesthesia or who have neurologic deficits. Patients may present initially with coughing or shortness of breath or may appear well initially and then develop respiratory dysfunction during the next several hours.

Acute aspiration of acidic fluid into the lungs may produce fever, leukocytosis, purulent sputum, and radiographic infiltrates that mimic bacterial pneumonia. Although many of these patients go on to develop bacterial pneumonia, prophylactic administration of antibiotics is controversial. Antibiotics should be initiated if the patient develops signs of bacterial pneumonia, including new fever, expanding infiltrate appearing more than 36 hr after aspiration, or unexplained deterioration. Systemic corticosteroids for acute aspiration are of no benefit.

MANAGEMENT

The possibility of communicable disease should suggest early isolation. Patients with a history of TB exposure, suggestive symptoms (e.g., persistent cough, weight loss, night sweats, and hemoptysis), or belonging to a group at high risk for TB (e.g., homeless, intravenous drug user, alcoholic, HIV risk, and immigrant from high-risk area) should be given a mask and placed in respiratory isolation before evaluation. ED that frequently care for patients at risk for TB should consider triage protocols to identify these individuals rapidly before patients, visitors, or staff are unnecessarily exposed.

Empirical antimicrobial therapy

Antimicrobials should be administered in the ED for patients who are being admitted to the hospital. Timely administration of antimicrobials has been associated with improved outcomes for hospitalized pneumonia patients, but a rush to treatment without a diagnosis of pneumonia can result in inappropriate antibiotic use. The antibiotics selected should cover the likely etiologies based on clinical, laboratory, radiologic, and epidemiologic information. However, the regimen should also be as selective as possible to avoid drug toxicity, emergence of resistance to broad-spectrum agents, and excessive cost.

The prevalence of drug-resistant S. pneumoniae (DRSP) is increasing. DRSP that is resistant to penicillin is usually resistant to other β-lactams, macrolides, tetracyclines, and trimethoprim-sulfamethoxazole(TMP-SMX). Many extended-spectrum or "respiratory" fluoroquinolones are available, such as levofloxacin, moxifloxacin, and gemifloxacin. These agents are active against DRSP and other typical or atypical pneumonia pathogens. It is not clear that in vitro resistance is related to adverse clinical outcome. Hence, individualized treatment is recommended.

CA-MRSA has rapidly emerged as the most common pathogen isolated in community-acquired skin and soft tissue infections. It is also increasingly recognized as a cause of severe, rapidly progressing pneumonia with sepsis, often in healthy young adults with influenza. Antimicrobials with consistent in vitro activity against CA-MRSA isolates include vancomycin, TMP-SMX, daptomycin, tigecycline, linezolid, and ceftaroline.

Appropriate agents for outpatient treatment of adults with CAP include macrolides, doxycycline, and fluoroquinolones with enhanced activity against *S. pneumoniae* (Table 19-1).

Table 19-1 CAP in Adults: Outpatient Treatment

CLINICAL SETTING	ANTIBIOTIC REGIMEN	COMMENTS
Previously healthy, no antimicrobials in last 3 mo	Doxycycline 100 mg PO bid	Preferred for adolescent/young adult when likelihood of mycoplasma is high; variable activity vs. *S. pneumoniae*.
	Azithromycin	Treats common typical bacterial and atypical pathogens. Variety of dosing regimens: 500 mg once followed by 250 mg daily for 4 d; 500 mg PO daily for 3 d; 2 g PO extended-release suspension once. Can substitute clarithromycin.
Comorbidities, or antimicrobials in last 3 mo	Levofloxacin 750 mg PO daily for 5 d	Can substitute moxifloxacin or gemifloxacin Treats common typical and atypical bacterial pathogens; active vs.DRSP. Use if recently received -lactam or macrolide.
	Cefpodoxime 200 mg PO bid azithromycin 500 mg PO daily	Use if recently received fluoroquinolones. Can substitute cefdinir,cefprozil, or amoxicillin/clavulanate for cefpodoxime. Variable activity against DRSP

Many ED initiate outpatient therapy in moderately ill patients with an initial parenteral dose of a long-acting antibiotic, such as ceftriaxone, and employ extended observation (i.e., 12–24 hr) while administering supportive care, such as hydration, antipyretics, and bronchodilators, before discharge on an oral regimen.

Outpatient treatment for pneumonia is generally 10 to 14 d. A 5 d treatment course is possible with azithromycin or levofloxacin (750 mg daily).

Combined antibiotic therapy

For patients who have received a fluoroquinolone within the previous few months, a combination of a macrolide plus a β-lactam agent (e.g., high-dose amoxicillin [1 g three times daily], amoxicillin-clavulanate [2 g orally twice daily], or cefpodoxime) is appropriate.

For patients whose illness is severe enough to require hospital admission and parenteral antibiotics, options include a combination of a β-lactam agent (e.g., ceftriaxone, cefotaxime, ampicillin-sulbactam, or ertapenem) and a macrolide (e.g., intravenous or oral azithromycin) or an extended-spectrum fluoroquinolone alone. These regimens treat the most common bacterial pathogens, such as *S. pneumoniae*, *M. catarrhalis*, and *H. influenzae*, and atypical pathogens, such as *Mycoplasma*, *Chlamydophila*, and *Legionella* spp. Azithromycin alone might be an appropriate choice for people with milder illness who are less likely to be bacteremic. If anaerobic organisms are suspected (e.g., aspiration), clindamycin or metronidazole could be added to the regimen, or the regimen could include an antibiotic with anaerobic activity, such as ertapenem, ampicillin-sulbactam, or piperacillin-tazobactam. Some quinolones, such as moxifloxacin, are also active against anaerobes (Table 19-2).

Table 19-2 CAP in Adults: Inpatient Antimicrobial Treatment

CLINICAL SETTING	ANTIBIOTIC REGIMEN	COMMENTS
Community-acquired,nonimmunocompromised	Ceftriaxone 1 g q24h + azithromycin 500 mg q24h IV or PO	Could substitute cefotaxime, ampicillinsulbactam, or ertapenem for ceftriaxone.
	Respiratory fluoroquinolone (levofloxacin 750 mg IV q24h or moxifloxacin 400 mg IV q24h)	Treats most common bacterial and atypical pathogens. Active vs. DRSP
Severe pneumonia (ICU)	Ceftriaxone 1 g IV q24h+levofloxacin 750 mg IV q24h+vancomycin 1 g IV q12h	Can substitute cefotaxime, cefepime, ertapenem,or β-lactam/β-lactamase inhibitor for ceftriaxone. Can substitute moxifloxacin for levofloxacin. Can substitute linezolid for vancomycin.
Health care–associated pneumonia or severe pneumonia with neutropenia, bronchiectasis (risk for *Pseudomonas*)	Cefepime 2 g IV q12h + ciprofloxacin 500 mg IV q12h + vancomycin 1 g IV q12h	Can substitute other antipseudomonal β-lactam,such as piperacillin-tazobactam, imipenem, or meropenem, for cefepime. Can substitute aminoglycoside plus macrolide for ciprofloxacin.
Presumed PCP	Trimethoprim-sulfamethoxazole 240/1200 mg IV q6h	Add ceftriaxone to TMP/SMX if severe, until PCP confirmed. Alternatives for sulfa allergy include pentamidine + third-generation cephalosporin; clindamycin + primaquine; or atovaquone + ceftriaxone.

IV, intravenous

Patients with severe pneumonia, who present with severe sepsis or septic shock, require aggressive fluid resuscitation and may benefit from more intensive management with vasopressors, transfusion, and inotropic agents as part of early goal-directed therapy. For pneumonia patients admitted to an ICU, adequate activity against DRSP may be more important. Outcomes with severe pneumococcal pneumonia may be better with combination therapy compared with a single agent such as a fluoroquinolone alone. A third-generation cephalosporin or β-lactam/β-lactamase inhibitor can be combined with a fluoroquinolone. Addition of an aminoglycoside should be considered if septic shock is present.

Patients with recent hospitalization, neutropenia, or underlying bronchiectasis are at increased risk of infection with *P. aeruginosa*. Empirical therapy should include two agents with extended gram-negative activity, including *P. aeruginosa*. Empirical regimens include cefepime, imipenem, meropenem, or piperacillin-tazobactam, plus either ciprofloxacin (high dose) or an aminoglycoside and a macrolide. For life-threatening pneumonia in populations at risk for MRSA, and for patients recently exposed to fluoroquinolones who may have fluoroquinolone-resistant *S. pneumoniae*, consider vancomycin or linezolid. The regimen should also cover atypical pathogens and gram-negative bacilli. Improved severe pneumonia survival was associated with earlier antibiotic prescription and increased use of combined antibiotic therapy.

Since health care–associated pneumonia is associated with higher mortality and a greater likelihood of unusual pathogens, it is appropriate to give broader spectrum empirical therapy, usually with a combination of antimicrobials to increase the chance that at least one antibiotic will be active against the causative pathogen. Appropriate combinations include an antipseudomonal β-lactam agent, such as piperacillin-tazobactam, cefepime, imipenem, or meropenem, with either an aminoglycoside or a fluoroquinolone and vancomycin or linezolid for MRSA.

For patients with AIDS, it is important to treat *P. jirovecii* and bacterial pathogens such as *S. pneumoniae*. TMP-SMX is the treatment of choice; the usual regimen is 20 mg/kg of TMP and 100 mg/kg of SMX daily in four divided doses, to be continued for 21 d. For most adult patients, a regimen of three ampules (80 mg of TMP and 400 mg of SMX per ampule) every 6 hr is appropriate.

Antiviral treatment

Patients with a positive influenza antigen test or culture may benefit from antiviral treatment. Empirical antiviral treatment is reasonable with compatible clinical findings when influenza is in the community, and it may be associated with reduced mortality when started early in the course of influenza. Neuraminidase inhibitors such as oseltamivir are recommended instead of amantadine and rimantadine because they are active against influenza A and B and because many circulating strains are resistant to these older agents.

DISPOSITION

There is tremendous variability in physician admission decisions for pneumonia. The more common tendency is overestimation of disease severity, leading to hospitalization of patients at low risk for death or serious complications.

Scoring of Disease Severity

Scoring systems may predict the severity of disease and help determine whether a patient with CAP requires hospitalization or admission to an ICU.

One commonly used system is based on the Pneumonia Patient Outcomes Research Team study, a prospectively validated predictive rule for mortality among immunocompetent adults with CAP. This model (also known as the PSI) suggests a two-step approach to assess risk. Patients in the lowest risk class who are recommended for outpatient management are those younger than age 50 yr, without significant comorbid conditions (neoplasm, CHF, cerebrovascular disease, renal disease, liver disease, and HIV), and without the following findings on physical examination: altered mental status, pulse 125 beats/min or greater, respiratory rate 30 breaths/min or greater, SBP less than 90 mmHg, or temperature less than 35 or 40℃ or greater. Patients who do not fit the lowest risk category are classified into categories based on a scoring system that accounts for age, comorbid illness, physical examination findings, and laboratory abnormalities (Table 19-3). Hospitalization is recommended for patients with a score greater than 91, and brief admission or observation may be considered for patients with a score of 71 to 90. Although this method of assessing the likelihood of successful outpatient management is helpful, it is not modeled to predict acute life-threatening events.

Table 19-3 Scoring System for Pneumonia Mortality Prediction

PATIENT CHARACTERISTICS	POINTS
Demographic factor	
Age	
Male	No. years of age
Female	No. years of age-10
Nursing home resident	10
Comorbid illness	
Neoplastic disease	30
Liver disease	20
CHF	10

Continued

PATIENT CHARACTERISTICS	POINTS
Cerebrovascular disease	10
Renal disease	10
Physical examination finding	
Altered mental status	20
Respiratory rate ⩾ 30	20
SBP ⩽90 mm Hg	20
Temperature < 35℃ or > 40℃	15
Pulse ⩾ 125 beats/min	10
Laboratory or radiographic finding	
Arterial pH < 7.35	30
Blood urea nitrogen >30 mg/dL	20
Sodium <130 mEq/L	20
Glucose > 250 mg/dL	10
Hematocrit < 30%	10
Arterial PO_2 < 60 mm Hg	10
Pleural effusion	10

A similar tool that is easier to use is the CURB-65 rule. This rule uses only five simple criteria to determine patients at lower risk for adverse events: confusion, uremia (BUN > 20 mg/dL), respiratory rate greater than 30, SBP less than 90 or DBP less than 60 , and age 65 or greater. Patients with zero or one feature can receive outpatient care, those with two should be admitted, and ICU care should be considered for those with three or more.

The disposition of HIV-infected patients with possible PCP is dictated by the likelihood of progression to severe disease and by the feasibility of close outpatient follow-up. Factors associated with decreased survival in AIDS patients with PCP include a history of prior PCP, anemia, hypoxemia, and medical comorbidity. Patients without multiple poor prognostic factors may be discharged from the ED with close outpatient follow-up, ideally within 2 or 3 d. An empirical trial of a macrolide may be indicated for treatment of bronchitis or mild CAP in a patient at low risk for PCP (e.g., recent CD4 count >350/mm^3). Any deterioration on outpatient oral antibiotics should prompt admission for a more extensive evaluation.

The decision to admit a patient to the ICU is straightforward when patients are intubated or require vasopressors. It is more difficult to identify patients who do not require these interventions initially but may be at greater risk for deterioration and require a level of monitoring that may be beyond that available on the typical hospital ward.

Above all, the decision to hospitalize or admission a patient to an ICU ultimately depends on the physician's judgment, but all factors that are contained in these scoring systems should be considered.

Most patients with CAP do not need respiratory isolation. Patients who could pose a threat of transmission to other patients (e.g., influenza, varicella, TB, and plague) should be isolated. People with fever and respiratory symptoms who have been traveling in an area with SARS or avian influenza should also be isolated. Neutropenic patients generally are placed in reverse isolation. HIV-infected patients who present with pneumonia should be isolated until TB can be evaluated by sputum acid-fast bacilli smears; this is particularly true for patients with other risk factors for TB. Isolation should be strongly considered for others at high risk for TB, such as inner-city homeless people and intravenous drug users.

ACUTE RESPIRATORY DISTRESS SYNDROME

ARDS is a form of noncardiogenic pulmonary edema that is a result of the nonspecific response of the lung to a variety of insults. The American-European Consensus Conference (AECC) has published diagnostic criteria for ARDS: acute onset; P_AO_2/F_iO_2 of 200 or less, regardless of PEEP; bilateral infiltrates seen on frontal chest radiograph; and pulmonary artery wedge pressure of 18 mmHg or less when measured, or no clinical evidence of left atrial hypertension.

The pathophysiology of ARDS is not completely understood. A direct pulmonary or indirect extrapulmonary insult is believed to cause a proliferation of inflammatory mediators that promote neutrophil accumulation in the microcirculation of the lung. (Box 19-1). A variety of mediators are implicated in the development of ARDS, including neutrophil production of proteases and oxygen radicals, interleukins and other cytokines, tumor necrosis factor, and complement factors. This inflammatory cells and cytokine mediator release lead to pathologic vascular permeability, gaps in the alveolar epithelial barrier, and necrosis of type I and Ⅱ alveolar cells. This, in turn, leads to the pulmonary edema, hyaline membrane formation, and loss of surfactant that decrease pulmonary compliance and make air exchange difficult. Subsequent infiltration of fibroblasts can lead to collagen deposition, fibrosis, and worsening disease.

Treatment of ARDS is primarily supportive. When mechanical ventilation is required, patients with ARDS should be started at lower tidal volumes (6 mL per kg) instead of at traditional volumes (10 to 15 mL per kg). Higher PEEP values (12 to 18 or more cm H_2O) should be considered for initial mechanical ventilation in patients with ARDS. Other ventilator techniques that may be beneficial include inverse-ratio ventilation with prolonged inspiratory time and use of a high-frequency oscillatory ventilator. Fluid balance must avoid increased pulmonary capillary pressure while maintaining organ perfusion. Prone positioning during ventilation may improve distribution of perfusion to ventilated lung regions. Inhaled nitric oxide, *N*-acetylcysteine, prostaglandin E_1, ketoconazole, and nonsteroidal anti-inflammatory drugs produce variable results. Corticosteroids do not reduce mortality in early ARDS but may have benefit in the late fibroproliferative phase. Although lung function approaches normal in some survivors, not all of the deleterious health effects of hospitalization for ARDS resolve over time.

Box 19-1 Conditions Associated with ARDS

- Sepsis
- Shock
- Toxic gas or smoke inhalation
- Aspiration
  - Gastric contents
  - Near-drowning
  - Hydrocarbons/solvents
- Pneumonia
- Drug reaction
  - Salicylates
  - Opiates
  - Tricyclic antidepressants
  - Cyclosporine
  - Amiodarone
  - Cancer chemotherapeutic agents (e.g., bleomycin)
  - Hydrochlorothiazide
- Trauma
- Burns
- Transfusion reaction
- Radiation injury
- Pancreatitis
- Thromboembolism
- Fat embolism
- Air embolism
- Amniotic fluid embolism
- Eclampsia
- Neurogenic (e.g., subarachnoid hemorrhage, head trauma)
- DIC
- High-altitude exposure
- Oxygen toxicity
- CPB

(ZHANG Hong)

Chapter 20

Pulmonary Embolism and Deep Vein Thrombosis

KEY CONCEPTS

PE results from a clot in the deep veins and dislodged, traveled through the venous system, and traversed the RV into the pulmonary vasculature. What the patient experiences varies widely, ranging from no symptom to cardiovascular collapse.

An ELISA or immunoturbidimetric D-dimer concentration below 500 ng/mL can rule out PE or DVT in all but high-risk patients.

CTPA usually used as the primary method of evaluating for PE.

Massive PE is defined by hypotension with a SBP below 90 mmHg for more than 15 min.In the absence of contraindications, patients with proven massive PE probably benefit from fibrinolysis.

Patients who cannot be given anticoagulants or who have a recurrence of VTE despite anticoagulation therapy should be considered for vena caval intervention.

Surgical embolectomy may be the best option for patients who have severe PE with a contraindication to fibrinolysis.

PERSPECTIVE

This chapter discusses the diagnosis and treatment of venous thromboembolism (VTE), including DVT and PE, from the perspective of the emergency physician and provides a functional resource for the evaluation and treatment of VTE in the ED.

Pathophysiology of Thrombosis

VTE forms as a result of excessive fibrin production from the action of thrombin on fibrinogen. Factors that enhance fibrinogen synthesis and promote its catalysis to fibrin include systemic inflammation, traumatic or immune-related vascular trauma, inherited thrombophilias and hemoglobinopathies, cancer, pregnancy, and sluggish blood flow. Venous injury, slow blood flow, and hypercoagulability are the cardinal inciting mechanisms for VTE.

DEEP VEIN THROMBOSIS

DVT represents a disease spectrum ranging from a minimally symptomatic isolated calf vein thrombosis to a limb-threatening iliofemoral venous obstruction.

Anatomy

The venous anatomy of the lower extremity is divided into the deep and superficial systems.The deep venous system includes the anterior tibial, posterior tibial, and peroneal veins, collectively called the calf veins. The calf veins join together at the knee to form the popliteal vein. The femoral vein sometimes is called the superficial femoral vein. A clot in the superficial femoral vein is indeed a DVT . The femoral vein joins with the deep femoral vein to form the common femoral vein. Proximal DVT refers to a clot in the popliteal vein or higher, whereas distal clot refers to an isolated calf vein thrombosis.

Clinical Presentation

The initial symptoms of DVT can be as subtle and nonspecific as a mild cramping sensation or sense of fullness in the calf, without objective swelling, and may be difficult to differentiate clinically from myriad other, unrelated disorders (Box 20-1).The clinical signs of DVT vary and may include unilateral swelling, edema, erythema, and warmth of the

Box 20-1 Differential Diagnosis of DVT

- Muscle strain, hematoma
- Popliteal (Baker's) cyst
- Lymphedema
- Cellulitis
- Vasculitis
- Fracture
- Superficial thrombophlebitis
- Chronic venous insufficiency
- Proximal venous compression (e.g., tumor, gravid uterus)
- Congestive heart failure (swelling usually bilateral)
- Hypoalbuminemia (swelling usually bilateral)

affected extremity; tenderness to palpation along the distribution of the deep venous system; dilation of superficial collateral veins; and a palpable venous "cord".Upper extremity DVT refers to a thrombosis in the axillary vein and causes arm swelling on the same side as an indwelling catheter or recent intravenous infusion site.

Diagnosis

Diagnosis of DVT and PE starts with an estimation of the pretest probability (PTP). This estimation may be accomplished either by the clinical gestalt of an experienced practitioner or in conjunction with a clinical decision tool, such as that derived and validated by Wells and colleagues (Table 20-1). Patients with a low PTP can have DVT excluded with a normal quantitative D-dimer.

Table 20-1 Clinical Model for Estimating the PTP of DVT

CLINICAL FEATURE	SCORE*
Active cancer (treated within the previous 6 mo or currently receiving palliative treatment)	1
Paralysis, paresis, or recent plaster immobilization of the lower extremities	1
Recently bedridden for ≥3 d or major surgery within 12 w requiring general or regional anesthesia	1
Localized tenderness along the distribution of the deep venous system	1
Entire leg swollen	1
Calf swelling at least 3 cm larger than on the asymptomatic side (measured 10 cm below the tibial tuberosity)	1
Pitting edema confined to the symptomatic leg	1
Collateral superficial veins (nonvaricose)	1
Previously documented deep vein thrombosis	1
Alternative diagnosis at least as likely as deep vein thrombosis	−2

*A score of <2 indicates that the probability of DVT is low.

Laboratory Evaluation

The D-dimer is a protein derived from enzymatic breakdown of cross-linked fibrin, and an elevated plasma concentration indicates the presence of a clot formed somewhere in the body within the previous 72 hr. D-dimer concentration may be elevated with any condition that causes fibrin deposition, including malignancy, pregnancy, advanced age, prolonged bed rest, recent surgery, infection, inflammation, new indwelling catheters, stroke, and MI. D-dimer concentration is proportionate to the size of the clot and decreases as the clot matures, so the test is less sensitive with small or chronic clots.

The D-dimer less than 500 ng/mL is a negative test result .

Radiographic Evaluation

DVT evaluation is by a combination of D-dimer testing and duplex venous ultrasonography.

Venous duplex ultrasonography has a sensitivity and specificity of approximately 95% for proximal DVT.A single normal whole-leg ultrasound is sufficient to exclude DVT with any PTP. A negative three-point ultrasound together with a negative quantitative D-dimer is sufficient to exclude DVT with any PTP. An expertly performed and interpreted positive ultrasound is sufficient to confirm the diagnosis of DVT. Ultrasound cannot be used to rule out iliac or pelvic vein thrombosis.

Indirect CT venography is not a primary imaging modality for DVT but may be performed in conjunction with computed tomography pulmonary angiography(CTPA) of the chest during the evaluation of suggested PE.

MRI can evaluate the pelvic vasculature and vena cava. MRI is not a primary diagnostic test for patients with suspected DVT.

Treatment

When the diagnosis of DVT has been established, anticoagulation should be initiated, with a LMWH (e.g., enoxaparin 1 mg/kg subcutaneously [SQ] every 12 hr), fondaparinux (5-10 mg SQ once daily, depending on patient weight), or unfractionated heparin (70-80 units/kg intravenous bolus followed by 17-18 units/kg/hr infusion).Treatment requires transition to oral anticoagulation with warfarin for at least 3 mo.If admission is contemplated, after heparin has been given, the first dose of warfarin can be given in the ED to help reduce overall length of stay in the inpatient unit.Patients who cannot be given anticoagulants or who have a recurrence of VTE despite anticoagulation therapy should be considered for vena caval intervention.

Superficial Leg Thrombophlebitis

Patients with a clot in the greater saphenous vein that extends above the knee are at risk for progression to DVT via the saphenous-femoral vein junction and may require an abbreviated course of anticoagulation. The saphenous vein thrombophlebitis can adequately be treated with nonsteroidal anti-inflammatory drugs, heat, and graded compression stockings (fitted to exert 30-40 mmHg of pressure at the ankle) followed by a mandatory repeat ultrasound in 2 to 5 d. If the clot is extending, then anticoagulation is indicated.

Isolated Calf Vein Thrombosis

Approximately 25% of isolated calf vein thromboses propagate proximally, prompting recommendations for treatment with anticoagulation as for proximal leg DVT.For tibial or peroneal vein thrombosis in an otherwise healthy, ambulatory patient with no other indication for anticoagulation, antiplatelet therapy with aspirin and close follow-up with repeat duplex ultrasound scan at 2 to 5 d to evaluate for clot propagation.

Phlegmasia Cerulea Dolens (Painful Blue Leg)

Patients with phlegmasia cerulea dolens may require emergent thrombectomy.Early thrombolytic therapy may be a limb-salvaging procedure in the absence of contraindications. One strategy is to infuse alteplase (1 mg/min to a total dose of 50 mg) via a peripheral intravenous catheter placed distal to the thrombus.

Upper Extremity Venous Thromboses

DVT of the upper extremity have become more common in association with increased use of indwelling venous catheters and wires for electronic cardiac devices. Upper extremity DVT can cause PE, and all patients with DVT above the elbow require definitive treatment.

Patients with catheter-associated DVT should receive anticoagulation if they do not have contraindications.

Complications

Although the most feared complication of DVT is fatal PE, DVT damages venous valves, causing venous insufficiency.

PULMONARY EMBOLISM

PE results from a clot that formed hours, days, or weeks earlier in the deep veins and dislodged, traveled through the venous system, and traversed the right ventricle into the pulmonary vasculature. What the patient experiences during this process varies widely, ranging from no symptom to cardiovascular collapse.

Pathophysiology of Pulmonary Vascular Occlusion

The pulmonary vascular tree normally has a low resistance to fluid flow, and young persons without cardiopulmonary disease can tolerate at least 30% obstruction, often with minimal symptoms or signs. Although a segmental pulmonary artery constitutes only about one sixteenth of the entire pulmonary vascular circuit, a clot lodged deeply in a segmental artery can obstruct blood flow to a sufficient degree to cause tissue necrosis.Over several days the infarcted segment becomes consolidated on chest radiography and exudes a pleural effusion, manifesting an intense underlying inflammatory process.

Dyspnea of patients with noninfarcting emboli may be constant and oppressive or may be intermittent and perceived only with exertion.The presence of hypoxemia increases the probability of PE. Conversely, a normal oxygen saturation can be used only when considered together with multiple other clinical features and should not alone or independently be used to forego testing for PE (Box 20-2).

Box 20-2 PE Rule-Out Criteria (PERC Rule)

Low PTP for PE by the treating clinician's unstructured estimate, plus:
- Age less than 50
- Pulse rate less than 100 beats/min
- Oxygen saturation greater than 94%
- No hemoptysis
- No unilateral leg swelling
- No recent major surgery or trauma
- No prior pulmonary embolism or DVT
- No hormone use

In the ED, about half of all patients with PE have a heart rate greater than 100 beats/min. Tachycardia from PE probably results from impaired left ventricular filling, leading to a pathophysiologic process that parallels that of hemorrhagic shock.When PE obstructs more than 50% of the vasculature, it usually causes an acute increase in right ventricular pressure. Arterial hypotension represents an ominous hemodynamic consequence of PE. In its most extreme form, PE can obstruct the right ventricular outflow entirely, either by casting the entire pulmonary vascular tree (Fig. 20-1 see color illustration) or by acutely occluding the main pulmonary artery. PEA is the most common ECG result from obstructive PE.

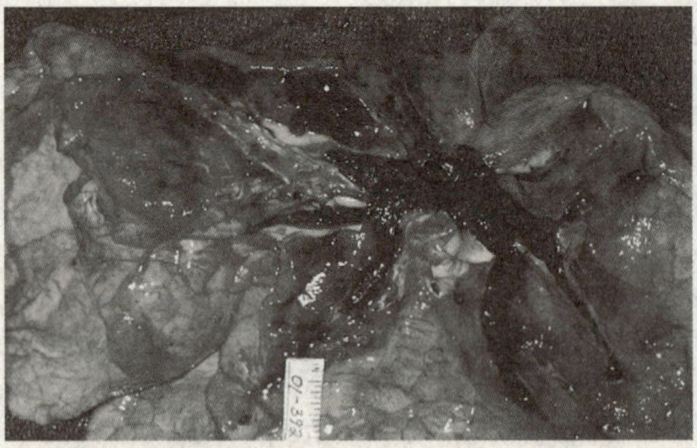

Fig. 20-1 Massive PE on autopsy

Clinical Presentation

Table 20-2 presents a listing of factors that significantly increase the probability of PE in the ED population.

Table. 20-2 Classic Risk Factors and Physiologic Findings for PE

FACTOR	MECHANISMS	STRENGTH OF ASSOCIATION WITH PE IN ED OPULATIONS
Inherited thrombophilia	Hypercoagulability	++
Connective tissue disease	Inflammation	Unknown
Acquired thrombophilia	Hypercoagulability	Unknown
Active cancer (under treatment)	Hypercoagulability	+
Inactive cancer (considered in remission)	Presumed hypercoagulability	Not significant
Limb or generalized immobility	Stasis	++
Prior PE or DVT	Multiple	+
Trauma within previous 4 w requiring hospitalization	Inflammation, venous injury and stasis	+++
Surgery within previous 4 w requiring general anesthesia	Inflammation, venous injury and stasis	++++
Smoking	Inflammation	Not significant
Estrogen	Hypercoagulability	++
Pregnancy or postpartum	Hypercoagulability	Minimal
Family history of VTE	Inherited condition	Not significant
Symptoms		
Pleuritic chest pain	Lung ischemia, muscle strain	
Substernal chest Pain	Presumed cardiac ischemia	Not significant
Dyspnea	$\dot{V}/\dot{Q}$ mismatch	+
Sudden onset of symptoms	Vascular obstruction	Not significant
Hemoptysis	Infarction	+++
Syncope	Vascular obstruction	Minimal

Continued

FACTOR	MECHANISMS	STRENGTH OF ASSOCIATION WITH PE IN ED OPULATIONS
Signs		
Pulse rate >100 beats/min	Cardiac stress, baroreceptors	+++
Pulse oximetry reading <95%	$\dot{V}/\dot{Q}$ mismatch	+++
Unilateral leg or arm swelling	Venous obstruction	++++
Normalization of vital signs	Presumptive from treatment or Hawthorne effect	Not significant

clinical picture of any ED patient related to weakness, shortness of breath, dizziness or syncope, pain, extremity discomfort, or nonspecific malaise or functional deterioration could represent a potential PE.A patient with PE typically presents with 2 to 3 d of shortness of breath, now worsened enough to seek care. The chest pain usually is vaguely described. A few patients have focal pleuritic chest pain with breathing.PE with lung infarction can result in a clinical picture that is similar to lobar pneumonia, including focal chest pain, fever, and unilateral rales on auscultation. However, a temperature greater than 101.5°F suggests infection rather than infarction.An occasional clue to pulmonary infarction is the onset of pain and blood-red hemoptysis on the same day, whereas lobar pneumonia usually causes productive cough for a few days before rust-tinged sputum.

The physical examination can sometimes provide specific information about the presence of PE, including unilateral leg asymmetry, suggesting presence of DVT. Massive PE is defined by hypotension with a SBP below 90 mmHg for more than 15 min.Jugular venous distention in a patient with severe dyspnea and clear lung fields on auscultation suggests pure right-sided HF. Bilateral rales suggest the diagnosis of LV failure.

Diagnosis

Chest radiography seldom provides specific information of PE diagnoses. Unilateral basilar atelectasis on the chest radiograph increases the probability of PE. If symptoms have been present for 3 d or more, pulmonary infarction sometimes shows an apex-central, pleural-based, wedge-shaped area of infiltrate, producing the Hampton's hump finding. Unilateral lung oligemia (Westermark's sign) is a rare radiographic manifestation of a large PE.

When PE causes ECG changes, this is usually a result of acute or subacute pulmonary hypertension. The most common effects of pulmonary hypertension on ECG are rapid heart rate, symmetrical T-wave inversion in the anterior leads (V_1-V_4), the McGinn-White $S_1Q_3T_3$ pattern, and incomplete or complete RBBB (Fig. 20-2).

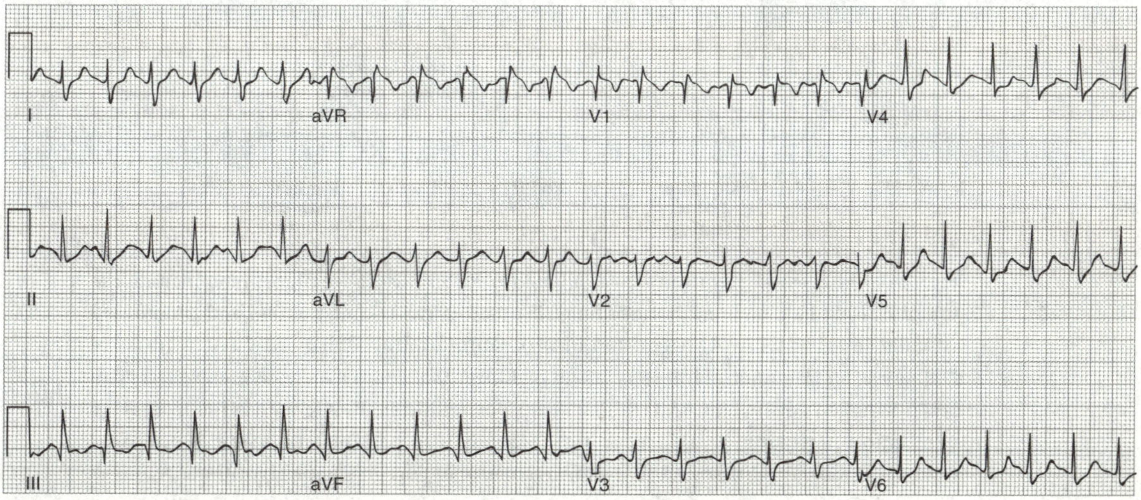

Fig. 20-2 Initial ECG tracing from an 18 yr-old woman on oral contraceptives in the ED with syncope. Several findings consistent with PE are shown, including tachycardia, the $S_1Q_3T_3$ pattern, and an incomplete RBBB. CTA revealed extensive bilateral pulmonary emboli, and ECG showed severe right heart dysfunction.

Specific risks include exposure to the ionizing radiation and intravenous contrast necessary for CTPA and CT venography and the risk of false-positive interpretation, which may occur in as many as 10% of scans read as positive for PE. The appropriate use of D-dimer testing decreases the need for imaging in all but patients at high risk.

To identify the very low-risk group in whom PE could be safely excluded at the bedside with no diagnostic testing, the PE rule-out criteria (the PERC rule) were derived and prospectively validated in 8138 patients in 13 different hospitals across the United States and in New Zealand (Box 20-2).

PE also is less likely when some other disease process can explain the patient's complaints and findings in a patient otherwise not believed to be at high risk for PE.The flow algorithms provided here are predicated on the following goals: (1) to identify as many ED patients as possible who have PE; (2) to avoid mislabeling (and administering anticoagulants to) patients who do not have PE; and (3) to use available resources efficiently and effectively (Fig. 20-3).

For a patient for whom suspicion is implicit or with explicit score suggesting a PTP over 40%, clinicians should skip the D-dimer, order pulmonary vascular imaging, and strongly

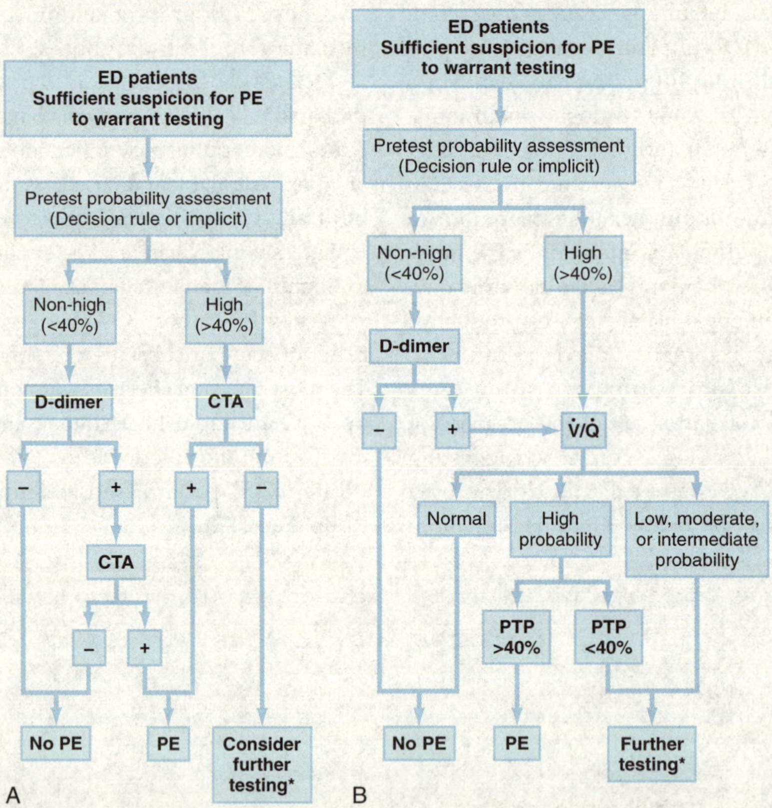

Fig. 20-3 Suggested algorithms to evaluate for PE in ED. These algorithms include the use of PTP, ELISA, or immunoturbidimetric quantitative D-dimer assay, and pulmonary vascular imaging CTA. A, Algorithm incorporating contrast-enhanced CTA. A negative D-dimer is an immunoturbidimetric assay or ELISA that returns a concentration less than 500 fibrinogen equivalent units (FEUs) (ng) per milliliter. B, Algorithm incorporating ventilation-perfusion ($\dot{V}/\dot{Q}$) scanning. *May require patient admission. Additional testing—Option 1: "Crossover" to perform either scanning or CT for algorithms A and B. Option 2: Perform lower extremity venous ultrasound, and if initial venous ultrasound is negative, repeat the lower extremity venous ultrasound in 1 week. Option 3: Perform formal pulmonary angiography.

consider initiating anticoagulation in the absence of contraindications.

The PTP to safely exclude the diagnosis of PE must be equal to 1%, which is at least equivalent to that of a normal scan or a negative CTPA. This combination can be achieved by the combination of a PTP assessment less than 40% and a quantitative D-dimer concentration less than 500 ng/mL. When the PTP is high or the screening D-dimer is positive, pulmonary vascular imaging by CTPA or scanning is advised. Although CTPA is not perfect, it has multiple advantages over scanning and usually can confirm or exclude the presence of PE.

Most academic centers now use CTPA as the primary method of evaluating for PE.

CTPA can provide additional information to enhance its usefulness in the ED. CTPA often provides information about alternative processes that might explain the patient's symptoms (Box 20-3). Pneumonia is the most common alternative diagnosis found in ED patients. In about 10% of ED patients evaluated for PE, CT as a single test could (1) show absence of PE; (2) provide evidence of alternative disease, which can be used with other evidence to reduce the probability of PE to a reasonably low level to stop the workup; and (3) facilitate treatment for the alternative disease.

Box 20-3 Frequency of Nonpulmonary Embolism Diagnoses Discovered on CT

Pneumonia (6%)*
Unsuspected pericardial effusion (1%)
Mass suggesting new carcinoma (1%)
Aortic dissection (0.5%)
Pneumothorax (0.5%)

* Percentage of all 1025 ED patients who underwent CT to evaluate for PE.

The scintillation scan remains a good diagnostic option for patients with contraindications to iodinated intravenous contrast. The accuracy and precision of the scan were shown in the PIOPED study, which compared the results of scanning with the most accurate criterion standard test available at the time—formal pulmonary angiography (Table 20-3). A moderate probability or indeterminate scan requires additional formal pulmonary angiography or a CTPA. Even in patients with a low PTP, a low probability scan usually indicates a need for additional testing, such as either CTPA or venous duplex ultrasonography of the legs.

Table 20-3 Prevalence of PE Stratified by Ventilation-Perfusion Scan Result and PTP Estimate

V/Q RATIO SCAN RESULT	Clinician Estimate of PTP for PE			
	80%-100%	20%-79%	0%-19%	ALL
High probability	28/29 (96%)	70/80 (88%)	5/9 (56%)	103/118 (87%)
Intermediate probability	27/41 (66%)	66/236 (28%)	11/68 (16%)	104/345 (30%)
Low probability	6/15 (40%)	30/191 (16%)	4/90(4%)	40/296 (14%)
Near-normal or normal	0/5 (0%)	4/62(6%)	1/61(2%)	5/128(4%)
Total	61/90 (68%)	170/569 (30%)	21/228 (9%)	252/887 (28%)

Management

Anticoagulation

Either unfractionated heparin (80 units/kg intravenous bolus, followed by 18 units/kg/hr intravenous infusion), fractionated LMWH (e.g., enoxaparin, 1 mg/kg SQ or IV every 12 hr), or the pentasaccharide factor Xa inhibitor fondaparinux (5-10 mg, depending on body mass) can be used for treatment of most patients with PE. LMWH is recommended over unfractionated heparin.Heparin provides several immediate benefits, including the reduction in clot extension; reduces the transient hypercoagulable effect of warfarin treatment; and over a period of days to weeks allows the natural fibrinolytic system to reduce clot size.

All patients with a high PTP, no contraind-ication to anticoagulation, and evidence of hemodynamic instability, including recent syncope, any hypotension, hypoxemia, or clinical evidence of right-sided heart strain, should receive immediate empirical heparin.

For a patient diagnosed with PE in the presence of a major contraindication to anticoagulation, such as a recent cerebral hemorrhage or large cerebral infarction, the appropriate consultant should be contacted for urgent placement of an inferior vena cava filter. If vena caval interruption cannot be performed within 12 hr, one option is to perform a baseline head CT scan, then start an unfractionated heparin infusion at 18 units/kg/hr and admit the patient to the ICU for close neurologic monitoring and frequent partial thromboplastin time determinations.

Table 20-4 summarizes the criteria that can be used to risk stratify patients with PE into four groups.

Table 20-4 Risk-Stratification and Associated Treatment Recommendations for Acute PE

CATEGORY	CRITERIA	ACTION
Low-risk PE	SBP>90 mmHg at all times and all of the following: Shock index <1 SaO_2 almost always > 94% Daniel score <3 Normal troponin or BNP or proBNP level PESI score <66	Begin LMWH Optional admission to unmonitored regular bed Consider outpatient treatment if adequate compliance and follow-up can be ensured
Moderate-risk PE	SBP>90 mmHg at all times and any one of the following: Shock index 1 or greater at any time SaO_2 persistently <94% Daniel score >3 Elevated troponin or BNP or proBNP level PESI score >65 and <125 Echocardiography with any degree of right ventricular hypokinesis	Begin heparin treatment Fibrinolytics in the minority of cases Admission to a telemetry bed
More severe (submassive) mode rate-risk PE	Appearance of at least moderate distress AND Shock index >1 and severe right ventricular hypokinesis on echocardiography Worsening Daniel score, particularly a new incomplete right bundle branch block (iRBBB) or progression of iRBBB to complete RBBB SaO_2 <90% and serum troponin level clearly elevated PESI score >124	Begin heparin treatment Fibrinolytic treatment in the majority of patients without contraindications in the ED Admission to a step-down or intensive care unit
High risk (major) PE	Any SBP<90 mmHg or <20 mmHg below documented baseline and appearance of distress Any persistent SBP<90 mmHg regardless of appearance	Begin heparin treatment Fibrinolytic treatment in all patients without contraindications in the ED Admission to intensive care unit

Thrombolytic Therapy

Administration of alteplase to patients with PE results in more rapid symptomatic improvement than standard antithrombotic therapy alone. Alteplase also increases the risk of hemorrhage.In patients with preexisting hypertension, the threshold is adjusted to below 100 mmHg or a reduction in the baseline SBP of more than 60 mmHg. In the absence of contraindications, patients with proven massive PE probably benefit from fibrinolysis.

A subset of patients with submassive PE may benefit from fibrinolysis, including those with moderate-to-severe respiratory distress and hypoxia and those with echocardiographic evidence of right ventricular dysfunction. When echocardiography is unavailable in a timely manner, surrogate laboratory markers of right ventricular dysfunction may be useful, including an elevated troponin level or a BNP level greater than 90 pg/mL (Table 20-4). The FDA-approved regimens for thrombolysis are shown in Table 20-5.

Table 20-5 Food and Drug Administration–Approved Fibrinolytic Regimens for Acute Treatment of PE

Streptokinase	1 million units infused over 24 hr
Urokinase	1 million–unit bolus followed by 24-hr infusion at 300,000 units/hr
Alteplase	15-mg bolus followed by 2-hr infusion of 85 mg; discontinue heparin during infusion

A patient can be stable and then hypotensive within minutes because of the highly variable effect of the clot on right ventricular outflow obstruction, especially when it is perched in the main pulmonary artery (Fig. 20-4). Additional mechanisms of rapid instability include new embolization of clot material, release of mediators of pulmonary vasospasm, sudden bradycardiac or asystolic arrhythmias, and respiratory failure. A particularly ominous finding is the evolution on ECG from a narrow-complex tachycardia to iRBBB to a complete RBBB (Fig. 20-5) as evidence of life-threatening pulmonary hypertension and incipient cardiac arrest.

Clinical evidence of impending or actual respiratory failure indicates the need for prompt endotracheal intubation. Other induction agents that depress cardiac function or reduce preload may precipitate severe hypotension. In the case of impending respiratory or cardiac arrest, fibrinolytic therapy should be strongly considered.

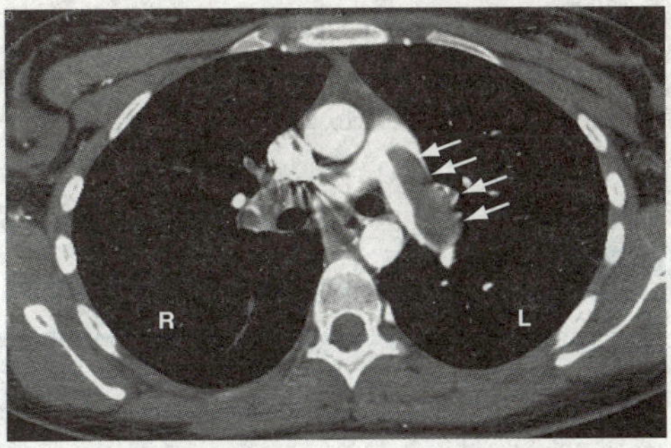

Fig. 20-4 Massive PE on a contrast-enhanced CT scan of the chest. This CT scan is at the level of the bifurcation of the main pulmonary artery. The left main branch of the pulmonary artery shows a massive filling defect (arrows). The patient was a young woman who recently began taking oral contraceptives. The patient had cyanosis, hypoxemia, and worsened hemodynamic findings when supine but was normotensive when sitting upright. She was given anticoagulant therapy, had emergent surgical embolectomy, and survived with excellent outcome. Her DNA had factor V Leiden mutation, by polymerase chain reaction testing in both alleles.

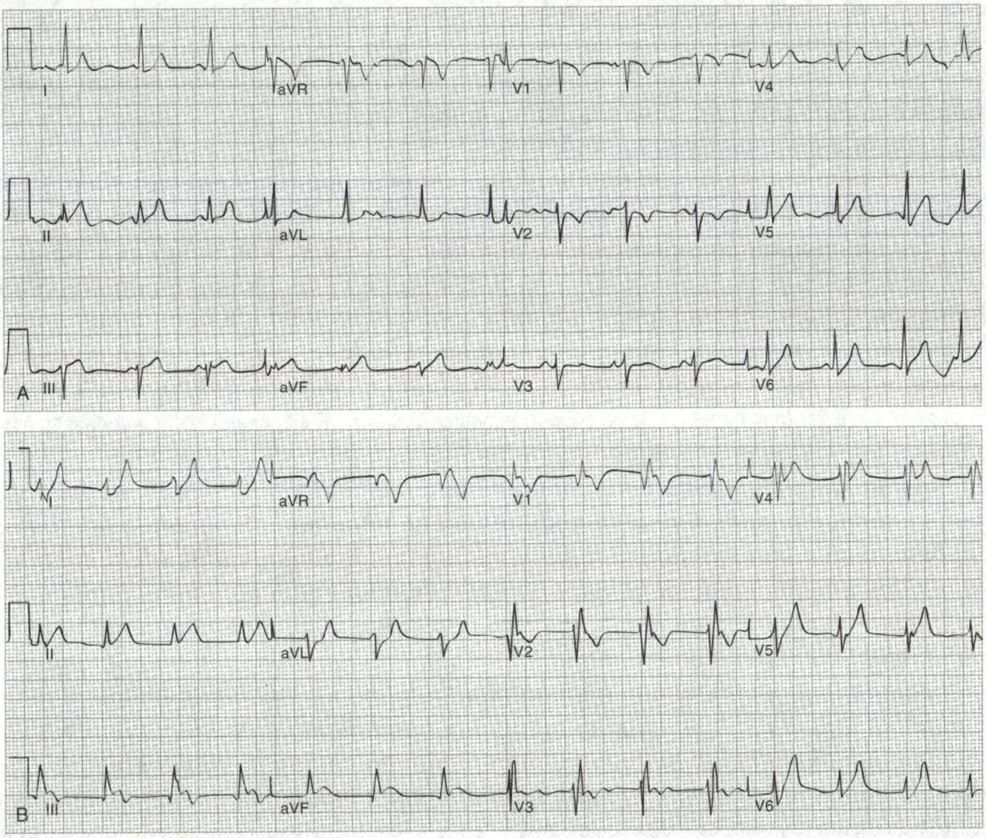

Fig. 20-5 Serial electrocardiograms obtained 2 min apart show the progression from a narrow complex rhythm (A) to a RBBB pattern (B) in a patient with massive bilateral pulmonary emboli. Shortly after the second tracing was obtained, the patient developed cardiovascular collapse refractory to vigorous resuscitation efforts.

Surgical Embolectomy

For patients with known floating thrombi in the right side of the heart or for patients with severe refractory hypotension, surgery is the most likely intervention to save the patient's life.Surgical embolectomy may be the best option for patients who have severe PE with a contraindication to fibrinolysis.

Box 20-4 details questions that commonly arise regarding the diagnosis and treatment of PE in the ED.

Box 20-4 Unique Questions That Commonly Arise in ED

1. I cannot get imaging at night. Is it reasonable to treat the patient with heparin until morning?
   The short answer to this question is yes, if the patient has no contraindications. Many smaller hospitals routinely use this method and use a single dose of enoxaparin.
2. How do I manage the patient who is being treated for PE who returns to the ED for chest pain?
   If the patient has a therapeutic international normalized ratio(1.5-2.5) and returns with symptoms only (e.g., chest pain, dyspnea) and without syncope, appears relatively comfortable, has normal vital signs, and has no new changes suggesting pulmonary hypertension on ECG (in particular, no $S_1Q_3T_3$ pattern and no T wave inversion in leads V_1 through V_4), follow-up imaging is probably not needed. Other causes of chest pain (especially acute coronary syndrome) should be considered. In the absence of an identified alternative diagnosis, symptomatic care with an anti-inflammatory agent is safe and reasonable therapy for the return complaint of chest pain. Persistent dyspnea at rest raises more concerns of unresolved or recurrent thrombosis with secondary effects, including bronchospasm or, worse, pulmonary vascular hyperplasia with pulmonary hypertension. Repeat pulmonary vascular imaging may provide evidence of an unresolved or new clot. More important, a transthoracic echocardiogram can disclose evidence of persistent right ventricular dysfunction and pulmonary hypertension. Symptomatic patients with unresolved filling defects and pulmonary hypertension can progress to chronic thromboembolic pulmonary hypertension. For prevention of this decline, patients who return to the ED with persistent rest dyspnea and have unresolved filling defects and pulmonary hypertension should be admitted or referred to a program that offers the option of pulmonary thrombectomy.
3. How can I rule out pulmonary embolism in a pregnant patient without use of ionizing radiation?
   One clinical conundrum is the fact the pregnancy is accompanied by both an increased risk of PE and a predictable elevation in D-dimer, even in the absence of PE. Given that PE is the most common nontraumatic cause of death in pregnant women, clinicians are justified in adopting a liberal *rule-out PE* approach to all pregnant women with dyspnea. To evaluated suspected PE in pregnancy, I recommend the following sequence. First, assess the PERC rule criteria and apply a modified version of the PERC rule with a slightly elevated top limit for the pulse rate (normal up to 104 beats/min instead of 99 beats/min). If the result of this modified PERC rule is negative, then order a quantitative D-dimer. Use thresholds to define a normal D-dimer that is elevated on the basis of trimester (first trimester, 1.5×; second trimester, 2×; and third trimester, 2.5× standard threshold). If the result of the modified PERC rule is positive or the D-dimer is above the adjusted threshold, then order bilateral lower extremity ultrasound; if this is positive for DVT, then treat for PE. If the bilateral ultrasound is negative, proceed to pulmonary vascular imaging. The issue of the optimal imaging procedure in pregnancy remains controversial. A 2003 survey of radiologists indicated an almost equal split (53% in favor of CTPA, 47% in favor of $\dot{V}/\dot{Q}$ scanning) in their choice for imaging for PE in pregnancy.
4. How do I evaluate the patient with possible PE who is too obese to fit in a CT scanner?
   Each CT scanner has a maximum patient weight that it will accommodate. When a patient's weight exceeds the scanner limit and a larger capacity scanner is not available, I recommend duplex venous ultrasonography of the lower extremities to rule out DVT. Although often technically suboptimal in a massively obese patient, venous ultrasound occasionally provides positive evidence of DVT, ostensibly clinching the diagnosis. Another option is to anticoagulate empirically based on a moderate-to-high PTP and a D-dimer concentration that exceeds 1000 ng/mL. The adequate regimen for anticoagulation is uncertain, but many experts recommend subcutaneous enoxaparin, 1 mg/kg of actual body weight up to a maximum of 200 μg/kg.

(YUAN Zhiming)

Chapter 21

Nontraumatic Pleural Problems

KEY CONCEPTS

The most common condition associated with secondary spontaneous pneumothorax is COPD. While in developing countries, tuberculosis and lung abscess remain the leading causes.

Point of care thoracic ultrasound can be used to rule out pneumothorax with greater sensitivity than a portable supine chest X-ray examination. Chest CT is the gold standard for diagnosis of pneumothorax.

Tension pneumothorax is a life-threatening condition. The pleural space should be decompressed as soon as it is believed to be present.

In most cases of secondary spontaneous pneumothorax, tube thoracostomy should be considered.

The clearest indication for diagnostic thoracentesis in the ED is to diagnose immediately life-threatening conditions.

This chapter reviews the two most common nontraumatic pleural problems: spontaneous pneumothorax and pleural inflammation with effusion.

Presentations of nontraumatic pleural problems range in severity from asymptomatic pleural effusion to tension pneumothorax.

SPONTANEOUS PNEUMOTHORAX

Pneumothorax is defined as the presence of free air in the intrapleural space. Pneumothorax could be divided into two types: spontaneous pneumothorax and traumatic pneumothorax. A *spontaneous pneumothorax* occurs in the absence of any external precipitating factor, either traumatic or iatrogenic.

Etiology and pathogenesis

According to the presence of primary pulmonary disease, spontaneous pneumothorax is usually divided into primary spontaneous pneumothorax and secondary spontaneous pneumothorax. *Primary spontaneous pneumothorax* occurs in individuals without clinically apparent lung disease. *Secondary spontaneous pneumothorax* arises in the context of an underlying pulmonary disease process.

Primary spontaneous pneumothorax

Primary spontaneous pneumothorax typically occurs in healthy young men of taller than average height. Factors associated with primary spontaneous pneumothorax include cigarette smoking and changes in ambient atmospheric pressure. Familial patterns suggest an inherited propensity in some cases of primary spontaneous pneumothorax. Mitral valve prolapse and Marfan's syndrome are associated with spontaneous pneumothorax in the absence of clinically apparent lung disease.

Secondary spontaneous pneumothorax

Approximately one third of spontaneous pneumothoraces occur in the context of underlying pulmonary disease (Box 21-1). The incidence of secondary spontaneous pneumothorax is three times higher in men. The most common condition associated with secondary spontaneous pneumothorax is COPD, which accounts for nearly 70% of cases. Patients with severe COPD (e.g., with forced expiratory volume in 1 s<1 L) are at highest risk.

Spontaneous pneumothorax occurs in approximately 2% of patients with AIDS, almost always in the setting of *Pneumocystis jiroveci* (previously known as *Pneumocystis carinii*) pneumonia. Bilateral pneumothoraces are common with *P. jiroveci* pneumonia, as are problems with delayed reexpansion and recurrences. Mortality in these patients is high.

Box 21-1 Causes of Secondary Spontaneous Pneumothorax

Airway Disease
- COPD
- Asthma
- Cystic fibrosis

Infections
- Necrotizing bacterial pneumonia, lung abscess
- *Pneumocystis jiroveci* pneumonia
- Tuberculosis

Interstitial Lung Disease
- Sarcoidosis
- Idiopathic pulmonary fibrosis
- Lymphangiomyomatosis
- Tuberous sclerosis
- Pneumoconioses

Neoplasms
- Primary lung cancers
- Pulmonary or pleural metastases

Miscellaneous
- Connective tissue diseases
- Pulmonary infarction
- Endometriosis, catamenial pneumothorax

Malignancy is another common etiology of secondary spontaneous pneumothorax. In developing countries, tuberculosis and lung abscess remain leading causes of secondary spontaneous pneumothorax.

Catamenial pneumothorax is a rare condition in which recurrent spontaneous pneumothorax occurs in association with menses (typically within 72 hr of onset).

Pathophysiologic Principles

Normally, intrapleural pressure is negative, fluctuating from −10 mm Hg to −12 mm Hg during inspiration to approximately −4 mm Hg during expiration. Intrabronchial and intra-alveolar pressures are negative during inspiration (−1 to −3 mm Hg) and positive during expiration (+1 to +3 mm Hg). The alveolar walls and visceral pleura form a barrier that separates the intrapleural and intra-alveolar spaces and maintains the pressure gradient. If a defect occurs in this barrier, air enters the pleural space until either the pressures equalize or the communication seals.

With the loss of negative intrapleural pressure in one hemithorax, the ipsilateral lung collapses. A large pneumothorax results in restrictive ventilation impairment, with reduced vital capacity, functional residual capacity, and total lung capacity. Shunting of blood through nonventilated lung tissue may result in acute hypoxemia, although over time this effect is mitigated by compensatory vasoconstriction in the collapsed lung.

In tension pneumothorax, the alveolar-pleural defect acts as a one-way valve, allowing air to pass into the pleural space during inspiration and trapping it there during expiration (Fig. 21-1). This trapping leads to progressive accumulation of intrapleural air and increasingly positive intrapleural pressure, causing compression of the contralateral lung with asphyxia and worsening hypoxia. Intrapleural pressure exceeding 15 to 20 mm Hg impairs venous return to the heart. If allowed to progress, cardiovascular collapse and death ensue.

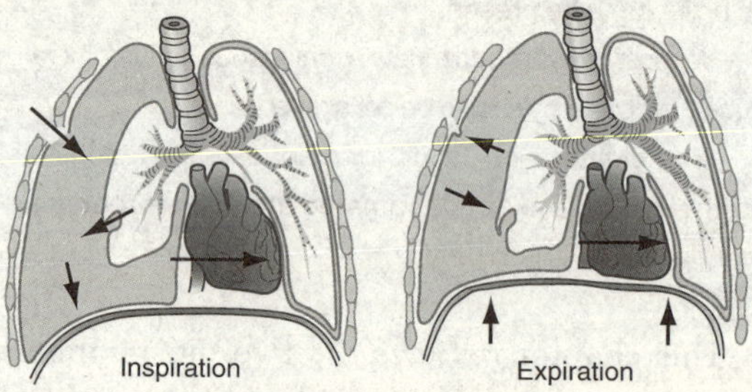

Fig. 21-1 Tension pneumothorax with total collapse of the right lung and shift of mediastinal structures to the left. Air is forced into the pleural space during expiration and cannot escape during inspiration.

In primary spontaneous pneumothorax, disruption of the alveolar-pleural barrier occurs when a subpleural bulla (or bleb), typically located at the lung apex, ruptures into the pleural space. The etiology of these bullae may be related to degradation of elastic fibers within the lung and an imbalance in the protease-antiprotease and oxidant-antioxidant systems.

In the case of secondary spontaneous pneumothorax, the underlying lung disease weakens the alveolar-pleural barrier. In patients with COPD, chronic exposure to cigarette smoke results in the development of large, thin-walled bullae that are at an increased risk for rupture. Other factors, including increased intrabronchial and intra-alveolar pressures generated by bronchospasm and coughing, also play a role.

Clinical Features

Symptoms of primary spontaneous pneumothorax typically begin suddenly while at rest. Ipsilateral chest pain and dyspnea are the most common symptoms. At the outset, the pain is typically "pleuritic" in nature (i.e., often described as sharp and made worse with deep inspiration), but it often evolves over time into a dull, steady ache. Although patients frequently describe shortness of breath, extreme dyspnea is uncommon in the absence of underlying lung disease or tension pneumothorax. Cough is present in a few individuals. Occasionally, patients are asymptomatic or have only nonspecific complaints. Without treatment, symptoms often resolve spontaneously within 24 to 72 hr, although the pneumothorax is still present.

Physical findings tend to correlate with the degree of symptoms. A mild sinus tachycardia is the most common physical finding. With a large pneumothorax, decreased or absent breath sounds with hyperresonance to percussion may be present. Other classic signs include unilateral enlargement of the hemithorax, decreased excursion with respirations, absent tactile fremitus, and inferior displacement of the liver or spleen. Absence of any or all of these findings does not exclude pneumothorax, however, and a chest radiograph should be obtained when pneumothorax is suspected.

With tension pneumothorax, signs of asphyxia and decreased cardiac output develop. Tachycardia (often >120 beats/min) and hypoxia are common. Hypotension is a late and ominous finding. Distention of the jugular veins is common but may be difficult to detect. Displacement of the trachea to the contralateral side is classically described but is an uncommon finding, usually occurring only in the immediately preterminal phase of the pneumothorax.

In patients with significant underlying lung disease, pneumothorax presents differently. Because of poor pulmonary reserve, dyspnea is nearly universal, even when the pneumothorax is small, and symptoms tend not to resolve on their own. Physical findings, such as hyperexpansion and distant breath sounds, often overlap considerably with the underlying lung disease, making the clinical diagnosis difficult.

Auxiliary Examination

The diagnosis of pneumothorax is generally made with the chest radiograph. The classic radiographic appearance is that of a thin, visceral pleural line lying parallel to the chest wall, separated by a radiolucent band devoid of lung markings. The average width of this band can be used to estimate the size of the pneumothorax with a fair degree of accuracy (Fig. 21-2), but in general, it is more reasonable simply to characterize the pneumothorax as small, moderate, large, or total. The estimated size of the pneumothorax and the patient's clinical status can be useful in guiding management decisions.

Tension pneumothorax is a clinical diagnosis, and delaying treatment to obtain radiographic

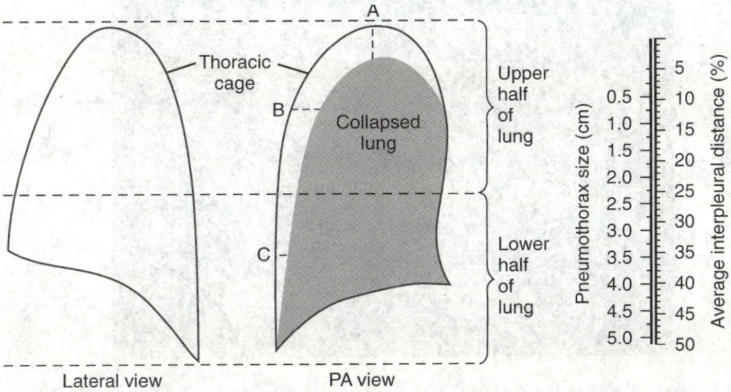

Fig. 21-2 Determining the size of a pneumothorax. Calculation of average interpleural distance to predict pneumothorax size. PA, posteroanterior.

confirmation is inadvisable. When the diagnosis of tension pneumothorax is not apparent clinically and a chest radiograph is obtained, the classic appearance is one of complete lung collapse with gross distention of the thoracic cavity on the affected side and shift of mediastinal structures across the midline (Fig. 21-3A). In patients with underlying pulmonary disease, however, pleural adhesions and lack of lung elasticity may mask the fact that a pneumothorax is under significant positive pressure.

When pneumothorax is suspected but not seen on a standard chest radiograph, an expiratory film may be obtained. Theoretically, the volumes of the lungs and the chest cavity are reduced during expiration so that the relative size of the pneumothorax is enhanced. In critically ill patients for whom only a supine chest radiograph can be obtained, the finding of a "deep sulcus" (i.e., a deep lateral costophrenic angle) can suggest the presence of pneumothorax on that side (Fig. 21-3A).

In patients with COPD, the clue to differen-

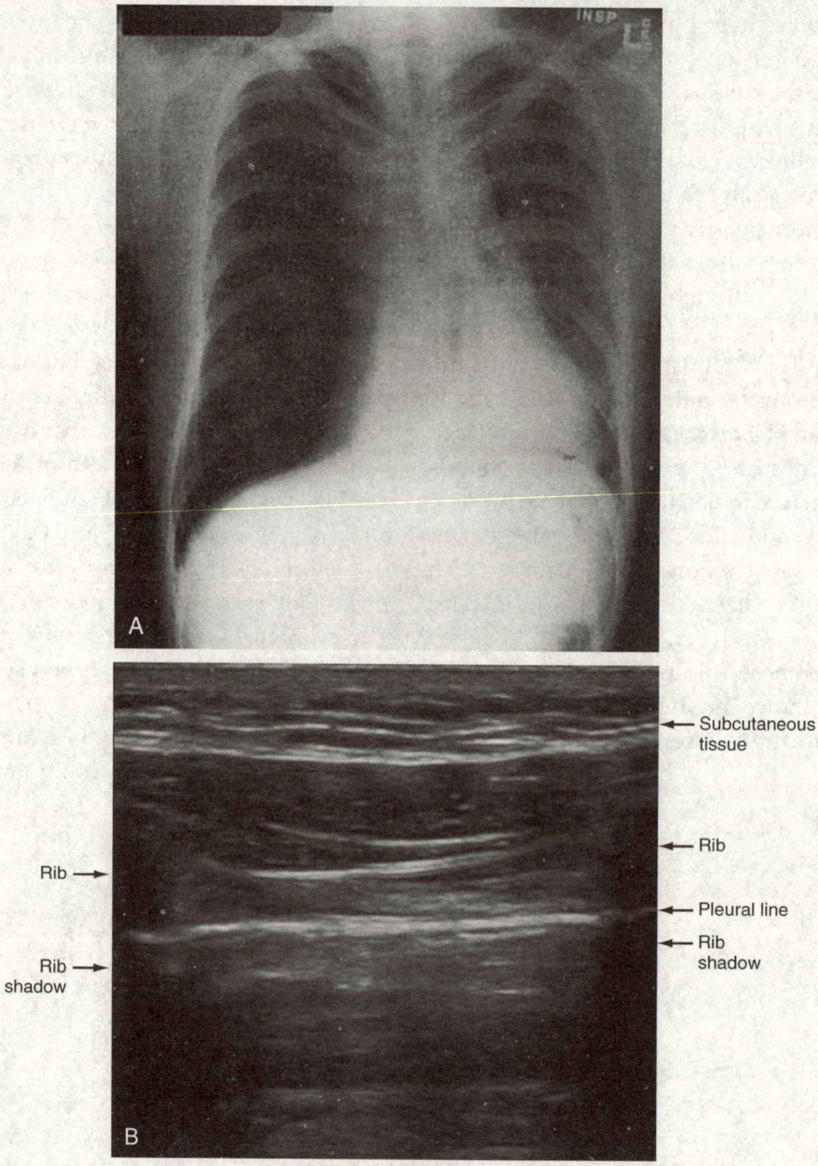

Fig. 21-3 A.Radiograph of tension pneumothorax with mediastinal shift to left.B, Ultrasound demonstrating location of pleural line.Lung sliding is dynamic and visualized in real time as shimmering or sliding of the pleural line.

tiating a pneumothorax from a giant bulla is that the former tends to run parallel to the chest wall, whereas the latter tends to have a more concave appearance. When the diagnosis is unclear, CT can differentiate between the two entities.

Chest CT is considered the gold standard for the diagnosis of pneumothorax; however, it requires that patients be stable enough for transport. Although portable chest radiography is convenient and commonly used, it has poor overall sensitivity. Bedside thoracic ultrasound is more rapid and sensitive than a supine chest radiograph for the diagnosis of pneumothorax and avoids ionizing radiation. In normal lung the closely opposed visceral and parietal pleura create the appearance of shimmering or sliding of the pleural interface during respiration. Assessment for pneumothorax is optimally performed with a high-frequency linear probe to most accurately visualize the lung sliding at the pleural line (Fig. 21-3B). In supine patients, air rises; scanning a few interspaces on the anterior chest wall along the midclavicular line can effectively evaluate the most likely areas for pneumothorax. Extending the examination to the lateral chest wall can help identify the "lung point" or boundary between normal lung and pneumothorax and is highly specific for the detection of pneumothorax. Visualization of lung sliding at the pleural line effectively rules out pneumothorax in the area being scanned. A small pneumothorax may not be detected with ultrasound, and false-positive results can occur in patients with blebs, pleural scarring, or severe ARDS or in single-lung intubation.

The differential diagnosis of pneumothorax includes pulmonary embolism, most pleural-based processes (pneumonia, embolism, tumor) and AMI .

Complication

Spontaneous pneumomediastinum is diagnosed by the presence of subcutaneous emphysema and the finding of mediastinal air on chest radiography. Spontaneous pneumomediastinum typically occurs during exertion, particularly after a strenuous Valsalva maneuver.

Spontaneous hemopneumothorax is a rare but potentially serious condition that occurs when collapse of the lung is associated with rupture of a vessel in a parietopleural adhesion. The clinical presentation is similar to that of spontaneous pneumothorax but may be accompanied by symptoms and signs of hemorrhagic shock.

Management

Whether in the field or in the ED, if the clinical circumstances suggest tension pneumothorax, treatment should not be delayed by awaiting further cardiovascular compromise or definitive diagnosis by chest radiography. As soon as tension pneumothorax is believed to be present, the pleural space should be decompressed. This decompression may be accomplished by insertion of an intravenous catheter or by immediate tube thoracostomy. The diagnosis is confirmed by the hiss of air escaping under positive pressure as the needle or chest tube enters the pleural space. Needle decompression is only a temporizing procedure, and definitive management requires prompt tube thoracostomy.

The management of spontaneous pneumothorax has two goals: (1) to evacuate air from the pleural space, and (2) to prevent recurrence. Therapeutic options for treatment of pneumothorax range from simple observation or aspiration with a catheter to video-assisted thoracoscopic surgery or thoracotomy. Decisions must be individualized and consider several factors, including size of the pneumothorax, severity of signs, presence of underlying pulmonary disease, other comorbidities, history of previous pneumothoraces, patient reliability, degree and persistence of the air leak, and available follow-up monitoring.

For otherwise healthy, young patients with a small primary spontaneous pneumothorax (i.e., <20% of the hemithorax), observation alone may be appropriate. The intrinsic reabsorption rate ranges from 1% to 2% per day, a rate that is accelerated by a factor of 4 with the administration of 100% oxygen. By lowering the alveolar partial pressure of nitrogen, supplemental oxygen increases the rate at which air diffuses across the pleural-alveolar barrier. Most physicians admit these patients for at least 6 hr of observation. A repeat chest radiograph can be obtained before discharge. Air travel and underwater diving must be avoided until the pneumothorax has completely resolved.

For primary spontaneous pneumothoraces that are larger in size (i.e., ⩾20% of the hemithorax), aspiration with an intravenous catheter may be attempted. If 6 hr after aspiration the chest radiograph shows no reaccumulation of the pneumothorax, the catheter is removed, and the patient can be discharged home.

If aspiration fails to reexpand the lung fully, the catheter can be attached to a water-seal device or to a one-way Heimlich valve and managed like a small-caliber chest tube.

Most secondary spontaneous pneumothoraces should be managed with tube thoracostomy . Similarly, patients who present with respiratory distress, have tension pneumothorax, or are likely to require mechanical ventilation should undergo tube thoracostomy to reexpand the lung definitively. Also, if there is detectable pleural fluid (hemothorax or hydrothorax), tube thoracostomy is required. Finally, tube thoracostomy may be considered in uncomplicated cases of primary spontaneous pneumothorax either as a first-line intervention or after a less invasive approach (i.e., observation or simple aspiration) fails.

For most primary spontaneous pneumothoraces, placement of a small-caliber (7–14F) tube is generally sufficient. Complications associated with small-caliber tubes include kinking, malposition, inadvertent removal, occlusion by pleural fluid or clotted blood, and large persistent air leaks. For secondary spontaneous pneumothorax, a standard size (20–28F) thoracostomy tube is recommended. When there is detectable pleural fluid or an anticipated need for mechanical ventilation, a larger tube size (≥28F) is required.

After insertion, the tube is attached to a water-seal device and left in place until the lung has reexpanded fully and the air leak has ceased. A Heimlich valve, which consists of a one-way flutter valve covered in transparent plastic, can be used in place of a water-seal device and allows unhindered ambulation. Specific complications associated with the use of a Heimlich valve include accidental disconnection and occlusion by fluid.

The use of suction (with a pressure of 20 cm H_2O) is reserved for situations in which the lung fails to reexpand after drainage through a water-seal device or Heimlich valve for 24 to 48 hr.

In most cases, chest tube management requires hospital admission. Common complications of chest tube placement include incorrect placement, pleural infection, and prolonged pain. Reexpansion pulmonary edema and reexpansion hypotension are rare occurrences after rapid evacuation of large pneumothoraces.

Outcome

Most spontaneous pneumothoraces resolve within 7 d of tube thoracostomy. If an air leak persists beyond 4 to 7 d, surgical intervention generally is recommended.

Recurrences of spontaneous pneumothorax are common.

A variety of operative and nonoperative interventions prevent recurrences. One strategy promotes adherence of parietal and visceral pleura, which obliterates the pleural space. Pleurodesis can be accomplished by mechanical pleural abrasion or by instillation of sclerosing agents. Another strategy involves resection of apical bullae or other lesions at risk for causing recurrences.

PLEURAL INFLAMMATION AND EFFUSION

The most common cause of pleural effusions in Western countries is CHF, followed by malignancy, bacterial pneumonia, and pulmonary embolism. In other countries, tuberculosis is the leading cause of pleural effusions. Other conditions commonly associated with pleural effusions include viral infections of the lung parenchyma or pleura, uremia, myxedema, cirrhosis, nephrotic syndrome, ovarian hyperstimulation syndrome, collagen vascular diseases (e.g., SLE, RA), and intra-abdominal processes (e.g., acute pancreatitis, subphrenic abscess, ascites). Esophageal perforation is a rare but uniquely morbid cause of a pleural effusion.

Pleuritis (also referred to as *pleurisy*) is a nonspecific term denoting inflammation of the pleura. Pleuritis can occur with or without significant exudation of fluid into the pleural space. Pleuritis is a common presentation for a range of disease processes, from self-limited viral syndromes to more serious acute conditions, such as pneumonia and pulmonary embolism, to chronic illnesses, such as SLE and other connective tissue diseases.

A pleural effusion associated with bacterial pneumonia, bronchiectasis, or lung abscess is called a *parapneumonic effusion*. The term *complicated parapneumonic effusion* refers to parapneumonic effusions that require tube thoracostomy for their resolution. The diagnosis of empyema (or pus in the pleural space) requires the presence of bacteria on Gram staining of the pleural fluid.

Fluid anatomically confined and not freely flowing in the pleural space is termed a *loculated effusion*. Loculated effusions occur when there are adhesions between the visceral and the parietal pleurae. Hemothorax and chylothorax (i.e., from rupture of the thoracic duct) are special instances of pleural effusion that are approached separately.

Pathophysiologic Principles

Pleural fluid is produced from systemic capillaries at the parietal pleural surface and absorbed into pulmonary capillaries at the visceral pleural surface. Lymphatics also play an important role in removing pleural fluid. Movement of fluid across the pleural surfaces is governed by Starling's law. Under normal circumstances, the direction of pleural fluid flow is largely governed by the difference in hydrostatic pressure between the systemic and the pulmonary circulations (Fig. 21-4). Pleural fluid exists in a dynamic equilibrium in which influx equals efflux, with approximately 1 L of fluid traversing the pleural space in 24 hr. Under normal conditions, the amount of fluid that remains in the pleural space is small (0.1-0.2 mL/kg body weight) and clinically or radiographically undetectable. Pleural effusion develops whenever influx of fluid into the pleural space exceeds efflux. Numerous disorders can lead to formation of a pleural effusion. Pleural effusions classically are divided into two groups— *transudates* and *exudates*—according to the composition of the pleural fluid (Box 21-2).

Box 21-2 Causes of Pleural Effusion

Transudates
- CHF
- Cirrhosis with ascites
- Nephrotic syndrome
- Hypoalbuminemia
- Myxedema
- Peritoneal dialysis
- Glomerulonephritis
- Superior vena cava obstruction
- PE

Exudates

Infections
- Bacterial pneumonia
- Bronchiectasis
- Lung abscess
- Tuberculosis
- Viral illness

Neoplasms
- Primary lung cancer
- Mesothelioma
- Pulmonary or pleural metastases
- Lymphoma

Connective Tissue Disease
- Rheumatoid arthritis
- Systemic lupus erythematosus

Abdominal or Gastrointestinal Disorders
- Pancreatitis

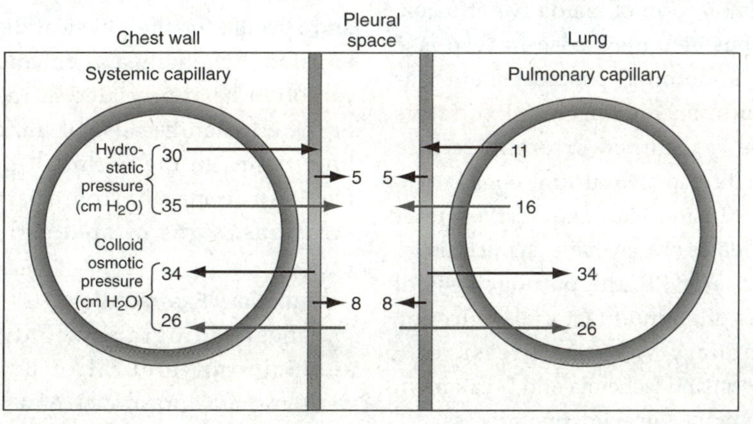

Fig. 21-4 Diagram representing pressures involved in formation and absorption of pleural fluid.

Subphrenic abscess
Esophageal rupture
Abdominal surgery

Miscellaneous Conditions

Pulmonary infarction
Uremia
Drug reactions
Postpartum
Chylothorax

Transudates are essentially ultrafiltrates of plasma, containing very little protein. A *transudative effusion* develops when there is an increase in the hydrostatic pressure or decrease in the oncotic pressure within pleural microvessels. The primary cause of increased hydrostatic pressure is CHF. In hepatic cirrhosis and nephrotic syndrome, increased hydrostatic pressure is combined with loss of plasma oncotic pressure because of significant decreases in serum albumin. Patients with severe malnutrition may develop transudative effusions resulting from severe isolated hypoalbuminemia.

Exudates contain relatively high amounts of protein, reflecting an abnormality of the pleura itself. An *exudative effusion* is the result of increased membrane permeability or defective lymphatic drainage. Any pulmonary or pleural process associated with inflammation can result in an exudative effusion.Pleurisy without pleural effusion is typical of most viral pleuritis. The most common form of an exudative effusion is a parapneumonic effusion, in which infection of the adjacent lung elicits an intense inflammatory response in pleura. Malignant effusions are the second most common form of exudative effusion. Exudative effusions also may arise in response to inflammatory abdominal processes, such as pancreatitis or subphrenic abscess. Exudative effusions may be reabsorbed or organize into fibrous tissue, resulting in pleural adhesions.

Some pleural effusions can manifest as either transudates or exudates or may have characteristics of both. In the case of PE, the pathogenesis of pleural effusion is often multifactorial, reflecting increased pulmonary vascular pressure (a transudative process) and ischemia and breakdown of the pleural membrane (an exudative process).

Massive effusions (>1.5-2 L) are most commonly associated with malignancy but also can arise in the setting of congestive heart failure, cirrhosis, and other conditions. Massive effusions may restrict respiratory movement, compress the lungs, and result in intrapulmonary shunting. In extremely rare cases, tension hydrothorax can develop, with mediastinal shift and circulatory embarrassment.

Clinical Features

Symptoms associated with pleural effusion are most often caused by the underlying disease process and not the effusion itself. Small pleural effusions often are entirely asymptomatic. A new or enlarging pleural effusion may be heralded by localized pain or pain referred to the shoulder. Viral pleuritis and pulmonary infarction commonly are associated with pleuritic chest pain. When the volume of pleural fluid reaches 500 mL, dyspnea on exertion or at rest may occur as a result of compromised pulmonary function.

The pain of viral pleuritis usually is preceded by several days of a typical viral prodrome, with low-grade fever, sore throat, and other upper respiratory or constitutional symptoms.

Physical findings depend on the size of the effusion but are often either dominated or obscured by the underlying disease process. Classic physical signs of pleural effusion include diminished breath sounds, dullness to percussion, decreased tactile fremitus, and occasionally a localized pleural friction rub. The simple technique of auscultatory percussion (i.e., percussing the chest while listening for a dullness with the stethoscope) may be even more sensitive and specific for the physical diagnosis of pleural effusion. Egophony and enhanced breath sounds can often be appreciated at the superior border of the effusion because of underlying atelectatic lung tissue. In the setting of pleuritis, a pleural friction rub may be appreciated. With massive effusions, signs of mediastinal shift may be present.

Auxiliary Examination

Chest radiography confirms the clinical suspicion of pleural effusion. The classic radiographic appearance of a pleural effusion is blunting of the costophrenic angle on the upright chest radiograph. On a frontal (anteroposterior or posteroanterior) projection, a volume of 250 to 500 mL of pleural fluid is required before radiographic demonstration is possible. A lesser amount of fluid may be visible in the posterior costophrenic gutter on a lateral projection. With larger effusions, the hemidiaphragm is obscured, and an upwardly concave meniscus may be seen because pleural fluid has a tendency to layer higher laterally than centrally. Pleural fluid can extend up a major fissure and appear as a homogeneous density in the lower two thirds of the lung field. Massive pleural effusion can appear as a totally opacified hemithorax.

In the recumbent patient, free pleural fluid gravitates superiorly, laterally, and posteriorly and may not be clearly discernible on a supine radiograph. If the effusion is large enough, diffuse haziness or partial opacification of a hemithorax may be seen. Other findings on the supine radiograph may include apical capping, obliteration of the hemidiaphragm, and a widened minor fissure.Clues to the presence of a subpulmonic effusion include shifting of the apparent dome of the diaphragm toward the lateral chest wall and, when located on the left side, an increase in the distance between the gastric bubble and aerated lung. Loculated fluid in a fissure may assume a fusiform appearance and can simulate a mass (Fig. 21-5A and B). Such "fluid pseudotumors" are common in patients with CHF.

Other imaging techniques, such as ultrasound and CT, may be helpful in localizing and quantifying effusions and characterizing underlying lung processes. Bedside thoracic ultrasound is particularly helpful because it is more sensitive than chest radiography and can be used to guide thoracentesis

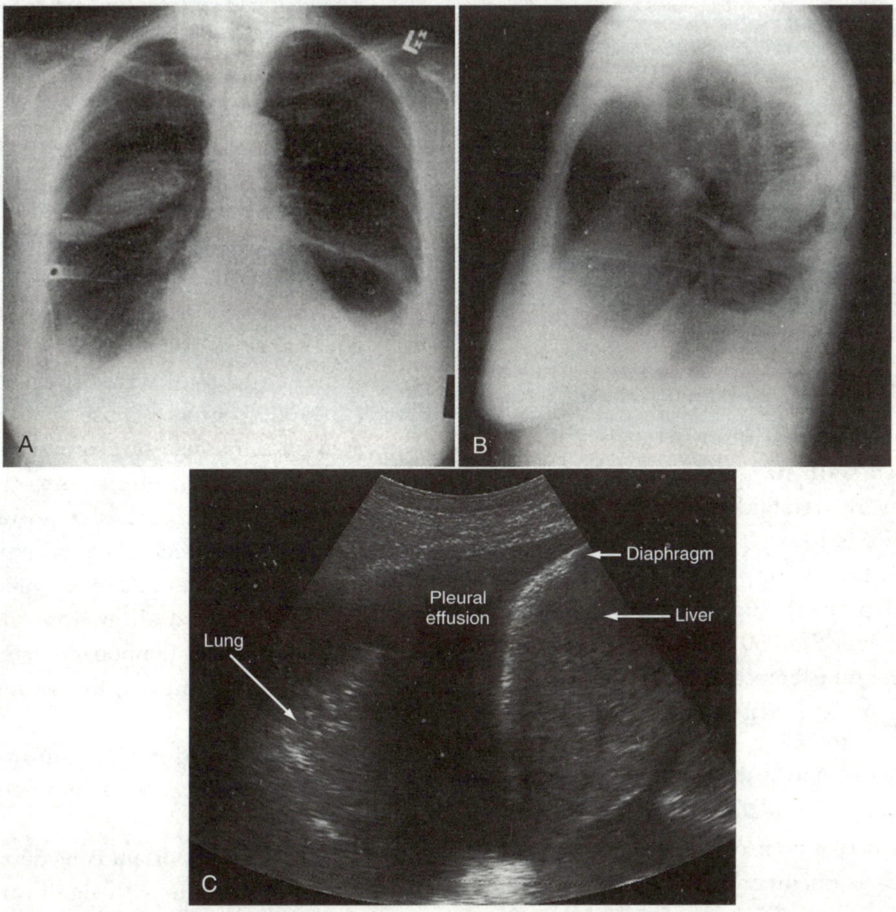

Fig. 21-5 A and B, Radiographs of pleural effusion along major and minor fissures. C, Ultrasound image of the right upper quadrant demonstrating the typical hypoechoic appearance of a pleural effusion.

in real time.Sonographically, pleural effusions are typically visualized as hypoechoic fluid located above the diaphragm and can be visualized with a curvilinear probe in the midaxillary line (Fig. 21-5C). Not all pleural fluid is hypoechoic, however, and both hemothorax and pyothorax can appear heterogeneous.

The primary goal of pleural fluid analysis is to distinguish between transudative and exudative effusions. Transudative effusion usually is found in patients with known underlying disorders (e.g., CHF, nephrotic syndrome), whereas the presence of an exudate requires a detailed diagnostic evaluation. Light's criteria remain a widely accepted means of differentiating transudates and exudates (Box 21-3).

Box 21-3 Light's Criteria for Differentiating Transudates from Exudates

Pleural fluid is considered an exudate if one or more of the following conditions are met:

1. Pleural fluid protein level: serum protein level exceeds 0.5
2. Pleural fluid LDH level: serum LDH level exceeds 0.6
3. Pleural fluid LDH level exceeds 2/3 × (upper limit of normal for serum LDH level)

In the presence of an exudative effusion, additional pleural fluid analyses further classify the effusion. A pleural fluid pH of less than 7.3 is associated with parapneumonic effusions, malignancies, rheumatoid effusions, tuberculosis, and systemic acidosis. A pH of less than 7.0 strongly suggests empyema (or esophageal rupture). A pleural fluid pH of less than 7.0 and glucose less than 50 mg/dL are reasonable indications for tube thoracostomy.

Normal pleural fluid contains less than 1000 WBC/mm^3; exudative pleural fluid may contain over 10,000 WBC/mm^3. Although the absolute cell count has limited diagnostic value, a predominance of neutrophils suggests an acute process, such as pneumonia, pulmonary embolus, or acute tuberculous pleuritis. A predominance of monocytes or lymphocytes suggests a more chronic process, such as malignancy or established tuberculosis. Pleural fluid from any patient with an undiagnosed exudative pleural effusion should undergo Gram staining and culture for bacteria (aerobic and anaerobic), mycobacteria, and fungi.

In the absence of a traumatic tap, bloody fluid suggests trauma, neoplasm, or pulmonary infarction. If the hematocrit of the pleural fluid is more than 50% that of the peripheral blood, the effusion is, by definition, a hemothorax.

Cytologic analysis provides the diagnosis of cancer in a majority of malignant effusions.

Diagnosis

Determine the presence of pleural effusion

According to the symptoms such as chest tightness, shortness of breath, the signs such as the diminished breath sounds, dullness to percussion, combined with the auxiliary examination such as CXR, B ultrasound, it is not difficult to determine the presence of pleural effusion.

Distinguish transudates and exudates

We can distinguish transudates and exudates according to Light's criteria (Box 21-3).

Identify the cause of pleural effusion

Management

In patients with large effusions, urgent therapeutic thoracentesis may stabilize respiratory or circulatory status. The presence of empyema necessitates insertion of a chest tube to drain the pleural space adequately and prevent the development of loculations. If an effusion is already loculated, streptokinase or urokinase can be injected by a thoracic surgeon, pulmonologist, or interventional radiologist into the pleural space in an attempt to dissolve adhesions and allow fluid to drain freely. Hemothorax requires tube thoracostomy to evacuate the pleural space, quantify bleeding, and allow apposition of the two pleural surfaces to tamponade hemorrhage. If bleeding exceeds 200 mL/hr, thoracotomy should be considered.

Thoracentesis under ultrasound guidance decreases complications and should be used when possible.

Pain relief is an important consideration in the management of patients with significant pleuritic pain. NSAID are relatively successful in treating pleural pain. Opioid analgesia is safe and effective.

Relative contraindications to thoracentesis

include coagulopathy and other bleeding disorders.

After thoracentesis has been completed, a chest radiograph should be obtained to evaluate for an iatrogenic pneumothorax. Other potential complications of thoracentesis include hemothorax, lung laceration, shearing of the catheter tip, and infection. Transient hypoxia caused by ventilation-perfusion mismatch often occurs, whereas unilateral, postexpansion pulmonary edema is rare except when large volumes (>1500 mL) are drained in one session. Hypotension also can occur after removal of a large volume of fluid, particularly in patients who are already intravascularly volume depleted.

Outcome

Small pleural effusions after abdominal surgery and in the postpartum state resolve spontaneously within a few days. Viral pleuritis, with or without effusion, is generally self-limited and resolves without specific treatment.

For patients with CHF, pleural effusions generally respond well to diuretic therapy.

Pleural effusions associated with malignancy are a significant cause of morbidity in patients with advanced cancer.Therapeutic thoracentesis can relieve dyspnea in the short term, but malignant effusions tend to be recurrent, often rapidly so.

Parapneumonic effusions contribute significantly to the morbidity and mortality of pneumonia. Empyema can develop in 5% to 10% of patients with a parapneumonic effusion, but in most cases, it responds well to parenteral antibiotics and pleural drainage. In nearly 20% of pleural effusions, no definitive diagnosis can be established even after extensive investigation. A sizable percentage of these effusions may be caused by viral infections, and most resolve spontaneously without sequelae.

(HAN Jiyuan)

Chapter 22

Acute Pancreatitis

KEY CONCEPTS

Most cases of acute pancreatitis are caused by gallstones and alcoholism. Other causes include medications, toxins, and trauma.

The clinical spectrum of acute pancreatitis ranges from mild to life-threatening. The mortality rate for severe pancreatitis approaches 30%.

Serum amylase and lipase assays are highly specific for pancreatitis when serum levels are elevated five times above the upper limits of normal.

Emergent abdominal CT should be performed in patients with clinically suspected pancreatitis who appear acutely ill and in patients with an uncertain diagnosis.

Patients with severe pancreatitis usually need EICU admission.

BACKGROUND

The pancreas is a retroperitoneal organ extending across the posterior abdomen in the epigastrium that provides essential endocrine and exocrine functions (Fig. 22-1, see color illustration).Acute pancreatitis is an inflammatory process of the pancreas usually associated with abdominal pain, elevated pancreatic enzymes, and variable involvement of other regional tissues or remote organ systems.Both local and systemic complications may occur.

The pancreas has both essential exocrine and endocrine functions. Exocrine products include

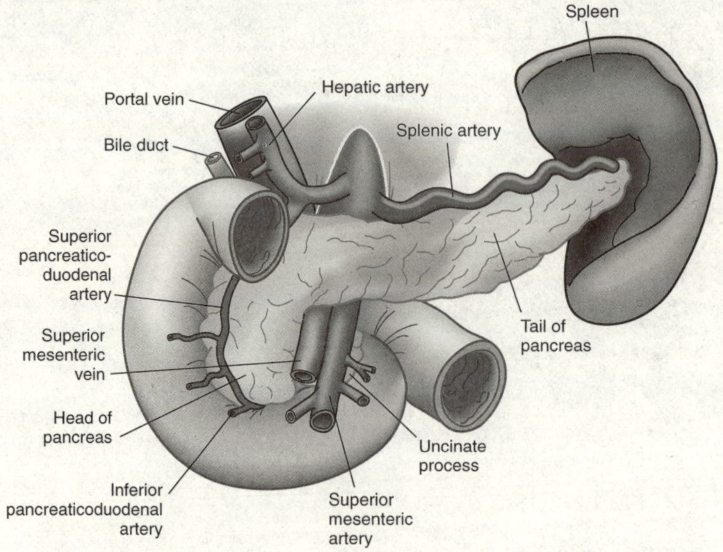

Fig. 22-1 Diagrammatic representation of the pancreas, anterior view.

amylase, lipase, trypsin, chymotrypsin, elastase, carboxypeptidase, phospholipase, and other enzymes. In addition, bicarbonate is produced in greatest quantity from this organ. The bicarbonate serves to neutralize gastric acids as well as the enzymes that break down proteins, carbohydrates, and fats. Cholecystokinin, pancreozymin, and secretin, as well as other factors, control secretion of these enzymes. The endocrine functions of the pancreas are managed by insulin, glucagon, pancreatic polypeptide, and somatostatin.

PERSPECTIVE

The first reports of pancreatitis date to the 1700s, and the first accurate study and description were completed by Fitz in 1889. He noted that performing surgery in the early stages of this disease was "extremely hazardous." Since then, the understanding of pancreatitis has evolved; however, treatment remains largely supportive rather than curative. Advances in care have decreased hospital mortality for all patients with pancreatitis, from 10% to 15% as reported 20 yr ago to 4% to 7% more recently. Most patients with pancreatitis have a mild course; however, 10% to 15% of cases will progress to severe disease, with a mortality rate in this subset of 20% to 50%. Severity also is increased in obese patients.

Pancreatitis can be classified as mild or severe, the latter category of the disease being defined by the presence of organ failure or local complications, such as necrosis, pseudocysts, or abscess. The gravity of the impending illness may not be apparent at the initial presentation, and in all patients, disease progression and outcome are difficult to predict at onset. Death in the first week usually is from pulmonary failure, MOF, or cardiovascular collapse. Later deaths are more likely to be from infective complications. In approximately 40% of cases, fatal pancreatitis on autopsy was undiagnosed. Therefore pancreatitis should be suspected in moribund patients with MOF, particularly elders.

The incidence appears to be increasing, although the increase may be related to both improved diagnosis and greater prevalence of risk factors. Gallstones are the most common obstructive cause of pancreatitis and occur more commonly in women than in men, with peak symptomatic incidence between the ages of 50 and 60 yr. Some variations of ductal anatomy are associated with increased risk of obstruction. Many gallstones are asymptomatic; however, among people with gallstones, pancreatitis occurs with a frequency of 8 to 20 per 1000 person-years. Alcoholic pancreatitis is more common in men than in women. In most (but not all) populations, this is the second leading cause of pancreatitis after obstructive causes.

PRINCIPLES OF DISEASE

Pathophysiology

Many of the pathobiologic responses that occur in acute pancreatitis, such as edema, inflammation, and parenchymal cell death, are easy to conceptualize.

Acute pancreatitis may be divided into three pathologic phases.

Local inflammation. The first phase is the local inflammation from obstruction of the pancreatic or bile ducts, direct toxicity of the pancreatic cells, toxins, infections, trauma, or idiopathic causes. Local inflammation subsequently causes premature activation of pancreatic enzymes, such as trypsinogen and zymogen, either in the ducts or in the acinar cells. This activation causes the release of enzymes that are intended to digest dietary proteins and fats; instead they produce cellular breakdown and pancreatic tissue autodigestion. Initially the inflammatory process is localized, creating focal pancreatic injury and edema.

Generalized injury. With increasing severity, the inflammation becomes generalized and causes necrosis of the pancreas and spreads to the surrounding fat and tissues. During this second phase of generalized injury, there may be necrosis of the pancreatic ducts as well as the vascular structures, leading to hemorrhage. Necrosis involving more than 30% of the pancreas increases both morbidity and mortality.

Enzyme activation, inflammation, and necrosis cause a variety of complications. For example, fluid collections develop in 30% to 50% of patients with severe pancreatitis. Over time, a fibrinous or granulation wall may form around this fluid collection, creating a pseudocyst. Thus, pseudocysts are not present in the initial phases of pancreatitis but instead develop over 4 to 6 w. Fluid collections, necrotic areas, or pseudocysts may become infected in a small number of cases, usually after several weeks. In addition, irritation of the surrounding bowel is common, creating bowel wall edema, ileus, and third-spacing of fluid. Formation of ascites is common and, together with bowel edema, can lead to significant intravascular fluid loss and hypotension.

Multiorgan damage. The final stage of injury occurs with the development of multiorgan damage. Because of the release of inflammatory mediators, the initial localized inflammatory response may cause a SIRS, resulting in MOF. This is a sepsis-like response, and any organ system can be involved, potentially resulting in myocardial depression, ARDS, DIC, or renal failure.

Etiology

Pancreatitis has several causes, but the vast majority of cases(80%) will be a result of either gallstones or alcohol, with gallstones the most common cause in most series (approximately 45% vs. 35%) (Box 22-1). The exact pathomechanism of biliary pancreatitis is not clear. Either a stone within

Box 22-1 Etiology of Pancreatitis

Toxic
- Alcohol, methanol
- Drugs
- Scorpion bites (in Trinidad)

Metabolic
- Hypercalcemia (often from hyperparathyroidism)
- Hyperlipidemia and hypertriglyceridemia (triglyceride levels>1000 mg/dL)

Obstructive
- Biliary tract disease
- Ampullary tumors
- Pancreas divisum with obstruction of the accessory duct
- Periampullary duodenal diverticula
- ERCP and postpancreatography
- Pancreatic neuroendocrine tumors
- Pancreatic carcinoma
- Sphincter of Oddi fibrosis, stricture, tumor, or hypertension

Infectious

Viral
- Adenovirus
- Coxsackievirus
- CMV
- EBV
- Echovirus
- Hepatitis A, B, C viruses
- HIV
- Varicella
- Rubella

Other Infections
- *Aspergillus*
- *Campylobacter*
- Clonorchiasis
- Cryptococcus
- *Cryptosporidium*
- Dysentery
- MAI
- Mumps
- *Mycobacterium* TB
- *Mycoplasma* species
- *Legionella* species
- Leptospirosis
- *Salmonella typhimurium*
- Scarlet fever
- Streptococcal food poisoning
- *Toxoplasma* infection
- Tuberculosis
- Ascariasis

Other Causative Disorders and Conditions
- Diabetic mellitus, DKA
- Crohn's disease
- Cystic fibrosis
- Emboli (atherosclerotic)
- Hemochromatosis
- Hereditary pancreatitis
- Hypothermia
- Vasculitis
- Lupus
- Polyarteritis nodosa, malignant hypertension
- Ischemia from hypoperfusion
- Perforated ulcer
- Postoperative
- Pregnancy
- Reye's syndrome
- Trauma
- Uremia
- Idiopathic causes

CMV, cytomegalovirus; *EBV*, Epstein-Barr virus;*MAI, Mycobacterium avium-intracellulare*

the bile duct applies transmural pressure on the pancreatic duct, or a stone in the common channel of the pancreatic duct or common bile duct causes obstruction. Obstruction or pressure on the pancreatic duct causes bile reflux or increased pressure of pancreatic secretions. Either mechanism leads to the activation of pancreatic enzymes, setting off the cascade of pancreatitis. Many cases presumed to be idiopathic probably are caused by small stones, sludge, or crystals that are too small to be detected on ultrasound examination but may be seen on endoscopic retrograde cholangiopancreatography(ERCP). This cause of pancreatitis is potentially correctable; if it is missed, recurrences are likely.

Alcohol is the cause of approximately 35% of pancreatitis cases. As with the other causes of pancreatitis, the mechanism by which alcohol is toxic to the pancreas is not well understood. Possible mechanisms include toxic effects of the ethanol metabolite acetaldehyde, ethanol-related lipid metabolism, or spasm of the sphincter of Oddi. Patients with alcoholic pancreatitis usually have 5 to 10 yr of chronic alcohol use before the onset of pancreatitis.

In addition to alcohol, many medications and toxins may cause pancreatitis, including didanosine, pentamidine, oral contraceptives, and selected scorpion venoms(Box 22-2). Pancreatitis can be caused by hypertriglyceridemia, with levels more than 500 mg/dL being implicated. In pregnancy, both gallstones and increased triglyceride levels can cause pancreatitis. When this occurs, both maternal and fetal mortality rates are high.

Blunt and penetrating abdominal trauma can disrupt the ductal system and the pancreatic cells, setting off the enzyme cascade that will result in acute pancreatitis. Pancreatitis also may result from iatrogenic ductal injury in 1% to 10% of ERCP procedures. Likewise, postoperative pancreatitis is well recognized and carries a higher mortality than that associated with other causative disorders.

Although both viral and bacterial disorders may precipitate pancreatitis, the two most common viral causes of pancreatitis are mumps and Coxsackievirus B infection. Pancreatitis is more common in patients with HIV infectionthan in the general population. In addition to the common etiologic risk factors for pancreatitis, this population is at additional risk because of the risk of opportunistic infections, toxicity from HIV-specific medications , and AIDS–related cancers. Acute pancreatitis is ultimately classified as idiopathic in approximately 10% of cases.

Box 22-2 Drug-Induced Pancreatitis

Definite	Possible
Acetaminophen	Bumetanide
Azathioprine	Carbamazepine
Cimetidine	Chlorthalidone
Cisplatin	Clonidine
Corticosteroids	Colchicine
Didanosine	Cyclosporine
Erythromycin	Cytarabine
Estrogens	Diazoxide
Ethyl alcohol	Enalapril
Furosemide	Ergotamine
L-Asparaginase	Ethacrynic acid
Mercaptopurine	Indomethacin
Methyldopa	Isoniazid
Metronidazole	Isotretinoin
Nitrofurantoin	Mefenamic acid
Octreotide	Opiates
Organophosphates	Phenformin
Pentamidine	Piroxicam
Ranitidine	Procainamide
Tetracycline	Rifampin
Salicylates	Thiazides
Sulfonamides, trimethoprim-sulfamethoxazole, sulfasalazine	
Sulindac	
Valproic acid	

The etiologies of pancreatitis in adults and children are similar, although incidence rates for specific causative disorders are different. Other causes include infections and congenital anomalies.

CLINICAL FEATURES

Pancreatitis should be suspected in all patients with epigastric abdominal pain, regardless of age. Once the diagnosis has been made, the underlying cause and presence of complications related to the disease should be sought.

Almost all patients with pancreatitis give a history of abdominal pain, most commonly in the midepigastric area; however, the pain also can be in the right or left upper quadrant. If significant inflammation is present, the pain may be diffuse and the patient may have difficulty localizing the discomfort. Typically, onset of symptoms is relatively rapid, increasing in severity over a few hours. The pain generally is described as constant and severe and may radiate to the midback. The degree of pain does not correlate with the severity of disease. Even though gallstones are frequently the cause of pancreatitis, the onset of pain is not usually related to eating. Nausea and vomiting often will accompany the pain. Although the discomfort may be lessened by lying on the side or sitting up, more typically little relief is obtained with position change, moving, eating, vomiting, or bowel movement. Colicky pain or pain that waxes and wanes suggests another diagnosis. Approximately 50% of patients will have a history of similar abdominal pain that may represent a previous episode of biliary colic or mild pancreatitis.

On physical examination, vital signs may be stable but frequently are abnormal. Hypotension, tachycardia, and shock indicate severe disease with complications or an alternate diagnosis. Vital signs also may be influenced by pain (tachycardia, tachypnea, hypertension) or alcohol withdrawal (tachycardia, hypertension, fever). A low-grade fever is present in approximately half of patients with pancreatitis, both at presentation and for the first several days thereafter, even in the absence of infection. A high fever is uncommon during the acute phase of pancreatitis; infection is usually a late complication. Ongoing evaluation should include pulse oximetry because acute hypoxia is an indicator of systemic complications and severe disease.

Patients with pancreatitis generally appear restless and in moderate distress as they search to find a position to relieve their discomfort. They may be jaundiced if an obstructing stone is present. The cardiopulmonary examination may be significant for rales or diminished breath sounds if the patient is hypoventilating from pain or if a pleural effusion (developing more commonly on the left) is present. On inspection, the abdomen may appear normal or may be notably distended. Only rarely will there be evidence of blood within the peritoneum or retroperitoneum resulting from severe hemorrhagic pancreatitis. Presence of blood within these areas is classically manifested as Cullen's sign (discoloration around the umbilicus) or Grey Turner's sign (discoloration of the flank). Auscultation of the abdomen may reveal normal, decreased, or absent bowel sounds, depending on whether the patient has a concomitant ileus. Because the pancreas is a retroperitoneal organ, palpation of the abdomen generally reveals epigastric guarding, with rebound tenderness being a less common finding. Murphy's sign may be present if the pancreatitis is secondary to a biliary source. Very rarely the physician may see evidence of subcutaneous fat necrosis: red nodules most prominent on the extremities. Other physical findings, such as the stigmata of alcoholism or xanthomas of hyperlipidemia, may help point to the cause of the pancreatitis.

Complications

The patient with acute pancreatitis will often have low grade fever, tachycardia, and leukocytosis; these findings represent three of the four criteria for SIRS. These patients may progress to fulminant sepsis or other severe illness related to the intense localized inflammation of pancreatitis.

Shock may result from volume loss. Fluid sequestration occurs in the pancreas and the bowel lumen and wall. Hemorrhage into necrotic pancreatic tissue also may occur. In addition, release of vasodilator and cardiodepressive substances may occur and worsen hypoperfusion.

Approximately 18% to 30% of patients may have pulmonary complications, including degradation of surfactant by pancreatic phospholipases; pleural effusions (more commonly noted on the left and frequently with elevated amylase levels); hypoxia from atelectasis, hypoventilation, and intrapulmonary shunting; and ARDS. ARDS, caused by the loss of surfactant as well as capillary leak caused by the inflammatory mediators, is rare but carries a 60% mortality rate.

Metabolic complications of pancreatitis include hyperglycemia and hypocalcemia. Hyperglycemia is caused by decreased insulin and increased glucagon. The mechanisms for hypocalcemia are sequestration or saponification of calcium in areas of fat necrosis; hypoalbuminemia, hypomagnesemia, or hyperglucagonemia; and inactivation of parathyroid hormone.

Coagulopathy develops from circulating proteases that affect the coagulation cascade. ATN can cause acute renal failure and results from the effects of circulating inflammatory mediators or from hypotension and hypoperfusion. Ultimately, MOF will occur if the balance of proinflammatory cytokine production overwhelms the anti-inflammatory response, which seeks to restrict the inappropriate movement of proinflammatory agents into the circulation.

Late complications occur after the second week of illness and include involvement of local structures, abscess formation (1%-4%), gastrointestinal bleeding from stress ulcers, splenic vein thrombosis, rupture of pancreatic pseudoaneurysms, fistula formation, splenic rupture, venous thrombosis, and right hydronephrosis. Pancreatic pseudocysts develop in 1% to 8% of patients after 4 to 6 w and are more common with alcoholic pancreatitis (Fig.22-2). Long-term complications of acute pancreatitis include recurrent or chronic pancreatitis, diabetes mellitus, and digestive and malabsorption problems.

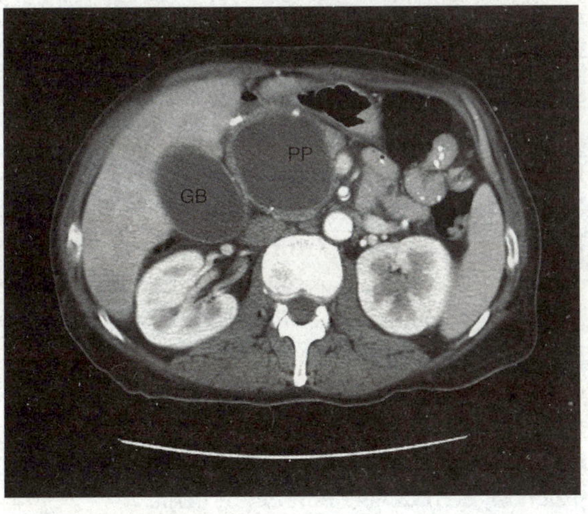

Fig. 22-2 CT scan showing pancreatic pseudocyst *(PP)*. In this patient the pseudocyst was so large that it compressed the common bile duct, causing obstructive jaundice. *GB*, gallbladder.

DIAGNOSTIC STRATEGIES

Laboratory Tests

The diagnosis of acute pancreatitis and the differentiation from other abdominal disorders depend on careful clinical assessment in conjunction with abnormalities on certain laboratory tests and supportive radiographic findings. Three enzymes are derived from pancreatic acinar cells: amylase, lipase, and the proenzyme trypsinogen. Each has been tested as a biochemical marker of acute pancreatitis.

Amylase Assay

Amylase is an enzyme that cleaves carbohydrates. It is produced primarily in the salivary glands and pancreas, although it also can be found in small amounts in the fallopian tubes, ovary, testis, muscle, intestines, and other organs. Elevations of amylase may be seen in healthy persons, patients with ectopic pregnancy, macroamylasemia, parotitis, renal failure (decreased clearance), mesenteric ischemia, bowel obstruction or infarction, perforated duodenal ulcer, acute peritonitis from other causes, and many other diseases. In acute pancreatitis, amylase rises within 6 to 24 hr, peaks in 48 hr, and normalizes in 3 to 7 d. Thus the sensitivity of amylase decreases after the first 24 to 48 hr.

The sensitivity of amylase for the diagnosis of pancreatitis ranges widely, depending on the comparative choice of the standard test. In up to 25% of patients with pancreatitis, especially in alcoholics and patients with hypertriglyceridemia (which interferes with the assay) or chronic pancreatitis, the amylase level can be normal. Mild amylase elevations in patients with severe acute abdominal pain of unclear cause, particularly in elders, should raise suspicion for another serious abdominal pathology. Thus the amylase assay, although recognized as an imperfect standard with which to make the diagnosis of pancreatitis, is used by default in some circumstances because of its low cost and rapid availability. However, its precise value is unclear in the initial diagnosis of pancreatitis, particularly in cases with an atypical clinical presentation. Amylase levels alone, whether normal, mildly elevated, or extremely elevated, are not diagnostic for pancreatitis unless accompanied by the appropriate clinical picture.

Lipase Assay

In the presence of pancreatic inflammation, lipase levels increase within 4 to 8 hr and peak at 24 hr. The levels stay elevated longer than amylase levels, falling over 8 to 14 d, thus providing greater sensitivity in patients with delayed presentations.

Lipase, like amylase, is present in other tissues and tends to be elevated in similar clinical situations. At values five times the upper limits of normal, lipase is 60% sensitive and 100% specific. The use of twice the upper limit of normal has been recommended to decrease the possibility of missing the diagnosis of pancreatitis. Expert guidelines recommend the use of lipase over amylase in the diagnosis of pancreatitis.

The degree of elevation of amylase or lipase is not a marker of disease severity. For example, compared with nonalcoholic patients, alcoholics will frequently have lower amylase levels but may have more severe disease. In a patient with prolonged abdominal pain or a history of pancreatitis, elevated biomarkers for longer than a week may suggest pseudocyst or pancreatic absess. Use of the amylase-to-lipase ratio has not proved helpful in the determination of a specific cause of pancreatitis.

Additional Laboratory Evaluation

In evaluating a patient with abdominal pain, amylase or lipase assays, along with other blood tests, are necessary to narrow the differential diagnosis, detect complications, and determine prognosis. Ranson developed a two-step list of primarily laboratory parameters, performed at hospital admission and after 48 hr, to determine the risk of death from pancreatitis (Box 22-3). Additional testing should consist of a CBC, LDH determination, and a comprehensive metabolic panel (including measurement of liver enzymes, calcium, renal function, and glucose). In patients with liver disease, coagulation studies should be performed to determine the degree of liver dysfunction. Arterial blood gas analysis should be done selectively in patients who are acidotic or hypoxic. This information can be used for treatment decisions and to determine prognosis based on Ranson's criteria. Magnesium should be checked in alcoholic patients and in those patients with electrolyte abnormalities. Both hypocalcemia and hyperglycemia are common in pancreatitis, with the hyperglycemia resulting from glucagon and insulin abnormalities. Calcium is best determined with use of the ionized calcium level. Serum calcium is falsely low in the presence of low albumin levels, as may be seen in patients with pancreatitis. Elevations of creatinine and BUN may indicate the presence of hypovolemia or renal involvement, or both.

Box 22-3 Ranson's Criteria for Pancreatitis-Associated Mortality

At Admission	Within 48 Hours of Admission
Age >55 yr	Hematocrit fall >10%
WBC >16,000/mm^3	BUN rise >5 mg/dL
Glucose >200 mg/dL	Calcium <8 mg/dL
LDH >350 U/L	PO_2 <60 mm Hg
AST >250 SF units	Base deficit >4 mEq/L
	Fluid sequestration >6 L
Substitute if Gallstone Induced Admission:	**Within 48 Hours of Admission**
Age >70 yr	Hematocrit fall >10%
WBC >18,000/mm^3	BUN rise > mg/dL
Glucose >220 mg/dL	Calcium <8 mg/dL
LDH >400 U/L	Base deficit >5 mEq/L
AST >250 SF units	Fluid sequestration >4 L
Add the total number of signs at 48 hr:	
Number	**Associated Mortality Rate**
0-3	1%
3-4	15%
5-6	40%
>7	100%

Elevation in liver enzymes may result from biliary-induced pancreatitis or from other diseases of the liver or biliary tract. In addition, liver enzyme levels may increase from the pressure on the common bile duct that results from the surrounding pancreatic inflammation. Mild elevations of bilirubin are common in all types of pancreatitis, as well as in many other liver disorders. For the patient diagnosed with pancreatitis, higher elevations of aspartate transaminase(AST) and LDH are related to worse prognosis according to Ranson's criteria.

When liver enzymes are elevated, the pattern of elevation may help determine the underlying cause of the pancreatitis (Table 22-1). Alanine aminotransferase (ALT) is the best single marker for a biliary cause; levels greater than three times baseline support the diagnosis of biliary pancreatitis. The higher the elevation of ALT, the greater the specificity and predictive value for gallstones. ALT levels higher than 150 U/L have 96% specificity, positive predictive value (PPV) of 95%, and 48% sensitivity for gallstone pancreatitis. Significant rises in AST, alkaline phosphatase, and bilirubin also are more likely to be related to biliary pancreatitis but are not as sensitive as ALT. The CBC may be notable for an elevated white blood cell count; the hematocrit may be either high or low. Early in the disease course, the hematocrit may be elevated because of third-space volume loss. A decrease in hematocrit is a poor predictor of prognosis because it indicates intra-abdominal hemorrhage and severe pancreatitis. An ECG also should be included early in the workup to determine whether the patient's abdominal pain may be cardiac in origin.

Table 22-1 Sensitivity and Specificity of Liver Enzymes for the Cause of Pancreatitis

ENZYME AND LEVEL	SENSITIVITY(%)	SPECIFICITY(%)	PPV (%)
ALT >150 mmol/L	48	96	95
AST >150 mmol/L	44	95	87
Alkaline phosphatase >300 units/L	24	95	87
Bilirubin>2.8 mg/dL	38	93	89

PROGNOSIS

At present, a variety of markers are available to aid in the detection of severe pancreatitis, including specific laboratory values that measure the systemic inflammatory response, scoring systems that tabulate the extent of inflammation or organ failure, and findings on imaging studies. The most commonly used scoring system is Ranson's criteria (Box 22-3). In this system, the five criteria evaluated on hospital admission indicate the degree of local inflammation; the six criteria assessed at 48 hr reflect the development of systemic complications. Although Ranson's criteria constitute a simple and well-known scoring system, reliance on these criteria alone may result in delayed recognition of illness severity; therefore the APACHE II system also may be used to judge severity. This system uses 12 physiologic variables, age, and chronic health status to generate a total point score (Box 22-4). Many online medical calculators are available to allow easy calculation of the APACHE score by summing the weighed values of the measured physiologic parameters. Scoring can be performed on admission and throughout the hospital stay. An APACHE score of 8 or higher indicates severe disease. A score greater than 13 is associated with high likelihood of death. An APACHE III scoring system also has been developed and includes additional physiologic variables, but this system has not proved to be better at predicting outcomes in patients with acute pancreatitis.

Box 22-4 APACHE II Clinical and Laboratory Parameters for Scoring*

Age	pH or serum HCO_3
Chronic health problems	Sodium
Temperature	Potassium
Mean arterial pressure	Creatinine
Heart rate	Hematocrit
Respiratory rate	White blood cell count
P_aO_2 or A-a gradient	Glasgow Coma Scale score

* Each clinical or laboratory parameter is assigned points with 0 being normal and 4 being most abnormal (high or low). Use either table or medical calculator to calculate the score. The score is then used to predict mortality.

CRP level above 150 mg/L at 48 hr after symptom onset are poor prognostic predictors of disease severity. To account for the various factors that indicate the severity of disease in patients with acute pancreatitis, the Atlanta criteria for severity are widely accepted (Box 22-5). Finally, a fourvariable predictive model that uses BUN, age, LDH, and interleukin-6 has been proposed; initial analysis indicates that it is as accurate as other scoring systems. This scoring system will need further validation, however. Given the limitations in the ability to accurately predict severity of illness, patients with acute pancreatitis should initially be treated as though the disease is severe.

Box 22-5 Atlanta Criteria for Predicting Severe Acute Pancreatitis

Criteria for severe acute pancreatitis—one or more of thefollowing:

1. Ranson score 3 or higher on admission (or during the first 48 hr)
2. APACHE II score 8 or higher at any time during course
3. Presence of organ failure
   - Shock (systolic blood pressure <90 mm Hg) *or*
   - Pulmonary insufficiency (P_aO_2 60 mm Hg or less on room air) *or*

- Renal failure (serum creatinine >2 mg/dL after fluid resuscitation)

4. Systemic complications
   - DIC (thrombocytopenia and hypofibrinogenemia and fibrin split products) *or*
   - Metabolic complications (serum calcium 7.5 mg/dL or less) *or*
5. Presence of one or more local complications (pancreatic necrosis, pancreatic abscess, pancreatic pseudocyst)

RADIOGRAPHIC STUDIES

In pancreatitis, plain abdominal radiographs may reveal an ileus with a sentinel jejunal loop or spasm of the transverse colon and dilation of the ascending colon. Pancreatic calcifications of chronic pancreatitis or gallstones may rarely be seen. The portion of the chest seen as part of the abdominal series may show left-sided or bilateral pleural effusions, atelectasis, or ARDS. Up to 80% of radiographs obtained in patients with pancreatitis will demonstrate some abnormality. Unfortunately, many of these findings are nonspecific, and plain radiography has largely been replaced by more advanced imaging.

CT and ultrasound imaging are complementary studies in the evaluation of pancreatitis. MRI offers no significant advantages over CT. Ultrasonography provides more accurate images of the biliary tract than CT; however, the pancreas itself, as well as local complications, are less well visualized by ultrasound. If a biliary cause is suspected, an ultrasound study performed within the first 24 hr of admission may help determine whether gallstones or dilation of the common bile duct is present.CT was 39% sensitive for biliary disease, whereas ultrasonography was 83% sensitive. In another study, ultrasound imaging was 94% sensitive for gallstones but only 19% for common duct stones and 38% for common duct dilation. Because of these limitations, when gallstone pancreatitis is highly suspected, an endoscopic ultrasound study may be more accurate and can help guide the emergency use of ERCP. MRCP is a noninvasive test that may be used to help determine the cause of acute pancreatitis. Although ultrasound imaging is more sensitive than CT for investigating biliary causes of pancreatitis, CT may be useful in evaluating for other causes of abdominal pain, the presence of peripancreatic complications (such as hemorrhage, pseudocyst, abscess, or vascular abnormalities), and the extent of any pancreatic necrosis. The Atlanta International Symposium recommended CT in patients with (1) an uncertain diagnosis; (2) severe clinical pancreatitis, abdominal distention, tenderness, fever with temperatures higher than 102°C, and leukocytosis; (3) a Ranson score greater than 3 or APACHE score greater than 8; (4) no improvement within 72 hr; and (5) acute deterioration. If the diagnosis is clear and evidence of obstruction is lacking, CT or ultrasound imaging can be delayed until after the patient has been admitted to the hospital. The main indication for obtaining a CT in the ED is to exclude other diagnoses; if the patient is significantly ill and can tolerate the procedure, early CT may determine whether complications are already present.

CT also may be used to stage the severity and prognosis of acute pancreatitis. The CT severity index is an additional grading system that uses the CT to evaluate how the pancreas looks, as well as evidence of fluid collections or gas adjacent to the pancreas. Grades A (no abnormality) and B (focal or diffuse pancreatic enlargement) indicate lower levels of inflammation. Grade C shows mild peripancreatic inflammation and is associated with an increased risk of complications. Grade D (enlarged pancreas with fluid in the anterior pararenal space) and grade E (enlarged pancreas with two or more fluid collections) are associated with significant risk of infection, with mortality rates of up to 15%. Another CT-based scoring system, the extrapancreatic inflammation on CT scan score, is based on the presence of pleural effusion, ascites, and retroperitoneal fluid collection. The initial study was small but showed this system to be superior to the CT severity index in prediction of outcome.

DIFFERENTIAL CONSIDERATIONS

Pancreatitis should be differentiated from other abdominal processes, cardiopulmonary disorders, and systemic diseases (Box 22-6). A number of acute surgical conditions may mimic pancreatitis in presentation and also may cause elevated biomarkers. Examples are bowel perforation, peritonitis, ischemic bowel, small and large bowel obstruction, and ruptured ectopic pregnancy.

Box 22-6 Differential Diagnosis for Pancreatitis

Abdominal Disorders

- Perforated viscus
- Peptic ulcer disease
- Cholecystitis, gallbladder colic
- Cholangitis
- Gastroenteritis
- Nephrolithiasis or pyelonephritis
- Bowel obstruction
- Mesenteric ischemia
- Abdominal aortic aneurysm
- Ectopic pregnancy

Cardiopulmonary Disorders

- Myocardial infarction
- Pericarditis
- Pneumonia
- ARDS
- Pleural effusion

Systemic Disease

- Sickle cell crisis

MANAGEMENT

The management of pancreatitis is primarily supportive; rehydration, pain and nausea control, nutritional supplementation, and monitoring for complications constitute the foundations of care. The supportive care given to the patient with acute pancreatitis has multiple objectives. Because of vomiting and fluid sequestration, most patients with pancreatitis are dehydrated. Fluids should be replaced with normal saline; several liters may be required. Vital signs and urine output should be used to judge the adequacy of volume replacement. Electrolytes should be monitored and replenished.

Abdominal pain associated with pancreatitis is severe and will generally necessitate use of narcotic analgesia. Meperidine has been used historically in pancreatitis and biliary disease. Although morphine may increase the tone of the sphincter of Oddi, evidence that it worsens the disease process in pancreatitis is lacking. Patient-controlled analgesia may be the most effective method of pain control. Antiemetics are indicated to control nausea or vomiting.

In the past, patients with pancreatitis were allowed nothing by mouth and nasogastric suctioning was initiated out of concern that oral intake would stimulate the release of pancreatic enzymes. However, randomized clinical trials in patients with mild-to-moderate pancreatitis have shown no benefit from either fasting or use of nasogastric suctioning. Currently, nasogastric suctioning is indicated only in cases of intractable vomiting or ileus, and some enteral feeding should begin as soon as it is tolerable. Some evidence suggests that early enteral nutrition (delivered by feeding tubes placed beyond the ligament of Treitz) may improve outcomes even in severe pancreatitis; however, if oral feedings are not tolerated or are inadequate, then parenteral feedings should be initiated.

A key management principle is frequent reevaluation for complications of pancreatitis. Hypotension should be corrected with large volumes of normal saline (up to 6 L). In fact, hemodynamic instability in severe pancreatitis results from similar processes seen in sepsis, and management approaches used in septic patients (early goal-directed therapy) are appropriate. Invasive hemodynamic monitoring may be necessary. Respiratory support is appropriate for respiratory failure or continued shock. Hyperglycemia should be treated cautiously because it may self-correct as the pancreatitis resolves. Hypocalcemia may be the result of decreased albumin or hypomagnesemia; ionized calcium and magnesium levels should be checked before replacement therapy is initiated. If true hypocalcemia is present and the patient is experiencing symptoms, treatment is appropriate. Calcium gluconate should be used if calcium needs to be replenished. The serum potassium should be normalized before calcium replacement, however, because calcium will cause intravascular potassium shifts.

In the case of gallstone pancreatitis, gastroenterology consultation is appropriate to discuss the use of ERCP. Early operative removal of gallstones and the gallbladder has been shown to increase mortality; however, early removal of common bile duct stones by ERCP may reduce morbidity. At present, consensus is lacking regarding the optimal timing of ERCP in the presence of gallstone pancreatitis. Early endoscopic sphincterotomy (in 24-48 hr) and stone removal are recommended in the setting of cholangitis, sepsis, and severe obstructive pancreatitis. In mild pancreatitis, early ERCP has not consistently been shown to decrease morbidity. In addition, there is approximately a 5% rate of pancreatitis with ERCP and papillotomy, as well as other complications associated with the procedure (bleeding and perforation). In view of the ongoing controversy, it is appropriate to involve the consultant early in the case so that a well-coordinated management plan can be created.

Theoretically, certain medications should moderate the course of pancreatitis; histamine H_2 receptor blockers decrease the release of secretin by inhibition of gastric acid, glucagon directly suppresses pancreatic exocrine secretion, and octreotide inhibits pancreatic secretion. However, these therapies have not been shown to be clinically effective. Other approaches that use inhibitors of inflammatory mediators also have failed to produce clinical improvement. For patients with severe pancreatitis, an H_2 blocker, although not helpful for the acute disease, may decrease stress-induced ulcers.

Use of antibiotics in patients with severe pancreatitis with or without evidence of necrosis of pancreatic tissue is controversial. Prophylactic antibiotics have been reported to be effective in reducing subsequent infection. These positive effects have not been consistently observed, however, and some evidence indicates that use of prophylactic antibiotics in patients with severe pancreatitis may increase the risk of fungal infection. Two recent studies found no difference with respect to the development of infected pancreatic necrosis with the use of prophylactic antibiotics. The usefulness of early antibiotic treatment remains unclear, although there appears to be a consensus to withhold antibiotics until clear evidence of infection is present.

Surgical intervention or percutaneous drainage may be necessary for cases of infected pancreatic necrosis, infected pseudocyst, or unresolved pseudocyst. Surgery is preferred when percutaneous drainage is not effective or not possible (as with extensive pancreatic necrosis or deteriorating clinical status).

DISPOSITION

The course of acute pancreatitis is unpredictable, and complications may occur hours or days after the onset of illness; therefore almost all patients with acute pancreatitis should be admitted to the hospital. Patients with evidence of severe pancreatitis should be admitted to the EICU, especially if findings include agitation, confusion, rising hematocrit, pulmonary insufficiency, or cardiovascular problems such as hypotension, progressive tachycardia, or poor urine output. Specifically, patients with a score greater than 2 on Ranson's criteria on admission or other evidence of organ failure, local complications, or significant comorbid illness will also require EICU management.

(WANG Xiujie)

Chapter 23

Gastrointestinal Bleeding

KEY CONCEPTS

GIB is traditionally classified by the bleeding source—UGIB is proximal and LGIB is distal to the ligament of Treitz in the terminal duodenum.

UGIB can routinely manifest as bloody or coffee-ground-like vomit known as *hematemesis* or as dark, tarry stools known as *melena*. LGIB usually produces bright red or maroon blood per rectum, known as *hematochezia*.

The diagnostic approach to the GIB patient involves a number of key decision points. First, the clinician should assess the patient's general appearance, vital signs, and volume status. The second decision point involves use of the historical facts and physical examination findings to determine if the patient has UGIB or LGIB. The third decision point relies on the severity of the UGIB or LGIB.

Upper endoscopy is the most effective diagnostic and therapeutic intervention for UGIB, achieving hemostasis in more than 90% of cases.

Continued hemodynamic instability and/or ongoing hemorrhage dictates the need for blood transfusion.

PERSPECTIVE

Epidemiology

Gastrointestinal bleeding (GIB) accounts for more than 1 million hospitalizations annually in the United States, with significant morbidity, mortality, and economic burden. GIB is traditionally classified by the bleeding source – upper gastrointestinal bleeding (UGIB) is proximal and lower gastrointestinal bleeding (LGIB) is distal to the ligament of Treitz in the terminal duodenum. Bleeding between the ligament of Treitz and ileocecal junction is middle GI tract.

UGIB accounts for more than 500,000 U.S. hospital admissions annually, with approximately 165 incidents per 100,000 patients. Mortality rates have remained consistent at 13% to 14% over the past two decades. An increasing proportion of elderly patients, who may die owing to comorbid conditions, and increases in the number of cirrhotic and variceal patients may contribute to the lack of change in mortality rates. Age greater than 70 yr, intestinal ischemia, comorbid illness, coagulation defects, transfusion of PRBC, and male gender are the predictors of increased LGIB mortality.

DIAGNOSTIC APPROACH

Differential Considerations

The characteristics of the bleed and the age of the patient can help determine the cause of the GIB. UGIB can routinely manifest as bloody or coffee-ground-like vomit known as *hematemesis* or as dark, tarry stools known as *melena*. Peptic ulcer disease, erosive gastritis, and esophageal varices account for the majority of these cases (Table 23-1). In fact, peptic ulcers make up more than half of all acute cases of UGIB seen in the ED. However, in inner city populations, varices and gastritis are more prevalent. Contrary to this, LGIB usually produces bright red or maroon blood per rectum, known as *hematochezia*. Anorectal sources, such as hemorrhoids, are the most common causes of LGIB in all age groups. The most common sources of hematochezia are colonic diverticula and angiodysplasia. Other noteworthy causes

Table 23-1 Common Causes of GIB in Adults and Children

	ADULTS	CHILDREN
Common causes of UGIB	Peptic ulcers (gastric more than duodenal) Gastric erosion Esophagogastric varices Mallory-Weiss tears Esophagitis Gastric cancer	Duodenal ulcers Gastric ulcers Esophagitis Gastric erosion Esophageal varices Mallory-Weiss tears
Common causes of LGIB	Diverticular disease Angiodysplasia Colitis (inflammatory, infectious, ischemic) Anorectal sources Neoplasm UGIB	Anorectal fissure Infectious colitis Inflammatory bowel disease Juvenile polyps Intussusception Meckel's diverticulum

include colitis caused by ischemia, infection, and inflammatory bowel disease.The source of GIB is not identified in 8% to 14% of patients.

Death from exsanguination resulting from GIB is rare. However, there are two causes of GIB that may rapidly cause death if not recognized and mitigated: esophageal varices and aortoenteric fistula. The former is the single most common source of massive UGIB and has a mortality rate of 30%. The latter is caused when an abdominal aortic aneurysm or, more commonly, an aortic graft adheres to and erodes through a bowel wall. Aortoenteric fistula is a rare but rapidly fatal cause of LGIB. As is the case for any patient with acute massive hemorrhage, prompt consultation with a surgeon is warranted when aortoenteric fistula is a likely diagnosis.

Finally, in the differential considerations, one must determine if in fact the patient is having actual GIB. Epistaxis, dental bleeding, or red food coloring can mimic the appearance of hematemesis. Bismuth-containing medications and iron supplements can create melanotic-appearing (but guaiac-negative) stools. Vaginal bleeding, gross hematuria, and partially digested red foods (such as beets) can all be mistaken for hematochezia. Unless an alternative diagnosis is clearly evident, the appropriate approach is to continue with the workup for GIB.

Pivotal Findings

The approach to the GIB patient requires a thorough history centering on the gastrointestinal tract and on the timing, quantity, and appearance of the bleeding. Relevant comorbid conditions should be reviewed as well. The extent of the history will be dictated by the severity of the complaint and the hemodynamic stability of the patient on ED arrival. Reviewing the patient's vital signs, appearance of the stool, and basic laboratory studies will help in triaging and initiating the workup of the bleeding source.

Medical History

A useful starting point for the clinician is to determine the time of onset, duration of symptoms, and relevant supporting historical facts.

1. *Context:* The context of the bleeding can help explain its cause. For instance, if a patient complains of bright red blood per rectum after several days of constipation and straining, that presentation suggests an anorectal source for the bleeding. Alternatively, a patient with hematemesis after several earlier episodes of retching would lead one to suspect an esophageal tear. Finally, a patient with easy bruising and recurrent gingival bleeding might suggest a long-standing, underlying coagulopathy.
2. *Quantity:* Efforts should also be made to quantify the amount of blood lost during the bleeding event. Patients may describe the passage of large clots, blood changing the toilet bowl water red, or simply streaks of blood on the toilet paper. The patient's recollection of the bleed and its amount is usually poorly quantified and inaccurate. Often, the degree of bleeding is better gauged by assessing symptoms associated with significant intravascular loss such as dyspnea, lightheadedness, or chest pain.
3. *Appearance:* Classifying the blood as hematemesis, melena, or hematochezia provides the initial clues to the source of bleeding. Vomiting of fresh blood or blood with the appearance of coffee grounds

strongly suggests an UGIB. The passage of melena, dark digested stools, also suggests likely UGIB. In contrast, the presence of hematochezia, bright red or maroon stools, usually signifies LGIB. There are exceptions, however. In a hemodynamically unstable patient, bright red blood per rectum can represent brisk UGIB. Hematemesis rarely can arise from a source in the lower GI (LGI) tract that is proximal to an obstruction. The emergency clinician uses the history to make a rough estimate of the source and help guide the initial workup.

4. *Relevant medical history:* A review of the patient's relevant medical history and risk factors for bleeding should note whether a patient has had similar bleeding before and the location of the causative lesion (Table 23-2). This is especially important with UGIB, as the majority of these presentations are caused by rebleeding of previously identified sources. Next, identification of relevant comorbid diseases helps to risk stratify these patients in the context of their bleed. Patients with GIB and a history of CAD, congestive heart failure, liver disease, or diabetes have a higher mortality. A review of the patient's medications should pay particular attention to gastrotoxic substances, anticoagulants, and antiplatelet drugs. Medications such as NSAID, aspirin, warfarin, clopidogrel, corticosteroids, and certain chemotherapeutic agents are known to increase the risk of GIB. Alcohol abuse is associated with gastritis and peptic ulcer disease. It can also result in cirrhosis, portal hypertension, and ultimately esophageal variceal bleeding. Smoking cigarettes results in slower healing and greater recurrence of ulcers.

Table 23-2 Characteristics of Patients with High-Risk GIB

Medication use
• Aspirin
• NSAID
• Steroids
• Anticoagulants (warfarin, heparin)
• Chemotherapeutic agents
History of peptic ulcer disease
Known liver disease, cirrhosis
Advanced age (older than 60 yr)
Alcoholism
Current smoker
Chronic medical comorbidities
• Congestive heart failure
• Diabetes
• Chronic renal failure
• Malignancy
• CAD
History of abdominal aortic aneurysm graft

Physical Examination

Vital Signs. Hypotension and tachycardia can suggest moderate hypovolemia and can be the early indicators of impending shock.

General Examination. Eye examination may show conjunctival pallor, suggesting blood loss anemia. In similar fashion, dermatologic changes can lend supporting evidence to the presence and cause of a GIB. Generalized pallor in a hemodynamically stable patient might indicate the anemia of a subacute or chronic GIB; in the unstable patient, pallor might reinforce the impression of massive blood loss. Cold, clammy skin on the extremities might signal significant volume loss consistent with hemorrhagic shock. Ecchymoses or petechiae suggest a coagulopathy. Finally, jaundice, palmar erythema, or spider angiomata suggests the possibility of UGIB from esophageal varices.

The abdomen should be carefully examined for subtle findings that can help identify the source of bleeding. Hyperactive bowel sounds are a nonspecific finding, but might indicate UGIB, as intraluminal blood is a known cathartic that can stimulate peristalsis. Tenderness to palpation can be seen in many cases of peptic ulcer disease. Severe, diffuse tenderness on examination warrants the consideration of bowel ischemia, mechanical obstruction, ileus, or bowel perforation. The abdominal examination may also show further signs of portal hypertension with the presence of hepatomegaly, ascites, or caput medusae. A rectal examination, with determination of the type of bleeding, should be performed in most patients with GIB. The examination should include evaluation of the external anus, a digital rectal examination, and anoscopy looking to identify possible bleeding sources such as hemorrhoids, polyps, or fisures.

Emergency Department Studies

Occult Blood and Guaiac Bedside Testing. In patients with suspected UGIB, guaiac testing can be performed at the bedside to evaluate for occult blood even when stool appears normal. The test makes use of the pseudoperoxidase activity found in hemoglobin. When hydrogen peroxide is dripped onto the guaiac paper containing the stool sample, an oxidative reaction rapidly turns the paper blue. The test can actually be positive for up to 2 w after an acute bleed and thus is more useful at diagnosing chronic occult bleeding. False positives can be triggered by ingestions of red meat, turnips, horseradish, vitamin C, methylene blue, and bromide preparations. Iron-and bismuth-containing medications can cause dark stools that will be guaiac negative. Similar testing is available for gastric contents but can be unreliable if minor trauma from the passage of a nasogastric tube (NGT) or vomiting has caused occult bleeding.

Clinical Laboratory Testing

Laboratory studies can assist in the risk stratification of GIB. Minimum testing should include evaluation of the patient's hemoglobin, BUN, coagulation studies, and platelets. Hemoglobin does not immediately decline in the setting of an acute bleed, as whole blood is initially lost. In general, a hemoglobin less than 8 to 10 g/dL in a patient with GIB should prompt strong consideration of blood transfusion, with greater attention and a much lower threshold to transfuse in elders and those with significant comorbidities such as CAD.

BUN levels can be elevated in the setting of UGIB owing to the absorption of digested blood into the circulatory system during intestinal transit. The BUN can also be elevated from prerenal azotemia in the setting of hypovolemia. A BUN-to-Cr ratio greater than 36 in the setting of no renal failure can be highly suggestive of UGIB.

Coagulation studies, particularly PT, should be undertaken to ensure that coagulopathy is not worsening the patient's blood loss. This becomes especially important in patients with liver disease or those taking therapeutic anticoagulants such as warfarin.

Leukocytosis may represent the stress of the acute bleed, but the possibility of underlying infection should also be considered. A lactate level may be elevated in the setting of bowel ischemia or secondary to shock from hypovolemia and the resultant hypoperfusion. Laboratory findings may help guide risk stratification, resuscitation, and ultimate disposition.

Electrocardiogram

An ECG is recommended and is especially relevant in elders and those with known CAD.

Radiographic Imaging

Emergent imaging of the chest and abdomen in the ED setting is rarely indicated in the patient with acute GIB, and abdominal CT scan is the preferred imaging modality. Identification of subdiaphragmatic air and peritoneal findings on abdominal examination suggest the possibility of bowel perforation.Multidetector CT may have a role in identifying angiodysplasia and other localized bleeding sites throughout the GI tract. Scintigraphy and angiography can also be used to localize the source of bleeding, and angiography may allow for therapeutic options via embolization. These imaging modalities are rarely used in the acute ED setting, and their use is often based on hospital availability and consultant preference.

DIAGNOSTIC ALGORITHM

The diagnostic approach to the GIB patient involves a number of key decision points. First, the clinician should assess the patient's general appearance, vital signs, and volume status. This initial assessment can help triage the patient into a stable or unstable category.

The second decision point involves use of the historical facts and physical examination findings to determine if the patient has UGIB or LGIB.

The third decision point relies on the severity of the UGIB or LGIB to determine the ED management and disposition.

EMPIRICAL MANAGEMENT

Rapid identification of the bleeding source (i.e., UGI versus LGI tract), risk stratification, resuscitation, consultation, and disposition are the integral elements of this process. Initial management includes an assessment of airway, breathing, and circulation. Massive bleeding, active hematemesis, hypoxia, severe tachypnea, or altered mental status may necessitate tracheal intubation for protection and to supplement tissue oxygenation. Fig. 23-1 outlines both diagnostic and management guidelines.

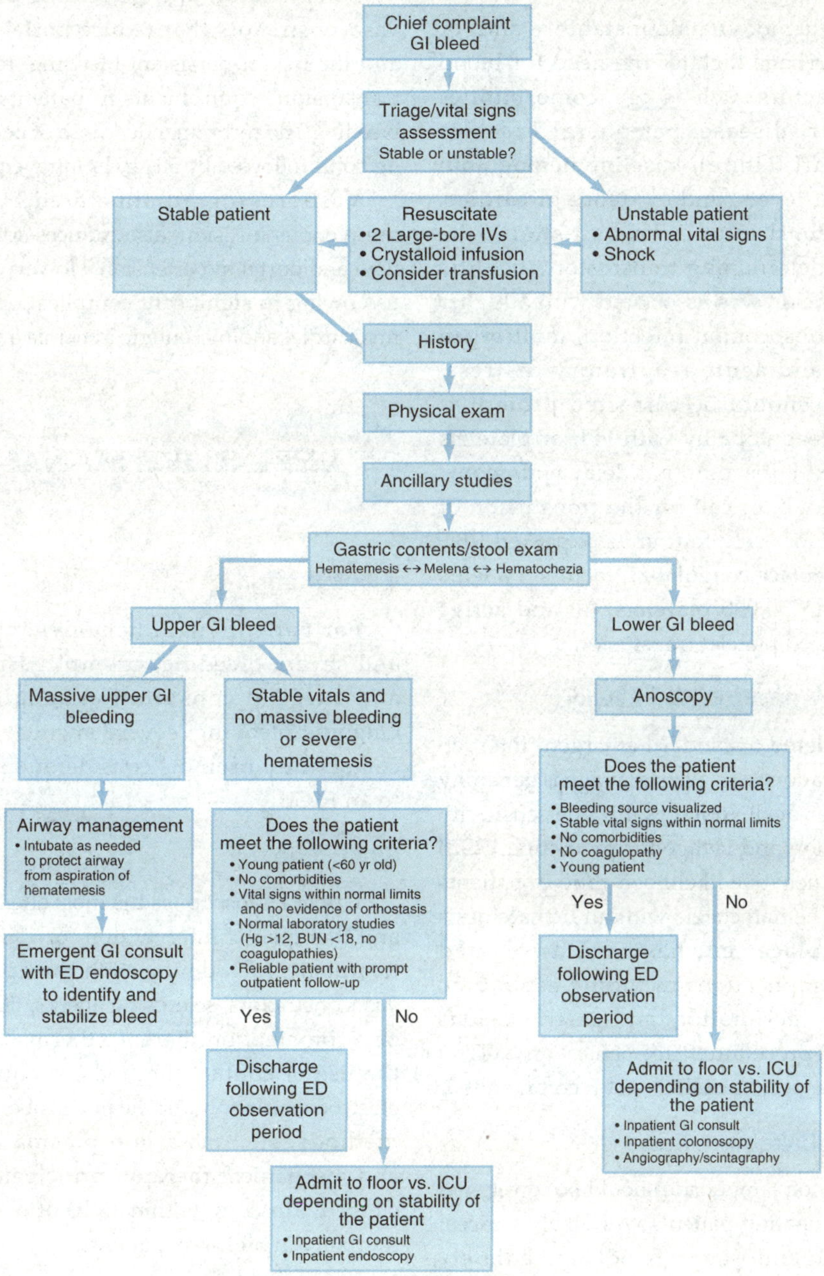

Fig. 23-1 Diagnostic and management strategies for GIB.

Resuscitation

Hemodynamic instability and estimated volume loss should guide initial resuscitation. Patients should be placed on pulse oximetry, be administered supplemental oxygen, and receive early aggressive crystalloid resuscitation with two peripheral large-bore intravenous catheters. Cardiac telemetry should be initiated because demand ischemia and MI may occur in patients with GIB.Endpoints of adequate resuscitation would include appropriate vital signs, urine output greater than 1 mL/kg/hr, and appropriate mental status. Prompt blood transfusion is also considered.

Blood Product Transfusion

Continued hemodynamic instability and/or ongoing hemorrhage dictates the need for blood transfusion. Factors such as age, comorbidities (ischemic heart disease, peripheral vascular disease, or heart failure), baseline hemoglobin and hematocrit levels, and evidence of cardiac, renal, or cerebral hypoperfusion should be considered in determining transfusion quantity. Massive transfusion was associated with a higher risk of death, nosocomial infection, multiorgan dysfunction, and acute respiratory distress. Coagulopathy should be corrected promptly. Correction of coagulopathy with FFP or platelets is recommended but should not delay endoscopy. Consensus guidelines call for the transfusion of one unit of FFP for every four units of packed RBC transfused to replace coagulation factors. Patients with fewer than 50,000 platelets/μL and active bleeding may need platelet transfusion.

Nasogastric Aspiration and Lavage

Once considered a standard emergent interven tion, NGT aspiration with gastric lavage is generally not indicated for evaluation of GIB. The sensitivity of NGT aspiration and lavage for predicting UGIB is low, and the negative likelihood ratio in patients with melena or hematochezia without hematemesis is poor.NGT placement has been associated with severe complications including aspiration, pneumothorax, perforation, and gastric lesions and is a painful procedure.Placement of an NGT in patients with suspected UGIB is not recommended.

Sengstaken–Blakemore Tube

Bedside balloon tamponade should be considered only in exsanguinating patients with likely variceal bleeding when endoscopy is not immediately available. Complications are common and significant, but intervention is indicated in the appropriate patient population owing to the high mortality associated with uncontrolled bleeding.

Medications

Infusion of high-dose PPI before endoscopy accelerates the resolution of signs of bleeding in ulcers and reduces the need for endoscopic therapy. The recommended dosage is an 80 mg bolus of omeprazole intravenously, followed by 8 mg/hr for 3 d.

Somatostatin and octreotide are splanchnic vasoconstrictors that reduce portal hypertension and the risk of persistent bleeding, rebleeding, and transfusion requirements in patients with variceal bleeding.The recommended dose of octreotide is a 50-μg bolus followed by 50 μg/hr intravenously.

Vasopressin, administered by continuous intravenous infusion, also reduces splanchnic blood flow and portal hypertension. However, it has limited use owing to significant complications that include myocardial and mesenteric ischemia and MI.

DEFINITIVE MANAGEMENT

Consultation

For patients with hemodynamic instability and severe bleeding, prompt gastroenterology and surgical consultation should be sought. Ongoing bleeding, severe anemia, or significant comorbidity prompts consideration of admission to an EICU.

Endoscopy

Upper endoscopy is the most effective diagnostic and therapeutic intervention for UGIB.Endoscopic treatments include injection therapy (e.g., saline, vasoconstrictors, sclerosing agents, tissue adhesives, or a combination thereof), thermal therapy (with the use of contact methods, such as multipolar electrocoagulation and heater probe, or noncontact methods, such as argon plasma coagulation), and mechanical therapy (principally endoscopic clips). Endoscopy within 13 hr of bleeding reduces mortality in high-risk patients.

Colonoscopy

Urgent colonoscopy has variable diagnostic value for identification of a bleeding source in LGIB. Lesion visualization is maximized by bowel preparation with polyethylene glycol in brisk but not in severe hemorrhage.

Angiography

Angiography is used in a very small proportion of cases of GIB and requires a hemorrhage rate of greater than 0.5 mL/min to optimize detection of acute bleed. Although also potentially therapeutic, angiography has a high rate of complications, including acute renal failure, contrast reactions, and bowel infarction. CT angiography also has variable sensitivities reported for the detection of acute GIB.

Tagged Red Blood Cell Imaging

Tagged RBC imaging or nuclear scintigraphy involves erythrocyte injection to detect indolent or elusive bleeding and is primarily useful in the inpatient setting. Timing is essential—95% to 100% of scans performed within 2 hr of injection correctly localize bleeding sites, whereas substantially fewer scans performed after 2 hr localize bleeding accurately.

DISPOSITION

Several scoring systems to risk stratify UGIB patients into low-and high-risk groups have been developed.These groups are based on adverse outcomes that are usually defied as a risk of recurrent bleeding of greater than 5% and greater than 1% mortality. Unfortunately, many of these scores rely on both clinical and endoscopic variables.

A consensus panel of 34 multidisciplinary experts from 34 countries identified the following clinical predictors as high risk: age older than 65 yr; shock; poor overall health status; comorbid illness; low initial hemoglobin levels; melena; transfusion requirement; fresh red blood on rectal examination, in the emesis, or in the NGT aspirate; sepsis; and elevated urea, creatinine, or serum aminotransferase levels.

The Blatchford score (Table 23-3) and clinical (or preendoscopic) Rockall score (Table 23-4) use only clinical and laboratory data to risk stratify patients.

Table 23-3 Blatchford Score

ADMISSION RISK MARKER	SCORE COMPONENT VALUE
Blood urea nitrogen level (mg/dL)	
≥18.2 to <22.4	2
>22.4 to <28	3
>28 to <70	4
>70	6
Hemoglobin level for men (g/dL)	
>12 to <13	1
≥10 to <12	3
<10	6
Hemoglobin level for women (g/dL)	
≥10 to <12	1
<10	6
Systolic blood pressure (mm Hg)	
≥100 to <109	1
>90 to <99	2
<90	3
Other markers	
Pulse rate ≥100 beats/min	1
Presentation with melena	1
Presentation with syncope	2
Hepatic disease	2
Heart failure	2

Table 23-4 Clinical Rockall Risk Score

VARIABLE	Score			
	0	1	2	3
Age (years)	<60	60-79	≥80	
Shock		HR>100 beats/min	SBP<100 mm Hg, IHD, CHF,any maj or comorbidity	Renal failure,liver failure,metastatic malignancy

Once identified, high-risk UGIB patients require admission for inpatient monitoring, assessment, and consultation for definitive diagnosis and treatment.

Through use of these scores and others, low-risk UGIB patients can be identified as those with no comorbid diseases, normal vital signs, normal or trace positive result on stool guaiac testing, negative findings on gastric aspiration, normal hemoglobin and hematocrit, good support systems, proper understanding of signs and symptoms of significant bleeding, immediate access to emergent care, and follow-up within 24 hr.

There are no clear guidelines on risk stratification for outpatient management of LGIB patients.Patients with LGIB not clearly caused by hemorrhoids, fissure, or proctitis should be admitted for nuclear medicine imaging or colonoscopy.

(LIU Zhi)

Renal Emergency

Chapter 24

Acute Kidney Injury

KEY CONCEPTS

The hallmark of AKI is progressive azotemia, depending on the severity and duration of renal dysfunction. These include metabolic derangements, disturbances of body fluid balance, and a variety of effects on almost every organ system.

The causes of AKI can be classified as prerenal, postrenal, and intrinsic renal disorders.

Management of AKI is directed first at potentially lethal complications such as hyperkalemia or volume overload and then at reversal of the underlying cause of renal dysfunction. It is important to avoid any further hemodynamic or toxic insults to the kidneys.

The patient's impaired renal function must be considered when fluid is administered and drugs are prescribed.

Dialysis is usually initiated when the BUN level exceeds 100 mg/dL or the serum Cr level exceeds 10 mg/dL.

Patients with renal failure often have varying degrees of volume overload. Volume overload generally is the first diagnostic consideration when dyspnea is the presenting complaint.

The hallmark of AKI is progressive azotemia, depending on the severity and duration of renal dysfunction. These include metabolic derangements, disturbances of body fluid balance,and a variety of effects on almost every organ system (Box 24-1).

Box 24-1 Clinical Features of AKI

Cardiovascular
- Pulmonary edema
- Arrhythmia
- HTN
- Pericarditis
- Pericardial effusion
- Myocardial infarction
- Pulmonary embolism

Metabolic
- Hyponatremia
- Hyperkalemia
- Acidosis
- Hypocalcemia
- Hyperphosphatemia
- Hypermagnesemia
- Hyperuricemia

Neurologic
- Asterixis
- Neuromuscular irritability
- Mental status changes
- Somnolence
- Coma
- Seizures

Gastrointestinal
- Nausea
- Vomiting
- Gastritis
- Gastroduodenal ulcer
- Gastrointestinal bleeding
- Pancreatitis
- Malnutrition

Hematologic
- Anemia
- Hemorrhagic diathesis

Infectious
- Pneumonia
- Septicemia
- Urinary tract infection
- Wound infection

The causes of AKI may be divided into those that decrease renal blood flow (prerenal), produce a renal parenchymal insult (intrarenal), or obstruct urine flow (obstructive or postrenal). The renal parenchymal causes of AKI can be usefully subdivided into those primarily affecting the glomeruli, the intrarenal vasculature, or the renal interstitium. The term ATN denotes another broad category of intrinsic renal failure(Fig. 24-1).

PRINCIPLES OF DISEASE

Prerenal Azotemia

The possible causes can be grouped into entities

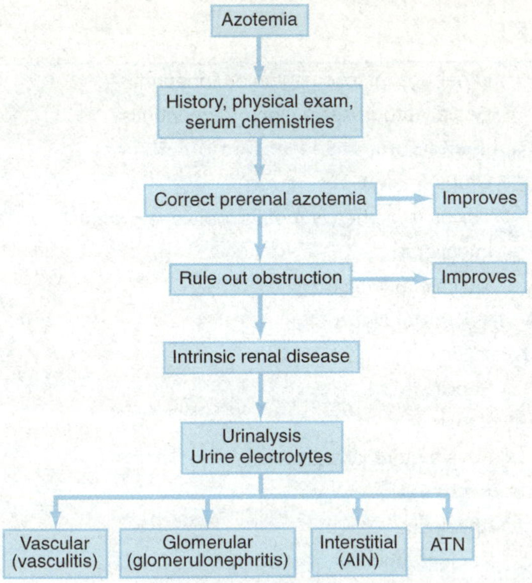

Fig. 24-1 Evaluation of azotemia.

causing intravascular volume depletion, volume redistribution, or decreased CO (Box 24-2).

Box 24-2 Causes of Prerenal Azotemia

Volume Loss
- Gastrointestinal: vomiting, diarrhea, nasogastric drainage
- Renal: diuresis
- Blood loss
- Insensible losses
- Third-space sequestration
- Pancreatitis
- Peritonitis
- Trauma
- Burns

Cardiac Causes
- Myocardial infa-rction
- Valvular disease
- Cardiomyopathy
- Decreased effective arterial volume
- Antihypertensive medication
- Nitrates

Neurogenic Causes
- Sepsis
- Anaphylaxis
- Hypoalbuminemia
- Nephrotic syndrome
- Liver disease

Prerenal azotemia is characterized by increased urine specific gravity, BUN/Cr ratio generally between 10 : 1 and 20 : 1, urine sodium concentration less than 20mEq/dL, and FENa less than 1%. However, severe prolonged prerenal azotemia can eventuate in ATN.

Postrenal (Obstructive) Acute Renal Injury

Obstruction may occur at any level of the urinary tract but most commonly is produced by prostatic hypertrophy or by functional bladder neck obstruction(Box 24-3).

Box 24-3 Causes of Postrenal Renal Failure

Intrarenal and Ureteral Causes
- Kidney stone
- Sloughed papilla
- Malignancy
- Retroperitoneal fibrosis
- Uric acid, oxalic acid, or phosphate crystal precipitation
- Sulfonamide, methotrexate, acyclovir,or indinavir precipitation

Bladder
- Kidney stone
- Blood clot
- Prostatic hypertrophy
- Bladder carcinoma
- Neurogenic bladder

Urethra
- Phimosis
- Stricture

Treatment of postrenal AKI consists of relief of the obstruction.

Intrinsic Acute Renal Failure

Glomerulonephritis, interstitial nephritis, and abnormalities of the intrarenal vasculature are responsible for only 5% to 10% of cases of AKI (Box 24-4) in adult inpatients; most are caused by ATN.

Glomerular Disease(Box 24-4)

Patients may have dark urine, HTN, edema, or CHF. The hematuria associated with glomerular disease may be microscopic or gross and may be persistent or intermittent.Proteinuria not uncommonly is in the nephrotic range. The presence of hematuria, proteinuria, or red cell casts is highly suggestive of glomerulonephritis.

The specific diagnosis of acute glomerulonephritis caused by primary renal disease often is ultimately made by renal biopsy.

Interstitial Disease

Acute interstitial nephritis most commonly is precipitated by drug exposure or by infection. The most commonly incriminated drugs are the penicillins, diuretics, and NSAID. Acute interstitial nephritis has been reported in association with bacterial, fungal, protozoan, and rickettsial infections.

Patients with acute interstitial nephritis classically have rash, fever, eosinophilia, and eosinophiluria. Pyuria, gross or microscopic hematuria, and mild proteinuria are observed in some cases. A definite diagnosis sometimes can be made only on renal biopsy.

Intrarenal Vascular Disease

Disorders such as renal arterial thrombosis or

Box 24-4 Intrinsic Renal Diseases That Cause AKI

Vascular Diseases

Large-Vessel Diseases

- Renal artery throm-bosis or stenosis
- Renal vein thrombosis
- Atheroembolic disease

Small-and Medium-Vessel Diseases

- Scleroderma
- Malignant HTN
- Hemolytic uremic syndrome
- TTP
- HIV-associated microangiopathy

Glomerular Diseases

Systemic Diseases

- Systemic lupus erythematosus
- Infective endocarditis
- Systemic vasculitis (e.g., periarteritis nodosa, Wegener's granulomatosis)
- Henoch-Scholein purpura
- HIV-associated nephropathy
- Essential mixed cryoglobulinemia
- Goodpasture's syndome

Primary Renal Diseases

- Poststreptococcal glomerulonephritis
- Other postinfectious glomerulonephritis
- Rapidly progressive glomerulonephritis

Tubulointerstitial Diseases and Conditions

- Drugs (many)
- Toxins (e.g., heavy metals, ethylene glycol)
- Infections
- Multiple myeloma

Acute Tubular Necrosis

Ischemia

- Shock
- Sepsis
- Severe prerenal azotemia

Nephrotoxins

- Antibiotics
- Radiographic contrast agents
- Myoglobinuria
- Hemoglobinuria

Other Diseases and Conditions

- Severe liver disease
- Allergic reactions
- NSAID

embolism must be bilateral to produce AKI. The most common cause of thrombosis probably is trauma; thrombosis also may occur after angiography or may be secondary to aortic or renal arterial dissection. Renal arterial embolism can cause acute renal infarction, generally manifested by sudden flank, back, chest, or upper abdominal pain. Urinary findings, including hematuria, are variable. Fever, nausea, and vomiting are not uncommon. The diagnosis usually is made by renal flow scanning or arteriography.

Several diseases that affect the smaller intrarenal vessels can cause AKI (Box 24-4).

Patients with scleroderma (systemic sclerosis) may have "scleroderma renal crisis," characterized by malignant HTN and rapidly progressive renal failure.

In patients with scleroderma renal crisis, specific therapy with ACEI has been shown to result in improvement in renal function.

Acute Tubular Necrosis

The term ATN refers to a generally reversible deterioration of kidney function associated with a variety of renal insults. Oliguria may or may not be a feature. The diagnosis is made after prerenal and postrenal causes of ARF and disorders of glomeruli, interstitium, and intrarenal vasculature have been excluded.

The most common precipitant of ATN is renal ischemia occurring during surgery or after trauma and sepsis. The remainder of cases occur in the administration of nephrotoxic aminoglycoside antibiotics or radiocontrast agents or in association with rhabdomyolysis.

Postischemic ATN can occur in the setting of volume loss from the GI tract (upper or lower), skin, or kidneys or can result from severe hemorrhage or major burns. Heatstroke commonly is associated with the development of ATN.Another cause of ATN is hyperglycemic hyperosmolar nonketotic coma. ATN also is seen in the setting of cardiogenic shock, sepsis, and third spacing of fluids in pancreatitis and peritonitis.

ATN is common in postoperative patients. Concomitant sepsis, increased age, preexisting renal disease, and other comorbid conditions are associated with a worse outcome.

Nephrotoxins constitute the other major cause of ATN. Among the most prominent of these are the endogenous pigments myoglobin and hemoglobin. Rhabdomyolysis and ARF resulting from crush injuries many other causes of pigment nephropathy have been reported (Box 24-5).

Box 24-5 Causes of Pigment-Induced AKI

Rhabdomyolysis and myoglobinuria	Alcoholism
Vigorous exercise	Hypokalemia
Arterial embolization	Hypophosphatemia
Status epilepticus	Hemoglobinuria
Status asthmaticus	Transfusion reactions
Coma-induced and pressure-induced myonecrosis	Snake envenomation
Heat stress	Malaria
Diabetic ketoacidosis	Mechanical destruction of RBCs by prosthetic valves
Myopathy	G6PD deficiency

ATN associated with rhabdomyolysis is often oliguric; it is characterized by rapid increases in the serum Cr, potassium, phosphorus, and uric acid levels. Creatine released from muscle is metabolized to Cr, which may result in serum Cr increases of more than 2 mg/dL/day, in contrast to the increase of 0.5 to 1.0 mg/dL/day typically seen in other forms of AKI. The BUN/Cr ratio often is less than 10 : 1. Intracellular potassium released from damaged muscle may raise the serum potassium by 1 to 2 mEq/L in several hours.

Urine dipstick testing yields a positive result for heme in only 50% of patients with rhabdomyolysis, because myoglobin is rapidly cleared from the serum. Measurement of serum CK levels is a more sensitive test.

Aminoglycosides and radiographic contrast agents are other nephrotoxins implicated in the development of ATN.

The most important risk factors for radiocontrast agent-induced ATN are preexisting renal insufficiency, diabetes mellitus, multiple myeloma, age older than 60 yr, volume depletion, and higher doses of contrast material.

CLINICAL FEATURES

The clinical distinction between AKI and chronic kidney disease often is difficult.The finding of small kidneys on abdominal radiography or bone changes of secondary hyperparathyroidism on hand films suggests that the renal failure is chronic. Anemia, hypocalcemia, and hyperphosphatemia, on the other hand, should not be relied on to identify patients who have chronic kidney disease because these abnormalities can develop rapidly in AKI.

In evaluating the patient with azotemia, the clinician uses history, physical examination, and laboratory studies to seek clue to the cause and to identify signs and symptoms of uremia, volume overload, or other complications of renal failure. A history of acute anuria is most often the result of high-grade urinary tract obstruction.Intermittent anuria, on the other hand, is characteristic of obstructive disease.

A history of HTN, dark-colored urine, rash, fever, or arthritis suggests intrinsic renal disease or a multisystem disorder. In older patients the presence of symptoms suggestive of multiple myeloma should be elicited.

The physical examination focuses on signs of volume depletion.

Ultrasonography can be used to detect bladder distention.

Prostate examination in adult men and pelvic examination in adult women are necessary components of the examination.

DIAGNOSTIC STRATEGY

Laboratory Findings

The laboratory evaluation begins with a dipstick and microscopic urinalysis and measurement of urine output. BUN, serum Cr, urine sodium, and FENa levels are determined to help evaluate renal function and to provide clues to the cause of AKI. CBC, serum electrolyte panel, ECG, and chest radiograph help to establish the patient's baseline status and to provide information about possible complications.

Urethral or bladder neck obstruction is documented by the finding of significant amounts of residual urine in the bladder by catheterization or ultrasound examination. A renal parenchymal disorder often can be diagnosed by its manifestations on microscopic urinalysis or by associated extrarenal manifestations or the clinical setting.

Radiography and Ultrasonography

Significant hydronephrosis usually is readily demonstrable by ultrasonography and may indicate either upper or lower tract obstruction.

MANAGEMENT

ED management of AKI is directed at reversing decreases in GFR and urine output (if possible) while minimizing further hemodynamic and toxic insults, maintaining normal fluid and electrolyte balance, and managing other complications of AKI as required.

After ensuring that the vital signs are adequate and that the patient is in no immediate danger from volume or metabolic derangements, the next step is to correct prerenal and postrenal factors. Intravascular volume is repleted in hypovolemic patients. Postrenal or obstructive ARF is treated by restoration of normal urine outflow. Bladder outlet obstruction may be relieved by passage of a Foley catheter, whereas upper tract obstruction may require percutaneous nephrostomy.

The challenge to the emergency physician is to identify the cause of intrinsic renal AKI (Box 24-4).

Use of loop diuretics or mannitol often is effective in increasing urine flow when intravascular volume deficits have been corrected.

Dopamine also has been used, with and without furosemide,but has not proven effective. Pigment-induced ATN may be prevented by avoidance of hemolysis and muscle injury and by correction of the factors.

Mannitol has been shown to prevent AKI in experimental models of myoglobinuria.Furosemide has not consistently shown a beneficial effect. Myoglobin precipitates in an acid urine but not in an alkaline urine. Thus, aggressive volume repletion, alkalinization, and mannitol infusion have traditionally been recommended after crush injuries to reduce the likelihood or severity of AKI.

Patients who have radiocontrast agent-induced ATN usually require only supportive therapy.

Volume and Metabolic Complications

An important component of the management of AKI is the prevention or control of systemic complications(e.g., hyperkalemia, hypocalcemia, hyperphosphatemia, metabolic acidosis) and complications of volume overload (e.g., HTN, CHF).

Uremia patients associated infection is a significant cause of morbidity and mortality in AKI. Thus patients with fever require aggressive treatment.

Pericarditis also may occur in patients with AKI. Pericarditis or pericardial effusion in the setting of AKI generally is an indication for the urgent initiation of dialysis.Neurologic abnormalities in AKI may be precipitated by electrolyte abnormalities, medications, or uremia.

DISPOSITION

Patients with new-onset AKI should be hospitalized.

Decisions regarding dialysis generally are made by intensivist and take into account many factors, including laboratory test abnormalities and the presence or absence of signs and symptoms of uremia. Many intensivist choose to initiate dialysis when the BUN level exceeds 100 mg/dL or the serum Cr level exceeds 10 mg/dL. Intractable volume overload and life-threatening hyperkalemia are the two most common indications for emergency dialysis.

Complications of Hemodialysis

Vascular Access-Related Complications

Bleeding from the dialysis puncture site can occur hours after a hemodialysis treatment. Such bleeding almost always can be stopped by applying firm pressure to the access site; possibly cause thrombosis of the vessel by compressing it too vigorously.

Infection of the vascular access can result in persistent or recurrent bacteremia. Most infections are caused by staphylococci typical of skin flora.For this reason, it is common practice to obtain blood cultures for all patients on hemodialysis who have a fever without an obvious source of infection.

Vancomycin 1 to 1.5 g given IV as a single loading dose is the drug of choice in this situation. If a gram-negative infection also is thought to be likely, a loading dose of a second drug (e.g., a third-generation cephalosporin or an aminoglycoside) also can be administered.

Non-Vascular Access-Related Complications

The hemodialysis procedure itself often is associated with acute complications such as hypotension, shortness of breath, chest pain, and neurologic abnormalities.

Hypotension

With rapid removal of extracellular fluid, there is inadequate time for transcellular fluid shifts to replace intravascular volume. Antihypertensive medications can contribute to the hypotension when intravascular volume is normalized.

Patients with significant hypotension on dialysis should be considered to be at risk for AMI, acute dysrhythmias, and sepsis. These are common causes of hypotension among all patients in the ED, and consideration should first be given to these entities (Box 24-6).

Box 24-6 Differential Diagnosis of Hypotension in Hemodialysis Patients

Hypovolemia	Hypercalcemia or hypocalcemia
Excessive fluid removal	Hypermagnesemia
Hemorrhage	Vascular instability
Septicemia	Drug-related
Cardiogenic shock	Dialysate-related
Dysrhythmia	Autonomic neuropathy
Pericardial tamponade	Excessive access arteriovenous flow
Myocardial infarction	Anaphylactoid reaction
Myocardial or valvular dysfunction	Air embolism
Electrolyte disorders	
Hyperkalemia or hypokalemia	

Occasionally, acute hypotension may be caused by anaphylaxis or an anaphylactoid reaction to some component of the dialyzer or the dialysate.

Life-threatening hyperkalemia can occur in the presence of underlying catabolic illness or with a prolonged period of hypotension.Patients who are hyperkalemic can have profoundly slow heart rates, particularly if they have been treated with beta-blockers or calcium channel blockers. If a dialysis patient is in cardiac arrest, it should be assumed that hyperkalemia is present, and intravenous calcium should be given immediately.

Shortness of Breath

Shortness of breath in dialysis patients generally is caused by volume overload,primarily sudden cardiac failure, or pleural hemorrhage. Often, pneumonia or underlying reactive airway disease is responsible.

Chest Pain

Most dialysis patients have risk factors for coronary artery disease. During hemodialysis,these underlying factors may be added to acute physiologic stresses such as transient hypotension and hypoxemia, thereby increasing myocardial oxygen demand while decreasing oxygen delivery.

Among nonischemic causes of chest pain, pericarditis should always be a consideration.The presentation is essentially the same as in nonrenal patients; fever, a friction rub, or atrial dysrhythmias may be associated findings.Indomethacin often is effective in relieving pain.

(CHAI Yanfen WANG Lijun)

Hematologic Emergency

Chapter 25

Disorders of Hemostasis

KEY CONCEPTS

Hemostasis is a balance between the excessive bleeding state and thrombosis, and depends on normal function and integration of the vasculature, platelets, and coagulation pathway.

Platelet dysfunction is often equated with low platelet counts.

The patient with chronic form of ITP may have petechiae or purpura, and platelet counts between 30,000/mm^3 and 100,000/mm^3 are common.

TTP is classically seen as the constellation of thrombocytopenic purpura, microangiopathic hemolytic anemia, fluctuating neurologic symptoms, renal disease, and fever. The diagnosis is currently considered for unexplained thrombocytopenia in association with microangiopathic hemolytic anemia.

DIC is a relatively common acquired coagulopathy. It needs to be considered in any patient in whom purpura, a bleeding tendency, and signs of organ injury, particularly of the CNS and kidney, develop.

PERSPECTIVE

Hemostasis is the process of blood clot formation and represents a coordinated response to vessel injury. It requires an orchestrated response from platelets, the clotting cascade, blood vessel endothelium, and fibrinolysis. Thrombin-stimulated clot formation and plasmin-induced clot lysis are closely related and regulated. This dynamic process is often viewed in phases: formation of a platelet plug, propagation of the coagulation cascade, formation of a clot, and fibrinolysis of the clot.

Most hemostatic abnormalities are acquired and result from drugs (e.g., aspirin or warfarin), from associated disease (e.g., hepatic insufficiency), or from iatrogenic causes (e.g., multiple transfusions).

PATHOPHYSIOLOGY

Hemostasis depends on normal function and integration of the vasculature, platelets, and coagulation pathway.

Vasculature

Vascular integrity is maintained by a lining of nonreactive over-lapping endothelial cells supported by a basement membrane, connective tissue, and smooth muscle. These cells are important in maintaining a barrier to macromolecules and, when injured, in contributing to the metabolic response and local vasoconstriction. The vascular endothelium contributes to both clot formation and regulation.

Platelets

Platelets have multiple and ever-expanding roles in our understanding of hemostasis. Platelets contain lysosomes, granules, a trilaminar plasma membrane, microtubules, and a canalicular system. Granules are an important component of hemostasis and contain platelet factor, adhesive and aggregation glycoproteins, coagulation factors, and fibrinolytic inhibitors. Each participates in the process of coagulation. The platelet's role is termed primary hemostasis, and it serves as the initial defense against blood loss. Platelet activity is summarized in Box 25-1.

Box 25-1 Role of Platelets in Hemostasis

Adhesion to subendothelial connective tissue: collagen, basement membrane, and noncollagenous microfibrils; serumfactor Ⅷ (von Willebrand's) permits this function; adhesioncreates the initial bleeding arrest plug

Release of adenosine diphosphate, the primary mediator andamplifier of aggregation; release of thromboxane A, another aggregator and potent vasoconstrictor; release of calcium, serotonin, epinephrine, and trace thrombin

Platelet aggregation over the area of endothelial injury

Stabilization of the hemostatic plug by interaction with thecoagulation system:

Platelet factor 3, a phospholipid that helps accelerate certainsteps in the coagulation system

Platelet factor 4, a protein that neutralizes heparin

Pathway initiation and acceleration by thrombin production

Possible secretion of active forms of coagulation proteins

Stimulation of limiting reactions of platelet activity

Coagulation Pathway

The coagulation pathway is a complex system of checks and balances that results in controlled formation of a fibrin clot. Coagulation factors have been given standard Roman numerals matching their order of discovery (Box 25-2).

Box 25-2 Coagulation Factors

Ⅰ. Fibrinogens
Ⅱ. Prothrombin
Ⅲ. Tissue thromboplastin
Ⅳ. Calcium
Ⅴ. Labile factor (proaccelerin)
Ⅵ. Not assigned
Ⅶ. Proconvertin
Ⅷ. Antihemophilic A factor
Ⅸ. Antihemophilic B factor (plasma thromboplastin component, Christmas factor)
Ⅹ. Stuart-Prower factor
Ⅺ. Plasma thromboplastin antecedent
Ⅻ. Hageman factor (contact factor)
XIII. Fibrin-stabilizing factor

A simplified version of the coagulation pathway is presented in Fig. 25-1. The clotting cascade is traditionally depicted as consisting of intrinsic and extrinsic pathways. The intrinsic pathway is initiated by exposure of blood to a negatively charged surface, such as a glass surface in the activated partial thromboplastin clotting time. The extrinsic pathway is activated by tissue factor exposed at the site of vessel injury or thromboplastin. Both pathways converge to activate factor X, which then activates prothrombin to thrombin.

The clinically important groups of coagulation factors are as follows:

Thrombin-sensitive factors contributing to the metabolic response and local vasoconstriction: Ⅰ, Ⅴ, Ⅷ, XIII

Vitamin K-sensitive factors: Ⅱ, Ⅶ, Ⅸ, Ⅹ

Sites of heparin activity: IIa, IXa, Xa (major site), XIa, platelet factor 3

Thrombin-sensitive factors are activated by thrombin and may give rise to a bleeding disorder if defective synthesis occurs. Vitamin K–sensitive factors may also cause bleeding from defective synthesis, as occurs with liver disease and warfarin anticoagulants. Heparin in combination with antithrombin Ⅲ affects the coagulation pathway at multiple sites.

Coagulation Control

All the components of the coagulation reaction are necessary to prevent excessive bleeding. Hemostasis is a balance between the excessive bleeding state and thrombosis. Once coagulation is initiated, controls are necessary to prevent local or generalized thrombosis. These controls include the following:

Removal and dilution of activated clotting factors through blood flow, which also mechanically opposes growth of the hemostatic plug

Modulation of platelet activity by endothelium-generated nitric oxide and prostacyclin

Removal of activated coagulation components by the reticuloendothelial system

Regulation of the clotting cascade by antithrombin Ⅲ, protein C, protein S, and tissue factor pathway inhibitor

Activation of the fibrinolytic system

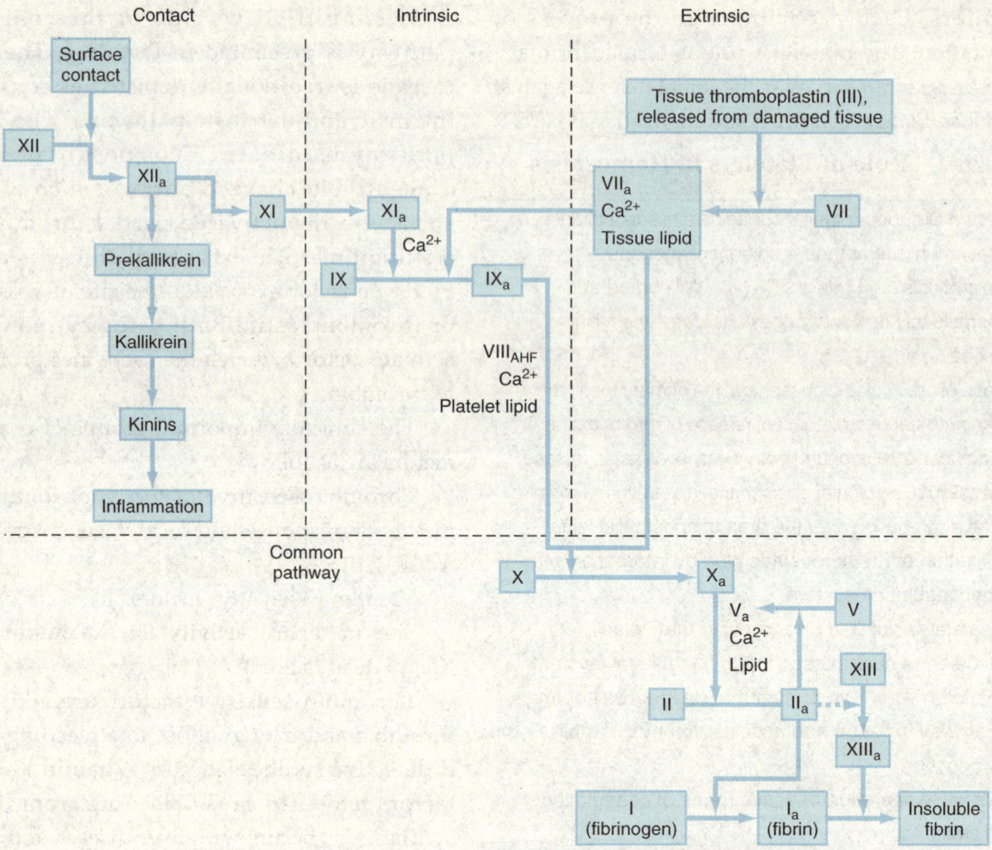

Fig. 25-1 Coagulation pathway

CLINICAL FEATURES

Patients who do not respond quickly to the usual measures of hemostasis should be considered to have a potential bleeding disorder.

History and Physical Examination

An outline of the history and physical examination is presented in Box 25-3. Platelet disorders are usually manifested as acquired petechiae, purpura, or mucosal bleeding and are more common in women. Coagulation problems are commonly congenital, are characterized by delayed deep muscle or joint bleeding, and are seen more often in men.

Ancillary Evaluation

A definitive diagnosis depends on laboratory

Box 25-3 Clinical Evaluation of a Bleeding Patient

History

Nature of bleeding
- Petechiae
- Purpura
- Ecchymosis
- Significant bleeding episodes

Sites of bleeding
- Skin
- Mucosa: oral or nasal
- Muscle
- Gastrointestinal
- Genitourinary
- Joints

Patterns of bleeding
- Recent onset or lifelong
- Frequency and severity
- Spontaneous or after injury

Challenges to hemostasis
- Tooth extraction

Operative procedures
Association with medication, particularly aspirin
Medications
Associated diseases
Uremia
Liver disease
Infection
Malignant neoplasm
Previous transfusion
Family history

Physical Examination
Vital signs
Skin: nature of bleeding, signs of liver disease
Mucosa: oral or nasal
Lymphadenopathy
Abdomen: liver size and shape, splenomegaly
Joints: signs of previous bleeding
Other sites of blood loss: pelvic, rectal, urinary tract

evaluation. Tests pertinent to the ED are discussed and listed in Box 25-4.

Box 25-4 Coagulation Studies

CBC and smear (EDTA—purple top)
Platelet count (EDTA—purple top)
Bleeding time
Prothrombin time (citrate—blue top)
Partial thromboplastin time (citrate—blue top)
Other coagulation studies: fibrinogen level, thrombin time, clotsolubility, factor levels, inhibitor screens
As necessary: electrolyte values; glucose, BUN, and creatinineconcentrations; type and crossmatch

CBC and Blood Smear

CBC assesses the degree of anemia associated with the bleeding episode. The peripheral blood smear may demonstrate schistocytes or fragmented RBC in DIC. Teardrop-shaped or nucleated RBC may refect myelophthisic disease. A characteristic WBC morphologic condition is seen with thrombocytopenia associated with infectious mononucleosis, folate or vitamin B_{12} defciency, or leukemia.

Platelet Count

Normally, one platelet is present per 10 to 20 RBC. Often, the normal range being 150,000 to 400,000/mm^3. Platelet counts less than 100,000/mm^{3}define thrombocytopenia. Levels below 20,000/mm^3 may be associated with serious spontaneous hemorrhage. However, the count gives no information about the functional capability of platelets.

Bleeding Time

Bleeding time is the best test to determine both vascular integrity and platelet function that can be performed in the ED. A normal time is 8 min, a time of 8 to 10 min is borderline, and a time longer than 10 min is typically abnormal. The high incidence of drug-induced platelet dysfunction.A prolonged bleeding time associated with platelet counts above 100,000/mm^3 suggests impaired function.

Prothrombin Time

PT tests the factors of the extrinsic and common pathways. The PT detects deficiencies in fibrinogen, prothrombin (factor Ⅱ), factor Ⅴ, factor Ⅶ, and factor Ⅹ. It is used to test the extrinsic pathway. A PT of 2 s or more above the control time is considered signifcant. Results are usually reported as the INR.

Partial Thromboplastin Time

PTT tests the components of the intrinsic and common pathways, that is, essentially all factors but Ⅶ and ⅩⅢ in the entire clotting cascade. The average time is 25 to 29 s. Inappropriately high values may occur if the plasma is too turbid or icteric. APTT is most sensitive to abnormalities in the sequence of the coagulation cascade that precedes activation of factor X.

Fibrinogen

Fibrinogen is present in suffcient concentration to be measured directly. Because it is the final coagulation substrate, its level refects the balance between production and consumption. It may be decreased by low production, as in severe liver disease, or by overconsumption, as in DIC. Low levels and altered function increase the PT, PTT, and thrombin clotting time. Because fibrinogen is an acute-phase reactant, certain conditions, including malignant disease, sepsis, infammation, and pregnancy, may alter the test result.

Thrombin Time

Measurement of the thrombin clotting time bypasses the intrinsic and extrinsic pathways by directly converting fibrinogen to fibrin. It is a useful screening test for both qualitative and quantitative abnormalities of fibrinogen and inhibitors such as heparin and fbrin split products.

Clot Solubility

The result of clot solubility testing may be the only abnormality in disorders involving factor XIII defciency and some abnormal fibrinogen. A washed clot is incubated in acetic acid or urea. If the clot is not properly cross-linked, it dissolves.

Factor Level Assays

Factor levels are determined either by bioassay or by immunologic assay. Inhibitor screening tests reveal antibodies in plasma that prolong the normal plasma clotting time when mixed.

DIFFERENTIAL DIAGNOSIS AND MANAGEMENT

When a bleeding disorder is diagnosed or suggested, the assessment initially includes stabilization, which may necessitate volume, RBC, and coagulation factor replacement.A clinically useful scheme approaches bleeding disorders in terms of three constituents: vascular integrity, platelets, and coagulation factors. This differential diagnostic approach can be further divided into inherited and acquired disorders.

Vascular Disorders

Vascular disorders have signs and symptoms similar to those of thrombocytopenic states. The inherited forms are rare. Acquired forms are usually associated with connective tissue changes or endothelial damage. The differential diagnosis of vascular disorders is listed in Box 25-5.

Box 25-5 Differential Diagnosis of Vascular Disorders

Inherited

Disorders of connective tissue
- Pseudoxanthoma elasticum
- Ehlers-Danlos syndrome
- Osteogenesis imperfecta

Disorders of blood vessels
- Hemorrhagic telangiectasia

Acquired

Scurvy (vitamin C deficiency)

Simple or senile purpura

Purpura secondary to steroid use

Vascular damage
- Infection (meningococcemia)
- Hemolytic-uremic syndrome
- Hypoxemia
- Thrombotic thrombocytopenic purpura
- Snakebite
- Dysproteinemic purpura

Platelet Disorders

General Approach

Platelet abnormalities can be caused by congenital disorders, but most are from acquired conditions. The bleeding source is usually capillary, with resultant cutaneous and mucosal petechiae or ecchymosis. Epistaxis, menorrhagia, and gastrointestinal bleeding are common initial symptoms. The bleeding is generally mild and occurs immediately after surgery or dental extractions. Petechiae and purpura may be noted on physical examination, and superficial ecchymoses may be found around a venipuncture site. The purpura associated with platelet disorders is typically asymptomatic and not palpable. This is in contrast to purpura associated with vasculitis, which can burn or itch and is palpable. Deep muscle hematomas and hemarthroses are not aspects of the clinical picture. The bleeding time is prolonged, and the platelet count may be low, normal, or high. The differential diagnosis of platelet disorders is listed in Box 25-6.

Box 25-6 Differential Diagnosis of Platelet Disorders

Thrombocytopenia

Decreased production
- Decreased megakaryocytes secondary to drugs, toxins, or infection
- Normal megakaryocytes with megaloblastic hematopoiesis or hereditary origin
- Platelet pooling and splenic sequestration

Increased destruction
- Immunologic
  - Related to collagen vascular disease, lymphoma, leukemia

Drug related
Infection
Posttransfusion
Idiopathic (autoimmune) thrombocytopenic purpura
Mechanical
DIC
Thrombotic thrombocytopenic purpura
Hemolytic-uremic syndrome
Vasculitis
Dilutional secondary to massive blood transfusion
Thrombocytopathy
Adhesion defects such as von Willebrand's disease
Release defects: acquired and drug related
Aggregation defects such as in thrombasthenia
Thrombocytosis
Autonomous (primary thrombocythemia)
Reactive (secondary thrombocythemia)
Iron deficiency
Infection or inflammation
Trauma
Non hematologic malignant disease
Postsplenectomy
Rebound from alcohol, cytotoxic drug therapy, folate or vitaminB_{12} deficiency

Thrombocytopenia

Decreased Production. Thrombocytopenia from decreased bone marrow production is usually caused by the effects of chemotherapeutic drugs, myelophthisic disease, or direct bone marrow effects of agents such as alcohol or thiazides.

Splenic Sequestration. Splenic sequestration is rare. It is seen primarily with hypersplenism resulting from hematologic malignant disease, portal hypertension, or disorders involving increased splenic RBC destruction.

Increased Destruction

Immune Thrombocytopenia. Thrombocytopenia associated with increased peripheral destruction of platelets and shortened platelet survival caused by an antiplatelet antibody is seen in a number of diseases.

SLE may cause an antiplatelet antibody-related platelet decrease. Similar associations have been noted with leukemia and lymphoma, particularly lymphocytic lymphoma. All evaluations of suggested immune thrombocytopenia should include CBC, peripheral smear, antinuclear antibody test, and bone marrow examination. Quinine and quinidine are common offenders that affect platelets through an "innocent by stander" mechanism. Heparin is an important cause of drug-induced thrombocytopenia in hospitalized patients.

LMWH may be associated with less thrombocytopenia than standard, unfractionated heparin is. Heparin-induced thrombocytopenia (HIT) is a serious immune-mediated side effect associated with heparin. It usually occurs 5 to 7 d after the initiation of heparin treatment. Thrombus develops in approximately half the patients with HIT. The diagnosis is suggested in the presence of absolute thrombocytopenia or a greater than 50% reduction in platelets after the initiation of heparin. The most specific diagnostic tests for HIT are serotonin release assays, heparin-induced platelet aggregation assays, and solid-phase immunoassays. Platelet-associated IgG levels are commonly elevated, but this finding is less specifc or sensitive. This form of HIT occurs a median of 14 d after the initiation of heparin, but it has been reported to occur up to 40 d after heparin is started. The administration of heparin can result in the development of antibodies to the heparin and platelet factor 4 complex. The heparin–platelet factor 4 antibody complex is removed from the circulation, resulting in thrombocytopenia; this complex also results in the generation of microparticles. Treatment of thrombotic complications in these patients involves the use of direct thrombin inhibitors (lepi-rudin, argatroban), factor Xa inhibitors (fondaparinux), or hepa-rinoids (danaparoid).

Digitoxin, sulfonamides, phenytoin, and aspirin are other drugs that may be associated with a thrombocytopenia. An idiopathic thrombocytopenic purpura type of syndrome has been reported in intravenous cocaine users. The platelet count may fall below 10,000/mm^3 and be complicated by serious bleeding. Laboratory testing may confirm the presence of anti-body, especially with the use of quinine and quinidine. After administration of the drug is stopped, the platelet count improves slowly during a period of 3 to 7 d. A short course of corticosteroid therapy, such as prednisone in a dose of 1 mg/kg with rapid tapering, may facilitate recovery.

Postinfectious immune thrombocytopenia is usually associated with viral diseases. Although many cases associated with sepsis have a mechanical origin, some immune mechanisms have been demonstrated.

Post-transfusion thrombocytopenia is a rare

disorder that causes a precipitous fall in platelets approximately 1 w after the transfusion. The platelet count often falls precipitously below 10,000/ mm^3, with a signifcant risk for major bleeding. Intracranial hemorrhage occurs in approximately 10% of such cases. Patients are usually middle-aged women with a history of pregnancy who may have been previously sensitized to the PLA1 antigen during pregnancy. Plasma exchange therapy is an effective intervention.

Idiopathic Thrombocytopenic Purpura. Idiop- athic thrombocytopenic purpura (ITP) is associated with an IgG antiplatelet antibody.

The chronic form of ITP is primarily an adult disease found three times more often in women than in men. The patient may have petechiae or purpura, and platelet counts between 30,000/mm^3 and 100,000/mm^3 are common. Splenomegaly is unusual in either acute or chronic ITP.

Management includes stopping of all nones sential drugs. The initial treatment of chronic ITP is typically corticosteroids (prednisone 1 mg/ kg per day). Intravenous immune globulin and anti-D immunoglobulin, in conjunction with steroids, have also been used as frst-line therapy. Splenectomy, monoclonal antibody therapy, and immunosuppressives are considered in steroid-failure cases.Life-threatening bleeding is treated with platelet transfusions, intravenous immune globulin (0.7 g/kg), and methylprednisolone (15 mg/kg intravenously). Recombinant factor VIIa used in ITP showed that the agent helped stop bleeding.

Nonimmune Thrombocytopenia. Nonimmune platelet destruction is usually consumptive or mechanical. Consumption occurs as part of the process of intravascular coagulation. TTP, hemolytic-uremic syndrome, and vasculitis all initiate platelet destruction through endothelial damage. The most striking difference between the first two is the age at onset and the prognosis.

Thrombotic Thrombocytopenic Purpura. The pathologic state of TTP is the result of subendothelial and intraluminal deposits of fibrin and platelet aggregates in capillaries and arterioles. Hemolytic-uremic syndrome is considered to be similar to TTP; however, hemolytic-uremic syndrome is associated with less CNS and more renal involvement than TTP is. Prostacyclin and abnormal platelet aggregation are believed to play a central role in pathogenesis of the disease. 60% of cases occur in women. Most cases of TTP are idiopathic. However, TTP can be associated with medications. Quinine is the most common drug associated with the disease. The antiplatelet drugs ticlopidine and clopidogrel have also been associated with TTP. It is classically seen as the constellation of thrombocytopenic purpura, microangiopathic hemolytic anemia, fluctuating neurologic symptoms, renal disease, and fever. The diagnosis is currently considered for unexplained thrombocytopenia in association with microangiopathic hemolytic anemia.

Therapy has included corticosteroids, splenectomy, anticoagulation(such as aspirin and dipyridamole), plasma exchange transfusion, and dextran. With the exception of life-threatening bleeding, platelet transfusion is avoided.

Dilutional Thrombocytopenia. Dilutional thrombocytopenia occurs in cases of massive transfusion, exchange transfusion, or extracorporeal circulation.

Thrombocytopathy

The drug-induced form may be one of the most commonly seen causes of abnormal bleeding. Defects may occur at any level of platelet function, including adhesion, release, and aggregation.

Adhesion Defects. The representative adhesion disorder is von Willebrand's disease, which is a factor Ⅷ problem more than a platelet deficiency. Platelets are normal in terms of their morphologic condition, number, release, and aggregation.

Release Defects. Release defects may be congenital or acquired, as in SLE, alcoholism, or lymphoma. Drugs induce the most common release problem. Testing for this risk has been suggested by development of the post-aspirin bleeding time as a screening test for hemostatic disorders. Phenylbutazone and indomethacin affect function only while they are present in the circulation.

Aggregation Defects. This platelet membrane abnormality may be detected by the lack of clot retraction during a 2 hr clot retraction test.

Platelet Transfusions. Platelet transfusions are commonly indicated for primary bone marrow disorders (e.g., aplastic anemia or acute leukemia). At counts higher than 50,000/ mm^3, hemorrhage caused by platelet deficiency is unlikely. Spontaneous bleeding may occur in patients with platelet counts below 5000 to 10,000/mm^3, and prophylactic platelet infusions should be reserved for this level of thrombocytopenia.

Thrombocytosis

Thrombocytosis is a platelet count higher than 600,000/mm^3; Box 25-6 presents the list of potential causes. It is often caused by infection or iron deficiency. The primary or autonomous state may be associated with bleeding or thrombosis. It is often an associated finding in patients with polycythemia vera, myelofibrosis, or chronic myelogenous leukemia.

Disorders of the Coagulation Pathway

The clinically significant disorders have a number of characteristic features that help differentiate them from platelet disorders, including the following:

The bleeding source is often an intramuscular or deep soft tissue hematoma from small arterioles.

The congenital form of the disease occurs predo minantly in men, often as a sex-linked inheritance.

Bleeding may occur after surgery or trauma but is delayed in onset up to 72 hr.

Epistaxis, menorrhagia, and gastrointestinal sources of bleeding are rare, whereas hematuria and hemarthrosis are common in severe cases.

The bleeding time is normal except in patients with von Willebrand's disease.

The PT and PTT are the basic laboratory diagnostic tools for the evaluation of coagulation disorders and can be used to organize the approach to their diagnosis.

Abnormal Prothrombin Time and Other Test Results Normal

An elevated PT reflects an extrinsic pathway abnormality mediated through deficiency of factor Ⅶ. The acquired form is commonly seen and may be a result of vitamin K deficiency, warfarin use, or liver disease. The PT is a sensitive gauge of hepatic function and the efficacy of warfarin administration. INRs calculate the prothrombin ratio raised to the power of an international sensitivity index for specific thromboplastin reagents. It is recommended with most warfarin therapy that the INR be maintained between 2.0 and 3.0, except in the setting of cardiac valvular disease, in which the target INR is 2.5 to 3.5.

Abnormal Partial Thromboplastin Time and Other Test Results Normal

Two groups of inherited disorders manifest an isolated elevation in the PTT. The first group consists of the contact factors (e.g., Ⅻ [Hageman factor]), prekallikrein (Fletcher factor), and high-molecular-weight kininogen. They cause a benign disorder in which the PTT is elevated but the patient has no bleeding diathesis.

The second group causes significant bleeding problems resulting from deficiencies of factors within the intrinsic coagulation system. Deficiencies of factors Ⅷ, Ⅸ, and Ⅺ account for 99% of inherited bleeding disorders. Patients with active life-threatening bleeding can be supported with fresh frozen plasma, 15 mL/kg.

In a patient with a prolonged PTT and a lifelong history of bleeding, the most important test is assay of factor Ⅷ and factor IX. The two forms of this deficiency are hemophilia A and von Willebrand's disease.

Hemophilia A. Hemophilia A is caused by a variant form of factor Ⅷ that is present in normal levels but lacks a clot promoting property. Factor Ⅷ circulates in plasma in very low concentration and is normally bound to vWF. The source of factor Ⅷ production is uncertain, but hemophilia A can be corrected by liver transplantation. This severity may be directly related to the level of factor Ⅷ coagulant (factor Ⅷ:C) activity. Cases with less than 1% activity are severe, with a tendency toward spontaneous bleeding. Cases with 1% to 5% activity are moderate, with rare spontaneous bleeding. Cases with 5% to 10% activity and above are considered mild. The PTT may lack sensitivity for this group.

Bleeding can occur anywhere, but deep muscles, joints, the urinary tract, and intracranial sites are the most common. Recurrent hemarthrosis and progressive joint destruction are major causes of morbidity in hemophilia. Intracranial bleeding is the major cause of death in all age groups of hemophiliacs. Mucosal or gastrointestinal bleeding is rare. Trauma is a common initiator of bleeding in all stages of severity.

Management of Hemophilia A. Replacement

Therapy. The accepted therapy for hemophilia A is factor Ⅷ replacement with cryoprecipitate or factor Ⅷ:C concentrates.

As a general rule, 1 U/kg of factor Ⅷ will increase the circulating factor Ⅷ level by 2%. The dose of factor Ⅷ needed is the desired percentage increase in factor Ⅷ activity × 0.5 × the weight in kilograms. The typical percentage factor Ⅷ activity goals are 25% to 40% for minor bleeding or trauma, greater than 50% for moderate bleeding, and 80% to 100% for serious, life-threatening bleeding or trauma. Table 25-1 and Table 25-2 include guidelines for the recommended treatment in a variety of circumstances.

Table 25-1 Recommended Factor Ⅷ Therapy for Specific Problems in Hemophilia

TYPE OF BLEEDING	INITIAL DOSAGE	DURATION	COMMENT
Skin			
Abrasion	None	None	Treat with local pressure and topical thrombin
Laceration			
Superficial	Usually none; if necessary,treat as minor	None	Local pressure and anesthetic with epinephrine may benefit; watch 4 hr after suturing; reexamine in 24 hr
Deep	Minor bleeding (25 mg/kg)	Single-dose coverage	May need hospitalization for observation; repeated dose may be necessary for suture removal
Nasal epistaxis			
Spontaneous	Usually none; may need to be treated as mild bleeding	None	Uncommon; consider platelet inhibition; treat in usual manner
Traumatic	Moderate bleeding (25 mg/kg)	Up to 5-7 d	Trauma-related bleeding can be significant
Oral			
Mucosa or tongue bites	Usually none; treat as minor if persists	Single dose	Commonly seen
Traumatic (laceration) or dental extraction	Moderate (25 U/kg) to severe (50 U/kg)	Single dose; may need more	Saliva rich in fibrin lytic activity; oral ε-aminocaproic acid (Amicar) may be given at 100 mg every 6 hr for 7 d to block fibrinolysis; check contraindications; hospitalize patients with severe bleeding
Soft tissue or muscle hematomas	Moderate (25 U/kg) to severe (50 U/kg)	2-5 d	May be complicated by local pressure on nerves or vessels (e.g., iliopsoas, forearm, calf)
Hemarthrosis			
Early	Mild (25 mg/kg)	Single dose	Treat at earliest symptom (pain); knee, elbow, ankle more common
Late or unresponsive cases of early hemarthrosis	Mild to moderate (25 U/kg)	3-4 d	Arthrocentesis rarely necessary and only with 50% level coverage; immobilization is critical point of therapy
Hematuria	Mild (12.5 U/kg)	2-3 d	Urokinase, the fibrinolytic enzyme, is in urine; with persistent hematuria, an organic cause should be ruled out
Major or life-threatening bleeding	Major bleeding (50 U/kg)	7-10 d or 3-5 d after bleeding ceases	In head trauma, therapy should be given prophylactically; early computed tomography scan of head is recommended for all

Table 25-2 Dosage of Factor VIII (Antihemophilic Factor)

BLEEDING RISK	DESIRED FACTOR VIII LEVEL (%)	INITIAL DOSE (U/kg)
Mild	5-10	12.5
Moderate	20-30	25
Severe	50 or greater	50

Standard Calculation

1. Patient's plasma volume (50 mL/kg × weight in kg) × (desired level of factor VIII [percent]) − (present level of factor VIII [percent]) =number of units for initial dose.
2. In emergency therapy, the present level of factor VIII is assumed to be zero.
3. One unit is the activity of the coagulation factor present in 1 mL of normal human plasma.
4. Because the half-life of factor VIII is 8 to 12 hr, the desired level is maintained by giving half the initial dose every 8 to 12 hr.
5. Cryoprecipitate is assumed to have 80 to 100 U of factor VIII:C per bag; factor VIII:C concentrates list the units per bottle on the label.

The response to therapy can be monitored by clinical improvement, a decreasing PTT, and, optimally, serial factor VIII:C activity levels. The lack of a response to factor VIII administration should raise the possibility of circulating IgG antibodies. A variety of therapies have been considered, including "overwhelming" factor VIII doses, exchange plasmapheresis, immuno-suppressive therapy, and the infusion of prothrombin complexes containing activated clotting factors. Other recommended therapies include porcine factor VIII and recombinant activated factor VIIa. Acquired IgG antihemophilic factor antibodies may exist in nonhemophiliac patients.

Desmopressin acetate has been shown to increase levels of factors VIII:C and VIII:Ag in patients with hemophilia A and in some with von Willebrand's disease. It is given intravenously at 0.3 μg/kg per dose. Benefits are primarily noted in patients with mild to moderate disease, and the effects of a single dose last for 4 to 6 hr.

Prophylaxis. It is recommended that patients who sustain head trauma but who have normal CT scans have factor VIII therapy initiated to greater than 50% activity level. Gene therapy represents a potential development in the treatment of hemophilia.

VON Willebrand's Disease. Factor VIII has at least three activities. First is its antihemophilic, or coagulant, activity, VIII:C. A second activity supports platelet adhesion ; it is called von Wille brand's factor activity, or VIII/vWF. A third component reacts with rabbit antibodies to factor VIII; it is termed the factor VIII antigen, or VIII:Ag, and relates to the measured plasma level rather than to the activity of factor VIII. The antigen and cofactor activity for platelet function are structurally related. von Willebrand's disease has both decreased factor VIII:Ag levels and decreased VIII:C activity secondary to underproduction. The patient's platelets are normal in number, morphologic condition, and other functions, but in the absence of circulating factor VIII/vWF, their adhering properties are diminished. The disease occurs as an autosomal dominant trait with a variable penetrance pattern.

Manifestations of von Willebrand's disease are usually milder and less crippling than those of hemophilia. The factor VIII:C level is in the 6% to 50% range. Bleeding sites are predominantly mucosal (e.g., epistaxis) and cutaneous. Menorrhagia and gastrointestinal bleeding are common. Laboratory differentiation from hemophilia A includes abnormal bleeding time, decreased level of factor VIII:Ag, and abnormal platelet aggregation with ristocetin. In patients with severe disease, replacement therapy with factor VIII in the form of intermediate purity factor VIII concentrate is the method of choice. The initial dose is 25 to 50 U/kg every 12 hr to keep vWF levels at 50% or to control bleeding. After the initial dose, fewer units are necessary, and longer dosage schedules may be followed by a clinical response and a combination of factor VIII:C activity and serial bleeding times.

In extreme circumstances without alternatives, fresh frozen plasma may be used. A factor VIII concentrate (Humate-P) has also demonstrated sufficient VIII/vWF to treat the disease. Drug therapy with desmopressin is of benefit in patients with mild to moderately severe von Willebrand's disease.

Hemophilia B (Christmas Disease). Hemophilia B is a deficiency of factor IX activity. Factor IX is a vitamin K–dependent glycoprotein. Its deficiency is diagnosed by a factor IX assay, usually after the factor VIII:C assay is found to be normal. Clinical concerns and treatment strategies associated with hemophilia A also apply to hemophilia B.

Miscellaneous Coagulation Disorders

Disseminated Intravascular Coagulation. DIC is a relatively common acquired coagulopathy. Hemostasis is achieved by a fine balance between procoagulants and inhibitors and thrombus formation and lysis. The balance may be disturbed by pathologic processes that result in an out-of-control coagulation and fibrinolytic cascade within the systemic circulation . The following occurs in this abnormal clotting sequence:

Platelets and coagulation factors are consumed, especially fibrinogen and factors V, Ⅷ, and XIII.

Thrombin is formed, and it overwhelms its inhibitor system and acts to accelerate the coagulation process and directly activate fibrinogen.

Fibrin is deposited in small vessels in multiple organs.

The fibrinolytic system by means of plasmin may lyse fibrin and impair thrombin formation.

FDP are released and affect platelet function and inhibit fibrin polymerization.

Coagulation inhibition levels (e.g., antithrombin III, protein C, and tissue factor pathway inhibitor) are decreased.

The clinical consequence of these processes is the life-threatening combination of a bleeding diathesis. The condition needs to be considered in any patient in whom purpura, a bleeding tendency, and signs of organ injury, particularly of the CNS and kidney, develop. The clinical diagnosis of DIC is confrmed by laboratory tests (Table 25-3).

Table 25-3 Laboratory Diagnosis of DIC

TEST	FINDING	PATHOPHYSIOLOGY
Peripheral smear	Low platelets, schistocytes, red blood cell fragments	Red blood cell fragmentation on fibrin strands; schistocytes not always seen
Platelet count	Low (usually <100,000/mm^3)	Consumed in clotting; lower numbers are reflected in the bleeding time
Prothrombin time	Prolonged	Factors Ⅱ and IV consumed
Partial thromboplastin time	Prolonged	Factors Ⅱ, V, and Ⅷ consumed
Thrombin time	Prolonged	Decrease in factor Ⅱ and fibrin degradation products
Fibrinogen level	Low	Factor Ⅱ consumed; may be difficult to interpret because it is an acute-phase reactant
Fibrin degradation products (D-dimer)	Zero to large	Dependent on the amount of secondary fibrinolysis
Serum creatinine or urinalysis	May be abnormal	Functional assessment of the organ most commonly injured by fibrin deposition

Two conditions that may simulate DIC are severe liver disease and primary fbrinolysis.

Many episodes of DIC are self-limited.

Replacement therapy is usually instituted simultaneously with attempts to control the primary process. If active bleeding is present, replacement therapy with platelets, FFP, and cryoprecipitate (Ⅰ, V, Ⅷ) is recommended. Selective replacement therapy can be based on the laboratory and clinical response. Retardation of bleeding, a decrease in FDP, and a rise in platelet counts and fibrinogen levels are useful monitors.

Heparin has selective use in the treatment of DIC when fibrin deposition and thrombosis dominate the pathologic picture. Examples include purpura fulminans, retained dead fetus before delivery, giant hemangioma, and acute promyelocytic leukemia. Low doses of heparin (300-500 units/hr) as a continuous infusion are currently recommended. LMWH may also be used instead of unfractionated heparin. Continuous monitoring of the clinical response, heparin levels, and bleeding status is necessary.

Recombinant activated protein C (drotrecogin alfa) has been associated with improved outcomes in septic shock, regardless of whether DIC was present.

DISPOSITION

All patients with bleeding disorders of unknown cause should be admitted to the hospital for further evaluation. Because of the delayed bleeding pattern in hemophiliacs, it may be especially hazardous to transfer them long distances.

(SHOU Songtao)

Metabolic Emergencies

Chapter 26

Diabetic Emergency

KEY CONCEPTS

Severe hypoglycemia is usually associated with a blood glucose level below 40 to 50 mg/dL and impaired cognitive function.

For patients with known or suspected ingestion of hypoglycemic agents, we recommend 23 hr of observation.

The essential treatment of DKA includes restoration of insulin, correction of dehydration, correction of potassium level, correction of acidosis, and treatment of the underlying cause.

Hyperglycemic hyperosmolar state is most commonly seen in elders with multiple comorbid conditions and is distinguished from DKA by lack of ketoacidosis.

DIABETES MELLITUS

Perspective

DM comprises a heterogeneous group of hyperglycemic disorders characterized by high serum glucose concentration and disturbances of carbohydrate and lipid metabolism.Acute complications include hypoglycemia, DKA, and hyperglycemic hyperosmolar state(HHS).

Pathophysiology and Etiology

Type 1 DM results from a chronic autoimmune process. The classic manifestations of type 1—hyperglycemia and ketosis occur late in the course of the disease, an overt sign of beta cell destruction. The exact cause of DM remains unclear.

Clinical Features

Type 1

The patient with type 1 DM is usually lean, younger than 40 yr, and ketosis prone. Onset of symptoms may be abrupt, with polydipsia, polyuria, polyphagia,and weight loss developing rapidly. In some cases the disease is heralded by ketoacidosis. Myriad problems related to type 1 DM include acute metabolic complications,such as DKA, and late complications, such as cardiovascular or circulatory abnormalities, retinopathy, nephropathy,neuropathy, foot ulcers, severe infections, and various skin lesions.

Type 2

The patient with type 2 DM is usually middle-aged or older and overweight.

Symptoms tend to begin more gradually in type 2 DM than in type 1. The diagnosis of type 2 is often made by the discovery of an elevated blood glucose level on routine laboratory examination. Decompensation of disease usually leads to HHS rather than to ketoacidosis.

Diagnostic Strategies

Serum Glucose

As a rule, any random plasma glucose level above 200 mg/dL, fasting plasma glucose concentration above 126 mg/dL, or 2 hr postload OGTT is sufficient to establish the diagnosis of DM.

Glycosylated Hemoglobin

Measurement of glycosylated hemoglobin

(HbA1c) is one of the most important ways to assess the level of glucose control. HbA1c value above 6.5%. Given the long half-life of red blood cells, the percentage of HbA1c is an index of glucose concentration of the preceding 6 to 8 w, with normal values approximately 4% to 6% of total hemoglobin. The ADA currently sets an HbA1c value of less than 7% as a treatment goal.

Urine Glucose

Urine glucose measurement methods are basically of two types:reagent tests and dipstick tests. The reagent tests (e.g., Clinitest) are copper reduction tests.Dipstick tests generally use glucose oxidase. Dipsticks may vary in their sensitivity and strength of reaction to a given concentration of glucose. With the "plus" system, 1+, 2+, 3+, and 4+ have different implications about urine glucose concentrations.

Urine Ketones

Urine ketone dipsticks is a good test for acetoacetate but does not measure β-hydroxybutyrate. Although the usual acetoacetate/β-hydroxybutyrate ratio in DKA is 1 : 2.8, it may be as high as 1 : 30, in which case the urine dipstick does not reflect the true level of ketosis.

Dipstick Blood Glucose

Dipsticks for testing of blood glucose are clearly more accurate than urine dipsticks as a means of monitoring blood glucose concentration. Hematocrits below 30% or above 55% cause unduly high or low readings, respectively. The largest errors are in the hyperglycemic range. Dipstick readings rarely err more than 30 mg/dL when actual concentrations are below 90 mg/dL.

HYPOGLYCEMIA

Hypoglycemia is a common problem in patients with type 1 DM. Severe hypoglycemia is usually associated with a blood glucose level below 40 to 50 mg/dL and impaired cognitive function and may be associated with significant mortality.

Principles of Disease

Hypoglycemia has many causes: missing a meal (decreased intake), increased energy output (exercise), and increased insulin dosage.Oral hypoglycemic agents have also been implicated in causing hypoglycemia.

Hypoglycemia is a dangerous complication of type 1 DM. Even a single hypoglycemic episode can reduce neurohumoralcounter-regulatory responses to subsequent episodes.Other factors associated with recurrent hypoglycemic attacks include overaggressive or intensified insulin therapy, longer history of DM, autonomic neuropathy, and decreased epinephrine secretion or sensitivity.

The Somogyi phenomenon is a common problem associated with iatrogenic hypoglycemia in the type 1 diabetic patient. The phenomenon is initiated by an excessive insulin dosage, which results in an unrecognized hypoglycemic episode that usually occurs in the early morning while the patient is sleeping. The counter-regulatory hormone response produces rebound hyperglycemia,evident when the patient awakens.

Clinical Features

Signs and symptoms of hypoglycemia include sweating, nervousness, tremor, tachycardia, hunger, and neurologic symptoms ranging from bizarre behavior and confusion to seizures and coma. Patients with hypoglycemia may have a seizure or show focal neurologic signs,which resolve with glucose administration.

Diagnostic Strategies

The cardinal laboratory test for hypoglycemia is the determination of blood glucose concentration.

If factitious hypoglycemia is suggested, testing for insulin antibodies or low levels of C peptide may be helpful. A patient who is surreptitiously administering exogenous insulin will have normal to low levels of C peptide and markedly elevated insulin levels.

Management

In alert patients with mild symptoms, oral consumption of sugar containing foods or beverages is often adequate. In other patients,after blood is drawn for glucose determination, one to three ampules of 50% dextrose in water ($D_{50}W$) is administered intravenously while the patient's airway, breathing, and circulation are assessed and maintained.

If intravenous access cannot be rapidly obtained, 1 to 2 mg of glucagon may be given intramuscularly or subcutaneously. The onset of action is 10 to 20 min, and peak response occurs in 30 to 60 min. It may be repeated as needed. Glucagon may also be administered intravenously; 1 mg has an effect similar to that of one ampule of $D_{50}W$.

Intranasal glucagon has not been widely used.

Although the response to intravenous administration of glucose is generally rapid, older patients may require several days for complete recovery.

Treatment of hypoglycemia secondary to oral hypoglycemic agents depends on the agent.Patients at risk, for hypoglycemia from oral sulfonylureas include patients with impaired renal function. However,onset of symptoms was delayed up to 18 hr in some patients.As a result, we recommend 23 hr of observation for patients with known or suspected ingestion of hypoglycemic agents.

Disposition

Type 1 diabetic patients with brief episodes of hypoglycemia uncomplicated by other disease may be discharged from the ED if a cause of the hypoglycemia can be identified and corrected by instruction or medication. All patients should be given a meal before discharge to ensure their ability to tolerate oral feedings.Patients who are discharged should receive short-term follow-up for ongoing evaluation. Patients with hypoglycemia caused by long-acting sulfonylurea medications should be observed in the hospital if they have recurrent hypoglycemia after a period of observation in the ED.

DIABETIC KETOACIDOSIS

Principles of Disease

Pathophysiology

DKA is a syndrome in which insulin deficiency and glucagon excess combine to produce a hyperglycemic, dehydrated, acidotic patient with profound electrolyte imbalance. All derangements producing DKA are interrelated and are based on insulin deficiency (Fig. 26-1). DKA may be caused by cessation of insulin intake or by physical or emotional stress.

When the hyperglycemia becomes sufficiently marked, the renal threshold is surpassed and glucose is excreted in the urine. The hyperosmolarity is the most important determinant of the patient's mental status.

This osmotic diuresis, combined with poor

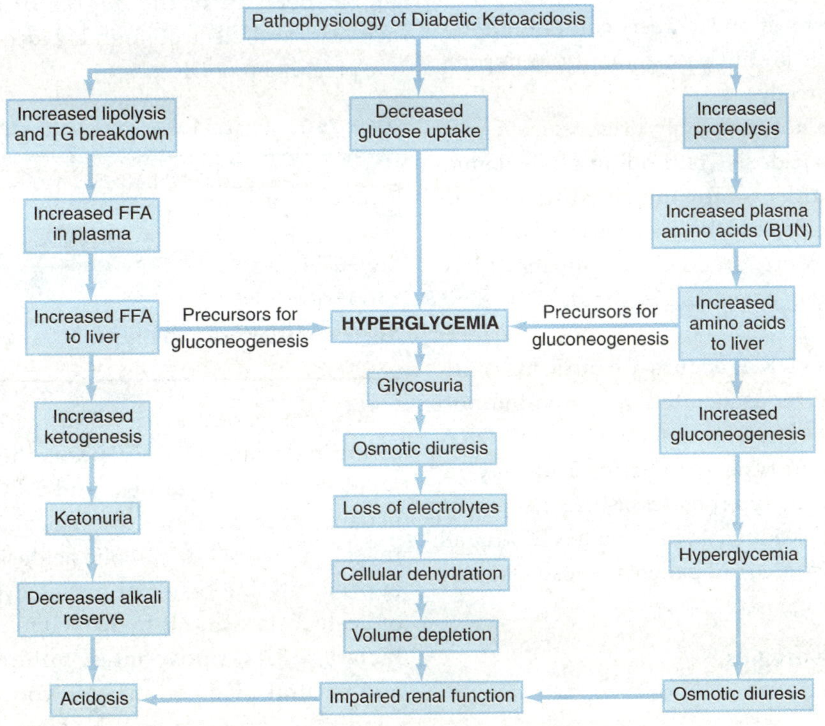

Fig. 26-1 Syndrome of diabetic ketoacidosis.

intake and vomiting, produces the profound dehydration and electrolyte imbalance associated with DKA (Table 26-1).

Potassium, magnesium, and phosphorus deficits of patients with DKA are usually marked. Hypokalemia may further inhibit insulin release.

Table 26-1 Average Fluid and Electrolyte Deficits in Severe DKA

WEI-GHT	WATER (mL/kg)	SODIUM (mEq/L)	POTASS-IUM (mEq/L)	CHLORIDE (mEq/L)	PHOSPHO RUS(mEq/L)
≤10 kg	100-120	8-10	5-7	6-8	3
10-20 kg	80-100	8-10	5-7	6-8	3
≥20 kg	70-80	8-10	5-7	6-8	3

Despite the increased pathologic glucagon-mediated production of ketones, the body acts as it does in any form of starvation to decrease the peripheral tissue's use of ketones as fuel. The combination of increased ketone production with decreased ketone use leads to ketoacidosis.

The degree of ketosis has been related to the magnitude of release of the counter-regulatory hormones epinephrine, glucagon,cortisol, and somatostatin. Glucagon is elevated fourfold to fivefold in DKA and is the most influential ketogenic hormone.Epinephrine,norepinephrine, cortisol, growth hormone, dopamine, and thyroxine enhance ketogenesis indirectly by stimulating lipolysis.

The acidotic patient attempts to increase lung ventilation to rid the body of excess acid with Kussmaul's respiration.Acidosis compounds the effects of ketosis and hyperosmolality to depress mental status directly.

Acidemia is not invariably present, even with significant ketoacidosis.The finding of alkalemia, however, should prompt the consideration of alcoholic ketoacidosis.If there is concern for mixed acid-base disorders, an ABG sample should be obtained instead of a venous gas sampl.

Etiology

Most often, DKA occurs in patients with type 1 DM and is associated with inadequate administration of insulin, infection, or MI. DKA can also occur in type 2 diabetics and may be associated with any type of stress, such as sepsis or gastrointestinal bleeding. Approximately 25% of all episodes of DKA occur in patients whose DM was previously undiagnosed.

Diagnostic Strategies

History

Clinically, most patients with DKA complain of a recent history of polydipsia, polyuria, polyphagia, visual blurring, weakness, weight loss, nausea, vomiting, and abdominal pain. Approximately half of these patients, report abdominal pain. In adults, however, abdominal pain more often signifies true abdominal disease.

Physical Examination

Typical findings of Physical examination include tachypnea with Kussmaul's respiration, tachycardia, frank hypotension or orthostatic BPchanges, the odor of acetone on the breath, and signs of dehydration. An elevated temperature suggests the presence of infection.

Laboratory Tests

Initial tests allow preliminary confirmation of the diagnosis and immediate initiation of therapy (Table 26-2).Subsequent tests are made to determine more specifically the degree of dehydration, acidosis, and electrolyte imbalance and to reveal the precipitant of DKA.

Table 26-2 Typical Laboratory Values in DKA and HHS

	DKA	HHS
Glucose (mg/dL)	>350	>700
Sodium (mEq)	low 130s	140s
Potassium (mEq)	≈4.5-6.0	≈5
Bicarbonate (mEq)	<10	>15
Blood urea nitrogen (mg/dL)	25-50	>50
Serum ketones	Present	Absent

On the patient's arrival to the ED, check the serum and urine glucose concentrations and ketone level, electrolyte values, and ABG. Glucose is usually elevated above 350 mg/dL. ABG usually reveals a low pH. Metabolic acidosis with an AG is primarily the result of elevated plasma levels of acetoacetate and β-hydroxybutyrate, although lactate, FFAs, phosphates, volume depletion, and several medications also contribute to this condition. Rarely, a well-hydrated patient with

DKA may have a pure hyperchloremic acidosis with no anion gap If an immediate potassium level is not available through blood gas analysis, an ECG may indicate elevated potassium levels. A CBC may be used to rule out other concomitant issues, such as anemia.Decisions about volume replacement need to be made irrespective of whether an azotemia is noted on blood chemistry testing.Urinalysis, in addition to the presence of ketones, may also help confirm a urinary tract infection as a precipitant of DKA. Sodium is often low in the presence of significant dehydration.When hyperglycemia is marked, thereby creating dilutional hyponatremia. Hypertriglyceridemia is common in DKA. In the absence of marked lipidemia, the true value of sodium may be approximated by adding 1.3 to 1.6 mEq/L to the sodium value on the laboratory report for every 100 mg/dL glucose above the norm.The effect of acidosis on the serum potassium determination can be corrected by subtracting 0.6 mEq/L from the laboratory potassium value for every 0.1 decrease in pH noted in the ABG analysis. Serum creatinine determinations may be falsely elevated. Leukocytosis more closely reflects the degree of ketosis than the presence of infection. Only the elevation of band neutrophils has been demonstrated to indicate the presence of infection.

Differential Considerations

Alcoholics with Kussmaul's respiration, a fruity odor to the breath, and acidemic ABG values may have alcoholic ketoacidosis. These patients may be euglycemic or hypoglycemic.The differential diagnosis for DKA includes any entity that may cause elevated AG acidosis, ketosis, or both. The presence of DKA should not exclude investigation for other causes of AG metabolic acidosis, such as sepsis, poisoning, or lactic acidosis.

Management

General Measures

The comatose patient with severe DKA, especially if vomiting, requires intubation.The patient in hypovolemic shock requires aggressive fluid resuscitation with 0.9% saline solution. Close monitoring of vital signs is essential. Bedside ultrasonography may be of benefit in excluding other causes of hypotension and evaluating the volume status of an individual patient. Likewise, evaluation of myocardial contractility and inferior vena cava diameter can help evaluate cardiac function and volume status noninvasively.When hyperglycemia, ketosis, and acidosis have been established, begin fluid, electrolyte, and insulin therapy (Box 26-1).

Box 26-1 Summary of Treatment of Diabetic Ketoacidosis

Identify diabetic ketoacidosis: serum glucose concentration,electrolyte values, ketone level, and arterial blood gas analysis;also obtain complete blood count with differential, urinalysis,chest radiograph, and electrocardiogram, if indicated.

Supplement insulin.
- Insulin replacement: 0.1 unit/kg/hr regular insulin IV
- Change IV solution to D5W/0.45% NS when glucose concentration is ≤300 mg/dL.

Rehydrate.
- 1-2 L NS IV during 1-3 hr
- Children: 20 mL/kg NS during first hour
- Follow with 0.45% NS

Correct electrolyte abnormalities.
- Sodium: Correct with administration of NS and 0.45% NS.
- Potassium: Ensure adequate renal function. Add 20-40 mEq KCl to each liter of fluid until ketoacidosis is corrected and potassium is normalized.
- Phosphorus: Usually unnecessary to replenish
- Magnesium: Correct with 1-2 g MgSO4. Serum magne sium levels may not correlate with body stores.

Correct acidosis.
- Correction of acidosis is done by administration of IV fluids and insulin.

Search for and correct underlying precipitant.

Monitor progress and keep meticulous flow sheets.
- Vital signs
- Fluid intake and urine output
- Serum glucose, K^+, Cl^-, HCO_3^-, CO_2, pH
- Amount of insulin administered

Admit to hospital or intensive care unit.
- Consider outpatient therapy in children with reliable caretaker

and
- Initial pH ≥ 7.35
- Initial HCO_3^- ≥ 20 mEq/L
- Can tolerate oral fluids
- Resolution of symptoms after treatment in emergency department
- No underlying precipitant requiring hospitalization

Insulin

Insulin therapy should be initiated as soon as the diagnosis of DKA is certain. In selected patients with mild DKA, the subcutaneous or intramuscular administration of insulin has been proved safe and as effective as the intravenous administration of insulin. The current therapy of choice as recommended by the ADA is regular insulin infused at 0.1 unit/kg/hr up to 5 to 10 units/kg/hr, mixed with the intravenous fluids. The use of higher doses of insulin and aggressive fluid resuscitation contributes to the development of cerebral edema comes .Because the half-life of regular insulin is 3 to 10 min, insulin should be administered intravenously by constant infusion.When the blood glucose concentration has dropped to 250 to 300 mg/dL, add dextrose to the intravenous fluids to prevent iatrogenic hypoglycemia and cerebral edema. In patients with euglycemic DKA, add dextrose to the intravenous fluids at the start of insulin therapy.

Dehydration

The severely dehydrated adult patient is likely to have a fluid deficit of 3 to 5 L. If the patient is in hypovolemic shock, administer NS as rapidly as possible in the adult until a SBP of 80 mm Hg is obtained. In the adult who has marked dehydration in the absence of clinical shock or heart failure, 1 L of NS may be administered in the first hour. In general, 2 L of NS during the first 1 to 3 hours is followed by a slower infusion of half-NS solution. Adjust the fluid rate according to age, cardiac status, and degree of dehydration to achieve a urine output of 1 to 2 mL/kg/hr.Fluid resuscitation alone may help lower hyperglycemia.In addition, a large volume of glucose may be cleared by the kidneys in response to improved renal perfusion. Thus, fluid resuscitation is an important factor in management of DKA. Acidosis also decreases after fluid infusion alone. Increased perfusion improves tissue oxygenation, thus diminishing the formation of lactate. Increased renal perfusion promotes renal hydrogen ion loss, and the improved action of insulin in the better-hydrated patient inhibits ketogenesis.

Potassium

In the patients with DKA, the initial potassium level is often normal or high . Potassium levels often plummet with correction of acidosis and administration of insulin.In patients with low serum potassium concentration at presentation, hypokalemia may become life-threatening when insulin therapy is administered; therefore, intravenous administration of potassium in concentrations of 20 to 40 mEq/L is required. If the measured serum phosphorus is low, it should be replaced with potassium phosphates.

Magnesium

Magnesium deficiency is a common problem in patients with DKA without renal disease. Magnesium deficiency may exacerbate vomiting and mental changes, promote hypokalemia and hypocalcemia, or induce fatal cardiac dysrhythmia. The normal person requires 0.30 to 0.35 mEq/kg/day. Thus, it is reasonable to include 0.35 mEq/kg of magnesium in the fluids of the first 3 to 4 hr.

Acidosis

Bicarbonate therapy may be indicated in severely acidemic patients (pH $\leqslant$ 7.0). Overly rapid correction of acidosis is contraindicated because the blood-brain barrier is much more permeable to carbon dioxide than to bicarbonate.In the short term, however, as the blood acidosis is corrected, the acidity of the fluid surrounding the brain increases, causing paradoxical cerebrospinal fluid acidosis. The administration of bicarbonate increases the potassium requirement. The overaggressive use of bicarbonate may produce alkalosis, which induces dysrhythmias.Bicarbonate can increase ketonuria and delay the fall in serum ketones compared with saline infusion alone. Bicarbonate worsens the prognosis even in patients with severe acidosis and pH values in the range 6.9 to 7.1. It is possible to manage severe DKA with fluids and insulin alone.

Complications

Morbidity in DKA is largely iatrogenic: hypokalemia from inadequate potassium replacement, hypoglycemia from failure to replenish glucose in intravenous solutions when serum glucose concentration drops below 250 to 300 mg/dL, alkalosis from overaggressive bicarbonate replacement, and pulmonary edema from overaggressive hydration. The primary causes of death of patients with DKA remain infection , arterial thromboses, and shock.

Disposition

Most patients with DKA require hospital admission, often to ICU.

HYPERGLYCEMIC HYPEROSMOLAR STATE

HHS characterized by marked hyperglycemia, hyperosmolarity and dehydration, and decreased mental functioning that may progress to frank coma.Ketoacidosis is generally minimal or absent, although metabolic acidosis from another source, such as lactic acidosis from sepsis or uremia from acute renal failure, may be present. Focal neurologic signs may be present, or there may be a global encephalopathy. DKA and HHS may occur together.

Principles of Disease

Pathophysiology

As with DKA, the pathophysiologic mechanism of HHS varies with the particular patient. Because most patients with HHS are elders, decreased renal clearance of glucose produced by the decline of renal function with age often contributes to the illness. As with DKA, decreased insulin action results in glycogenolysis, gluconeogenesis, and decreased peripheral uptake of glucose. The hyperglycemia pulls fluid from the intracellular space into the extracellular space. Soon, however, this fluid is lost in a profound osmotic diuresis, limited finally by hypotension and a subsequent drop in the GFR. The urine is extremely hypotonic. This hypotonic diuresis produces profound dehydration, leading to hyperglycemia, hypernatremia, and associated hypertonicity.The reason for the absence of ketoacidosis in HHS is unknown. FFA levels are lower than in DKA, thus limiting substrates needed to form ketones. The most likely reason for the blunted counter-regulatory hormone release and lack of ketosis seems to be the continued secretion of tiny amounts of insulin that block ketogenesis.

Etiology

HHS is a syndrome of severe dehydration that results from a sustained hyperglycemic diuresis under circumstances in which the patient is unable to drink sufficient fluids to offset the urinary losses. HHS is most common in elders with type 2 DM. HHS may occur in patients who are not diabetic, especially after burns, parenteral hyperalimentation, peritoneal dialysis, or hemodialysis.

Clinical Features

If they are awake, patients may complain of fever, thirst, polyuria, or oliguria. Approximately 20% of patients have no known history of type 2 DM. The most common associated diseases are chronic renal insufficiency, gram-negative pneumonia, gastrointestinal bleeding, and gram-negative sepsis. Approximately 85% of patients have underlying renal or cardiac impairment. Arterial and venous thromboses are common. The patient often exhibits orthostatic hypotension or frank hypotension, tachycardia, and fever with signs of marked dehydration. The depression of the sensorium correlates directly with the degree and rate of development of hyperosmolarity. Neurologic issues are common in HHS. Whereas decreased level of consciousness is the most common neurologic finding, seizures, stroke syndromes, and movement disorders have been reported.

Diagnostic Strategies

Laboratory findings usually reveal a blood glucose level above 600 mg/dL and serum osmolarity above 350 mOsm/L. The blood urea nitrogen concentration is invariably elevated.The patient with HHS typically has a more profound electrolyte imbalance than the patient with DKA. Levels of potassium, magnesium, and phosphorus may seem initially high, even in the presence of marked total deficit.

Management

The fluid, electrolyte, and insulin regimens for the initial resuscitation in HHS are subject to the same controversies as the therapies for DKA (Box 26-1).Use of an isotonic crystalloid is a reasonable choice in the volume depleted patient.

Dehydration

For patients in coma or hypovolemic shock, initial intravenous fluid infusion is given as rapidly as possible. Add glucose to resuscitation fluids when the blood glucose level drops below

300 mg/ dL.

Electrolytes

Measurement of serum electrolytes should be used to guide replacement in the HHS patient. In particular, because the degree of acidosis is generally less, potassium levels more accurately reflect total body stores than they do in DKA.

Insulin

In patients with very high glucose levels (>700 mg/dL), in whom intramuscular or subcutaneous insulin absorption may be erratic. If an intravenous insulin infusion is used, it should be done at an infusion rate similar to that for DKA (0.1 unit/kg/hr).

Complications

Many patients with HHS are elders who have underlying cardiac and renal disease. The mortality rate of treated HHS patients ranges from 8% to 25%.

Disposition

In general, patients with HHS require hospitalization for intravenous hydration, glucose control, and evaluation of precipitating and complicating conditions.

CONTROL OF DIABETES

The common oral antidiabetic agents are presented in Table 26-3. There are several preparations of insulin available as well. Other newer agents include the incretin mimetics, such as exenatide, which is used for type 2 DM; it is injectable and used in conjunction with oral agents but not with insulin. Amylin analogues, such as pramlintide, are used with insulin but significantly increase the risk of hypoglycemia. The basic concepts of the diabetic diet remain unchanged. Various high-fiber diets have improved glycemic control. Exercise continues to be a cornerstone of DM management. Solid organ pancreas transplants have become more common.

Infections

Diabetic patients have an increased incidence of extremity infections and pyelonephritis compared with the general population.Treatment of diabetic patients with infection includes rapid culture and antibiotics (Table 26-4), glycemic control,and generally hospitalization.

Table 26-3 Common Oral Diabetic Medications

Biguanides (metformin)	Decrease hepatic glycogenolysis	500-1000 mg twice daily
Sulfonylureas (glipizide,glimepiride)	Stimulate pancreatic insulin release	2.5-5 mg daily
Thiazolidinediones(pioglitazone,rosiglitazone)	Insulin sensitizers,decrease hepatic gluconeogenesis	Increased risk of adverse cardiac events
Meglitinides(repaglinide, nateglinide)	Stimulate postprandial insulin release	Take with meals only
Dipeptidyl peptidase 4 inhibitors (sitagliptin)	Decrease insulin degradation and gluconeogenesis	Once a day; can be found in multiple combination medications
α-Glucosidase inhibitors (acarbose, miglitol)	Delay breakdown of carbohydrates in the intestines	Major side effect is diarrhea

Table 26-4 Common Serious Infections in Diabetics and Their Antimicrobial Therapy

INFECTIOUS CONDITION	ANTIMICROBIALS
Diabetic foot infection	Mild: consider trimethoprimsulfamethoxazole 800/160 twice daily or clindamycin 300 mg q6h Moderate to severe: clindamycin 600 mg IV q6h ± piperacillin-tazobactam (Zosyn) 3.375 g IV q6h and vancomycin 15 mg/kg IV q12h
Malignant otitis externa	Oral: ciprofloxacin 500 mg PO twice daily for 10-14 d IV: ceftazidime 2 g IV q8h ± gentamicin 2 mg/kg IV q8h

Continued

INFECTIOUS CONDITION	ANTIMICROBIALS
Mucormycosis	Amphotericin B 1-1.5 mg/kg/day Posaconazole 400 mg twice daily
Mucocutaneous candidiasis	Ketoconazole 200 mg PO daily; may need several weeks of therapy
Nonclostridial gas gangrene (including Fournier's)	Clindamycin 600 mg q6h + thirdgeneration cephalosporin + vancomycin 15 mg/kg q12h

Insulin Allergy

Insulin allergy is manifested by local itching or pain and delayed brawny edema, urticaria, or anaphylaxis. Systemic reactions are usually seen in patients who have previously discontinued insulin and then resumed therapy. Mild reactions may be treated with antihistamines, whereas anaphylaxis must be treated with epinephrine. Patients with significant reactions must be admitted for desensitization.

(SHOU Songtao ZHAI Jianhua)

Chapter 27

Electrolyte Disorders

KEY CONCEPTS

Renal failure is the most common cause of confirmed hyperkalemia.Rapid rises in serum potassium concentration may be seen in tumor lysis syndrome, rhabdomyolysis, or massive hemolysis. Nearly any cardiac arrhythmia can be seen with hyperkalemia.

Intravenous calcium should be used only for hyperkalemic emergencies.

After the critical decision about administration of calcium has been made, a beta$_2$-agonist, insulin and glucose, normal saline, and bicarbonate (if the patient is acidotic) can be given to shift potassium intracellularly..

Hypokalemia is often seen in association with hypomagnesemia.

Hypokalemia is a common adverse effect may cause fatal arrhythmias and increase the risk of digitalis toxicity.

Diabetes insipidus, a condition that results in insufficient production of or lack of response to antidiuretic hormone, can lead to lifethreatening hypernatremia.

Hyponatremia has many causes, they fall into four general categories: pseudohyponatremia, hyponatremia with dehydration and decreased extracellular volume, hyponatremia with increased extracellular volume, and euvolemic hyponatremia with increased total body water

CNS damage due to hyponatremia may be caused by cerebral edema and increased ICP.

It is also important to consider adrenal insufficiency when a dehydrated patient has both hyponatremia and hyperkalemia.

Patients in hypercalcemic crisis are usually dehydrated, often obtunded, and also predisposed to arrhythmias; thus they require intravenous access with a normal saline infusion and close monitoring.

PERSPECTIVE

Electrolyte abnormalities are common in emergency medicine and can vary greatly in importance, severity, and symptoms.

HYPERKALEMIA

Principles of Disease

Hyperkalemia is the most dangerous acute electrolyte abnormality, potentially leading to life-threatening arrhythmias and death. Hyperkalemia depends on risk factors for impaired potassium excretion, such as dehydration and renal failure, along with an awareness of medications that cause potassium retention. Upwards of 98% of potassium in the body is contained intracellularly, whereas less than 2% remains circulating in the blood. Serum potassium concentration is normally between 3.5 and 5.0 mEq/L and is tightly regulated by the kidney. In the healthy state, at least 90% of potassium excretion occurs through the kidney; in the renally impaired state, the gastrointestinal tract may account for roughly 25% of excretion. Hyperkalemia usually develops from impaired renal excretion or increased release from cells; however, in advanced chronic kidney disease or end-stage renal disease, dietary intake of potassium may be a significant factor in its development.Hyperkalemia causes cardiotoxicity.Nearly any cardiac arrhythmia can be seen with hyperkalemia, including heart blocks, bradydysrhythmias, pseudoinfarction ST segment elevation, and the classic "sine wave" pattern.

As hyperkalemia advances, the end result is cardiac arrest.A serum potassium level of 10.0 mEq/L is usually fatal. The most common cause of hyperkalemia is spurious elevation due to hemolysis. Renal failure is the most common cause of confirmed hyperkalemia. Box 27-1 organizes the most common causes of hyperkalemia.

BOX 27-1 Five Most Common Causes of Hyperkalemia

Spurious elevation	Hemolysis due to drawing or storing of the laboratory sample or post–blood sampling leak from markedly elevated white blood cells, red blood cells, or platelets
Renal failure	Acute or chronic
Acidosis	Diabetic ketoacidosis, Addison's disease,adrenal insufficiency, type 4 renal tubular acidosis
Cell death	Rhabdomyolysis, tumor lysis syndrome,massive hemolysis or transfusion, crush injury, burn
Drugs	Beta-blockers, acute digitalis overdose,succinylcholine, angiotensin-converting enzyme inhibitors, angiotension receptor blockers, nonsteroidal anti-inflammatory drugs, spironolactone, amiloride,potassium supplementation

Clinical Features

Patients with moderate to severe hyperkalemia may have gastrointestinal effects such as nausea, vomiting, and diarrhea often in association with their underlying disease. Neuromuscular findings, including muscle cramps, generalized weakness, paresthesias, tetany, and focal or global paralysis, may be seen in patients with severe hyperkalemia. The signs and symptoms of progressive muscle weakness, paresthesias, dyspnea, and depressed deep tendon reflexes are neither sensitive nor specific, nor do they appear reliably with a particular serum potassium level. Patients with severe hypokalemia may present with hemodynamic instability and cardiac arrhythmias.

Diagnostic Strategies

The ECG is helpful in making the diagnosis of hyperkalemia and can be used in unstable patients to initiate treatment (Fig. 27-1 to Fig. 27-3). Classic electrocardiographic changes–the peaked T wave, flattened P wave with prolonged PR interval or a totally absent P wave, wide QRS, and sine wave pattern, portending imminent cardiac arrest–have been well described as appearing sequentially with rising serum potassium levels.Peaked T waves usually appear as serum potassium levels exceed 5.5 to 6.5 mEq/L; P wave disappearance and PR prolongation are common with levels above 6.5 to 7.5 mEq/L; and QRS prolongation is seen with potassium levels above 7.0 to 8.0 mEq/L.A serum potassium level above 5.0 mEq/L is diagnostic of hyperkalemia.

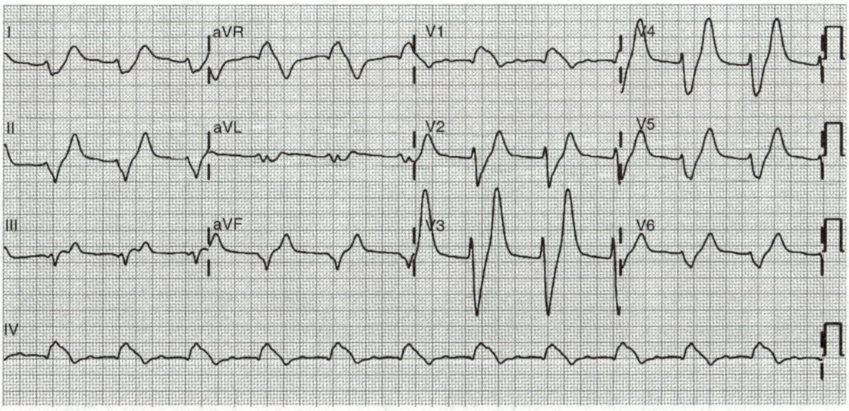

Fig. 27-1 Hyperkalemia with QRS widening merging into T wave,absent P wave.

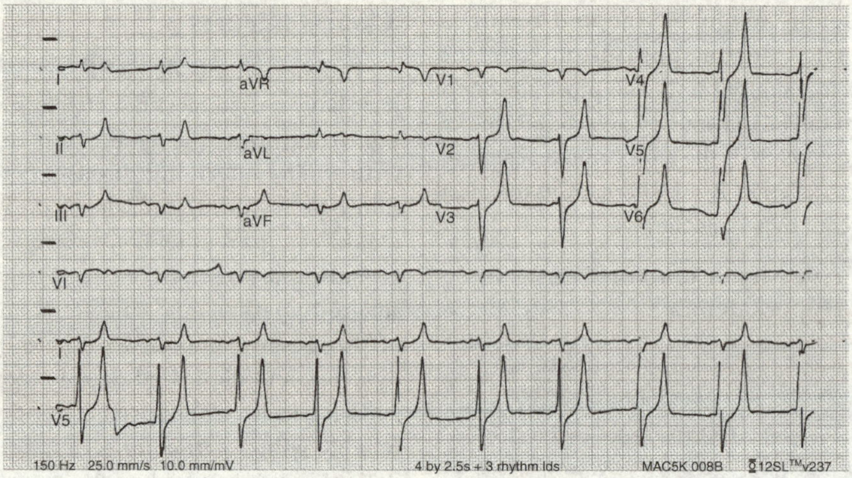

Fig. 27-2 Hyperkalemia in the same patient as in Fig 27-1 after potassium-lowering therapy has begun. Tall peaked T waves, decreased P wave.

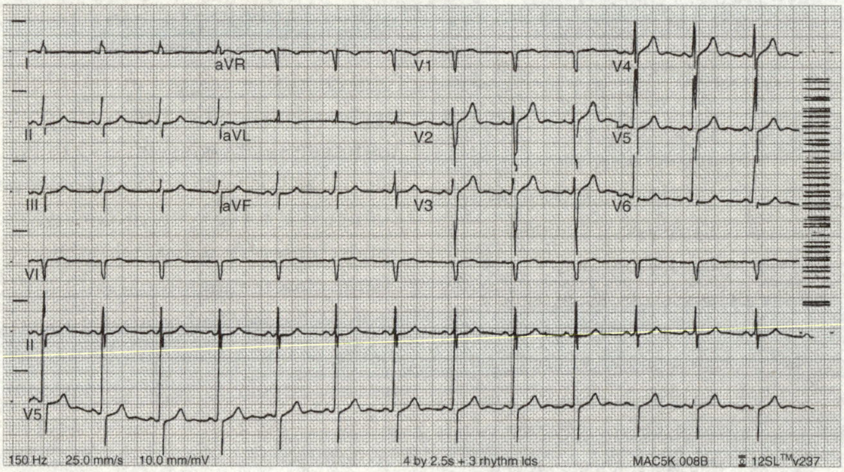

Fig. 27-3 The same patient as in Fig 27-1 and 27-2 after dialysis. The electrocardiogram is now normal.

Management

Patients with suspected or known hyperkalemia require intravenous access and continuous cardiac monitoring.The treatment strategy consists of three main steps (Table 27-1):

Stabilization of the cardiac membrane Intravenous calcium is used to stabilize the cardiac membrane by restoring the electrical gradient. Calcium does not decrease serum potassium levels, and its effect is rapid but transient.The dose is 10 mL of 10% calcium chloride solution or 10 mL of calcium gluconate as it contains only one third the calcium contained in calcium chloride.

Shifting of potassium into the cells Potassium can be shifted intracellularly with beta$_2$-agonists, insulin, saline, and potentially sodium bicarbonate.Insulin also shifts potassium into cells by stimulation of the Na^+, K^+-ATPase pump. The onset of action is less than 15 min, and the effect is maximal between 30 and 60 min, with a maximal drop of 0.6 mEq/L on average. Nebulized albuterol by face mask is effective in shifting potassium into cells by stimulation of the Na^+,K^+-ATPase pump. Nebulized albuterol begins to take measurable effect after 15 min and lowers the serum potassium level by 0.5 to 1 mEq/L. The effective dose is at least four times higher than that typically used for bronchodilation.The combination of nebulized albuterol and insulin with glucose appears to be additive, lowering

Table 27-1 **Treatment of Hyperkalemia**

TREATMENT	MEDICATION	FEATURES
Stabilize cardiac membrane	Calcium chloride(10 mL, maximum 20 mL) or calcium gluconate (10-30 mL),IV push	For wide QRS, restores the electrical gradient; does not decrease serum potassium
Shift potassium into cells	Insulin, 10 units, IV push, combined with 100 mL of 50% dextrose, IV push High-dose nebulized albuterol by face mask (15-25mg by continuous inhalation) Bicarbonate 50-100 Ml Normal saline 100-250 mL	If severely acidotic In conjunction with nephrologist if dialysis dependent
Remove potassium from the body	Hemodialysis Normal saline and furosemide Ion exchange resin	Emergently in cardiac arrest, urgently in renal failure; may delay if renal function is normal In patients with rhabdomyolysis or tumor lysis syndrome with intact urine output Not effective acutely

serum potassium by a mean of 1.2 mEq/L.Saline infusions also stimulate the Na^+,K^+-ATPase pump, and only a few hundred milliliters is required for beneficial effects. Sodium bicarbonate is effective only in hyperkalemic patients who are acidotic and has no benefit when it is used for hyperkalemia in nonacidotic patients.Although intravenous magnesium also can drive potassium intracellularly, it should never be used in hyperkalemia as most patients with elevated potassium levels are also at risk for concomitant hypermagnesemia.

Removal of potassium from the body Potassium can best be removed from the body acutely by hemodialysis. Hemodialysis effectively and reliably decreases serum potassium levels by at least 1 mEq/L in the first hour and another 1 mEq/L during the next 2 hr.In cases such as rhabdomyolysis or tumor lysis syndrome, it may be appropriate to use a normal saline infusion supplemented by furosemide to enhance diuresis and potassium excretion in the urine.

Hyperkalemia is seen in DKA,serum potassium levels rise because of cellular shifts.The mainstay of treatment of DKA—fluids and insulin— closely mirrors the treatment of hyperkalemia itself. Epinephrine has been shown to lower potassium by 0.25 mEq/L.Calcium chloride is given immediately by intravenous push, followed by insulin and glucose. Bicarbonate should be given by bolus dose if the patient is believed to be acidotic. Emergent hemodialysis is recommended if it is readily available.

HYPOKALEMIA

Principles of Disease

Hypokalemia is defined as a value of less than 3.5 mEq/L. Although hypokalemia is usually asymptomatic, severe cardiac dysrhythmias and rhabdomyolysis can occur secondary to potassium's effect on the heart and muscle. The five most common causes of hypokalemia are renal losses, increased nonrenal losses, decreased potassium intake, intracellular shift, and endocrine etiologies (Box 27-2). Hypokalemia is often seen in association with hypomagnesemia. Increased excretion of potassium, especially coupled with poor intake, is the most common cause of hypokalemia. Hypokalemia is a common adverse effect may cause fatal arrhythmias and increase the risk of digitalis toxicity.In addition to diuretics, other drugs and disorders can cause significant renal potassium losses, including hyperaldosteronism, steroid excess, metabolic acidosis, DKA, renal tubular acidosis, and alcohol consumption.Individuals with secondary hyperaldosteronism, whether it is due to CHF, hepatic insufficiency, or nephrotic syndrome, may also exhibit hypokalemia. Patients with renal tubular acidosis can become hypokalemic.Administration of insulin may cause a reduction in serum potassium.On occasion, excessive sweating can lead to hypokalemia from losses of potassium through the skin. In addition, patients with extensive burns can also suffer from hypokalemia.Dietary potassium deficiency should be considered in the severely malnourished patient and the chronic alcoholic. When poor potassium intake is combined with increased nonrenal losses, severe hypokalemia can result.Beta receptor stimulation can lead to hypokalemia, especially in patients using repetitive and high doses of beta-agonists for COPD. Albuterol induced hypokalemia can occur even at normal therapeutic doses.

Box 27-2 Five Most Common Causes of Hypokalemia

Renal losses	Diuretic use, drugs, steroid use, metabolic acidosis, hyperaldosteronism, renal tubular acidosis, diabetic ketoacidosis, alcohol consumption
Increased nonrenallosses	Sweating, diarrhea, vomiting, laxative use
Decreased intake	Ethanol, malnutrition
Intracellular shift	Hyperventilation, metabolic alkalosis, drugs
Endocrine	Cushing's disease, Bartter's syndrome, insulin therapy

Clinical Features

Hypokalemia is usually asymptomatic but can be manifested with nonspecific complaints, including palpitations, skeletal muscle weakness, easy fatigability, depression, and muscle pain. Although short periods of mild potassium depletion are typically well tolerated in healthy individuals, severe potassium depletion can result in serious cardiovascular instability, neurologic dysfunction, glucose intolerance, gastrointestinal symptoms, and renal failure as well as affect the acid-base balance in the body.In patients without underlying heart disease, abnormalities in cardiac conduction are extremely unusual, even when the serum potassium concentration is below 3.0 mEq/L. Paresthesias, depressed deep tendon reflexes, fasciculations, muscle weakness, and confusion can occur when the serum potassium level is less than 2.5 mEq/L. However, in patients with cardiac ischemia or heart failure, even mild to moderate hypokalemia increases the likelihood of cardiac arrhythmias. Hypokalemic patients can demonstrate first- and second-degree heart block, Af, Vf, and asystole. Hypokalemia can also promote metabolic acidosis. Hypokalemic periodic paralysis is a rare disorder characterized by potentially fatal episodes of muscle weakness through the involvement of the respiratory muscles.

Diagnostic Strategies

If there is any suspicion for hypokalemia or a patient presents with generalized weakness, palpitations, or arrhythmias, an ECG should be obtained. Just as a tall-peaked T wave is characteristic of hyperkalemia, a flattened T wave can be seen in hypokalemia. U waves, which are small deflections after the T wave, may also be seen (Figs. 27-4 and 27-5). The real danger of hypokalemia is that it may also cause a prolonged

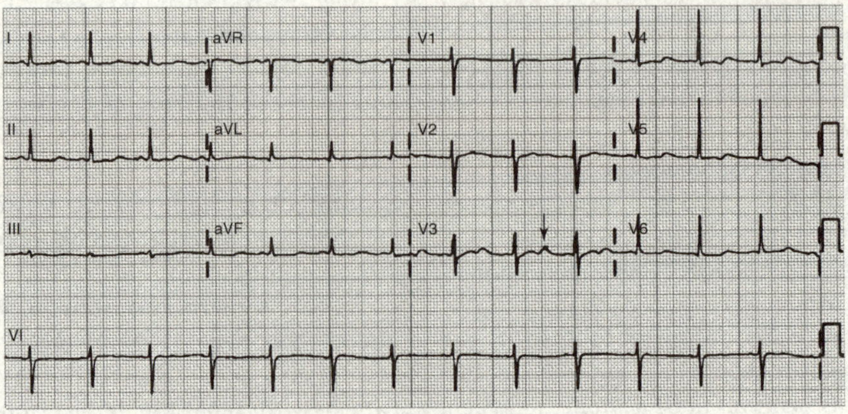

Fig. 27-4 Hypokalemic electrocardiographic changes, including flattened T wave,prolonged QT interval, nonspecific ST changes, and prominent U wave (*arrow*).

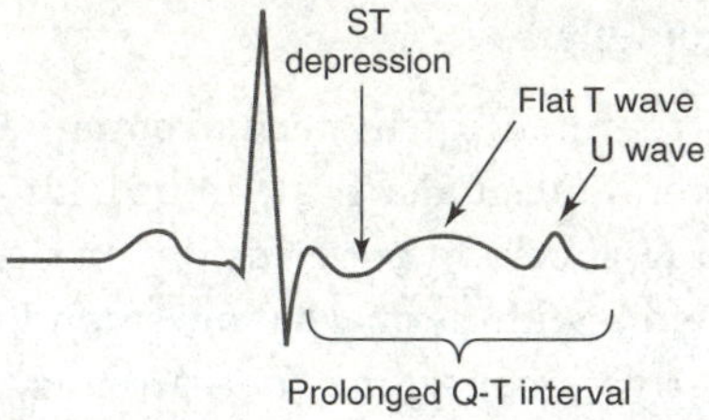

Fig. 27-5. Electrocardiographic changes in hypokalemia.

QT interval. Once the QT interval becomes longer than 500 ms, the risk of malignant ventricular arrhythmias and torsades de pointes increases dramatically.Hypokalemia is also notorious for causing nonspecific ST and T wave changes.A severe degree of hypokalemia with paralysis is a potentially life-threatening medical emergency; measurement of relative urinary potassium excretion and an assessment of the acid-base status might help narrow the differential diagnosis in the emergency setting.

Management

When treating hypokalemia, one should remember that each 0.3 mEq potassium drop below normal correlates with an approximately 100 mEq total body deficit.Patients who have mild or moderate hypokalemia may only need oral potassium replacement therapy if they do not have nausea or vomiting as the cause of their hypokalemia.Potassium chloride is the most commonly used supplementation, and 40 to 60 mEq orally every 2 to 4 hr is typically well tolerated. If the cause of hypokalemia is not clear or the hypokalemia is severe and associated with profound weakness.Patients in whom severe hypokalemia is suspected should be immediately placed on a cardiac monitor and intravenous access secured.If intravenous infusion is necessary, potassium chloride at a rate of 10 to 20 mEq/hr is considered safe. In the rare instance in which intravenous repletion is planned at more than 20 mEq/hr, closely monitor the patient with continuous cardiac monitoring and establish central line access. Hypokalemia is associated with hypomagnesemia, and the severity of the hypokalemia correlates with a similar degree of hypomagnesemia.Magnesium replacement should usually accompany potassium repletion.Correction of large potassium deficits may require several days, and oral and intravenous replacement can occur simultaneously.

HYPERNATREMIA

Principles of Disease

Hypernatremia is defined as a serum sodium concentration above 145 mEq/ L.Most hypernatremic patients have either an impaired sense of thirst or no access to water. Thus elders, patients in coma or with mental impairment.Hypernatremia can be divided into three physiologic pairings (Box 27-3). Diabetes insipidus, a condition that results in insufficient production of or lack of response to antidiuretic hormone, can lead to lifethreatening hypernatremia(Box 27-4).

Box 27-3 Three Types of Hypernatremia

Hypernatremia with dehydration and low total body sodium	Heatstroke Increased insensible losses: burns, sweating Gastrointestinal loss: diarrhea, protracted vomiting, continuous gastrointestinal suction Osmotic diuresis: glucose, mannitol, enteral feeding
Hypernatremia with low total body water and normal total body sodium	Diabetes insipidus Neurogenic Elderly with "reset" osmostat Hypothalamic dysfunction Suprasellar or infrasellar tumors Renal disease Drugs (amphotericin, phenytoin, lithium, aminoglycosides, methoxyflurane) Sickle cell disease
Hypernatremia with increased total body sodium	Salt tablet ingestion Salt water ingestion Saline infusions Saline enemas Intravenous sodium bicarbonate Poorly diluted interval feedings Primary hyperaldosteronism Hemodialysis Cushing's syndrome Conn's syndrome

Box 27-4 More Common Causes of Diabetes Insipidus

Central
Idiopathic
Familial disease
Cancer
Hypoxic encephalopathy
Infiltrative disorders
Postsupraventricular tachycardia
Anorexia nervosa

Nephrogenic
Chronic renal insufficiency
Polycystic kidney disease
Lithium toxicity
Hypercalcemia
Hypokalemia
Tubulointerstitial disease
Hereditary
Sickle cell disease

Clinical Features

Hypernatremia is a disease seen predominantly in elders. Patients may complain of polyuria or polydipsia or have obvious causes of extrarenal fluid losses. Hypernatremia should be considered in any patient presenting with altered mental status, especially individuals with severe mental retardation, cerebral palsy, and head injury.

Diagnostic Strategies

In addition to routine serum chemistries, serum osmolarity and urine sodium concentration and osmolality should be obtained.The patient's total body water (TBW) deficit can be estimated by the formula.

TBW deficit=TBW×(serum Na^+/140−1)

A patient's TBW is usually calculated by multiplying the patient's body weight in kilograms times 0.6. However, because of percentage body fat differences based on the age and sex of the patient, it is more accurate to use the correction factors listed in Table 27-2.

Table 27-2 Calculation of Body Water

POPULATION	TOTAL BODY WATER
Children and adult men	Body weight (kg) × 0.6
Adult women	Body weight (kg) × 0.5
Elderly men	Body weight (kg) × 0.5
Elderly women	Body weight (kg) × 0.45

Management

The treatment of hypernatremia has three interdependent goals: first, to quickly correct underlying shock, hypoperfusion, or significant hypovolemia with normal saline; second, to treat the underlying cause of hypernatremia, such as fever, vomiting, or diabetes insipidus; and third, to carefully lower the serum sodium level, usually by replacement of the body's total water deficit. The rate of correction in hypernatremia is extremely important to minimize morbidity and mortality. In adult patients who have had hypernatremia during a short time as a result of sodium loading, "rapid correction" at 1 to 2 mEq/hr lowering of serum sodium appears relatively safe.However, most adult patients have hypernatremia during days to weeks. In this group of patients, serum sodium concentration should be slowly corrected at no more than 0.5 mEq/hr or 10 to 12 mEq/day. Normal saline can typically be started for volume replacement until the patient is hemodynamically stable and then changed to half-normal saline at 100 mL/hr once vital signs have normalized. The treatment of central diabetes insipidus with desmopressin (DDAVP) is an effective means of improving polyuria and hypernatremia; initial doses in the acute setting range from 1 to 2 μg.

HYPONATREMIA

Principles of Disease

Hyponatremia, defined as serum sodium concentration of less than 135 mEq/L, is the second most common electrolyte abnormality. The most common causes of severe hyponatremia in adults are therapy with thiazides, the postoperative state including transurethral prostatectomy, the syndrome of inappropriate secretion of antidiuretic hormone (SIADH), polydipsia in psychiatric patients, and unintentional water intoxication. Gastrointestinal fluid loss, ingestion of overly dilute formula, accidental ingestion of excessive water. Symptoms of hyponatremic patients range from headache, nausea, and vomiting to confusion, seizures, and coma. There are two groups of hyponatremic patients that will require treatment with either normal saline or hypertonic saline: (1) severe but asymptomatic hyponatremia with a sodium level of 110 mEq/L or less and (2) acute symptomatic hyponatremia with a sodium level below 120 mEq/L. CNS damage due to hyponatremia may be caused by cerebral edema and increased intracranial pressure, by osmotic fluid shifts during overly aggressive treatment, or by both.If fluid therapy raises extracellular sodium levels too quickly, fluids shift out of neurons and diffuse demyelination may occur, leading to flaccid paralysis and often death due to a syndrome most commonly referred to as central pontine myelinolysis, although it is more accurately labeled the osmotic demyelinating syndrome.Although hyponatremia has many causes, they fall into four general categories: pseudohyponatremia, hyponatremia with dehydration and decreased extracellular volume, hyponatremia with increased extracellular volume, and euvolemic hyponatremia with increased total body water (Box 27-5).

Box 27-5 Causes of Hyponatremia

Pseudohyponatremia	Hyperlipidemia Hyperproteinemia (multiple myeloma, macroglobulinemia)
Dilutional	Hyperglycemia*
Hypovolemic hyponatremia: decreased total body water and sodium, with a relatively greater decrease in sodium	Body fluid losses: sweating,vomiting, diarrhea,gastrointestinal suction Third spacing: bowel obstruction,burns, pancreatitis,rhabdomyolysis Renal causes: diuretics,mineralocorticoid deficiency,osmotic diuresis, renal tubular acidosis, salt-wasting nephropathies
Hypervolemic hyponatremia: increased total body sodium with a relatively greater increase in total body water	Heart failure Chronic renal failure Hepatic failure or cirrhosis
Euvolemic hyponatremia: increased total body water with nearly normal total body sodium	SIADH Drugs causing SIADH (diuretics,barbiturates, carbamazepine,chlorpropamide, clofibrate,opioids, tolbutamide, vincri-stine) Psychogenic polydipsia Beer potomania Hypothyroidism Adrenal insufficiency MDMA (ecstasy) Accidental or intentional water intoxication

Pseudohyponatremia

Pseudohyponatremia is a falsely low sodium reading caused by the presence of other osmolar particles in the serum. The phenomenon of pseudohyponatremia is explained by the increased percentage of large molecular particles relative to sodium.Severe hypertriglyceridemia and hyperproteinemia are two common causes of this condition.Hyperglycemia is sometimes considered a cause of pseudohyponatremia; however, it actually causes a dilutional hyponatremia .One commonly used formula advocates the addition of 1.6 mEq/L to the measured sodium for every 100 mg/dL of glucose above 100. Another formula recommends use of 2.4 mEq as the correction factor because glucose values above 400 mg/dL may lower sodium values by 4 mEq/L per each 100 mg/dL of glucose rise.

Hypovolemic Hyponatremia

Hypovolemic hyponatremia, or hyponatremia in association with dehydration, occurs when there is decreased extracellular volume combined with an even greater loss of sodium. Hyponatremia secondary to body fluid losses must be differentiated from that due to renal losses. Hyponatremia with dehydration due to body fluid losses includes sweating, vomiting, diarrhea, and gastrointestinal suction. Hypovolemic hyponatremia is also seen with "third spacing" in bowel obstruction, burns, and intra-abdominal sepsis. Hypovolemic hyponatremia due to renal causes includes diuretic use, mineralocorticoid deficiency, renal tubular acidosis, and saltwasting nephropathy. Hypovolemic hyponatremia can be further exacerbated when fluid losses are replaced with hypotonic saline.

Hypervolemic Hyponatremia

Hypervolemic hyponatremia, or hyponatremia with increased extracellular volume, occurs when sodium and water are retained but water retention exceeds sodium retention. Most of these patients present with edema. Hyponatremia with increased total body sodium occurs in patients with heart failure, chronic renal failure, and hepatic failure. The fluid retention in these states is secondary to renal hypoperfusion, resulting in increased aldosterone secretion and a decrease in free water excretion.

Euvolemic Hyponatremia

Patients with euvolemic hyponatremia are euvolemic but have increased total body water. Causes of this type of hyponatremia include SIADH, psychogenic polydipsia,beer potomania, hypothyroidism, diuretic use in patients with mild CHF, and accidental or intentional water intoxication. These patients do not present with edema because most of the increased body water is intracellular and not intravascular. Hyponatremia without edema has also been described in patients after the use of the recreational drug *N*-methyl-3,4-methylenedioxyamphetamine (MDMA or ecstasy). MDMA-induced hyponatremia is multifactorial and is related to increased free water intake to avoid dehydration and rhabdomyolysis, along with the tendency to be very active while using the drug, leading to sweating and antidiuretic hormone secretion. SIADH is an important cause of hyponatremia that occurs when antidiuretic hormone is secreted independently of the body's need to conserve water.The three most common causes of SIADH are lung cancers (especially small cell cancer)and infections, CNS disorders, and drugs (Box 27-6).

Box 27-6 Three Most Common Causes of SIADH

- Lung masses
  - Cancer (especially small cell)
  - Pneumonia
  - Tuberculosis
  - Abscess
- Central nervous system disorders
  - Infection (meningitis, brain abscess)
  - Mass (subdural, postoperative, cerebrovascular accident)
  - Psychosis (with psychogenic polydipsia)
- Drugs
  - Thiazide diuretics
  - Narcotics
  - Oral hypoglycemic agents
  - Barbiturates
  - Antineoplastics

Diagnostic Strategies

A spot urinary sodium or urinary chloride level is useful to determine if hyponatremia of undetermined origin is renal in etiology.Patients with hypovolemic hyponatremia due to nonrenal causes typically have a low urinary sodium or chloride level (<20 mEq/L).Patients with hypovolemic hyponatremia due to renal causes will have elevated urine sodium and chloride levels above 20 mEq/L. Patients with euvolemic hyponatremia typically have a urinary sodium concentration greater than 20 mEq/L secondary to volume expansion caused by water retention. Patients with hypervolemic hyponatremia secondary to CHF or cirrhosis have urine sodium levels of less than 20 mEq/L because of renal hypoperfusion, whereas those with renal causes of hypervolemic hyponatremia or with SIADH have sodium levels in excess of 20 mEq/L.It is also important to consider adrenal insufficiency when a dehydrated patient has both hyponatremia and hyperkalemia.

Clinical Features

Nonspecific signs of hyponatremia include anorexia, nausea, vomiting, and generalized weakness. Acutely hyponatremic patients whose sodium level drops below 120 mEq/L during

24 to 48 hr may present with severe neurologic findings, including confusion, seizures, cerebral edema, coma, and brainstem herniation.The diagnosis of hypovolemic hyponatremia is more likely in the patient with diminished skin turgor, increased capillary refill, dry mucous membranes, and orthostasis. On the contrary, the patient with jugular venous distention, peripheral edema, or pulmonary congestion is much more likely to have hypervolemic hyponatremia. Patients with SIADH will have no edema and have normal skin turgor.

Management

Treatment of hyponatremia is guided by the patient's clinical presentation, severity of symptoms, estimated duration of illness, fluid status, and underlying cause of the sodium disturbance. Typically, sodium should be corrected during a time course of 48 to 72 hr. Central pontine myelinolysis can occur with too rapid correction of sodium.However, patients who have serum sodium levels of significantly less than 120 mEq/L and those who have acute alterations in mental status, seizures, or new focal findings due to hyponatremia need immediate intervention. Table 27-3 presents the sodium concentration of various infusates, and the following equation is helpful to estimate the effect of 1 L of any infusate on serum sodium:

Table 27-3 Characteristics of Infusates

INFUSATE	INFUSATE SODIUM (mmol/L)	EXTRACELLULAR FLUID DISTRIBUTION (%)
3% Hypertonic saline	513	100
0.9% Normal saline solution	154	100
Lactated Ringer's solution	130	97
Half-normal saline solution	77	73
0.2% Sodium chloride + 5% dextrose in water	34	55
5% Dextrose in water	0	45

Change in serum Na^+=infusate Na^+-serum Na^+/ total body water + 1

For relatively asymptomatic patients with sodium values of 115 to135 mEq/ L, free water restriction is typically the single most important treatment.Correction of hyponatremia by 4 to 6 mEq/L within 6 hr, with bolus infusions of 3% saline if necessary, is sufficient to manage the most severe manifestations of hyponatremia.It is recommendedthat critically ill hyponatremic patients with seizures,focal findings, or coma receive 100 mL of 3% hypertonic saline during 10 min. If a second bolus is required, an additional 100 mL of the 3% solution (513 mEq/L of sodium) may be administered during the next 50 min. Increased neurologic stability is highly likely once a symptomatic hyponatremic patient's serum sodium concentration has been raised by about 4 to 6 mEq acutely by the hypertonic saline. To minimize the likelihood of central pontine myelinolysis, it is essential that symptomatic patients with severe hyponatremia not have serum sodium levels rise by any more than a total of 10 to 12 mEq within the first 24 hr.If patients are retaining volume and diuresis is not adequate, furosemide can be used; D_5W is infused if the sodium level is rising too quickly. Demeclocycline in a dosage of 600 to 1200 mg daily is effective in patients with refractory hyponatremia.

Hypovolemic Hyponatremia

Hypotensive, dehydrated patients are volume resuscitated with normal saline.Typically, the normal saline is started at 500 to 1000 mL/hr until the blood pressure is stable and then slowed to 200 mL/hr with frequent sodium checks. If the sodium value is below 120 mEq/L, the sodium concentration should be allowed to rise only by an average of 0.5 mEq/hr or 10 to 12 mEq/d.It is essential to treat the underlying cause of hyponatremia.

Hypervolemic Hyponatremia

Restriction of fluid and sodium is the preferred treatment of patients with hypervolemic hyponatremia, although loop diuretics can be used in severe cases. Hemodialysis is an alternative in patients with renal impairment and will be required in significantly hyponatremic renal failure patients with volume overload. Patients with CHF will usually benefit from diuretics.In those patients with liver failure, albumin is a consideration, along with diuretics and possibly paracentesis to improve the underlying pathologic process. Water restriction may make the largest impact on the long-term care of these patients.

Euvolemic Hyponatremia

The mainstay of treatment of euvolemic hyponatremia is free water restriction.The only definitive treatment of SIADH is elimination of its underlying cause. Most cases of SIADH caused by malignant disease resolve with effective antineoplastic therapy.In patients with SIADH, normal saline may cause the serum sodium concentration to decrease If a patient is symptomatic because of a rapid decrease in serum sodium concentration, treatment with hypertonic saline is recommended. Demeclocycline and lithium are rarely used in the treatment of SIADH because of their many side effects and nephrotoxicity. Rapid correction of hyponatremia may occur during hemodialysis. To minimize the risks of central pontine myelinolysis, hemodialysis is reserved for patients with documented renal failure and used in a very careful manner.

HYPERCALCEMIA

Principles of Disease

Hypercalcemia is usually defined as a serum calcium level above 10.5 mg/dL; normal levels are usually defined as between 9 and 10.5 mg/dL. Hypercalcemia is considered mild if the total serum calcium level is between 10.5 and 12 mg/dL; levels higher than 14 mg/dL can be life-threatening. There are five major causes of hypercalcemia (Box 27-7). Primary hyperparathyroidism is the most common cause of hypercalcemia in outpatients, whereas malignant disease is the most common cause in hospitalized patients.

Box 27-7 Five Most Common Causes of Hypercalcemia

Malignant disease	Ectopic secretions of parathyroid hormone, multiple myeloma, cancer metastatic to bone Most common: breast, lung, hematologic, kidney, prostate
Endocrine	Hyperparathyroidism, multiple endocrine neoplasias, hyperthyroidism, pheochromocytoma, adrenal insufficiency
Granulomatous disease	Sarcoidosis, tuberculosis, histoplasmosis,beryliiosis, coccidioidomycosis
Pharmacologic agents	Vitamins A and D, thiazide diuretics,estrogens, milk-alkali syndrome
Miscellaneous	Dehydration, prolonged immobilization,iatrogenic, rhabdomyolysis, familial,laboratory error

Clinical Features

The clinical presentation of hypercalcemia is often vague and nonspecific. Symptoms include nonfocal abdominal pain, constipation, fatigue, diffuse body aches, anorexia, nausea, and vomiting. Symptom severity depends on the degree of hypercalcemia, the rapidity of onset, and the patient's baseline neurologic and renal function. In addition, some patients complain of polyuria or polydipsia. Neuropsychiatric disturbances include anxiety, depression, confusion, and hallucinations. The CNS manifestations that often predominate in more severe cases include lethargy, altered mental status, seizures, and coma. Death due to hypercalcemia is usually related to complications caused by coma, dehydration, or electrolyte disturbances. Cardiac conduction abnormalities may occur; bradydysrhythmias are the most common. Severe hypercalcemia has also been associated with sinus arrest,AVB, Af, and VT.

Diagnostic Strategies

Calcium is measured by determination of either a total serum calcium level or an ionized calcium level. The adjustment to serum albumin is accomplished by adding or subtracting 0.08 mg/dL to the measured total serum calcium for every 1.0 g/L of albumin below or above 4 g/L albumin, respectively. A short QT interval can be seen in hypercalcemia. The incidence and duration of QT shortening appear to be correlated with the degree of hypercalcemia (Fig. 27-6). ST segment elevation may be the least well documented but most consistent ECG finding, and hypercalcemia should be considered in the differential diagnosis of ST segment elevation caused by conditions other than MI.In severe cases of hypercalcemia, sinus bradycardia, bundle branch block, and high degree AVB may also been seen.

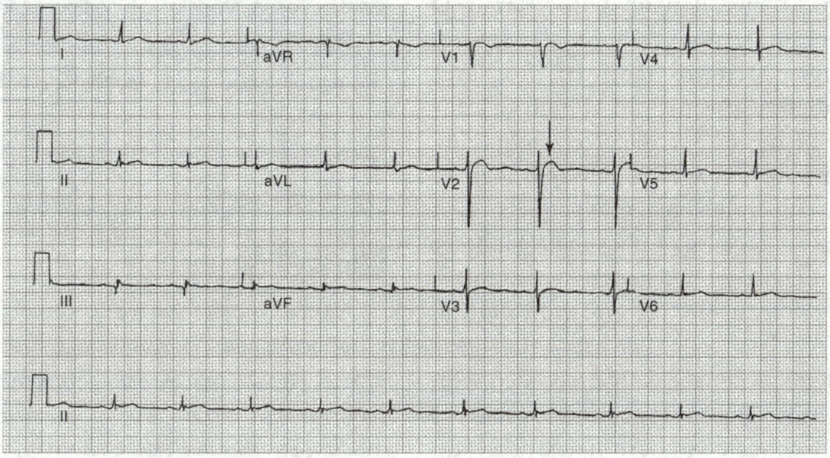

Fig. 27-6 Short QT interval *(arrow)* in a patient with multiple myeloma and a calcium level of 14.2 mg/dL.

Management

Patients in hypercalcemic crisis are usually dehydrated, often obtunded, and also predisposed to arrhythmias ; thus they require intravenous access with a normal saline infusion and close monitoring. After the initial bolus, the saline infusion is adjusted to a rate of approximately 200 to 300 mL/hr. Patients with underlying cardiac or renal disease may require lower infusion rates that are carefully titrated.The routine use of furosemide in the management of hypercalcemia is no longer recommended.The use of furosemide is reserved to augment saline diuresis and to avoid volume overload during the treatment of hypercalcemia. If it is given to patients who are not yet volume replete, this loop diuretic may worsen the hypercalcemia.Drugs that inhibit osteoclast-mediated bone resorption include the bisphosphonates, mithramycin, calcitonin, and glucocorticoids. Intravenous bisphosphonates are the most extensively studied and most efficacious agents for the treatment of malignancy-associated hypercalcemia.Zoledronic acid is the bisphosphonate of choice in hypercalcemia of malignancy. The infusion takes 15 min, and zoledronic acid may be more effective than other bisphosphonates at keeping the calcium level down over time. The use of intravenous bisphosphonates is restricted to the treatment of acute hypercalcemia associated with serum calcium concentrations above 15 mg/dL and rapid deterioration of CNS, cardiac, gastrointestinal, and renal function. In the rare case in which a patient has a life-threatening hypercalcemic arrhythmia or heart block, phosphates and hemodialysis are considered. In cases of hypercalcemic crisis resulting from primary hyperparathyroidism, urgent parathyroidectomy is potentially curative.

HYPOCALCEMIA

Principles of Disease

Calcium regulation is critical for normal cell function, neural transmission, membrane stability, bone structure, blood coagulation, and intracellular signaling. Total body calcium is controlled by a feedback system in which PTH induces the bone and the kidneys to increase serum calcium levels. Vitamin D facilitates intestinal calcium absorption. Conversely, elevated calcium levels normally inhibit PTH release. There are multiple causes of hypocalcemia, of which hypoalbuminemia is the most common (Box 27-8). Because calcium is bound to albumin and other serum proteins, hypoalbuminemia will cause a fall in the measured serum calcium by about 0.8 mg/ dL for every 1 g/dL reduction in serum albumin. The active form of calcium is the ionized calcium. Hypoparathyroidism is a common cause of hypocalcemia. Patients with vitamin D deficiency, including those with malabsorption syndromes, liver disease, malnutrition, and very little sunlight exposure, are at high risk for development of hypocalcemia. Derangements in magnesium and phosphate can also lead to hypocalcemia. Hyperphosphatemic patients often have hypocalcemia because of phosphate's affinity to bind calcium, whereas hypomagnesemia causes end-organ resistance to PTH and inhibits the hypocalcemic feedback loop. Patients with sepsis demonstrate hypocalcemia usually associated with hypoalbuminemia. The most common causes of symptomatic hypocalcemia are massive blood transfusions, toxins, pancreatitis, tumor lysis syndrome, and chronic malnutrition (Box 27-9). Hypocalcemia in acute pancreatitis is caused primarily by precipitation of calcium soaps in the abdominal cavity, but glucagon stimulated calcitonin release and decreased PTH secretion may play a role. Toxic exposures to hydrofluoric acid and ethylene glycol can cause profound hypocalcemia secondary to their abilities to complex and chelate with calcium. Hypocalcemia has been attributed to the precipitation of calcium phosphate salts. Finally, one should expect to encounter hypocalcemia in malnourished patients and chronic alcoholics.

Box 27-8 Most Common Causes of Hypocalcemia

- Hypoalbuminemia
- Hypoparathyroidism: inherited, postsurgical, autoimmune, infiltrative
- Vitamin D deficiency and vitamin D resistance: malabsorption syndrome, liver disease, malnutrition, sepsis, anticonvulsants, lack of sunlight exposure
- Chronic renal failure
- Hyperphosphatemia
- Hypomagnesemia
- Respiratory alkalosis
- Severe pancreatitis
- Drugs: bisphosphonates, phenytoin, phosphate, calcitonin
- Tumor lysis syndrome
- Rhabdomyolysis

Box 27-9 Five Most Common Symptomatic Causes of Hypocalcemia Seen in the Emergency Department

Hyperventilation	Anxiety, sympathomimetics
Ethanol abuse, chronic malnutrition	Hypoalbuminemia
Massive blood transfusion	More than 10 U
Toxins	Hydrofluoric acid, ethylene glycol
Severe pancreatitis	

Clinical Features

Although there are many clinical manifestations of hypocalcemia, neuromuscular and cardiovascular findings predominate. Severe, symptomatic hypocalcemia may result in cardiovascular collapse, hypotension, and dysrhythmias.The patient may complain of muscle cramping, perioral or finger paresthesias, shortness of breath secondary to bronchospasm, and tetanic contractions. More severe symptoms include hypotension, QT prolongation, angina, and CHF. Chronic hypocalcemia may be manifested with cataracts, poor dentition, dry skin, coarse hair, and pruritus. Chvostek's sign may be present. Trousseau's sign is relatively specific for hypocalcemia.

Diagnostic Strategies

A serum calcium level less than 8.5 mg/dL or an ionized calcium level less than 2.0 mEq/L is considered diagnostic. Total serum calcium is approximately 50% free (ionized) and 50% bound, primarily to albumin.The ionized calcium level is more accurate. It is best to perform the whole blood ionized calcium determination rapidly to avoid changes in chelation and pH. In select cases, a PTH level may be sent to assist the admitting or consulting physician.ECG and cardiac monitoring are recommended in suspected hypocalcemia patients to evaluate the QT interval and to provide continuous monitoring for potential dysrhythmias.

Management

Most asymptomatic patients and those with mild symptoms can be treated with oral calcium supplementation, such as calcium carbonate. Intravenous calcium is administered, either as calcium chloride or calcium gluconate, to patients with moderate to severe symptoms; 100 to 300 mg of elemental calcium given during 5 to 30 min will raise the ionized calcium level 0.5 to 1.5 mEq. Calcium chloride contains 272 mg of elemental calcium but can be caustic to veins. It is best given through a central line. Calcium gluconate contains 92 mg of elemental calcium. it is safer to administer and can be given peripherally. Most patients requiring intravenous calcium should be admitted to the hospital for monitoring and treatment of nausea, vomiting, hypertension, and bradycardia.Intravenous calcium administration is accompanied by continuous electrocardiographic monitoring.

HYPERMAGNESEMIA

Principles of Disease

Normal serum magnesium levels range from 1.5 to 3.0 mEq/L.Hypermagnesemia defined as a serum magnesium concentration above 2.2 mg/dL. Hypermagnesemia is most often seen in patients with renal insufficiency.Hypermagnesemia can also be caused iatrogenically in patients receiving intravenous magnesium for medical treatment or in patients taking over-the-counter laxatives and antacids. Even though most patients at risk for hypermagnesemia have underlying renal impairment, hypermagnesemia has been reported in patients with normal renal function, especially in elders. Box 27-10 lists the most common causes of increased serum magnesium levels.A healthy adult can excrete more than 6.0 g of magnesium daily, but renally impaired patients may not be able to tolerate a single dose of laxative syrup.

Box 27-10 Five Most Common Causes of Hypermagnesemia

Iatrogenic	Intravenous administration, dialysate
Oral administration	Laxatives, antacids, vitamins, cathartics,dialysate, parental
Impaired elimination: hypomotility	Bowel obstruction, chronic constipation
Impaired elimination: medications	Anticholinergics, narcotics, lithium therapy
Miscellaneous	Hypothyroidism, tumor lysis syndrome,adrenal insufficiency, milk-alkali syndrome, near-drowning in Dead Sea

Clinical Features

Patients with hypermagnesemia may present with flushing, nausea, vomiting, headache, and diminished deep tendon reflexes. Typically, symptoms begin to be manifested around magnesium levels of 4 mg/dL (Table 27-4).As magnesium levels rise, hypotension and ECG changes, including QRS widening and QT and PR prolongation, begin to occur. When serum magnesium levels rise above 7 mg/dL, patients can have signs and symptoms of hypotension, respiratory insufficiency, and heart block. Cardiac arrest and death have been reported in patients with serum magnesium levels above 10 mg/dL.Finally, hypermagnesemia causes suppression of PTH secretion and can be associated with hypocalcemia.

Table 27-4 Clinical Effects of Hypermagnesemia

EFFECT	LEVEL (mg/dL)
Decreased deep tendon reflexes	4-5
Hypotension	5-7
Respiratory insufficiency	10
Heart block	10-15
Cardiac arrest	10-24

Diagnostic Strategies

Measured plasma magnesium levels often do not reflect total magnesium content. Although there is some question of the role of measuring ionized magnesium in patients with hypomagnesemia, only total body magnesium needs to be followed in hypermagnesemic patients.

Management

Management of hypermagnesemia is dictated by the neuromuscular, cardiovascular, and CNS changes that occur. Most stable or asymptomatic hypermagnesemic patients can be treated with cessation of their magnesium therapy. As symptoms become more pronounced, intravenous isotonic fluids are adm}inistered to dilute the extracellular magnesium. Diuretics can be used to promote excretion of magnesium. In patients with higher levels of serum magnesium or more severe symptoms, it should be initiated immediately to arrange for dialysis. Intravenous calcium therapy to reverse magnesium toxicity should be reserved for patients with lifethreatening symptoms while dialysis is being arranged. Calcium directly antagonizes the neuromuscular and cardiovascular effects of magnesium and is recommended in hypotensive patients with respiratory depression and cardiac instability. In treating lifethreatening hypermagnesemia, initially administer 100 to 200 mg of intravenous calcium as either calcium chloride or calcium gluconate (1-2 mL of 10% calcium chloride or 5 mL of 1% calcium gluconate during 2-5 min) and then titrate to effect.One can then consider a continuous infusion at 2 to 4 mg/kg/hr if it is needed while dialysis is being arranged.

HYPOMAGNESEMIA

Principles of Disease

Symptoms of hypomagnesemia typically begin to be manifested at serum levels below 1.2 mEq/L, although symptoms are often not well correlated with the patient's serum level. Magnesium exists in three states: ionized magnesium, protein bound, and complexed to serum anions.There are many causes of hypomagnesemia (Box 27-11). The following are the five most common ED presentations of hypomagnesemia.Patients using either loop or thiazide diuretics are at increased risk for hypomagnesemia. Both types of diuretics can inhibit magnesium reabsorption.Malnourished and Alcoholic Patients. Healthy patients consume enough magnesium in green vegetables, legumes, fruits, shellfish, fresh meat, and cocoa on a regular basis to maintain normal total body magnesium stores. However, hypomagnesemia is common in patients with chronic protein-calorie malnutrition. This is especially true in chronic alcoholics, who may not eat foods rich in magnesium. Magnesium losses are further increased in chronic alcoholics because of alcohol's diuretic effects. Hypomagnesemia may also be seen in patients with malabsorption disorders and in patients with increased magnesium excretion (chronic diarrhea or inflammatory bowel conditions).

Box 27-11 Most Common Causes of Hypomagnesemia

- Dietary
- Gastrointestinal
- Renal
- Endocrine or metabolic
- Drug induced

Patients with Hypokalemia.Approximately 50% of patients with hypokalemia also have concomitant magnesium deficiency. Increasing degrees of hypokalemia are correlated with an increasing likelihood of a magnesium deficit. Hypokalemic patients who are refractory to potassium replacement are likely to also be hypomagnesemic.Patients who have a myocardial infarction are more likely than controls to be hypomagnesemic. At present, magnesium supplementation is recommended only for those ACS patients who have evidence of hypokalemia, prolonged QT, or known hypomagnesemia. Similarly, patients with AMI who have mild hypomagnesemia appear to have a twofold to threefold increase in the frequency of ventricular arrhythmias in the first 24 hr compared with those with normal magnesium levels.Dysrhythmia is the most common cardiovascular manifestation of hypomagnesemia. Patients Receiving Specific Medications.Many nephrotoxic drugs, including aminoglycosides, amphotericin B, cisplatin, and pentamidine, can produce magnesium wasting. however, longterm use of proton pump inhibitors may be associated with changes in intestinal absorption of magnesium.Severe hypomagnesemia can also be seen in patients preparing for colonoscopy with polyethylene glycol–based bowel preparations.

Clinical Features

Patients with hypomagnesemia typically have hypokalemia, hypocalcemia, and hyponatremia. However, many signs and symptoms are reported to correlate with hypomagnesemia, including muscle cramping, diffuse weakness, palpitations, vertigo, ataxia, depression, and seizures.Patients may present with hyperactive deep tendon reflexes, muscle cramps, Trousseau's and Chvostek's signs, and dysarthria and dysphagia from esophageal dysmotility. Cardiac conduction abnormalities secondary to magnesium depletion, and often coexisting hypokalemia, can result in PR as well as QT interval prolongation. Dysrhythmias including atrial fibrillation, multifocal atrial tachycardia, premature ventricular complexes, VT, torsades de pointes, and Vf are the most common cardiovascular manifestations of hypomagnesemia.

Diagnostic Strategies

Symptoms of hypomagnesemia begin to be manifested at serum levels below 1.2 mEq/L, but symptoms do not always correlate with the total serum magnesium level.However, the possibility of hypomagnesemia is considered in patients with malnourishment, significant or refractory hypokalemia, and ventricular arrhythmias. ECG findings in hypomagnesemia are nonspecific and may be caused by both the hypomagnesemia and concomitant hypokalemia. Hypomagnesemia should be suspected whenever ECG findings of hypokalemia are noted, including PR and QT interval prolongation, ST segment depression, flattening and widening of the T waves, and U waves.

Management

In patients with normal renal function, 1 to 2 g of magnesium sulfate is an appropriate loading dose. A stable patient with hypomagnesemia can be treated with a loading dose of 1 to 2 g of magnesium sulfate during 10 to 60 minutes, followed by a standard maintenance dose of 0.5 to 1 g/ hr until symptoms have resolved. However, patients in cardiac arrest should receive a bolus of 1 to 2 g magnesium sulfate by intravenous push. Magnesium administration is strongly encouraged for patients receiving intravenous potassium repletion. A dose of 0.5 g/hr is safe in patients who are well hydrated and have normal renal function. There are potential adverse effects to rapid aggressive magnesium replacement at more than 1 to 2 g/hr, including decreased deep tendon reflexes, respiratory depression, and heart block. Magnesium gluconate oral supplementation can be given if the patient is only mildly hypomagnesemic and asymptomatic.

HYPERPHOSPHATEMIA

Principles of Disease

Hyperphosphatemia is defined as a serum level above 2.5 mg/dL, but it is usually clinically significant only when levels are greater than 5 mg/dL.Hyperphosphatemia is extremely common in patients with renal insufficiency. Hyperphosphatemia can occur because of four major pathways: decreased phosphate excretion, excessive phosphate intake, increased renal tubular reabsorption, and shift of phosphate from intracellular to extracellular space. In addition, physicians must be aware of spurious elevations in phosphate (Box 27-12).When patients have GFR below 30 mL/min, the kidneys do not allow excretion of the full amount of ingested phosphate to maintain homeostasis.Hypoparathyroidism, vitamin D intoxication, and thyrotoxicosis increase renal phosphate reabsorption and may cause elevated phosphate levels. Hyperphosphatemia may also occur when there is a large shift of phosphate from the intracellular to the extracellular space and the kidney's ability to excrete phosphate is overwhelmed. This cause of hyperphosphatemia is seen in crush injuries and nontraumatic rhabdomyolysis, tumor lysis syndrome, and DKA. Hyperphosphatemia can be a spurious finding in cases of hyperproteinemia, such as multiple myeloma, hyperlipidemia, hemolysis, or hyperbilirubinemia. Drawing of a blood sample from a line containing heparin is another cause of a falsely elevated phosphate level.

Box 27-12 Five Most Common Causes of Hyperphosphatemia

Decreased phosphate excretion	Acute and chronic renal failure
Increased renal tubular reabsorption	Hypoparathyroidism Thyrotoxicosis Excess vitamin D administration
Excessive phosphate intake	Phosphate enemas or laxatives Intravenous or oral phosphate administration

Shift of phosphate from intracellular to extracellular space	Diabetic ketoacidosis Tumor lysis Rhabdomyolysis
Spurious hyperphosphatemia	Paraproteinemia Hyperbilirubinemia Hemolysis Hyperlipidemia

Clinical Features

Hyperphosphatemia causes hypocalcemia. It is this secondary hypocalcemia that can cause muscle cramping, tetany, and seizures. Chronic hyperphosphatemia can also lead to metastatic calcifications in joints, tissues, and arteries.

Management

Dietary restriction alone may suffice for control of hyperphosphatemia in persons with mild renal insufficiency. Most patients presenting with severe hyperphosphatemia also have hypocalcemia, treatment focuses on the correction of both electrolytes. In patients with normal renal function, phosphate excretion can be increased by saline infusion coupled with loop diuretics. Hyperphosphatemia usually resolves in 6 to 12 hr in patients with normal renal function.In patients with hyperphosphatemia with renal failure, hemodialysis or peritoneal dialysis should be considered early in the management.

HYPOPHOSPHATEMIA

Principles of Disease

Hypophosphatemia is defined as mild (2-2.5 mg/dL), moderate (1-2 mg/dL), or severe (<1 mg/dL). Mild to moderately severe hypophosphatemia is usually asymptomatic .Severe hypophosphatemia may result in potentially life-threatening complications. Symptoms of hypophosphatemia typically begin to be manifested at serum levels below 1.0 mg/dL. Acute hypophosphatemia is most commonly due to a rapid intracellular shift, but there are many other causes of clinical manifestations as well. Hyperventilation, glucose, insulin, volume, and resolving acidosis lead to hypophosphatemia by rapid intracellular shift. The many causes of hypophosphatemia include decreased phosphate intake or increased absorptive states, hyperventilatory states, hormonal and endocrine effects, medications, and disease states (Box 27-13).

Box 27-13 Five Most Common Causes of Hypophosphatemia in the ED

Decreased intake orincreased absorptive states	Chronic alcoholism Home parenteral nutrition AIDS Chemotherapy Vomiting Malabsorption syndromes Secretory diarrhea Vitamin D deficiency
Hyperventilatory states	Sepsis Alcohol withdrawal Salicylate poisoning Neuroleptic malignant syndrome Panic attacks Diabetic ketoacidosis Hepatic coma
Hormonal and endocrine effects	Insulin loading Glucose loading Exogenous epinephrine Hyperparathyroidism
Medications	Diuretics Chronic antacid ingestion Steroids Phosphate binders Xanthine derivatives $Beta_2$-agonists
Disease states	Trauma Severe thermal burns Acute renal failure Gout

Clinical Features

Mild to moderate hypophosphatemia is usually asymptomatic. Hypophosphatemia can affect a variety of organ systems and cause a wide variety of symptoms because phosphate is an essential component to adenosine triphosphate (Box 27-14). Patients with hypophosphatemia may present with nonspecific complaints including joint pain,

Box 27-14 Clinical Manifestations of Hypophosphatemia

Central nervous system	Irritability Confusion Paresthesias Depression Dysarthria Seizure Coma
Cardiovascular	Cardiomyopathy Depressed myocardial contractility Arrhythmias
Respiratory	Acute respiratory failure Depressed myocardial contractility
Gastrointestinal	Ileus, dysphagia
Hematologic	Depressed levels of 2,3-diphosphoglycerate and adenosine triphosphate Leukocyte dysfunction Hemolysis Platelet dysfunction
Renal	Acute tubular necrosis Metabolic acidosis Hypercalcemia
Endocrine	Insulin resistance Hyperparathyroidism

myalgias, irritability, and depression. Severe hypophosphatemia can be manifested as seizures, arrhythmias, cardiomyopathy, insulin resistance, acute tubular necrosis, rhabdomyolysis, and acute respiratory failure.

Management

Therapy for hypophosphatemia is recommended as levels drop below 1.5 to 2.0 mg/dL, and therapy is essential as levels fall below 1.0 mg/dL. Because hypophosphatemia often is manifested with hypokalemia, phosphate repletion is considered in conjunction with potassium administration. Oral phosphorous, 250 to 500 mg twice daily, can be given . Intravenous preparations are available as sodium phosphate (Na_2PO_4 and $NaPO_4$) or potassium phosphate (K_2PO_4 and KPO_4), and rate of infusion and choice of initial dosage should be based on severity of hypophosphatemia and presence of symptoms. If the serum phosphorus concentration is less than 1.5 mg/dL (0.48 mmol/L), 1.3 mmol/kg of elemental phosphorous (up to a maximum of 100 mmol) can be given in three or four divided doses in a 24 hr period. For routine replacement, give 0.5 mL/hr K_2PO_4; this may be increased to 1 mL/hr in severe symptomatic patients.Each milliliter of K_2PO_4 contains 3 mmol of phosphorus and 4.4 mEq of potassium. Typical replacement therapy provides approximately 1 g of phosphorus per day. Monitoring of patients for the development of hypocalcemia, hyperkalemia, and hyperphosphatemia is required while intravenous phosphate is administered, especially in patients with renal insufficiency.Risks of routine treatment with phosphate include hyperphosphatemia, renal failure, hypocalcemia, and hypomagnesemia.

(SHOU Songtao)

Chapter 28

Acid-Base Disorders

KEY CONSEPTS

Any condition that reduces minute ventilation may cause respiratory acidosis.

ABG analysis in Patients with COPD should be performed frequently and settings titrated to serum pH.

Metabolic acidoses are classically divided into normal AG and elevated AG to assist the clinician in determining their etiology.

When the cause of an elevated anion gap is determined to be lactate or ketones, diagnostic efforts are directed at identifying the cause of the lactic acidosis or ketoacidosis.

Severe metabolic alkalosis may cause hypocalcemic tetany, seizures, altered mental status, or dysrhythmias and require empirical therapy, with either acetazolamide or hydrochloric acid.

PERSPECTIVE

An acid-base disturbance may be the cause of a patient's symptoms and in some cases represents an immediate life threat. Treatment of many acid-base derangements is contingent on identification and treatment of the cause. Emergency physicians must therefore recognize when an acid-base disorder is present and have a diagnostic approach.

PRINCIPLES OF DISEASE

Many basic cellular processes are sensitive to small changes in serum pH; the kidneys, lungs, and physiologic buffers therefore defend serum pH, which is normally between 7.36 and 7.44. Serum pH is determined by the relative concentrations of bicarbonate (HCO_3^-) and carbon dioxide (P_aCO_2); when two of these variables are known. Most blood gas analyzers measure pH and $P_aCO_2$and report a calculated [HCO_3^-]; most laboratories, when they report a serum HCO_3^- concentration, are reporting a measured total carbon dioxide concentration,which is the sum of the serum bicarbonate and dissolved CO_2.

An acidosis is a process that lowers HCO_3^- or raises P_aCO_2 and tends to create an acidemia, which exists when serum pH is below 7.36. An alkalosis conversely represents a process that raises HCO_3^- or lowers P_aCO_2 and tends to create an alkalemia, which is present when serum pH is above 7.44. The terms acidemia and acidosis are not interchangeable; acidosis (or alkalosis) describes a process that pushes serum pH down (or up); acidemia and alkalemia describe the serum pH itself. A patient who is acidemic has at least one acidosis but may have two or more acidoses and may also have one or more alkaloses. Patients with normal serum pH, that is, without acidemia or alkalemia, may have acidoses and alkaloses whose net effect is serum neutrality.

HCO_3^- concentration is predominantly regulated by the kidneys and P_aCO_2 by lung ventilation. Diseases that affect kidney function may therefore produce a metabolic acidosis or alkalosis, for which the lungs will try to compensate by decreasing or increasing P_aCO_2, respectively. Likewise, pulmonary insults cause a respiratory acidosis or alkalosis, for which the kidneys will try to compensate by raising or lowering serum HCO_3^-, respectively.

In the majority of acid-base disturbances, the role of the emergency physician is to identify and manage dangerous causes of the disturbance. Uncommonly,serum pH below 6.7 or higher than 7.6

is considered unsustainable and may cause cardiac hypocontractility and irritability, seizures, cerebral edema, and a variety of metabolic disturbances.

A reduced serum HCO_3^- concentration defines a metabolic acidosis, which may be the primary disorder or a compensation for a primary respiratory alkalosis; an elevated serum HCO_3^- concentration defines a metabolic alkalosis, which may be the primary disorder or a compensation for a primary respiratory acidosis. Likewise, a reduced P_aCO_2 represents a respiratory alkalosis, and an elevated P_aCO_2 represents a respiratory acidosis. When only a primary disturbance and its corresponding compensation are present, it is described as a simple acid-base disorder. A mixed acid-base disorder exists when more than one primary disturbance occurs simultaneously.

Alterations in serum pH are resisted initially by intracellular and extracellular physiologic buffers, followed by specific responses from the lungs and the kidneys. Peripheral and central chemoreceptors adjust pulmonary minute ventilation in response to changes in serum pH. In a primary metabolic acidosis, an increase in minute ventilation lowers P_aCO_2 and pushes the serum pH closer to normal. A primary metabolic alkalosis likewise causes a reduction in minute ventilation to elevate P_aCO_2 in an attempt to restore physiologic serum pH.

The response of the kidneys to alterations in serum pH occurs over hours to days. A sustained acidemia promotes renal excretion of H^+ and retention of HCO_3^-, whereas alkalemia causes renal HCO_3^- excretion and H^+ retention.

DIAGNOSTIC STRATEGIES

An acid-base disturbance is often first identified when the results of laboratory tests ordered to evaluate the patient's symptoms demonstrate alterations in bicarbonate, pH, or P_aCO_2. The possibility of an acid-base disorder is suggested by clinical events such as toxic ingestions, severe vomiting, or diarrhea as well as in patients with diseases affecting the organs responsible for maintenance of acid-base balance—primarily the lungs and kidney. All critically ill patients and certainly all patients being mechanically ventilated require an assessment of acid-base status.

When the cause of an acid-base disturbance is not evident, the emergency evaluation begins with a full history and physical examination and proceeds with targeted laboratory studies.

Simple acid-base disorders are categorized by the serum pH, P_aCO_2, and HCO_3^- concentrations (Table 28-1). When the primary disturbance is identified, the next step is to determine its etiology and whether an appropriate compensation has occurred. An inappropriate compensation suggests that the process underlying the primary disturbance has hindered an appropriate response or that more than one primary disturbance is present. Simple formulas allow the calculation of an appropriate response once the primary disturbance has been categorized. Compensatory processes generally return pH toward normal but not to normal and never beyond normal; such an exaggerated "compensation" actually represents a second primary disorder.

Table 28-1 Categorization of Simple Acid-Base Disorders

	pH	P_aCO_2	HCO_3^-	EXPECTED COMPENSATION
Metabolic acidosis	↓	↓	↓	$\Delta P_aCO_2=1.2\ \Delta HCO_3^-$
Respiratory acidosis	↓	↑	↑	$\Delta HCO_3^-=0.10\ \Delta P_aCO_2$(acute) $\Delta HCO_3^-=0.35\ \Delta P_aCO_2$(chronic)
Metabolic alkalosis	↑	↑	↑	$\Delta P_aCO_2=0.9\ \Delta HCO_3^-$
Respiratory alkalosis	↑	↓	↓	$\Delta HCO_3^-=0.2\ \Delta P_aCO_2$(acute) $\Delta HCO_3^-=0.5\ \Delta P_aCO_2$(chronic)

ABG and serum chemistry analysis allows calculation and interpretation of the serum AG.

$$AG = Na^+ - (CL^- + HCO_3^-)$$

Plasma must remain electrically neutral: the sum of anions and cations must be equal. Because routinely measured cations exceed routinely measured anions, AG represents the concentration of anions other than chloride and bicarbonate in the blood. A variety of these anions are normally present, but serum albumin accounts for most of the physiologic (normal) AG, which is usually between 9 and 15. The higher AG, the more likely that one or more unmeasured anions is generating a metabolic acidosis. Besides albumin, classic unmeasured anions such as lactate and ketones are now also routinely measured and can be incorporated into a diagnostic pathway. Unmeasured cations are also present and may account for an elevated AG in cases of hypomagnesemia or hypocalcemia, often in combination with hypokalemia. Elevated concentrations of unmeasured cations may cause a low AG (<3 mEq/L), such as in cases of lithium toxicity and hypergammaglobulinemia seen in multiple myeloma. Bromide toxicity and hypertriglyceridemia may confound electrolyte measurements and also cause a low or negative AG.

The acute ketonemia therefore reduces serum HCO_3^- to "normal," and no AG is present. Patients at risk for hypoalbuminemia should have serum albumin measured, and if it is low, a normal serum HCO_3^- concentration represents a metabolic acidosis. AG can be adjusted to reflect hypoalbuminemia, when albumin is measured in grams per deciliter, by the following formula:

Adjusted AG=observed AG+2.5 (4.2-serum albumin)

A normal AG does not exclude clinically significant acidosis or high concentrations of unmeasured anions.

Independent of HCO_3^- levels, sodium and chloride play an important role in acid-base status. When $[Na^+] - [Cl^-]$, the so-called strong ion difference, is significantly less than 38, an acidosis is present. What remains is, in the case of metabolic acidosis, the unmeasured anions (e.g., lactate, ketones, uremic acids, toxic alcohols, or other toxins).

P_aCO_2, HCO_3^-, and pH values taken from peripheral venous, central venous, intraosseous, and capillary blood are all suitable for acid-base assessment.

RESPIRATORY ACIDOSIS

Respiratory acidosis occurs when hypoventilation leads to an inappropriately elevated P_aCO_2 and resulting acidemia. Any condition that reduces minute ventilation may cause respiratory acidosis (Box 28-1).When tissue oxygenation is adequate, hypercapnia which is better tolerated than hypoxemia tends to produce somnolence and obtundation with cerebral vasodilation and resulting elevation of intracranial pressure.

Beginning 6 to 12 hr after onset of the insult and progressing for 3 to 5 d, the kidneys respond to a respiratory acidosis by retaining HCO_3^- the resulting compensatory metabolic alkalosis, with an elevated serum HCO_3^-level, partially corrects serum pH. Chloride ions are excreted in the urine to increase serum HCO_3^-; patients with chronic respiratory acidosis are therefore often noted to have hypochloremia. An appropriate metabolic compensation for respiratory acidosis is an increase of approximately 3.5 mEq/L in serum HCO_3^- concentration for every increase of 10 mm Hg in $PacCO_2$; a patient with chronic respiratory disease resulting in a baseline P_aCO_2 of 60 mm Hg would therefore be expected to have a serum HCO_3^- level of approximately 30 mEq/L (and a slight acidemia).

Box 28-1 Causes of Respiratory Acidosis

Acute
- Airway obstruction
- Pulmonary disease
  - Pneumonia
  - Asthma
  - Pulmonary edema
  - Aspiration pneumonitis
- Central nervous system depression
  - Recreational drugs (opiates, barbiturates, benzodiazepines, alcohol, γ-hydroxybutyrate)
  - Intracranial catastrophe (intracerebral hemorrhage, subarachnoid hemorrhage, cerebrovascular accident)
  - Intravenous sedation
- Neuromuscular disorders
  - Myasthenia gravis
  - Guillain-Barré syndrome
- Thoracic trauma
  - Pneumothorax
  - Flail chest

Chronic
- Lung disease
  - COPD
  - Interstitial lung disease, idiopathic pulmonary fibrosis
- Neuromuscular disorders
  - Amyotrophic lateral sclerosis
  - Muscular dystrophy
- Obesity hypoventilation (pickwickian) syndrome

Acute respiratory acidosis is the most immediately dangerous of the acid-base disturbances.

Patients with chronic respiratory acidosis are often hypoxemic at baseline and may be susceptible to further hypoventilation if normal oxygen saturation levels are promptly restored.Typically, a patient with COPD being treated for an acute exacerbation receives high-flow oxygen and is later found to be obtunded with profound hypercapnia.However, supplemental oxygen must not be withheld from patients with dangerously low oxygen saturation or patients with end-organ hypoxic insults, such as myocardial or cerebral ischemia. In these cases, aggressive oxygenation therapies must be instituted, with preparations made to initiate mechanical ventilation if it is needed.

Patients with chronic respiratory acidosis who have been intubated should receive frequent blood gas analyses; standard ventilator settings applied to patients who chronically hypoventilate may precipitate posthypercapnic metabolic alkalosis. Correction of P_aCO_2 to normal levels (40 mm Hg) in this group can cause dangerous alkalemia; clinicians should target a slightly acidemic serum pH (~7.35), which, depending on the severity and chronicity of the patient's baseline respiratory acidosis, may correspond to remarkably high P_aCO_2 levels.

RESPIRATORY ALKALOSIS

Respiratory alkalosis occurs when increased minute ventilation causes a decreased P_aCO_2 and subsequent increase in serum pH. It is often associated with hysterical hyperventilation; however, as always, the emergency physician must consider dangerous conditions before arriving at a psychiatric diagnosis (Box 28-2).

Box 28-2 Causes of Respiratory Alkalosis

- Hyperventilation caused by hypoxia
  - High altitude
  - Severe anemia
  - Ventilation-perfusion mismatch
- Central hyperventilation
  - Voluntary or psychogenic
  - Cerebrovascular accident
  - Increased intracranial pressure (tumor, hemorrhage, trauma)
- Toxic or pharmacologic
  - Salicylates
  - Caffeine, nicotine
  - Catecholamines
  - Thyroxine
- Pulmonary
  - Pulmonary embolism
  - Pneumonia
  - Pulmonary edema
  - Asthma
  - Mechanical hyperventilation (iatrogenic)
- Endocrine
  - Pregnancy
  - Hyperthyroidism
- Septicemia
- Hepatic encephalopathy
- Hyponatremia

Of particular interest in the differential diagnosis of acute respiratory alkalosis is salicylate toxicity that may be manifested with hyperventilation as its most prominent feature. Suicidal aspirin ingestions often produce the classic syndrome of tinnitus, hyperthermia, confusion, and a variety of metabolic derangements ultimately leading to seizures, coma, and cardiovascular collapse.Emergency physicians should have a low threshold to obtain a serum salicylate level in cases of unexplained respiratory alkalosis.

Patients with respiratory alkalosis classically complain of lip and extremity paresthesias and may also experience muscle cramps and lightheadedness or even syncope as well as hypocalcemia symptoms, such as carpopedal spasm.If respiratory alkalosis persists, the kidneys excrete HCO_3^- and retain chloride, leading to a compensatory metabolic acidosis with reduced serum HCO_3^-, hypokalemia, and hyperchloremia.

As with other acid-base disorders, management of respiratory alkalosis is directed at the underlying cause.When organic causes of respiratory alkalosis have been excluded, hypocapnia symptoms can be relieved in patients with psychological hyperventilation by reassurance. The technique of using a paper bag to cause rebreathing probably works.

METABOLIC ACIDOSIS

Metabolic acidosis is defined by a reduced serum HCO_3^- concentration.

Etiology

Metabolic acidosis occurs when acids are added, acid excretion is impaired, or there is inappropriate loss of alkali. Metabolic acidoses are classically divided into normal AG and elevated AG to assist the clinician in determining their etiology.

Elevated AG Metabolic Acidosis

The causes of elevated AG metabolic acidosis are classically remembered by the mnemonic MUDPILES(methanol, uremia, DKA and alcoholic ketoacidosis, paraldehyde, INH and iron, lactic acidosis, ethylene glycol and salicylates); however, it is more useful to focus on the identity of the unmeasured anion (Box 28-3). If the cause of an elevated AG metabolic acidosis is found to be lactate or ketones, the next step is to determine the cause of the high serum lactate or ketone concentration.

Box 28-3 Causes of Elevated Anion Gap Metabolic Acidosis

Ketoacidosis
- DKA
- Alcoholic ketoacidosis
- Starvation ketoacidosis

Lactic acidosis
- Global tissue ischemia
  - Shock
  - Grand mal seizure (if persistent, consider isoniazid)
- Focal end-organ ischemia (limb ischemia, mesenteric ischemia)
- Inadequate blood oxygenation
  - Hypoxia (from airway or breathing disorder)
  - Carbon monoxide, methemoglobinemia
- Inability of tissues to use oxygen from cellular poisons
  - Cyanide (or nitroprusside therapy), hydrogen sulfide, aspirin, iron
- Impaired lactate clearance
  - Liver failure
  - Metformin or phenformin
  - Reverse transcriptase inhibitors (for HIV infection therapy)

Renal failure

Toxins metabolized to acids
- Toxic alcohols (methanol, ethylene glycol)
- Toluene
- Paraldehyde
- Aspirin

Severe rhabdomyolysis

Increased production of lactate is a common cause of elevated AG metabolic acidosis, and measurement of serum lactate is indicated. When the elevation of AG is accounted for by serum lactate concentration, the clinician next considers the causes of lactic acidosis; these may be divided into hypoxic or hypoperfusion states and exogenous cellular toxins, such as cyanide and carbon monoxide. Idiosyncratic causes of lactic acidosis include short gut syndrome (usually after bariatric surgery),reverse transcriptase inhibitor therapy for HIV infection,and metformin therapy. The likelihood of metformin causing lactic acidosis is thought to be enhanced by renal failure (serum creatinine >1.5 mg/dL), CHF, coexisting metabolic acidosis, and exposure to intravenous radiologic contrast media.

Common unmeasured anions other than lactate that cause an elevated AG metabolic acidosis include keto acids , acidic products of exogenous toxins , and organic acids that accumulate in renal failure.

Carbon Monoxide and Cyanide. Exposure to carbon monoxide and cyanide causes lactic acidosis through tissue hypoxia; both are important elements of the differential diagnosis of an elevated AG of unknown cause.Severity of carbon monoxide exposure and treatment requirements may be better predicted by the degree of initial acidemia than by carboxyhemoglobin level.

Diabetic Ketoacidosis. Patients with DKA classically complain of progressive polyuria, polydipsia, and malaise, but DKA may be manifested atypically with chief complaints of vomiting, abdominal pain, or altered mental status.DKA is often caused by medication noncompliance but may complicate any physiologic stress; when DKA is diagnosed, identification of the precipitant is a management priority. Treatment focuses on volume expansion with intravenous fluids, insulin therapy, and careful attention to and replacement of electrolytes, particularly potassium.

Alcoholic Ketoacidosis. Alcoholic ketoacidosis is usually seen when a long-standing ethanol user abruptly stops drinking; ketones are generated by a combination of malnutrition and dehydration. Patients with alcoholic ketoacidosis may demonstrate a high AG, but a mixed acid-base disorder can be due to concomitant ethanol withdrawal, which may cause a respiratory alkalosis, and vomiting, which produces a metabolic alkalosis. The resultant serum pH can therefore be acidemic, normal, or alkalemic. Like DKA, Alcoholic ketoacidosis includes the symptoms of vomiting, abdominal pain, dehydration, altered mental status, prostration, and lethargy. Alcoholic ketoacidosis patients generally do not demonstrate hyperglycemia or glycosuria. In alcoholic ketoacidosis, the ratio of the keto acid β-hydroxybutyrate to its metabolites acetoacetate and acetone is double the ratio seen in DKA. Urine dipsticks detect acetoacetate but not β-hydroxybutyrate.The treatment of alcoholic ketoacidosis is dextrose-containing fluids.

Methanol and Ethylene Glycol. Methanol and ethylene glycol, the toxic alcohols, represent an important element of the emergency differential for elevated AG metabolic acidosis. The first measurable sign of toxic alcohol poisoning is an *osmol gap*, which precedes the elevated AG; as the parent compounds are converted to their toxic metabolites, the *osmol gap* closes and AG widens. Treatment centers on prevention of the enzymatic conversion of methanol and ethylene glycol into their toxic metabolites by use of either ethanol or fomepizole. Many laboratories will report a spuriously elevated lactate concentration in the presence of glycolate, a byproduct of ethylene glycol poisoning. Isopropyl (rubbing) alcohol ingestion causes intoxication, ketosis, and an osmol gap but does not cause acidosis.

Renal Failure. Under normal circumstances, the body generates a net acid load that the kidneys must continuously excrete. Any condition that reduces GFR will undermine this function, and unmeasured anions such as sulfate, phosphate, urate, and hippurate will generate an elevated AG metabolic acidosis. Administration of sodium bicarbonate is used as a bridge to renal replacement therapy when uremia-associated metabolic acidosis is severe.

Isoniazid. Isoniazid (INH) toxicity is usually listed in the differential for metabolic acidosis, but consideration of INH toxicity should primarily be prompted by intractable seizures because it is the seizures that cause the lactic acidosis, not INH. Continuous seizure activity, in addition to cardio-respiratory embarrassment, causes a profound, life-threatening acidemia from lactate generation. The initial treatment of status epilepticus related to INH toxicity is the administration of vitamin B_6 (pyridoxine). Specific therapies targeting nonepileptic causes of seizures, such as hypoglycemia, eclampsia, hyponatremia, and cyanide toxicity, should also be considered in the patient with seizures unresponsive to standard therapy.

Salicylate Toxicity. Salicylate toxicity first produces a respiratory alkalosis,as described before.Untreated,the syndrome evolves into a complex acid-base disorder with paradoxical aciduria during the initial respiratory alkalosis, followed by an elevated AG metabolic acidosis and hyperthermia due to its interference with cellular metabolism. Serum pH can be normal during the initial phase of the disease—a false reassurance. Dehydration, electrolyte disturbances, fatigue, and lung injury ultimately lead to decompensation with respiratory acidosis—completing the so-called triple acid-base disturbance—followed by cardiovascular collapse. Management of aspirin toxicity includes gastrointestinal decontamination, urine alkalinization, meticulous supportive care, and hemodialysis.

Normal Anion Gap Metabolic Acidosis

The majority of cases encountered in the emergency department are caused by gastric loss of bicarbonate in the setting of diarrhea. A variety of other conditions and medications may cause a normal AG metabolic acidosis (Box 28-4).An important iatrogenic cause of normal AG metabolic acidosis is the rapid infusion of large volumes of normal saline.

Box 28-4 Causes of Normal Anion Gap Metabolic Acidosis

Gastrointestinal HCO_3^- loss
- Diarrhea
- Colostomy or ileostomy
- Enteric fistulas
- Ion exchange resins (e.g., sodium polystyrene sulfonate [Kayexalate])

Renal HCO_3^- loss
- Renal tubular acidosis
- Tubulointerstitial renal disease
- Hyperparathyroidism

Rapid normal saline infusion

Urologic procedures
- Ureterosigmoidostomy
- Ureteroileal conduit

Ingestions
- Acetazolamide
- Calcium chloride ($CaCl_2$)
- Magnesium sulfate ($MgSO_4$)

Other
- Hypoaldosteronism
- Hyperkalemia
- Toluene (after initial elevated anion gap metabolic acidosis)

Physiologic Compensation

Physiologic compensation for a metabolic acidosis occurs immediately by the extracellular HCO_3^--carbonic acid system and intracellular protein buffers. Medullary chemoreceptors augment alveolar ventilation to blow off CO_2, partially correcting serum pH. In severe metabolic acidosis (pH <7.1), hyperventilation is profound and assumes the appearance of Kussmaul's respirations.In cases of prolonged metabolic acidosis, the kidney generates a compensatory aciduria by secreting H^+ and retaining HCO_3^-.

Management

Management of metabolic acidosis is directed at identification and treatment of the underlying cause while appropriate resuscitative and supportive care is provided.

When to treat acidemia by actively correcting serum pH, with use of intravenous sodium bicarbonate, is controversial. Theoretic harms of using intravenous sodium bicarbonate to correct acidemia include the following:

- Paradoxical CNS acidosis. Because sodium bicarbonate does not readily cross the blood-brain barrier, serum alkalinizes much faster than the cerebrospinal fluid. As serum pH rises, minute ventilation slows and carbon dioxide, which readily crosses the blood-brain barrier, delivers an additional acid load to the CNS.
- Hypokalemia (which can cause respiratory muscle weakness, impairing respiratory compensation), hypocalcemia, hypernatremia
- Volume overload
- Hyperosmolality
- Overshoot alkalosis

It is commonly recommended to treat serum pH less than 7.1 empirically with sodium bicarbonate, 1 mEq/kg,unless the underlying acidosis is thought to be quickly responsive to therapy.Endpoints of therapy include pH above 7.1 and serum bicarbonate concentration above 10 mEq/L.

Bicarbonate has been variously recommended and used as an empirical therapy in cardiac arrest.

In summary, sodium bicarbonate should not routinely be used to treat undifferentiated acidemia or acidemia caused by lactic acidosis or ketoacidosis.Clinicians managing patients with acid-base disturbances should carefully monitor serum potassium concentration.

METABOLIC ALKALOSIS

Metabolic alkalosis occurs from the loss of H^+ or retention of HCO_3^-. Emergency physicians encounter metabolic alkalosis usually as a consequence of prolonged vomiting or nasogastric suction or as a compensation for chronic respiratory acidosis. The differential diagnosis includes a variety of predominantly endocrine and electrolyte disorders (Box 28-5). Patients taking diuretic medications may reduce their plasma volume around a steady concentration of HCO_3^-, causing a contraction alkalosis. Contraction alkalosis is often coincident with hypokalemia, which itself causes a metabolic alkalosis as intracellular K^+ is exchanged for H^+.

In the acute phase, the lungs compensate for a metabolic alkalosis by decreasing minute ventilation and retaining CO_2. Prolonged metabolic alkalosis leads to compensatory renal HCO_3^- excretion.

Metabolic alkalosis rarely causes dangerous alkalemia, and the emergency management of metabolic alkalosis is directed at identification and treatment of dangerous underlying causes. Usual management of patients who have volume loss, vomiting, or hypokalemia will address the resulting saline-responsive metabolic alkalosis. Severe metabolic alkalosis may cause hypocalcemic tetany, seizures, altered mental status, or dysrhythmias and require empirical therapy,with either acetazolamide or hydrochloric acid.

Box 28-5 Causes of Metabolic Alkalosis

Volume Contracted (saline responsive)
- Vomiting, gastric suction
- Diuretics (contraction alkalosis)
- Postrespiratory acidosis
- Ion-deficient baby formula
- Chloride-secreting colonic villous adenomas

Euvolemic/Volume Expanded (saline resistant)
- Hyperaldosteronism
- Hypercortisolemia
- Severe potassium depletion
- Adenocarcinoma
- Bartter's syndrome

Unclassified
- Hypoalbuminemia
- Milk-alkali syndrome
- Penicillin and related compounds
- Hypercalcemia of malignancy
- Massive transfusion (from citrate), especially with renal insufficiency

MIXED DISORDERS

Mixed acid-base disorders occur when two or more primary acid-base lesions coincide. These simultaneous conditions may push the serum pH in the same or opposite directions, and each will generate its own compensatory responses; mixed disorders may therefore be difficult to recognize by either clinical or laboratory features. Most patients with mixed acid-base disorders, there is a dominant, precipitating problem that either complicates an existing disease or causes failure of compensatory mechanisms.

Detailed acid-bases analysis is not typically performed in the emergency department; however, knowledge of frequently used acid-base assessment concepts and common conditions that cause a mixed disturbance is valuable. The body usually does not fully compensate for a primary acid-base disorder, so, for example, a primary metabolic acidosis should generate a compensatory respiratory alkalosis, but the serum pH is expected to still be below 7.36. Whether an appropriate respiratory compensation to a metabolic acidosis has occurred can be approximated by comparing the P_aCO_2 to the last two digits of the serum pH. In a primary metabolic acidosis with appropriate respiratory compensation, these two values should be similar, that is, a patient with a serum pH of 7.20 should have a P_aCO_2 of 20 mm Hg.If the serum pH is 7.17 and the P_aCO_2 is 30 mm Hg,the respiratory compensation is less than expected and a primary respiratory acidosisis present. This is commonly seen in patients whose dominant condition causes a metabolic acidosis but also impairs respiration, such as sepsis.

The delta gap(ΔG) describes the difference between the deviation of AG from normal and the deviation of the serum bicarbonate concentration from normal:

$$\Delta G=(AG-12)-(24-[HCO_3^-]).$$

Conceptually, calculation of the delta gap asks whether the AG is accounted for by the change in serum bicarbonate concentration. In patients with an elevated AG and a delta gap greater than +6, meaning that serum bicarbonate level is significantly higher than would be predicted by the number of unmeasured anions, a metabolic alkalosis in addition to a metabolic acidosis is likely to be present. This is commonly seen when the dominant acidosis condition causes severe vomiting (e.g., DKA). In patients with an elevated AG and delta gap more negative than −6, meaning that the serum bicarbonate level is significantly lower than expected given AG, a normal AG metabolic acidosis is likely be present in addition to the elevated anion gap metabolic acidosis. This is seen most commonly when a lactic acidosis complicates severe diarrhea.

(SHOU Songtao)

Neurologic Emergencies

Chapter 29

Acute Meningitis

KEY CONCEPTS

CNS infection should be considered in all patients with headache, neck stiffness, fever, altered sensorium, or diffuse or focal neurologic findings.

LP with sampling of CSF is the only reliable method of assessing the presence or absence of meningitis.

Antibiotic chemoprophylaxis should be ensured for close contacts of patients with meningitis resulting from Neisseria meningitidis or Haemophilus influenzae.

Concomitant CNS infection should be strongly considered in any patient with another severe systemic infection, such as urinary tract infection or pneumonia.

DEFINITION

Meningitis is defined as inflammation of the membranes of the brain or spinal cord and is also called *arachnoiditis* or *leptomeningitis*.

PRINCIPLES OF DISEASE

Etiology

Meningitis

Meningeal inflammation may be caused by a variety of disease processes, but the infectious causes predominate. Among the bacterial agents, *Streptococcus pneumoniae* remains the predominant pathogen in adult patients, followed by *Neisseria meningitides* and *Listeria monocytogenes. N. meningitidis* is the predominant organism in adults younger than 45 yr. Five major serogroups cause most meningococcal disease worldwide (A, B, C, Y, and W-135). Serogroup A accounts for the majority of cases of meningococcal meningitis in developing nations. A new vaccine for serogroup A may potentially reduce the impact of this disease in nearly half a billion individuals at risk. These pathogens account for the bulk of cases in nontraumatic meningitis, although virtually any organism can be encountered, particularly among patients who are elderly, alcoholic, or immunosuppressed and those who have cancer. Interestingly, higher case fatality has been observed in N. meningitidis outbreaks versus sporadic cases, probably because of increased virulence of outbreak-related strains. Causes of aseptic meningitis, simply defined as all cases with CSF cultures negative for bacteria, are listed in Box 29-1.

Box 29-1 Causes of Aseptic Meningitis

Infectious Causes	Noninfectious Causes
Viruses	***Postinfectious/postvaccinial***
Enteroviruses: polio, Coxsackie, ECHO virus	Rubeola
	Rubella
	Varicella
Herpes group of viruses	Variola
Herpes simplex virus types 1 and 2	Rabies vaccine
	Pertussis vaccine
Varicella-zoster virus	Influenza vaccine
Cytomegalovirus	Vaccinia
Epstein-Barr virus	Yellow fever vaccine
Human herpesvirus 6 (HHV-6)	***Drugs***
	NSAID

Respiratory viruses	Trimethoprim-sulfamethoxazole, amoxicillin
Adenovirus	
Rhinovirus	Muromonab CD3 (OKT3)
Influenza virus types A and B	Azathioprine
	Intravenous immune globulin
Arboviruses	Isoniazid
Mumps virus	Intrathecal methotrexate
Lymphocytic choriomeningitis	Intrathecal cytosine arabinoside
HIV	Allopurinol
Bacteria	Carbamazepine
Partially treated meningitis	Sulfasalazine
Parameningeal infection	***Systemic disease***
Endocarditis	Collagen vascular disorders
Mycoplasma pneumoniae	SLE
	Wegener's granulomatosis
Mycoplasma tuberculosis	Central nervous system vasculitis
Ehrlichiosis	
Borrelia burgdorferi	RA
Treponema pallidum	Kawasaki disease
Brucella	Sarcoidosis
Leptospirosis	Leptomeningeal cancer
Fungi	Post-transplantation lymphoproliferative disorder
Cryptococcus neoformans	
Histoplasma capsulatum	Behcet's disease
	Vogt-Koyanagi syndrome
Coccidioides immitis	***Neoplastic disorders***
Blastomyces dermatitidis	Leukemia
Candida	Carcinomatous meningitis *secondary to primary or secondary tumors of the brain*
Parasites	
Toxoplasma gondii	
Neurocysticercosis	
Trichinosis	***Inflammation of neighboring structures***
Naegleria	
Hartmannella	Brain abscess
Bartonella henselae	Epidural abscess
Rickettsiae	***Miscellaneous***
Rocky Mountain spotted fever	Arachnoiditis
	Migraine
Typhus	Urinary tract infection

Meningeal infection may also occur in association with a dural leak secondary to neurosurgery or neurotrauma. *S. pneumoniae*, *Staphylococcus aureus*, *Pseudomonas aeruginosa*, and coliform bacteria are seen most commonly in this population.

Viral meningitis may likewise be caused by a variety of etiologic agents. Enteroviruses are statistically encountered most commonly. Unfortunately, precise identification of the etiologic agent is often impossible. Fungal and parasitic meningitides are additional concerns, particularly among immunocompromised patients. Viral meningitis secondary to herpes simplex virus infection is actually relatively benign, especially in comparison with herpes simplex virus encephalitis.

Pathophysiology

Bacterial Meningitis

The pathogenetic sequence in bacterial meningitis has been well characterized. The first step is nasopharyngeal colonization and mucosal invasion. Although colonization rates vary, virulent microbes use secretion of immunoglobulin A proteases and induce ciliostasis of mucosal cells. After penetration occurs by a variety of mechanisms, bacterial intravascular survival occurs because of evasion of the complement pathway. The varying capsular properties of each organism protect the bacteria. The third step occurs when the bacteria cross the blood-brain barrier to enter the CSF. The dural venous sinuses, cribriform plate area, and choroid plexus have all been implicated as potential sites of invasion. Although the mechanism of invasion is not completely understood, host defense mechanisms within the CSF are often ineffective; there are low levels of complement, immunoglobulin, and opsonic activity. Bacterial proliferation then occurs, which stimulates a convergence of leukocytes into the CSF.

Meningeal and subarachnoid space inflammation is also associated with the release of cytokines into the CSF, most notably tumor necrosis factor and IL1 and IL6. This results in increased permeability of the blood-brain barrier, cerebral vasculitis, edema, and increased intracranial pressure. A subsequent decrease in cerebral blood flow leads to cerebral hypoxia. Glucose transport into the CSF is decreased concomitantly with an increased use of glucose by the brain, bacteria, and leukocytes, which depresses CSF glucose concentrations. The increased permeability leads to increased CSF proteins.

Viral Meningitis

Viruses enter the human host through the skin; through the respiratory, gastrointestinal, or urogenital tract; or by receipt of infected blood products.

Fungal Meningitis

Fungal meningitis probably develops in much

the same way as bacterial meningitis does.Immune system defects or immunosuppressive medications compromise host defense mechanisms, with ensuing development of CNS infection.

CLINICAL FEATURES

Symptoms and Signs

Numerous host factors have been implicated in the acquisition of meningitis (Box 29-2). Although these factors alone and in combination increase the risk of meningitis, the disease often occurs in patients with none of these factors.

Box 29-2 Host Factors Predisposing to Meningitis

- Age > 60 yr
- Male gender
- Low socioeconomic status
- Crowding (e.g., military recruits)
- Splenectomy
- Sickle cell disease
- Alcoholism and cirrhosis
- DM
- Immunologic defects
- Recent colonization
- Dural defect (e.g., traumatic, surgical, congenital)
- Continuous infection (e.g., sinusitis)
- Household contact with meningitis patient
- Thalassemia major
- Injection drug abuse
- Bacterial endocarditis
- Ventriculoperitoneal shunt
- Malignant disease

Many patients with meningitis present with advanced disease. The constellation of symptoms consists of fever, headache, photophobia, nuchal rigidity, lethargy, malaise, altered sensorium, seizures, vomiting, and chills.

Immunosuppressed and geriatric patients present a diagnostic challenge because the classic signs and symptoms of meningitis may not be present. Although some degree of fever is present in most patients, as are a headache and neck stiffness, meningitis should be carefully considered in any immunosuppressed patient with symptoms or signs of infectious disease. Often, the only presenting sign of meningitis in elders is an alteration of mental status.

The presentation of fungal meningitis can be obscure even in the healthy adult population. Headache, low-grade fever, lassitude, and weight loss may be present but often to such a mild degree that the correct diagnosis is not initially considered. This is also true of tuberculous meningitis, which often has a protracted course and a vague nonspecific presentation consisting of fever, weight loss, night sweats, and malaise, with or without headache and meningismus.

The systemic findings may include an obvious source of infection, such as sinusitis, otitis media, mastoiditis, pneumonia, or urinary tract infection.

Complications

Bacterial Meningitis

The immediate complications of bacterial meningitis include coma (with loss of protective airway reflexes), seizures, cerebral edema, vasomotor collapse, disseminated intravascular coagulation, respiratory arrest, dehydration, syndrome of inappropriate secretion of antidiuretic hormone, pericardial effusion, and death (Box 29-3). Various delayed complications include multiple seizures, focal paralysis, subdural effusions, hydrocephalus, intellectual deficits, sensorineural hearing loss, ataxia, blindness, bilateral adrenal hemorrhage (Waterhouse-Friderichsen syndrome), peripheral gangrene, and death.

Box 29-3 Complications of Bacterial Meningitis

Immediate

- Coma
- Loss of airway reflexes
- Seizures
- Cerebral edema
- Vasomotor collapse
- Disseminated intravascular coagulation
- Respiratory arrest
- Dehydration
- Pericardial effusion
- Death

Delayed

- Seizure disorde
- Focal paralysisSubdural effusion

Hydrocephalus
Intellectual deficits
Sensorineural hearing loss
Ataxia
Blindness
Bilateral adrenal hemorrhage
Cerebral venous thrombosis
Death

The case fatality rate for pneumococcal meningitis averages 20% to 25%; higher fatality rates occur in patients with serious underlying or concomitant disease or advanced age. The prognosis is related to the degree of neurologic impairment on presentation. Overall, 20% to 30% of the survivors of pneumococcal meningitis have some residual neurologic deficit. The case fatality rate for *Listeria* meningitis may be as high as 40%.

With the advent of antibiotic therapy, the mortality from meningococcal meningitis has markedly decreased to less than 20%, but it remains substantially higher in elders and those who have meningococcemia. Although most of the complications and sequelae are less common than with pneumococcal disease,the incidence of Waterhouse-Friderichsen syndrome is dramatically higher when meningococcemia is present. The overall mortality rate in community-acquired gram-negative meningitis has been less than 20% since the introduction of the third-generation cephalosporins.

Viral Meningitis

With rare exceptions, the overall prognosis for complete recovery from viral meningitis is excellent. Various complications related to the systemic effects of the particular virus include orchitis, parotitis, pancreatitis, and various dermatoses. Usually, all of these complications resolve without sequelae.

Tuberculous Meningitis

Death from tuberculous meningitis in the adult age group ranges from 10% to 50% of cases, with the incidence directly proportional to the patient's age and the duration of symptoms before presentation. Focal ischemic stroke may result from the associated cerebral vasculitis. In advanced disease, up to 25% of patients may require some neurosurgical procedure for obstruction (ventriculoperitoneal shunt or drainage). Some neurologic deficit develops in most patients, but severe long-term sequelae among survivors are unusual.

Fungal Meningitis

Common CNS complications with fungal meningitis include abscesses, papilledema, neurologic deficits, seizures, bone invasion, and fluid collections. Direct invasion of the optic nerve results in ocular abnormalities in up to 40% of patients with cryptococcal meningitis. The mortality rate is high but variable and is related to the timeliness of diagnosis, underlying illness, and therapeutic regimens.

DIAGNOSTIC STRATEGIES

Lumbar Puncture

The possibility of the diagnosis of meningitis mandates LP. Some patients have clinically obvious bacterial meningitis, and CSF examination serves primarily to help identify the organism.

Increased Intracranial Pressure

It is advisable to obtain a CT scan of the head before LP is performed. An algorithm for diagnostic and therapeutic decision-making is presented in Fig. 29-1.

It has been conventionally asserted that LP in the presence of increased intracranial pressure may be harmful or fatal to the patient.These patients may deteriorate precipitously during or after the procedure.

Patients with a markedly depressed sensorium that precludes careful neurologic examination or those with a focal neurologic deficit, papilledema, seizures, or evidence of head trauma must be considered to be at risk for a herniation syndrome that may be exacerbated by LP.The algorithmic alternatives are therefore (1) immediate LP followed by initiation of antibiotic treatment before the results are obtained (2) initiation of antibiotic treatment followed by a cranial CT scan and then LP. The latter choice of empirical treatment with antibiotics is now the routine in many institutions, although in some cases a third option could be considered:

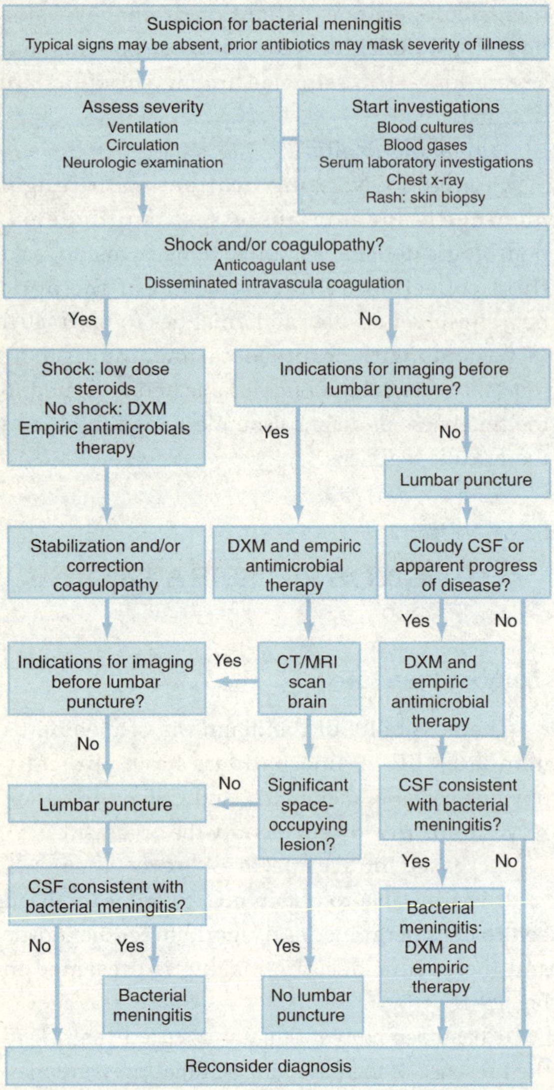

Fig. 29-1 Algorithm for diagnostic and therapeutic decisionmaking.

antibiotics and no LP despite an unremarkable CT scan.

Raised intracranial pressure may not be reliably detected by CT. Clinical signs of increased intracranial pressure, rapid change in consciousness, and recent seizures were identified as risk factors predicting deterioration despite a normal CT scan.

Cerebrospinal Fluid Analysis

The normal CSF pressure in an adult varies from 5 to 20 cm H_2O.

This value applies only to patients in the lateral recumbent position and may increase substantially when the patient is in the sitting position. The pressure is often elevated in bacterial, tuberculous, and fungal meningitides and a variety of noninfectious processes. Pressure may be falsely elevated when the patient is tense or obese or has marked muscle contraction.

At least three sterile tubes each containing at least 1 to 1.5 mL of CSF are obtained and numbered in sequence. A fourth tube may be desirable should later studies, such as viral cultures or a Venereal Disease Research Laboratory (VDRL) test for syphilis, become necessary. The fluid is sent to the laboratory for immediate analysis of turbidity, xanthochromia, glucose, protein, cell count and differential, Gram's stain, bacterial culture, and antigen testing (Table 29-1). In certain cases an India ink stain, a bacteriologic stain for acid-fast bacilli, or a VDRL test should be obtained.

Table 29-1 Analysis of Cerebrospinal Fluid

TEST	NORMAL VALUE	SIGNIFICANCE OF ABNORMALITY
Cell count	≤5 WBC/mm^3 ≤1 PMN/mm^3 ≤1 eosinophil/mm^3	Increased WBC counts are seen in all types of meningitis and encephalitis; increased PMN count suggests bacterial pathogen
Gram's stain	No organism	Offending organism identified 80% of the time in bacterial meningitis, 60% if patient has been pretreated
Turbidity	Clear	Increased turbidity with leukocytosis, blood, or high concentration of microorganisms
Xanthochromia	None	Presence of RBCs in spinal fluid for 4 hr before LP; occasionally caused by traumatic tap (if protein ≥150 mg/dL) or hypercarotenemia
CSF-to-serum glucose ratio	0.6 : 1	Depressed in pyogenic meningitis or hyperglycemia;lag time if glucose given intravenously

Continued

TEST	NORMAL VALUE	SIGNIFICANCE OF ABNORMALITY
Protein	15-45 mg/dL	Elevated with acute bacterial or fungal meningitis; also elevated with vasculitis,syphilis, encephalitis,neoplasms, and demyelination syndromes
India ink stain	Negative	Positive in one third of cases of cryptococcal meningitis
Cryptococcal antigen	Negative	90% accuracy for cryptococcal disease
Lactic acid	≤35 mg/dL	Elevated in bacterial and tubercular meningitis
Bacterial antigen tests	Negative	≥95% specific for organism tested; up to 50% falsenegative rate
Acid-fast stain	Negative	Positive in 80% of cases of tuberculous meningitis if ≥10 mL of fluid

Turbidity

Normal CSF is completely clear and colorless and is indistinguishable from water, any degree of turbidity is pathologic. Leukocytosis is the most common cause of CSF turbidity;counts greater than 200 cells/mm^3 usually cause clinically detectable changes in CSF clarity.

Cell Count and Differential

Normal adult CSF contains no more than 5 leukocytes/mm^3 with at most one granulocyte (polymorphonuclear [PMN] leukocyte); therefore, the presence of more than one PMN or a total cell count of more than 5 cells/mm^3 should be considered evidence of meningitis.

The cell counts in bacterial meningitis are usually markedly elevated, sometimes exceeding 10,000 cells/mm^3, and demonstrate a dramatic granulocytic shift. In general, counts exceed 500 cells/mm^3, with a preponderance of PMN leukocytes. However, the initial CSF analysis exhibits lymphocytosis (lymphocyte count greater than 50%) in 6% to 13% of all cases of bacterial meningitis.In addition, the same population of patients often has only a mild disturbance of CSF glucose and protein levels. In well-established viral meningitis, counts are usually less than 500 cells/mm^3, with nearly 100% of the cells being mononuclear. Early (48 hr) presentations may reveal significant PMN pleocytosis and hence be indistinguishable from presentations in early bacterial meningitis.

In some patients who have symptoms or signs of meningitis and have a normal initial CSF analysis, CSF pleocytosis may develop within 24 hr; the causative organism may be cultured from the original "normal" CSF.

Gram's stain

Gram's stain characteristics of the most commonly encountered organisms are described in Table 29-2. The yield from this procedure is diminished by 20% to 30% when there has been prior treatment with antibiotics.

Table 29-2 Gram's Stain Characteristics of Selected Meningeal Pathogens

PATHOGEN	TYPICAL CHARACTERISTICS
Staphylococci	Gram-positive cocci: singles, doubles,tetrads, clusters
Streptococcus pneumoniae	Gram-positive cocci: paired diplococci
Other streptococci	Gram-positive cocci: pairs and chains
Listeria monocytogenes	Gram-positive rods: single or chains
Neisseria meningitidis	Gram-negative cocci: negative paired diplococci; kidney or coffee bean appearance
Haemophilus influenzae	Gram-negative coccobacilli: "pleomorphic" bacilli
Enterobacteriaceae (including *Escherichia coli*)	Gram-negative rods
Pseudomonas aeruginosa	Gram-negative rods

Xanthochromia

Xanthochromia refers to the yellowish discoloration of the supernatant of a centrifuged CSF specimen. Xanthochromia is abnormal and results from the lysis of RBC.If the CSF protein level is less than 150 mg/dL, however, and systemic hypercarotenemia does not exist, xanthochromia of a centrifuged CSF specimen should suggest that subarachnoid hemorrhage has occurred.

Glucose

When the serum glucose concentration is

normal, the CSF glucose concentration is usually between 50 and 80 mg/dL.The CSF glucose concentration is normally in a ratio of 0.6 : 1 to the serum glucose concentration. Therefore, a CSF-to-serum glucose ratio of less than 0.5 in normoglycemic subjects or 0.3 in hyperglycemic subjects is abnormal and may represent the impaired glucose transport mechanisms and increased CNS glucose use associated with pyogenic meningitis.Mild decreases in the CSF glucose level may occur with certain viral and parameningeal processes. However, bacterial or fungal meningitis should be presumed to be the cause of low CSF glucose concentration, termed hypoglycorrhachia, until each is clearly excluded.

Protein

The normal CSF protein level in adults ranges from 15 to 45 mg/dL. An elevated CSF protein level, usually higher than 150 mg/dL, commonly occurs with acute bacterial meningitis. When a traumatic LP has occurred, the CSF protein level can be corrected for the presence of blood by subtracting 1 mg/dL of protein for each 1000 RBCs. Elevated CSF protein concentrations can result from any cause of meningitis, subarachnoid hemorrhage, CNS vasculitis, syphilis, viral encephalitis, neoplasms, and demyelination syndromes. A greatly elevated CSF protein level (>1000 mg/dL) in the presence of a relatively benign clinical presentation should suggest fungal disease.

India Ink Preparation

India ink staining of the CSF should be performed when a diagnosis of cryptococcal meningitis is being considered. The demonstration of budding organisms (Fig. 29-2) is virtually diagnostic for cryptococcal disease but occurs in only one third of the cases. A more definitive diagnostic test is the cryptococcal antigen.

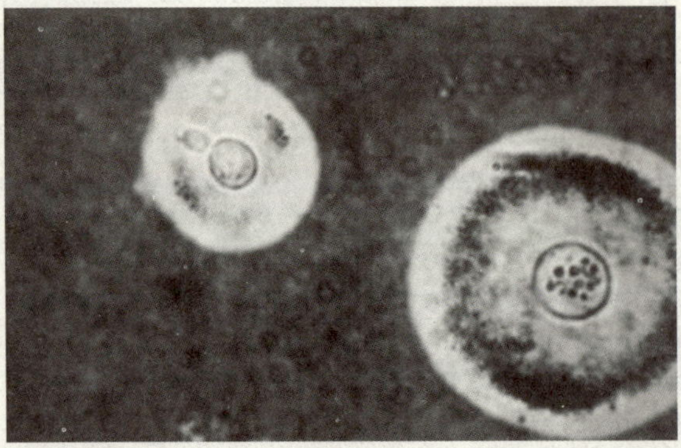

Fig. 29-2 India ink staining of cerebrospinal fluid showing cryptococcal meningitis.

Lactic Acid

Although nonspecific, elevations in CSF lactic acid concentrations (>35 mg/dL) are potentially indicative of bacterial meningitis, and lactate may rise before the decline in glucose. Normal lactate levels (<35 mg/dL) are usually seen in patients with viral meningitides.

Bacteriologic Cultures

Although results are not available for emergency management,bacteriologic cultures of CSF should be performed. Bacterial culture yields are significantly decreased in patients pretreated with antibiotics. Viral cultures may also be indicated.

Other Tests

A variety of additional, nonspecific tests of CSF have been advocated. These include measurement of CSF lactate dehydrogenase, CRP, and the limulus lysate test; however, none of these has demonstrated a high degree of clinical usefulness.

Neuroimaging Techniques

In the diagnostic evaluation of acute meningitis, however, a CT scan should not unnecessarily delay LP or antimicrobial therapy. MRI is also helpful in the evaluation of other infectious.

Additional Investigations

CBC with differential is a nonspecific adjunct in the diagnostic evaluation of a patient thought to have a CNS infection.Serum CRP is nonspecific, but a negative test result is potentially helpful. Procalcitonin is emerging as a promising serum marker in infectious disease; however, there is not convincing evidence at this point to advocate its use to attempt to rule out bacterial meningitis.

Two or three blood culture specimens should be obtained for all patients who are being evaluated for a CNS infection. The blood cultures can improve the identification of the causative organisms, especially with pneumococcus and, to a lesser degree, meningococcus.

As many as 50% of patients with pneumococcal meningitis also have evidence of pneumonia on an initial chest radiographic study.The identification of a pulmonary infection on chest radiography may assist in identification of causative organisms and appropriate antimicrobial therapy. Serum electrolyte, glucose, urea nitrogen, and creatinine levels should be measured to facilitate the interpretation of the CSF glucose level and to establish the level of renal function and the state of electrolyte balance. Although organism-specific abnormalities are uncommon, hyponatremia has been associated with tuberculous meningitis.

DIFFERENTIAL CONSIDERATIONS

Patients with meningitis may have symptoms and signs ranging from mild headache with fever to frank coma and shock. Meningitis may be divided into three clinical syndromes: acute meningitis, subacute meningitis, and chronic meningitis.

Acute meningitis encompasses patients with obvious signs and symptoms of meningitis who are evaluated in less than 24 hr after the onset of their symptoms and who rapidly deteriorate.The most likely pathogens in this syndrome are *S. pneumonia* and *N. meningitidis*.

In the syndrome of subacute meningitis, the symptoms and signs causing the patient to seek care have developed during a period of 1 to 7 d. This syndrome includes virtually all cases of viral meningitis along with most of the bacterial and some of the fungal causes. The differential diagnosis depends on the symptoms and signs at presentation.

The spectrum of chronic meningitis includes some of the viral meningitides as well as meningitis caused by tubercle bacilli, syphilis, and fungi.

MANAGEMENT

Assessment and Stabilization

Septic shock, hypoxemia, seizures, cerebral edema, and hypotension resulting from dehydration require aggressive management.

Hypotension or shock is treated with isotonic crystalloid infusion, high-flow oxygen, and pressors. Intravenous administration of dextrose may be required for hypoglycemia. Alcoholic or nutritionally compromised patients should also receive 50 to 100 mg of thiamine. In cases of moderate to severe hypotension, CVP monitoring should be initiated and used to determine additional intravenous fluids or vasopressors.

Active airway management with endotracheal intubation may be required in severely ill patients with meningitis, particularly in cases of coma, recurrent seizures, or severe accompanying pulmonary infection. Cardiac monitoring may also be necessary, particularly in elderly patients, those with known coronary disease, and those with an altered mental status.

If acute cerebral edema or an elevated ICP is present, it is managed by immediate intubation and adequate ventilation. Osmotic agents such as mannitol or diuretics such as furosemide may be used.

Definitive Therapy

Bacterial Meningitis

Therapy for bacterial meningitis requires antibiotics that penetrate the blood-brain barrier and achieve adequate CSF concentrations, are bactericidal against the offending organism in vivo, and maintain adequate tissue levels to treat the infection effectively.

Until the pathogenetic organism is identified, broad-spectrum coverage of the most common pathogens is necessary (Table 29-3). Many authorities recommend cefotaxime or ceftriaxone, plus vancomycin to cover potentially resistant organisms. High dose ampicillin is also added if concern exists about *Listeria*. In patients allergic to penicillin and cephalosporins, meropenem or chloramphenicol plus vancomycin may be effective while the outcome of desensitization techniques is awaited.

After the pathogen is identified, more targeted therapy can be instituted. It is prudent to refer to a current antimicrobial reference to guide therapy in all instances, given rapid changes in etiologic spectrum, drug resistance, and available agents. Duration of treatment varies, and in certain situations (namely, epidemics in sub-Saharan African), long-acting chloramphenicol or ceftriaxone is effective.

Table 29-3 Recommendations for Empirical Antimicrobial Therapy for Purulent Meningitis Based on Patient Age and Specific Predisposing Condition

PREDISPOSING FACTOR	COMMON BACTERIAL PATHOGENS	ANTIMICROBIAL THERAPY
Age		
<1 mo	*Streptococcus agalactiae, Escherichia coli, Listeria monocytogenes, Klebsiella* species	Ampicillin plus cefotaxime or ampicillin plus an aminoglycoside
1-23 mo	*Streptococcus pneumoniae, Neisseria meningitidis, S. agalactiae, Haemophilus influenzae, E. coli*	Vancomycin plus a third-generation cephalosporin
2-50 yr	*N. meningitidis, S. pneumoniae*	Vancomycin plus a third-generation cephalosporin
>50 yr	*S. pneumoniae, N. meningitidis, L. monocytogenes*, aerobic gramnegative bacilli	Vancomycin plus ampicillin plus a third-generation cephalosporin
Head trauma		
Basilar skull fracture	*S. pneumoniae, H. influenzae*, group A β-hemolytic streptococci	Vancomycin plus a third-generation cephalosporin
Penetrating trauma	*Staphylococcus aureus*, coagulase-negative staphylococci (especially *Staphylococcus epidermidis*), aerobic gram-negative bacilli (including *Pseudomonas aeruginosa*)	Vancomycin plus cefepime, vancomycin plus ceftazidime, or vancomycin plus meropenem
Postneurosurgery	Aerobic gram-negative bacilli (including *P. aeruginosa*), *S. aureus*, coagulase-negative staphylococci (especially *S. epidermidis*)	Vancomycin plus cefepime, vancomycin plus ceftazidime, or vancomycin plus meropenem
CSF shunt	Coagulase-negative staphylococci (especially *S. epidermidis*), *S.aureus*, aerobic gram-negative bacilli (including *P. aeruginosa*), *Propionibacterium acnes*	Vancomycin plus cefepime,vancomycin plus ceftazidime, or vancomycin plus meropenem

Corticosteroid treatment is additionally recommended in adult acute bacterial meningitis, although the evidence of efficacy is becoming less compelling over time. Studies demonstrate the salutary effects of the administration of corticosteroids in experimental pneumococcal meningitis, including reduced brain edema, CSF pressure, and CSF lactate levels. In adult bacterial meningitis, an absolute risk reduction of 10% for unfavorable outcome is seen when dexamethasone is given either 15 min before or concomitantly with antibiotics and continued for 4 d at 6 hr intervals. This benefit is greatest in those with *S. pneumoniae*. Subgroup analyses for different causative organisms did not establish a benefit; however, the study was not designed with adequate power to detect improved outcomes. In addition, amoxicillin and penicillin were the most commonly used initial therapy at the time of that study because of the process of health care delivery in Europe, in which nearly all patients were seen initially in an office based practice. A randomized controlled trial did not demonstrate a benefit of adjuvant dexamethasone in adult patients, even when only those with S. pneumoniae were included in a secondary analysis. In the current era of initial empirical parenteral therapy, rising β-lactam resistance, the possibility of the decreased CSF penetration of vancomycin after dexamethasone treatment, and shifts in the likely causative organisms secondary to vaccination campaigns, the true effectiveness of dexamethasone is unclear. The most recent meta-analysis suggests a benefit for patients in the developed (but not developing) world, but the included studies suffer from one or more of the aforementioned limitations.

Viral Meningitis

No specific agents are available to treat most types of viral meningitis. Investigational agents in development may reduce symptoms in enterovirus meningitis; however, with the exception of herpes simplex virus meningitis, the viral meningitides contracted in the United States are generally characterized by a short, benign, self-limited course followed by a complete recovery. The primary therapeutic consideration in cases of viral meningitis is therefore the validity of the diagnosis. Early cases of viral meningitis may be indistinguishable from bacterial meningitis, and this confusion may not be resolved by CSF analysis; therefore, when any doubt exists about the veracity of the diagnosis, appropriate culture specimens should be obtained and the patient admitted to the hospital. Antimicrobial therapy for presumed bacterial meningitis may be initiated on the basis of the clinical presentation or may be withheld pending the outcome of close clinical observation and repeated LP in 8 to 12 hr.

Tuberculous Meningitis

Early chemotherapeutic intervention in acute tuberculous meningitis improves the patient's prognosis. A strong clinical suggestion of this disease is an adequate indication to begin antituberculous therapy. A standard treatment regimen consists of isoniazid, rifampin, pyrazinamide, and ethambutol or streptomycin. Corticosteroids have also been shown to decrease secondary complications.

Fungal Meningitis

The treatment of fungal meningitis is complex. Four agents are commonly used: amphotericin B, flucytosine, miconazole, and fluconazole. Of these, amphotericin B, either alone or in combination with flucytosine, is the most commonly recommended initial therapeutic regimen. These diseases are rarely acutely lifethreatening but rather are slowly progressive. Prolonged therapy, often with multiple agents, is necessary. The initiation of antifungal therapy is rarely indicated in ED.

Chemoprophylaxis

Among household contacts, the incidence of transmission of meningococcus is approximately 5%; therefore, It is recommended that household contacts of bacteriologically confirmed cases receive rifampin (adults, 600 mg; children older than 1 month, 10 mg/kg; children younger than 1 month, 5 mg/kg) orally every 12 hr for a total of four doses. In addition, these contacts should be advised to watch for fever, sore throat, rash, or any symptoms of meningitis. They should be hospitalized with appropriate intravenous antimicrobial therapy if there are signs that active meningococcal disease is developing because rifampin is ineffective against invasive meningococcal disease. Intimate, nonhousehold contacts who have had mucosal exposure to the patient's oral secretions should also receive rifampin prophylaxis. Health care workers are not at increased risk for the disease and do not require prophylaxis unless they have had direct mucosal contact with the patient's secretions, as might occur during mouth-to-mouth resuscitation, endotracheal intubation, or nasotracheal suctioning. Ciprofloxacin 500 mg by mouth (adults only) and ceftriaxone 250 mg intramuscularly (125 mg intramuscularly for children younger than 15 yr) provide single-dose alternatives.

There is no indication for chemoprophylaxis in pneumococcal meningitis. Rifampin prophylaxis for the contacts of patients with *H. influenzae* type b meningitis is recommended for nonpregnant household contacts when there are children younger than 4 yr in the household (adults, 600 mg by mouth; children, 20 mg/kg by mouth daily for 4 d).

DISPOSITION

With the exception of viral meningitis, all but the most chronic CNS infections require initial inpatient evaluation and treatment. Bed rest, analgesics, and the institution of appropriate intravenous antimicrobials are indicated.

Some patients with suspected viral meningitides merit hospitalization. These include patients with more severe disease, immunocompromise, suspicion of herpes simplex virus meningitis, and potential nonviral causes. Some authorities manage patients with classic presentations of viral meningitis as outpatients and ensure close follow-up within 24 hr. Others admit all patients until the more serious causes, such as early bacterial meningitis and encephalitis, can be excluded with certainty.

(LI Li)

Chapter 30

Headache

KEY CONSEPTS

Headache commonly is divided into primary and secondary disorders. The primary headache disorders include migraine, cluster, and tension-type headaches. Secondary headache disorders include a variety of organic illnesses in which head pain is a symptom of an identifiable, distinct pathologic process.

Patients with the following headache presentations are at risk for serious underlying disease: sudden explosive headache; new-onset headache after the age of 50 yr; headache associated with papilledema,alteration in or loss of consciousness, or focal neurologic symptoms; subacute headache with increasing frequency or severity; headache associated with fever, or cancer.

The basic approach to secondary headache disorders includes CT and LP.

The sensitivity of CT for identifying SAH is reduced by nearly 10% for symptom onset greater than 12 hr and by almost 20% at 3 to 5 d.

PERSPECTIVE

Epidemiology

Headache as a primary complaint represents 3% to 5% of all ED visits. The vast majority of patients who have a primary complaint of headache do not have a serious medical cause for the problem. In addition, some patients present with headache as part of a constitutional illness.

Tension headache accounts for approximately 50% of patients visiting the ED, another 30% have headache of unidentified origin, 10% have migraine-type pain, and 8% have headache from other potentially serious causes (e.g., tumor, glaucoma). The most commonly encountered life-threatening cause of severe sudden head pain is SAH.

Meningitis, carbon monoxide poisoning, temporal arteritis, acute angle-closure glaucoma, ICH, cerebral venous sinus thrombosis, and increased ICP can often be linked with specific historical elements and physical findings that facilitate their diagnosis.

Pathophysiology

The brain parenchyma is insensitive to pain. The pain-sensitive areas of the head include the coverings of the brain (the meninges), the blood vessels and the various tissues lining the cavities within the skull. Much of the pain associated with headache, particularly with vascular headache and migraines, is mediated through the fifth cranial nerve. A specific inflammation in a specific structure (e.g., periapical abscess, sinusitis, or tic douloureux) is much easier to localize than the relatively diffuse pain.

DIAGNOSTIC APPROACH

Differential Considerations

The differential diagnosis of headache is complex because of the large number of potential disease entities and the diffuse nature of many types of pain in the head and neck region (Table 30-1). However, in evaluating the patient with a headache complaint, the top priority is to exclude the life-threatening causes: SAH and ICH, meningitis, encephalitis, and mass lesions.

Table 30-1 Differential Diagnosis

ORGAN SYSTEM	CRITICAL DIAGNOSES	EMERGENT DIAGNOSES	NONEMERGENT DIAGNOSES
Neurologic, CNS, vessels	SAH	Shunt failure Traction headaches Tumor or other masses Subdural hematomas	Migraine, various types Vascular, various types Trigeminal neuralgia Post-trauma Postlumbar puncture Headaches
Toxic or metabolic	Carbon monoxide poisoning	Mountain sickness	
Environmental			
Collagen vascular disease	Temporal arteritis		
Eye or ENT		Glaucoma or sinusitis	Dental problems, temporomandibular joint disease
Musculoskeletal			Tension headaches Cervical strain
Allergy			Cluster or histamine headaches
Infectious disease	Bacterial meningitis, encephalitis	Brain abscess	Febrile headaches, non-neurologic source of infection
Pulmonary or O_2		Anoxic headache Anemia	
Cardiovascular		Hypertensive crisis	Hypertension (rare)
Unspecified			Effort-dependent or coital headaches

Rapid Assessment and Stabilization

If the patient is in a critical or comatose state, initial stabilization, including airway management, is prioritized and, if at all possible, preceded by a neurologic examination. Headache can be divided into two categories: accompanied by altered mental status and without altered mental status.

Pivotal Findings

History

The history is the pivotal part of the workup for the patient with headache (Table 30-2).

Table 30-2 Significant Symptoms

SYMPTOM	FINDING	POSSIBLE DIAGNOSES
Sudden onset of pain	Lightning strike or thunder clap with any decreased mentation, any positive focal finding, or intractable pain	SAH
"Worst headache of my life"	Associated with sudden onset	SAH
Near syncope or syncope	Associated with sudden onset	SAH
Increase with jaw movement	Clicking or snapping; pain with jaw movement	Temporomandibular joint disease
Facial pain	Fulminant pain of the forehead and area of maxillary sinus; nasal congestion	Sinus pressure or dental infection
Forehead or temporal area pain (or both)	Tender temporal arteries	Temporal arteritis
Periorbital or retroorbital pain	Sudden onset with tearing	Temporal arteritis or acute angle-closure glaucoma

1. The patient should be asked to describe the pattern and onset of the pain. The rate of onset of pain may have significance. Pain with rapidonset of a few seconds to minutes

is more likely to be vascular in origin than pain that developed over several hours or days. However, a slow onset should not be solely relied on to rule out potential life-threatening causes for headache. A marked variation in headache pattern can signal a new or serious problem.

The "thunder clap" or "lightning strike" headache is common in acute presentations of SAH but is not highly specific. If the patient with moderate or severe headache can indicate the precise activity in which he or she was engaging at the time of the onset of the headache, the suddenness of onset should warrant consideration of SAH.

2. The patient's activity at the onset of the pain may be helpful. Headaches that come on during severe exertion have a relationship to vascular bleeding. The syndrome of postcoital headache is also a common time of onset for SAH.
3. If there is a history of head trauma, the differential diagnosis and emergent causes are narrowed significantly. The considerations now focus on epidural and subdural hematoma, traumatic SAH, skull fracture, and closed-head injury.
4. The intensity of head pain is difficult to quantify objectively. Rapid resolution of pain in the ED, either from time or therapy, also should not be relied on to rule out serious causes of headache.
5. The character of the pain (e.g., throbbing, steady), may not be adequate to differentiate one type of headache from another.
6. The location of head pain is helpful for diagnosis. Unilateral pain is more suggestive of migraine or a localized inflammatory process in the skull (e.g., sinus) or soft tissue. Occipital headaches are classically associated with hypertension. Temporal arteritis, temporomandibular joint (TMJ) disease, dental infections, and sinus infections frequently have a highly localized area of discomfort Meningitis, encephalitis, SAH, and even severe migraine, although intense in nature, are usually more diffuse in their localization.
7. Exacerbating or alleviating factors may be important. Headaches on awakening are typically described with brain tumors. Intracranial infections, dental infections, and other regional causes of head pain tend not to be improved or alleviated before therapy is given.

Box 30-1 Risk Factors Associated with Potentially Catastrophic Illness

1. Carbon monoxide poisoning
   a. Breathing in enclosed or confined spaces with engine exhaust or ventilation of heating equipment
   b. Multiple family members with the same symptoms
   c. Pattern of recurrence in one setting (where the exposure is occurring), relief when not in that setting
   d. Wintertime and working around machinery or equipment producing carbon monoxide (e.g., furnaces)
2. Meningitis, encephalitis, abscess
   a. History of sinus or ear infection or recent surgical procedure
   b. Immunocompromised state
   c. General debilitation with decreased immunologic system function
   d. Acute febrile illness—any type
   e. Extremes of age
   f. Impacted living conditions (e.g., military barracks, college dormitories)
   g. Lack of primary immunizations
3. Temporal arteritis
   a. Age >50
   b. Females more often than males (4 : 1)
   c. History of other collagen vascular diseases (e.g., systemic lupus)
   d. Previous chronic meningitis
   e. Previous chronic illness such as tuberculosis, parasitic or fungal infection
4. Glaucoma—sudden angle-closure
   a. Not associated with any usual or customary headache pattern
   b. History of previous glaucoma
   c. Age >30
   d. History of pain increasing in a dark environment
5. Increased intracranial pressure
   a. History of previous benign intracranial hypertension
   b. Presence of a cerebrospinal fluid shunt
   c. History of congenital brain or skull abnormalities
6. Cerebral venous sinus thrombosis
7. ICH
   a. SAH
      Ⅰ. Sudden severe pain; "worst headache of life"
      Ⅱ. Acute severe pain after sexual intercourse or straining (i.e., heavy lifting)

Ⅲ. History of SAH or cerebral aneurysm
Ⅳ. History of polycystic kidney disease
Ⅴ. Family history of subarachnoid hemorrhage
Ⅵ. Hypertension—severe
Ⅶ. Previous vascular lesions in other areas of the body
Ⅷ. Young and middle-aged

b. Subdural hematoma (SDH)
Ⅰ. History of alcohol dependency with or without trauma
Ⅱ. Current use of anticoagulants

c. Epidural hematoma (EDH)
Ⅰ. Traumatic injury
Ⅱ. Lucid mentation followed by acute altered mentation or somnolence
Ⅲ. Anisocoria on physical examination

8. Associated symptoms and risk factors may relate to the severity of headache but rarely point to the specific causes (Box 30-1). Nausea and vomiting are completely nonspecific. Migraine headaches, ICP, temporal arteritis, and glaucoma can all manifest with severe nausea and vomiting, as can some systemic viral infections with headache.
9. A prior history of headache, although helpful, does not rule out current serious problems.

Physical Examination

Physical findings associated with various forms of headache are listed in Table 30-3.

Ancillary Testing

The vast majority of headache patients do not require additional testing (Table 30-4). Brain CT can miss 6% to 8% of patients with SAH. The sensitivity

Table 30-3 Pivotal Findings on Physical Examination

SIGN	FINDING	POSSIBLE DIAGNOSES
General appearance	Alteration of mental status—nonfocal	Meningitis, encephalitis SAH Anoxia Increased CSF pressure
	Alterations of mental status with focal findings	Intraparenchymal bleed Tentorial herniation Stroke
	Severe nausea, vomiting	Increased CSF pressure Acute angle-closure glaucoma SAH
Vital signs	Hypertension with normal heart rate or bradycardia	Increased CSF pressure SAH Tentorial herniation Intraparenchymal bleed
	Tachycardia	Anoxia, anemia Febrile headache Exertional or coital headaches
	Fever	Febrile headaches Meningitis, encephalitis
HEENT	Tender temporal arteries	Temporal arteritis
Fundi—loss of spontaneous venous pulsa tions or presence of papilledema	Increased CSF pressure	Mass lesions
	Subhyaloid hemorrhage	Subarachnoid hemorrhage
	Acute red eye (severe ciliary flushing) and poorly reactive pupils	Acute angle-closure glaucoma
	Enlarged pupil with third nerve palsy	Tentorial pressure cone Mass effect (i.e., subdural or epidural hematoma, tumor, intraparenchymal hemorrhage)
Neurologic	Lateralized motor or sensory deficit	Stroke (rare) SDH, EDH, hemiplegic or anesthetic migraine (rare)
	Acute cerebellar ataxia	Acute cerebellar hemorrhage Acute cerebellitis (mostly children) Chemical intoxication—various types

Table 30-4 Diagnostic Adjuncts in Headache Assessment

TEST	FINDING	DIAGNOSIS
ESR	Significant elevation	Temporal arteritis
ECG	Nonspecific ST-T wave changes	Subarachnoid hemorrhage Increased CSF pressure
CBC	Severe anemia	Anoxia
CT-head	Increased ventricular size	Increased CSF pressure
	Blood in subarachnoid space	SAH
	Blood in epidural or subdural space	EDH or SDH
	Bleeding into parenchyma of brain	Intraparenchymal hemorrhage
	Areas of poor vascular flow	Pale infarct
	Structural, mass lesion	Traction headache secondary to mass effect
Lumbar puncture and CSF analysis	Increased pressure	Pseudotumor cerebri Mass lesions Shunt failure
	Increased protein	Tumor or other structural lesions
	Increased RBC	SAH
	Increased WBC	Infection
	Positive Gram's stain	Infection
	Decreased glucose	Infection

of CT for identifying SAH is reduced by nearly 10% for symptom onset greater than 12 hr and by almost 20% at 3 to 5 d. The basic approach to integrating CT and LP in the assessment of headache is outlined in Fig. 30-1.

Obtaining CSF should not delay antimicrobial treatment if intracranial infection is suggested. Intravenous antibiotics are given before LP. Abnormal mental status, signs of increased ICP, papilledema, focal findings on neurologic examination, or any other indication suggestive of a focal intracranial mass lesion requires CT before LP.

DIFFERENTIAL CONSIDERATIONS

Indications of patients at higher risk for serious causes of headache who are candidates for more comprehensive evaluation include (1) sudden onset of headache, (2) patient description of the headache as "the worst ever," (3) altered mental status, (4) meningismus, (5) unexplained fever, (6) focal neurologic deficit on examination, (7) symptoms refractory to appropriate treatment or worsening despite treatment, (8) onset of headache during exertion, or (9) history of HIV infection or immunosuppression.

Patients with a headache that is similar in

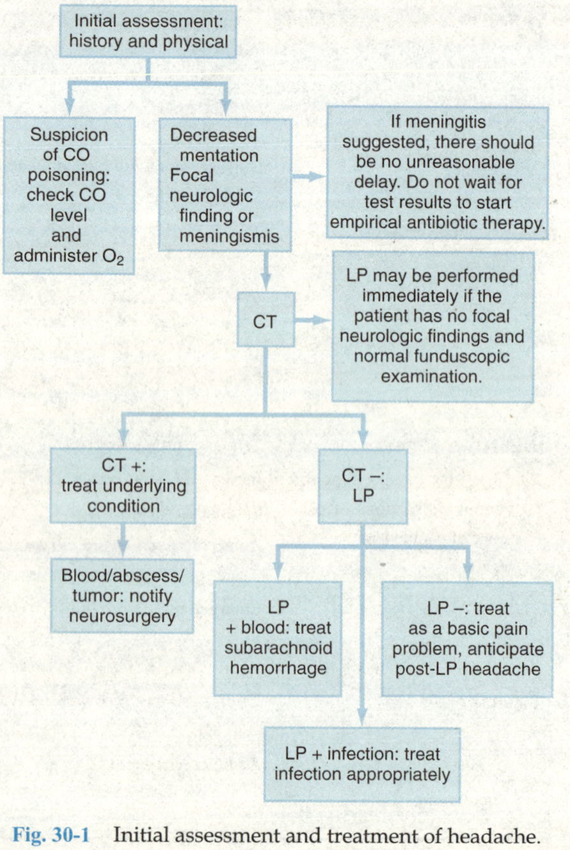

Fig. 30-1 Initial assessment and treatment of headache.

location and intensity to an established history of recurrent headache (e.g., migraine) or of minor severity and gradual onset (e.g., typical tension headache),with normal neurologic examination findings,with absence of fever or meningismus; and showing improvement with appropriate treatment generally require no laboratory testing or imaging.

Sequential evaluation of the patient's condition and response to therapy and assessment of ancillary data will confirm a working diagnosis or trigger a reconsideration of alternatives, including more serious conditions (Table 30-5).

SPECIAL MANAGEMENT

Headache commonly is divided into primary and secondary disorders. The primary headache disorders include migraine, cluster, and tension-type headaches. Secondary headache disorders include a variety of organic illnesses in which head pain is a symptom of an identifiable, distinct pathologic process. To facilitate a standardized approach to headache management, the International Headache Society published a classification system and diagnostic criteria for headache disorders, cranial neuralgias, and facial pain. This comprehensive and widely accepted system includes 14 major categories of headache disorders and uses specific operational diagnostic criteria to define each headache type (Box 30-2).

Box 30-2 International Headache Society Classification of Headache

1. Migraine
2. Tension-type headache
3. Cluster headache and trigeminal autonomic cephalalgias
4. Other primary headaches
5. Headache attributed to head and/or neck trauma
6. Headache attributed to nonvascular intracranial disorder
7. Headache associated with nonvascular intracranial disorder
8. Headache attributed to a substance or its withdrawal
9. Headache associated with noncephalic infection
10. Headache attributed to disorder of homeostasis
11. Headache or facial pain attributed to disorder of cranium,neck, eyes, ears, nose, sinuses, teeth, mouth, or other facial or cranial structures
12. Headache attributed to psychiatric disorder
13. Cranial neuralgias and central causes of facial pain
14. Other headache, cranial neuralgia, central or primary facial pain

PRIMARY HEADACHE DISORDERS

Migraine Headache

Principles of Disease

Migraine is a common, chronic neurovascular disease characterized by recurrent attacks of severe headache, autonomic nervous system dysfunction, and, in some patients, an aura causing visual, sensory, motor, or other neurologic symptoms.

Migraine attacks typically begin in the second decade of life and peak in prevalence in the fourth decade of life. Overall, migraine is more prevalent among women (18%) than among men (6%). After menarche, a correlation between migraine and menstruation is noted in half of female migraine sufferers. After menopause, the prevalence of migraine among women decreases.

Migraine is commonly thought of in two major categories: migraine without aura, or common migraine, which is the most frequent form of migraine and accounts for approximately 80% of all cases (Box 30-3); and migraine with aura, or classic migraine, which has specific reversible neurologic symptoms that precede the actual headache (Box 30-4) and is seen less frequently.

Box 30-3 Migraine without Aura (Common Migraine): International Headache Society Criteria

A. At least five attacks fulfilling criteria in B, C, D, and E

B. Attack lasts 4 to 72 hr (untreated or unsuccessfully treated)

C. Headache has at least two of the following characteristics:

1. Unilateral location

Table 30-5 Causes and Differentiation of Potentially Catastrophic Illness Manifesting with Nontraumatic Headache

DISEASE ENTITIES	PAIN HISTORY	ASSOCIATED SYMPTOMS	SUPPORT HISTORY	PREVA LENCE	PHYSICAL EXAMINATION	USEFUL TESTS	ATYPICAL OR IMPORTANT ASPECTS
Carbon monoxide poisoning	Usually gradual, subtle, dull, nonfocal throbbing pain	May wax and wane as individual leaves and enters the involved area of carbon monoxide; throbbing may vary considerably	Exposure to engine exhaust, old or defective heating systems, most common in winter months	Rare	No focal neurologic findings May need cognitive testing	Carbon monoxide level, cognitive testing	May improve on the way to the hospital Occurs in groups, may involve entire families or groups of people exposed to the carbon monoxid
SAH	Sudden onset,"thunder clap" or "lightning strike,"severe throbbing	Whenever altered mental status is present, the outcome is decidedly worse	History of polycystic kidney disease. History of chronic hypertension	Uncommon	Frequently decreased mentation—meningismus,increased blood pressure,decreased pulse, decreased spontaneous venous pulsations, rarely subhyaloid hemorrhage	CT, LP	If CT positive, immediate involvement of neurosurgery;if CT negative, lumbar puncture
Meningitis, encephalitis, abscess	Gradual—as general symptoms increase, headache increases—nonfocal	Decreased mentation prominent, irritability prominent With abscess, focal neurologic findings may be present	Recent infection Recent facial or dental surgery or other ENT surgery	Uncommon	Fever—late in course,decreased spontaneous venous pulsations	CT, LP	When such infection suspected, treat Do not delay antibiotics and steroids while awaiting laboratory results
Temporal arteritis	Often pain developing over a few hours from mild to severe Virtually always focal in nature	Decreased vision, nausea, vomiting intense—may confuse diagnosis	Age over 50 Other collagen vascular diseases or inflammatory diseases	Uncommon	Tender temporal arteries	Sedimentation rate	Usually unrelated and rapidly progressive
Acute angle-closure glaucoma	Sudden in onset	Nausea, vomiting, decreased vision	History of glaucoma History of pain going into dark area	Rare	"Steamy" cornea Midposition pupil poorly reactive Acute red eye	Measurement of intraocular pressure	Rapid intervention with medications required—if no relief, immediate surgery may be required
Increased intracranial pressure syndromes	Gradual, dull, nonfocal	Vomiting, decreased mentation	History of CSF shunt or other congenital brain or skull abnormality	Uncommon	Papilledema; loss of spontaneous venous pulsations	CT, shunt function study; if normal, lumbar puncture	Shunt failure or other cause of significant increased CSF pressure requires involvement of neurosurgery

2. Pulsating quality
3. Moderate to severe pain intensity
4. Aggravation by or causing avoidance of routine physical activity (e.g., walking or climbing stairs)

D. During headache, at least one of the following:
1. Nausea or vomiting (or both)
2. Photophobia and phonophobia

E. Not attributable to another disorder

Box 30-4 Migraine with Aura (Classic Migraine): International Headache Society Criteria

A. At least two attacks that fulfill criterion B

B. Presence of at least three of the following four characteristics for a diagnosis of classic migraine:
1. One or more fully reversible aura symptoms indicating focal cerebral cortical or brainstem dysfunction (or both)
2. At least one aura symptom developing gradually over more than 4 min, or two or more symptoms occurring in succession
3. No single aura symptom lasting longer than 60 min
4. Headache beginning during aura or afterward, with a symptom-free interval of less than 60 min (also may begin before aura)

C. Exclusion of related organic diseases by means of an appropriate history, physical examination, and neurologic examination with appropriate diagnostic tests

Clinical Features

Migraine is by definition a chronic and recurrent disease. The headache, characteristically, is unilateral, pulsating in quality, moderate to severe in intensity, and exacerbated by routine activities. The onset usually is gradual, and the attacks typically last 4 to 72 hr. Headache frequency is variable; those patients with more than 15 headache days per month are considered to have chronic migraine. Associated symptoms and signs include nausea, vomiting, anorexia, photophobia, phonophobia, osmophobia (aversion to odors), blurred vision, lightheadedness, and nasal congestion. Some patients experience premonitory cognitive impairment producing forgetfulness, irritability, and depression. Many patients have dramatic light and sound sensitivity and seek a cool, dark, and quiet room.

The aura of classic migraine consists of focal neurologic symptoms that precede and herald the migraine attack. By definition, the aura is fully reversible and typically lasts 10 to 20 min, although it may continue for as long as 1 hr. The most common aura is visual; features may include scintillating scotomas (bright rim around an area of visual loss), teichopsias (subjective visual image perceived with eyes open or closed), fortification spectrums (zigzagged wall of fortress slowly drifting across visual field), photopsias (poorly formed brief flashes or sparks of light), and blurred vision. Less common auras include somatosensory phenomena such as tingling or numbness, motor disturbances, and cognitive or language disorders.

Ophthalmoplegic migraine is a rare syndrome associated with paresis of one or more ocular nerves, most commonly the third cranial nerve. Patients typically present with ipsilateral headache associated with extraocular muscle paresis and occasionally pupillary changes.

Hemiplegic migraine is characterized by a motor aura consisting of hemiparesis or hemiplegia. The progression of the motor deficit is gradual and in most cases is accompanied by a visual, sensory, or speech disturbance. The neurologic symptoms last up to 60 min, followed by headache. A familial version of hemiplegic migraine is associated with genetic mutations of ion transporters.

Basilar-type migraines arise with an aura referable to the brainstem and are associated with multiple neurologic findings, including visual symptoms (often total blindness), dysarthria, tinnitus, vertigo, bilateral paresthesias, paresis, and altered level of consciousness. The symptoms are stereotypic and resolve spontaneously.

Status migrainosus is a severe migraine headache that persists for more than 72 hr. Associated symptoms are debilitating.

Many factors can trigger migraine headaches in predisposed persons. Common precipitants of migraine headaches include sleep deprivation, stress, hunger, hormonal changes including menstruation, and use of certain drugs including oral contraceptives and nitroglycerin. In addition, some patients report specific food sensitivities to chocolate, caffeine, and foods rich in tyramine, monosodium glutamate, and nitrates.

Differential Diagnosis

Other disorders that mimic migraine include nontraumatic subarachnoid hemorrhage, intracranial mass lesions, giant cell arteritis, cerebrovascular disease, and idiopathic intracranial hypertension.

Diagnostic Evaluation

Routine neuroimaging is not necessary for patients with typical recurrent migraine headaches.

Neuroimaging should be considered for older or immunocompromised patients with new-onset headaches, headaches with a progressive course, headaches worsened by Valsalva maneuver, headache causing awakening from sleep, or headaches associated with unexplained neurologic abnormalities. Such patients have a higher likelihood of having a secondary cause of headache, such as tumor, arteriovenous malformation, or structural lesion. In addition, patients who present with a thunderclap or abrupt-onset headache require a LP to rule out SAH.

Treatment

The goals of acute migraine therapy include rapid pain relief, minimization of headache recurrence and medication side effects, restoration of the patient's ability to function, and minimization of the use of backup and rescue medications.

There are several approaches to treatment of the acute headache episode (Table 30-6).

Table 30-6 Selected Medications for Acute Migraine Attacks

MEDICATION	DOSE AND ROUTE ADMINISTERED	COMMENTS
Mild to Moderate		
Acetaminophen	500-1000 mg PO	Gastrointestinal upset
Aspirin	650-1000 mg PO	Gastrointestinal upset
Ibuprofen	600-800 mg PO	Gastrointestinal upset
Naproxen sodium	275-550 mg PO	Gastrointestinal upset
Moderate to Severe		
Dihydroergotamine	1 mg IV or IM; may be repeated in 1 hr	Gastrointestinal upset (pretreat with antiemetic)
Triptans		Chest pain, throat tightness, flushing
Sumatriptan	6 mg SC; may be repeated once in 1 hr if partial response	Contraindicated with hypertension, coronary artery disease,peripheral vascular disease, and pregnancy
Sumatriptan	25-100 mg PO	
Rizatriptan	5-10 mg PO	Cannot be used within 24 hr of ergot use
Zolmitriptan	2.5-5 mg PO	
Naratriptan	1-2.5 mg PO	
Prochlorperazine	10 mg IV or IM; may be repeated in 30 to 60 min	Sedation and dystonic reaction
Metoclopramide	10 mg IV	Dystonic reaction
Droperidol	2.5 mg IV	QT prolongation; dystonic reaction
Ketorolac	30 mg IV or 30-60 mg IM	Gastrointestinal upset; avoid this medication in elderly and in patients with renal insufficiency
Morphine	4-8 mg IM or IV	Opioids less efficacious than other treatment modalities
Refractory Attack, Status Migrainosus		
Dihydroergotamine	1 mg IV q8h	Use in conjunction with antiemetic (e.g., metoclopramide,prochlorperazine)
Steroids	Various regimens	Gastrointestinal bleeding, infection, cataracts, aseptic necrosis,memory disturbances

For mild to moderate attacks, simple analgesics such as acetaminophen or NSAID are often effective.

For moderate to severe attacks, three classes of medications can be recommended as initial parenteral therapy: the antiemetic dopamine antagonists, such as metoclopramide, prochlorperazine, and droperidol; migraine-specific agents, such as the triptans and dihydroergotamine (DHE); and parenteral nonsteroidals, such as ketorolac.

Opioid analgesics such as morphine should be reserved for patients who do not respond to any of the medications listed or have contraindications to all standard migraine therapies.

Corticosteroids are effective at decreasing the rate of migraine recurrence after ED discharge. Oral naproxen 500 mg and sumatriptan 100 mg are reasonable treatment options for the recurrent headache.

Prophylactic Therapy

Prophylactic therapy is indicated for patients who have frequent attacks (more than two or three functionally disabling episodes per month), prolonged attacks lasting more than 48 hr, or attacks that are severe and debilitating. Several classes of medications are used for the prophylaxis of migraine, including beta-blockers, tricyclic antidepressants, and antiepileptic drugs.

Cluster Headache

Perspective

Cluster headache is more common in men than in women. It typically occurs in young to middle-aged adults who smoke, with a peak incidence in the late 20s. The headaches tend to occur repeatedly during a defined time interval, hence the term cluster. Several attacks can occur in 1 day, and a typical cluster period may last weeks to months. Several precipitating factors have been implicated, most notably the ingestion of alcohol. Stress and climatic changes may also play a role in susceptible persons.

Clinical Features

Cluster headaches occur suddenly, and multiple episodes can occur within a 24 hr period. Each headache lasts from 15 min up to 3 hr. The headache typically begins with a unilateral sharp, stabbing pain in the eye. The attacks occur exclusively in the territory of the trigeminal nerve. Unlike the migraineur, the patient with cluster headache predictably presents agitated and anxious, rocking, rubbing the head, and pacing. The attack subsides rapidly, often leaving the patient exhausted.

Accompanying the headache are ipsilateral autonomic symptoms such as ptosis, miosis, and forehead or facial sweating. The eye often is injected and tearing, and many patients have unilateral nasal congestion.

Differential Diagnosis

Other headache disorders that mimic cluster headache include carotid artery dissection, trigeminal neuralgia, and the rare trigeminal autonomic cephalalgia paroxysmal hemicrania. With trigeminal neuralgia, the pain peaks within seconds, lasts only a couple of minutes, and can be provoked by specific trigger points on the face or oral mucosa. The trigeminal autonomic cephalalgias are manifested by a brief unilateral headache that recurs dozens of times per day.

Treatment

High-flow oxygen should be considered first-line therapy. Delivered through a non-rebreather mask at a rate of 12 L/min. Subcutaneous sumatriptan is also an effective therapy for acute cluster headache and should be dosed at 6 mg. Alternatively, octreotide or intravenous dopamine antagonists may be effective.

A recommended regimen is 60 mg of prednisone daily for 10 d, followed by a 1 w taper. Verapamil, dosed at 120 mg three times a day, will decrease the frequency of attacks by the end of the first week of therapy.

Tension-type Headache

Perspective

Women are affected slightly more frequently than men are, with peak prevalence in the fourth decade of life. The median frequency of headaches is six per month, and stress and lack of sleep are implicated as triggering factors. By definition, episodic tension-type headache lasts as little as 30 min and as long as 7 d.

Clinical Features

Patients typically complain of a tight, bandlike discomfort around the head that is nonpulsating and dull. They also may experience tightening of the neck muscles. On occasion, the discomfort can build up slowly and fluctuate in severity for several days. Unlike in migraine, the headache does not worsen with physical activity, and accompanying symptoms are unusual. Anxiety and depression may coexist with chronic tension headache.

Differential Diagnosis

The most common disorders mimicking tension headache are migraine, idiopathic intracranial hypertension, oromandibular dysfunction, cervical spondylosis, sinus or eye disease, and intracranial masses.

Treatment

For a majority of patients with tension headaches, simple analgesics, such as acetaminophen or an NSAID, are adequate for pain control. Antiemetic dopamine antagonists may be useful therapy. Some nonpharmacologic regimens are meditation, massage, and biofeedback.

SECONDARY HEADACHE DISORDERS

Subarachnoid Hemorrhage

Principles of Disease

SAH refers to extravasated blood in the subarachnoid space. Presence of the blood activates meningeal nociceptors, leading to diffuse occipital pain along with signs of meningismus.

Approximately 80% of patients with nontraumatic SAH have ruptured saccular aneurysms. Other causes include arteriovenous malformations, cavernous angiomas, mycotic aneurysms, neoplasms, and blood dyscrasias. SAH may be caused secondarily by an intraparenchymal hematoma that dissects its way into the subarachnoid space.

The risk for aneurysmal SAH increases with age. The risk of rupture may increase with aneurysmal size. Other risk factors associated with SAH include HTN, smoking, excessive alcohol consumption, and sympathomimetic drugs. A familial association of cerebral aneurysms with several diseases, including autosomal dominant polycystic kidney disease, coarctation of the aorta, Marfan syndrome, and Ehlers-Danlos syndrome type IV, has been described.

Clinical Features

A majority of patients with SAH present with a sudden, cataclysmic thunderclap headache. The onset of headache may be associated with exertion, the Valsalva maneuver, or sexual intercourse. The headache of SAH classically peaks in intensity within seconds to minutes. Associated signs and symptoms include nausea and vomiting, neck stiffness, and seizures. Meningismus is present in more than 50% of patients, and up to 20% have focal neurologic abnormalities. Funduscopic examination may reveal retinal or subhyaloid hemorrhages, and patients also may have an isolated third or sixth nerve palsy. Oculomotor (third) nerve compression secondary to an expanding aneurysm leads to pupillary dilation. Approximately 50% of patients with a ruptured aneurysm are restless or have an altered level of consciousness. Focal neurologic signs may indicate the site of the aneurysm.

The Hunt and Hess scale stratifies patients according to their clinical signs and symptoms at the time of presentation and is predictive of outcome (Table 30-7). Patients who present with a grade 1 or grade 2 hemorrhage tend to have a good prognosis. Patients with grade 4 or grade 5 hemorrhage tend to do poorly, and these patients have an altered mental status, ranging from stupor to deep coma, together with focal neurologic signs and symptoms. Patients with grade 3 hemorrhage present with drowsiness or confusion and are at risk for rapid clinical deterioration.

Table 30-7 Hunt and Hess Clinical Grading Scale for Cerebral Aneurysms and SAH

GRADE	CONDITION
0	Unruptured aneurysm
1	Asymptomatic or minimal headache and slight nuchal rigidity
2	Moderate or severe headache, nuchal rigidity, no neurologic deficit other than cranial nerve palsy
3	Drowsiness, confusion, or mild focal deficit
4	Stupor, moderate to severe hemiparesis
5	Deep coma, decerebrate posturing, moribund appearance

Diagnostic Studies

A non-contrast-enhanced head CT scan is

the first-line test for the diagnosis of SAH (Fig. 30-2). Because the sensitivity of head CT is limited, particularly as the duration of headache increases, the CSF should be examined for blood or xanthochromia.

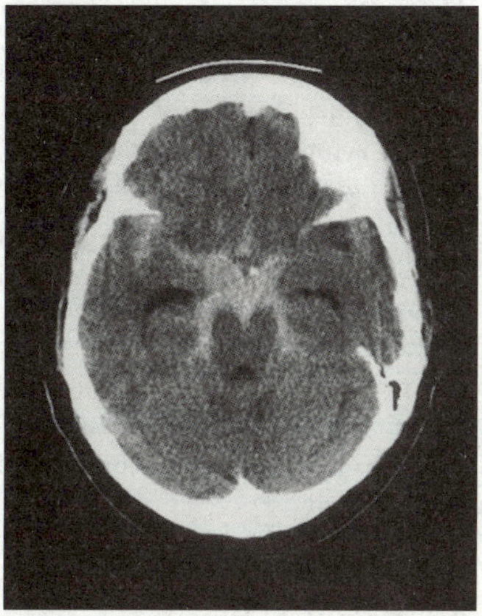

Fig. 30-2 Cerebral aneurysm. Shown is a CT scan of an aneurysmal SAH in a 55 yr-old woman. Subarachnoid blood can be seen within the nterpeduncular and ambient cisterns and the right sylvian fissure from a ruptured aneurysm at the junction of the right carotid artery and the posterior communicating artery.

CSF xanthochromia in association with normal findings on the CT scan is suggestive of SAH. After the diagnosis is established, angiography should be performed to study the vascular anatomy and to identify the source of hemorrhage.

A normal non-contrast-enhanced head CT scan followed by a normal spinal fluid analysis definitively rules out SAH and does not need to be followed with angiography. However, this strategy does not rule out other causes of thunderclap headache that may be in the differential diagnosis, such as carotid artery dissection, cerebral venous sinus thrombosis, and reversible cranial vasoconstrictor syndrome.

Up to 90% of patients with SAH have cardiac arrhythmias or electrocardiographic abnormalities. Typical electrocardiographic findings include ST-T wave changes, U waves, and QT prolongation.

Treatment

The management of SAH is complex and includes initial resuscitation, stabilization, and emergent neurosurgical consultation. The goals of management are to treat the acute medical and neurologic complications, to prevent recurrent hemorrhage, and to forestall the ischemic complications of vasospasm. Because of an altered level of consciousness, patients with SAH of grade 3 or higher are at risk for respiratory depression and hypercapnia, which can lead to further increases in ICP; therefore, these patients may require early endotracheal intubation. BP also should be closely monitored. The typical treatment goal of BP is a SBP below 160 mm Hg or MAP below 130 mm Hg.Nimodipin should be started soon after a diagnosis of aneurysmal SAH is made to lessen the likelihood of poor outcome. The recommended dose is 60 mg by mouth or nasogastric tube every 4 hr. Antifibrinolytics and corticosteroids do not improve overall outcome.

Analgesics, including opioids, should be used for persistent headache. In patients who are nauseated or at risk for vomiting, antiemetics should be administered. Agitated patients require sedation, and all patients should be placed at bed rest in a quiet and dark environment. Clinically evident seizures should be treated with anticonvulsants. A majority of patients require hemodynamic and ICP monitoring in EICU. For definitive management, endovascular coil embolization is preferable to neurosurgical clipping, but this decision is based on size, location, and morphologic features of the aneurysm as well as local expertise.

Intracranial Neoplasm

Headache, the most common presenting complaint among patients with brain tumor, is reported by approximately 50% of the patients. Headache can be caused by benign or malignant primary neoplasms of the CNS as well as by metastatic lesions. The most common causes of metastasis are lung and breast carcinoma, followed by malignant melanoma and carcinomas of the gastrointestinal tract.

The headache of intracranial neoplasms can be caused by several mechanisms, including direct involvement of and traction on pain-sensitive structures such as meninges or larger cerebral vessels, or it may be a symptom of increased ICP.

Clinical Presentation

The typical patient presents with complaints of a worsening headache that has been present for weeks to months. The classic triad of brain tumor headache (sleep disturbances, severe pain, and nausea and vomiting) is seen in a minority of patients. If increased ICP is present, the headache often is bilateral and worsened by coughing, sneezing, bending, defecation, and sexual intercourse. Other presentations of intracranial neoplasms include seizures, personality changes, and cognitive difficulties.

Diagnostic Evaluation

The diagnosis of brain tumor may be suspected from the history and neurologic examination. Neuroimaging with CT or MRI is the most efficient way to confirm the diagnosis. Contrast enhancement on CT often improves the identification of the underlying mass lesion and helps differentiate it from other causes, including abscess, hematoma, and vascular malformation.

Treatment

Management consists of urgent referral to neurosurgery and treatment of any acute complications, including increased ICP and seizures. Dexamethasone is the high-potency steroid used most often to treat edema associated with brain tumors. In general, most patients require between 8 and 16 mg of dexamethasone per day. An appropriate starting dose in the ED is 10 mg IV, followed by 4 mg every 6 hr.

Patients who have a seizure should receive anticonvulsant therapy.

Giant Cell Arteritis

Giant cell arteritis, or temporal arteritis, is a systemic inflammatory process of the small and medium-sized arteries. Extracranial branches of the aortic arch and the ophthalmic vessels most commonly are involved. The mean age at onset is 71 yr, and it is rare before the age of 50 yr. Women are affected more commonly than men are.

Clinical Presentation

The headache often is of 2 to 3 mo duration and can be continuous or intermittent and often worsens at night or on exposure to cold. The pain may be described as sharp, throbbing, boring, or aching and usually is localized to the temporal region but may occur anywhere in the head. The physical examination may reveal tenderness over the scalp in the area of the temporal artery. Patients also may experience jaw claudication secondary to vascular insufficiency of the masseter and temporalis muscles. Systemic signs and symptoms, including fever, anorexia, and weight loss, often are present. Patients develop symptoms of polymyalgia rheumatica, pain in their large proximal joints, with symptoms referable to the neck, torso, and lower back. Typically, pain and stiffness are worse in the morning and lessen as the day goes on.

The most serious complication of giant cell arteritis is permanent visual loss. Amaurosis fugax also can occur before permanent visual loss. Other complications include peripheral neuropathies, transient ischemic attacks, and stroke.

Diagnostic Evaluation

The physical examination may reveal abnormalities of the temporal arteries, including tenderness, reduced or absent pulsations, erythema, and nodularity or swelling. Visual acuity, visual field testing, and thorough funduscopic examination should be performed.

A majority of patients have a significant elevation of the ESR, often more than 100 mm/hr. Other abnormalities on laboratory studies include mild to moderate anemia, elevated CRP level, liver function abnormalities, and thrombocytosis.

Treatment

Steroids are the mainstay of therapy; the recommended initial dose of prednisone ranges from 60 mg/d. Symptomatic response usually occurs rapidly over days, although therapy should be continued for months, with close ESR monitoring.

Carotid and Vertebral Artery Dissection

Principles of Disease

Carotid and vertebral dissections are the most frequent cause of stroke in persons younger than 45 yr. Reported mechanisms include neck torsion, chiropractic manipulation, coughing, minor falls, and motor vehicle collisions.

The pathologic lesion is intramural hemorrhage within the media of the arterial wall. The hematoma can be localized or extend circumferentially along the length of the vessel. Platelet aggregation and thrombus formation also occur causing distal embolization.

Clinical Presentation

The presentation of the patient with carotid or vertebral dissection is the abrupt onset of pain in the neck or face. Neurologic findings usually occur within the first few hours.

Carotid Dissection. The classic triad of symptoms for carotid dissection includes unilateral headache, ipsilateral Horner's syndrome, and contralateral hemispheric findings that may include aphasia, neglect, visual disturbances, or hemiparesis. The headache is often severe and throbbing but may be subacute and similar to previous headaches. Most patients eventually develop signs of cerebral ischemia. Warning symptoms include transient ischemic attacks, amaurosis fugax, episodic lightheadedness, and syncope.

Vertebral Dissection. The classic presentation is that of a relatively young person with severe, unilateral posterior headache and neurologic findings. The majority of patients develop a rapidly progressive neurologic deficit with symptoms of brainstem and cerebellar ischemia. Common findings include vertigo, severe vomiting, ataxia, diplopia, hemiparesis, unilateral facial weakness, and tinnitus. For patients who survive, the prognosis is usually good.

Diagnosis and Treatment

The emergency physician should consider the diagnosis in any young patient who presents with head or neck pain with focal neurologic findings. CT angiography, MRI, and catheter angiography are required to confirm the diagnosis. Fig. 30-3 shows an example of carotid artery dissection on MRI. Treatment is aimed at prevention of strok.

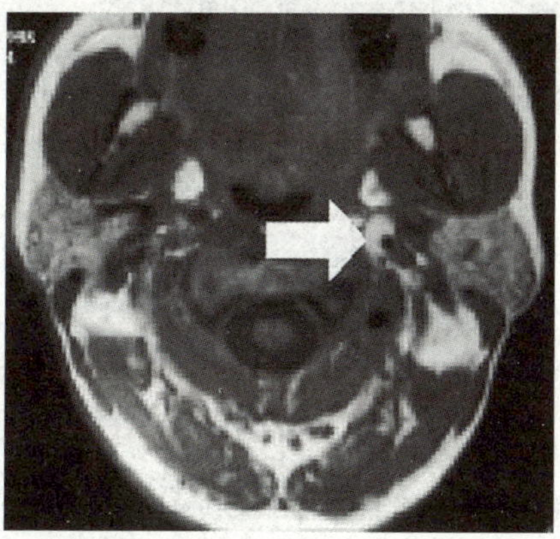

Fig. 30-3 Axial T1-weighted MRI demonstrating a crescent sign (*arrow*) in a patient with a left internal carotid artery dissection.

Cerebral Venous Sinus Thrombosis

Thrombophilia is usually identified in patients with cerebral venous sinus thrombosis,including genetic and hypercoagulable disorders, pregnancy and the puerperium, inflammatory systemic disorders including vasculitis, connective tissue disorders, and medications such as oral contraceptives. Other risk factors include head trauma, head and orofacial infections, and neurosurgical procedures.

Clinical Presentation

Common symptoms and signs include headache, seizures, decreased level of consciousness that may progress to coma, and focal neurologic deficits. With cavernous sinus thrombosis, the clinical picture is dominated by ocular findings including orbital pain, proptosis, and paralysis of extraocular movements.

Diagnostic Evaluation

An elevated D-dimer level is present. The key to diagnosis is to image the venous system itself. This is best accomplished by a combination of MRI to visualize the thrombosed vessel and magnetic resonance venography to detect nonvisualization of the same vessel. CT angiography and venography may also be used to visualize the cerebral venous system.

Treatment

Specific treatment of cerebral venous sinus thrombosis includes anticoagulation to prevent propagation of the thrombosis as well as complications Seizures should be treated with anticonvulsants.

Idiopathic Intracranial Hypertension

Although this disease is sometimes called pseudotumor cerebri or benign intracranial hypertension. Several predisposing factors have been identified, including the use of oral contraceptives, anabolic steroids, tetracyclines, and vitamin A.

Pathophysiology and Clinical Features

The pathophysiologic mechanism of IIH is often attributed to an imbalance between CSF production and reabsorption. The most prominent symptom is generalized headache, which often is gradual in onset and of moderate intensity. In some patients the headache is worsened by eye movement.

Patients may experience transient visual obscuration several times a day. These episodes can be followed by prolonged periods of visual loss. Patients also may complain of nausea, vomiting, dizziness, and pulsatile tinnitus. The physical examination will reveal papilledema and visual field defects. On occasion, a sixth nerve palsy is noted.

Diagnosis

The diagnosis of IIH should not be made without neuroimaging and measurement of ICP. Diagnostic criteria are listed in Box 30-5.

Box 30-5 ICHD-II Criteria for Diagnosis of IIH

1. Alert patient with neurologic examination that either yields normal findings or demonstrates any of the following abnormalities:
   A. Papilledema
   B. Enlarged blind spot
   C. Visual field defect (progressive if untreated)
2. Increased CSF pressure (>200 mm H_2O in nonobese patients,>250 mm H_2O in obese patients) measured by lumbar puncture in the recumbent position or by epidural or intraventricular pressure monitoring
3. Normal CSF chemistry (low CSF protein acceptable) and cellularity
4. Intracranial disease (including venous sinus thrombosis) ruled out by appropriate investigations
5. No metabolic, toxic, or hormonal cause of intracranial hypertension

ICHD-II, International Classification of Headache Disorders, 2nd ed

Treatment

Predisposing factors should be corrected. Symptomatic treatment often includes lowering of ICP and management of the headache. Acetazolamide can be used to decrease CSF production alone or with a loop diuretic such as furosemide. Steroids also have been used. Rebound headache often occurs when doses are tapered.

LP is commonly performed to alleviate acute symptoms.

Post-traumatic Headache

Headache is the most common symptom after minor head injury. It often is part of a complex syndrome that can include dizziness, fatigue, insomnia, irritability, memory loss, and difficulty with concentration.

Acute post-traumatic headache(PTHA) develops hours to days after the injury and resolves within 3 to 6 mo. Chronic PTHA may last several months to years and may mimic other forms of headache, including tension and migraine headaches. The presence of headache, dizziness, or nausea on initial presentation is strongly associated with the development of chronic PTHA.

Patients in whom PTHA develops after minor head injuries have normal findings on neurologic examination and neuroimaging studies. The pathophysiologic mechanism for their symptoms is unclear.

Treatment is symptomatic. For acute PTHA, analgesics such as acetaminophen or NSAIDs are adequate for pain control. Antidepressants and beta-blockers may be effective in selected patients.

Post-Dural Puncture Headache

Headache is the most common complication of LP. Although the onset often is immediate, patients may not report symptoms for several days. In a majority of affected persons, the duration of headache is less than 5 d.

The cause of post–dural puncture headache (PDPH) is not entirely clear.

PDPH typically is bilateral, throbbing, and exacerbated by the upright position. Associated signs and symptoms include neck stiffness, nausea, vomiting, auditory disturbances including tinnitus and hearing loss (hypoacusis), and ocular symptoms including blurred vision and diplopia.

Most PDPHs resolve spontaneously within a few days with bed rest, adequate hydration, and mild analgesics. For persistent headaches, methylxanthine agents may be useful. Caffeine sodium benzoate (500 mg in 1 L of fluid) may be effective.

Cervicogenic Headache

Cervicogenic headache refers to headache originating from disorders of the neck. Diagnosis is based on the presence of one of the following three distinct sets of symptoms:

1. Unilateral headache triggered by movements of the head or neck or certain head positions
2. Unilateral headache triggered by pressure on the neck
3. Unilateral headache spreading to the neck or possibly the ipsilateral shoulder or arm

Many of these headaches are reported after a whiplash injury. The pathophysiologic process of some headaches have not been adequately defined.

Reversible Cranial Vasoconstriction Syndrome

RCVS, also been called Call-Fleming syndrome, postpartum angiopathy or migrainous vasospasm, is a disorder of cerebral arteries characterized by segmental areas of vasoconstriction. It causes recurrent thunderclap headache in susceptible patients and is a cause of ischemic or hemorrhagic stroke. The headache is often described as severe and throbbing and is associated with nausea, vomiting, and photophobia. The headache may be provoked by use of vasoactive medications or substances. Typically, cerebral vascular imaging shows vasoconstriction of, abnormal areas, described as sausage on a string. Repeated vascular imaging within 3 mo shows resolution of the areas of vasoconstriction. Treatment with CCB has been described.

OTHER HEADACHE DISORDERS AND FACIAL PAIN

Nummular Headache

Nummular headache is a highly localized headache, rarely more than moderately painful, that is felt exclusively in a rounded, 2 to 6 cm area of the head. Epidemiology and pathogenesis are not yet well understood. Nummular headache is usually responsive to nonsteroidals, although a high frequency of headaches may be prevented with tricyclic antidepressants.

Trigeminal Neuralgia

Trigeminal neuralgia is a painful unilateral affliction of the face characterized by brief electric shock-like (lancinating) pains limited to the distribution of one or more divisions of the trigeminal nerve. Pain is commonly evoked by trivial stimuli (e.g., washing, shaving, smoking, talking, or brushing teeth) but also may occur spontaneously. Individual attacks are brief, lasting a few seconds to less than 2 min, and are stereotypic in the individual patient. The lightning-like pains and unilateral grimaces characteristic of trigeminal neuralgia led to the designation *tic douloureux*. The diagnosis is straightforward in most patients on the basis of clinical criteria. However, because these symptoms also can be caused by an underlying mass lesion or multiple sclerosis, MRI is indicated in previously undiagnosed patients and when sensory loss or motor dysfunction is present.

Several oral drugs have been effective in treatment of trigeminal neuralgia, including carbamazepine and oxcarbazepine. Phenytoin and baclofen may also be useful. However, approximately 30% of patients fail to respond to medical therapy. In these patients, surgical management, by alcohol or glycerol injection or microvascular decompression, may be indicated. For patients with acute severe pain, parenteral treatment with an antiepileptic drug such as phosphenytoin may be useful.

Coital Headache

Coital cephalgia is a recurrent, benign headache associated with sexual activity and is more common in men than in women. Different types have been described, including headaches that occur before, during, or immediately after orgasm. They typically are occipital in location and may increase in severity with mounting sexual excitement. Their duration can be minutes to hours. On occasion, some patients experience a sudden, explosive headache that occurs during orgasm. In these patients, SAH should be ruled out.

(YANG Lishan)

Chapter 31

Syncope

KEY CONSEPTS

Syncope is the sudden transient loss of consciousness with a loss of postural tone.

Risk factors for syncope include cerebrovascular disease, cardiac medications and hypertension.

Hospitalization is required for patients with chest pain, unexplained shortness of breath, a history of significant CHF, or valvular disease.

PERSPECTIVE

Syncope is the sudden transient loss of consciousness with a loss of postural tone. Diagnostic accuracy relies largely on the synthesis of patient risk factors and reported symptoms, with limited reliance on the physical examination and ancillary testing.

Epidemiology

The prevalence of syncope in the general population is approximately 19%. Patients come to the ED at a rate of 2.8 visits per 1000 population, which accounts for 0.8% of ED visits. Approximately 32% of these patients are admitted, and syncope accounts for 1% to 6% of all hospitalized patients.

Risk factors for syncope include cerebrovascular disease, cardiac medications, and hypertension. Age, congestive heart failure, and coronary artery disease are key predictors of mortality in patients with syncope, but syncope alone does not appear to alter risk. Recurrence of syncope may be as high as 50% and is not correlated with age or sex.

Pathophysiology

The final common pathway resulting in syncope is dysfunction of either both cerebral hemispheres or the brainstem (reticular activating system), usually from acute hypoperfusion. Reduced blood flow may be regional (cerebral vasoconstriction) or systemic (hypotension). By definition, the cause of CNS dysfunction should be transient. Persistent causes of significant CNS dysfunction result in coma or depressed consciousness.

Hypoperfusion resulting in approximately 35% or more reduction in cerebral blood flow usually produces unconsciousness, and any mechanism that adversely affects the components of perfusion (cardiac output, systemic vascular resistance, blood volume, regional vascular resistance) can cause or contribute to syncope. Other mechanisms of CNS dysfunction resulting in syncope include hypoglycemia, toxins, metabolic abnormalities, failure of autoregulation, and primary neurologic derangements.

DIAGNOSTIC APPROACH

Differential Considerations

The potential causes of syncope are numerous and can be categorized according to their primary mechanism (Box 31-1). The first differential diagnostic consideration is to distinguish syncope from seizure and uncommon disorders such as cataplexy. When syncope is established the life-threatening causes, primarily cardiovascular in origin, are considered first. The principal serious causes of syncope are dysrhythmias and myocardial ischemia. Cerebrovascular disease, principally SAH, is equally serious. Other important differential considerations should include toxic-metabolic abnormalities,critical aortic stenosis, PE and dissection of the thoracic aorta.

Box 31-1 Causes of Syncope

Focal Hypoperfusion of CNS Structures

- Cerebrovascular disease
- Hyperventilation
- Subclavian steal
- SAH
- Basilar artery migraine
- Cerebral syncope

Systemic Hypoperfusion Resulting in CNS Dysfunction

- Outflow obstruction
  - Mitral, aortic, or pulmonic stenosis
  - Hypertrophic cardiomyopathy
  - Atrial myxoma
  - PE
  - Pulmonary hypertension
  - Cardiac tamponade
  - CHF
- Reduced cardiac output
  - Tachycardia
    - Supraventricular tachycardia
    - VT
    - Vf
    - Wolff-Parkinson-White syndrome
    - Torsades de pointes
  - Bradycardia
    - Sinus node disease
    - Second-degree and third-degree AV block
    - Prolonged QT syndrome
    - Brugada's syndrome
    - Pacemaker malfunction
    - Implanted cardioverter-defibrillator malfunction
  - Other cardiovascular disease
    - Aortic dissection
    - MI
    - Cardiomyopathy
- Vasomotor—neurally mediated (reflex vasodepressor)
  - Neurocardiogenic (vasovagal)
  - Emotion
  - Pain
  - Situational
- Carotid sinus sensitivity
  - Necktie syncope
  - Shaving syncope
- Miscellaneous reflex
  - Tussive, sneeze
  - Exercise, postexercise
  - Gastrointestinal—swallowing, vomiting, defecation
  - Postmicturition
  - Elevated intrathoracic pressure (weightlifting)
- Other causes of hypoperfusion
  - Orthostatic hypotension—volume depletion
  - Anemia
  - Drug-induced

CNS Dysfunction with Normal Cerebral Perfusion

- Hypoglycemia
- Hypoxemia—asphyxiation
- Seizure
- Narcolepsy
- Psychogenic
  - Anxiety disorder
  - Conversion disorder
  - Somatization disorder
  - Panic disorder
  - Breath-holding spells
- Toxic
  - Drugs
  - Carbon monoxide
  - Other agents
  - Undetermined causes

Pivotal Findings

The majority of cases of syncope arise from benign causes, so the evaluation is largely focused on excluding serious pathology. The patient's history, particularly the setting of the syncope (e.g., postmicturition, venipuncture), patient position (e.g., sitting, standing), prior episodes, and the presence or absence of prodromal symptoms, is central to separating benign from serious causes of the syncopal episode. The yield of an ECG is generally low; however, it is broadly recommended.

Symptoms

The key characteristics of syncope include the rate of onset (gradual or abrupt), position on symptom onset (e.g., standing, sitting, or supine), and duration and rate of recovery. Abrupt onset, occurrence while sitting or supine, and duration of more than a few seconds are usually ascribed to serious, often cardiac, causes of syncope.

Additional history regarding the events preceding the syncope is helpful. Occurrence during significant exertion suggests outflow obstruction, whereas occurrence after exercise or a prolonged exposure to heat stress suggests orthostasis. The myriad mechanisms that may mediate a neurocardiogenic response, including significant emotional events, micturition, eating, bowel movements, emesis, and movement or manipulation of the neck causing stimulation of the carotid sinus, should be addressed. Occurrence in supine position or the presence of acute palpitations is relatively specific for syncope of cardiac origin. Seizures may be preceded by an aura and followed by a typical postictal state.

Events during the syncopal episode do not usually clarify the cause. Tonic-clonic movements should be differentiated from the prolonged activity with subsequent postictal depression of consciousness seen in seizure disorders. Trauma from a fall or other mechanism may distract the examiner from evaluating for the underlying syncope that caused the injury.

The postsyncopal events should be queried. Symptoms consistent with a postictal state are characteristic of seizures. Initial vital signs and cardiac monitoring by out-of-hospital medical providers may provide clues to primary cardiac dysrhythmias.Chest pain or dyspnea can suggest myocardial ischemia, aortic dissection, or PE. Diaphoresis and lightheadedness accompanied by a graying of vision may suggest orthostasis or vasovagal causes. Tongue biting and incontinence of urine or stool suggest seizures.

The past medical history is critical in stratifying risk. CHF is a key determinant of increased short- and long-term mortality in the setting of syncope. Prior coronary artery or cerebrovascular disease, diabetes, hypertension, and other significant chronic disease also appear to increase the risk of mortality after syncope. Certain medications are well established to be associated with syncope (Box 31-2). QT interval-prolonging agents, beta-blockers, insulin, and oral hypoglycemics, in particular, deserve attention.

Box 31-2 Medications That May Induce Syncope

Cardiovascular agents
Beta-blockers
Vasodilators (beta-blockers, calcium channel blockers, nitrates,hydralazine, ACEI, ARB, phenothiazines, phosphodiesterase inhibitors)
Diuretics
Central antihypertensives (clonidine, methyldopa)
Other antihypertensives (guanethidine)
QT-prolonging agents (amiodarone, disopyramide, flecainide,procainamide, quinidine, sotalol)
Other antidysrhythmics
Psychoactive agents
Anticonvulsants (carbamazepine, phenytoin)
Antiparkinsonian agents
CNS depressants (barbiturates, benzodiazepines)
Monoamine oxidase inhibitors
Antidepressants
Narcotic analgesics
Sedating and nonsedating antihistamines
Cholinesterase inhibitors (donepezil, tacrine, galantamine)
Drugs with other mechanisms
Drugs of abuse (cannabis, cocaine, alcohol, heroin)
Digitalis
Insulin and oral hypoglycemics
Neuropathic agents (vincristine)
Nonsteroidal anti-inflammatory drugs
Bromocriptine

Signs

The physical examination focuses primarily on the elements affecting the cardiovascular and neurologic systems. Specific findings are detailed in Table 31-1.

Table 31-1 Directed Physical Examination in Syncope

SYSTEM	PIVOTAL FINDING	SIGNIFICANCE
Vital signs	Pulse rate and rhythm	Tachycardia, bradycardia, other dysrhythmias
	Respiratory rate and depth	Tachypnea suggests hypoxia,hyperventilation, or pulmonary embolus
	Blood pressure	Shock may cause decreased cerebral perfusion;hypovolemia or medication use may lead to orthostasis
	Temperature	Fever from sepsis may cause volume depletion and orthostasis
Skin	Color, diaphoresis	Signs of decreased organ perfusion

Continued

SYSTEM	PIVOTAL FINDING	SIGNIFICANCE
HEENT	Tenderness and deformity	Signs of trauma
	Papilledema	Increased intracranial pressure,head injury
	Breath	Ketones from ketoacidosis
Neck	Bruits	Identify presence of cerebrovascular disease
	Jugular venous distention	Right-sided heart failure from myocardial ischemia,tamponade, PE
Lungs	Breath sounds, crackles, wheezes	Infection, left-sided heart failure from myocardial ischemia, rarely PE
Heart	Systolic murmur	Aortic stenosis, hypertrophic cardiomyopathy
	Rub	Pericarditis, tamponade
Abdomen	Pulsatile mass	Abdominal aortic aneurysm
Rectum	Stool for gross blood or melena	Anemia, gastrointestinal bleed
Pelvis	Uterine bleeding, adnexal tenderness	Anemia, ectopic pregnancy, hypovolemia
Extremities	Pulse equality in upper extremities	Subclavian steal, thoracic aortic dissection
Neurologic	Mental status, focal neurologic findings	Seizure, stroke, or other primary neurologic disease

HEENT, head, eyes, ears, nose, and throat.

Ancillary Studies

12-lead ECG (Table 31-2) is warranted in all cases of syncope except in young, otherwise healthy patients with a clear history and setting for benign neurocardiogenic (vasovagal) syncope. Dysrhythmias and shortened PR or prolonged QT intervals may be identified on the 12-lead ECG. A RBBB in association with ST elevation in leads V_1 through V_3 suggests Brugada's syndrome. Unanticipated cardiac hypertrophy may be revealed. Continuous limb-lead ECG monitoring in the ED may also identify transient dysrhythmias. An ECG showing RV strain pattern may suggest PE, whereas diffuse ST elevation or electrical alternans helps diagnose pericarditis associated with pericardial tamponade.

Table 31-2 Ancillary Studies in Syncope

STUDY	INDICATION
12-Lead ECG/limb-lead ECG monitoring	Cardiac dysrhythmia, ischemia, cardiomyopathy
Orthostatic vital signs	Orthostatic hypotension or bradycardia
Hemogram	Anemia
Electrolytes, serum	Metabolic abnormality, especially hyponatremia, hyperkalemia, or hypokalemia
Glucose, serum or blood	Hypoglycemia
D-dimer, serum	PE
Cardiac enzymes, serum	Myocardial infarction
β-hCG	Pregnancy

Continued

STUDY	INDICATION
Toxicologic screen	Drug-related syncope
ABG	Acid-base disturbance
Chest X-ray examination	Thoracic aortic dissection
Cranial CT or MRI	New-onset or focal seizure, trauma,intracranial hemorrhage
Echocardiogram	Cardiac outflow obstruction, tamponade, thoracic dissection
Ventilation-perfusion scan	PE
CT pulmonary angiogram	PE, thoracic aortic dissection
Abdominal ultrasound or CT	AAA
Pelvic ultrasound	Ectopic pregnancy
Tests Usually Performed as Part of an Inpatient or Outpatient Evaluation	
Holter or loop ECG	Dysrhythmia
Echocardiogram	Cardiomyopathy, valvular disease
Exercise and ^{99m}Tc sestamibi ECG	Myocardial ischemia
Electrophysiologic study	Dysrhythmia
Carotid ultrasound	Stroke, TIA
Head-up tilt-table test	Orthostatic hypotension
Electroencephalogram	Seizures

When suggested by the history and physical examination findings, however, selective use of the hemogram, serum electrolytes and glucose, urine drug screen, and pregnancy test may identify or exclude some uncommon causes of syncope (Table 31-2). Chest radiography and serum BNP testing are warranted if HF is suspected or known by history.Cranial CT is indicated only when intracerebral hemorrhage is suspected on the basis of sudden syncope with accompanying headache, particularly of sudden onset, or in the presence of abnormalities on neurologic examination.

In otherwise healthy patients in whom a benign dysrhythmia, such as episodic SVT or Af, is suspected, Holter or event ECG monitoring may be helpful. In patients with significant underlying cardiac disease or when a significant dysrhythmia is a possible cause of the syncope, echocardiography, continuous monitoring, or cardiovascular stress testing may be helpful. Electroencephalography is useful only when a seizure episode is suspected. Orthostatic vital signs, may be helpful when positional changes are accompanied by typical presyncopal symptoms and a significant rise in heart rate or fall in BP. A schematic of selected diagnostic testing strategies for syncope is depicted in Fig. 31-1.

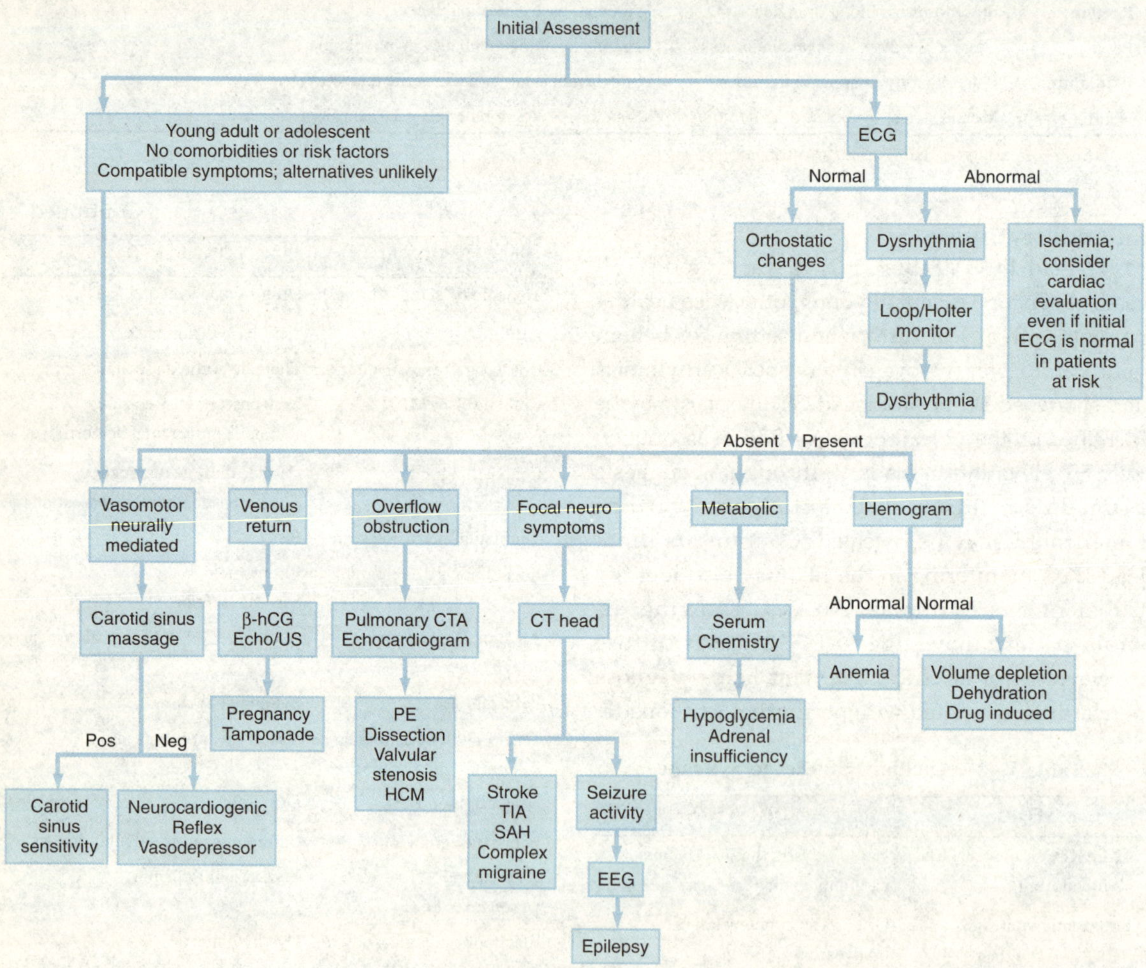

Fig. 31-1 Management algorithm for patients with syncope.

DIAGNOSTIC ALGORITHM

The critical diagnoses to consider are listed in Table 31-3.The emergent causes of syncope are included in Box 31-1. Many other causes such as neurocardiogenic and reflex-mediated syncope have benign mechanisms.

After stabilization and assessment, the clinical features coupled with onset and recovery can suggest the cause (Table 31-4). A logical approach to the history, physical examination, and diagnostic

Table 31-3 Critical Diagnoses to Consider in Syncope

Myocardial infarction
Life-threatening dysrhythmias
Thoracic aortic dissection
Critical aortic stenosis
Hypertrophic cardiomyopathy
Pericardial tamponade
AAA
PE
SAH
Stroke
Toxic-metabolic derangements
Severe hypovolemia or hemorrhage

testing is depicted in Fig. 31-2. The emphasis is on risk stratification because short-term mortality risk in syncope is related to structural cardiac disease, HF, and dysrhythmias.

Table 31-4 Clinical Features of Common and Serious Causes of Syncope

CAUSE	ONSET AND RECOVERY	FEATURES
Dysrhythmia	Classically abrupt onset and rapid recovery	Classic presentation uncommon; past cardiac history, risk factors for CAD more common in elderly; implanted pacemaker or cardioverter-defibrillator
Cardiac outflow obstruction	Exertion causes abrupt symptoms; rapid recovery with rest	Murmurs not always audible; mechanical valves warrant close monitoring
Myocardial infarction	Exertion or at rest; recovery often incomplete with chest pain persisting	Past cardiac history, risk factors for CAD; chest pain and shortness of breath common but frequently absent in diabetics and the elderly
PE	Abrupt onset; recovery often incomplete with dyspnea persisting	Chest pain, dyspnea, hypercoagulable state, DVT, pregnancy
Thoracic aortic dissection	Spontaneous; recovery often incomplete with chest or upper back pain persisting	Tearing chest pain; associated with hypertension, Marfan syndrome, cystic medial necrosis
AAA	Spontaneous onset; recovery often incomplete with abdominal pain persisting	Abdominal or low back pain; associated with peripheral vascular disease
Pericardial tamponade	Penetrating chest trauma or thoracic cancers	Beck's triad of hypotension, JVD, muffled heart sounds
Anomalous left coronary artery	Onset with exercise, Valsalva maneuver	Left coronary artery arises from pulmonary artery; usually detected in childhood
SAH	Rapid onset; sentinel event may resolve	Focal neurologic findings; "thunderclap" worst headache; nuchal rigidity
Vertebrobasilar insufficiency	Posture change or neck movement	Vertigo, nausea, dysphagia, dysarthria, blurry vision common associated symptoms
Hypovolemia	Bleeding, emesis, heat stress, dehydration; gradual onset	Orthostatic hypotension
Anemia	Bleeding, often occult or gradual from menses or gastrointestinal sources; iron deficiency or decreased red blood cell production	Orthostatic hypotension commonly associated
Hypoglycemia	Gradual onset; incomplete spontaneous recovery common	Diabetes, ingestion or injection of hypoglycemics or insulin; diaphoresis, anxiety, jitteriness
Hypoxemia	Usually gradual onset; spontaneous recovery if asphyxiating circumstance is reversed	Carbon monoxide, natural gas, sewer gas, bleach-ammonia mix
Subdural hematoma	Onset with or after trauma (which may be trivial in high-risk patients)	Elderly, alcoholics, patients on anticoagulants at greater risk
Air embolus	Diving	Hyperbaric oxygen a key treatment
Pulmonary hypertension	Associated with MI or PE	Risk factors for MI or PE

Continued

CAUSE	ONSET AND RECOVERY	FEATURES
Drug syncope	Medication associated with syncope	Consider illicit and alternative drug use; elderly at risk for polypharmacy and drug interactions
Ruptured ectopic pregnancy	Patient often unaware of pregnancy	Abdominal pain, abnormal tenderness; positive β-hCG test
Seizure	Abrupt or with aura; postictal state common	Past history common
Carotid sinus sensitivity	Carotid sinus sensitivity; rapid onset and recovery	Shaving, necktie, sudden neck movement; carotid massage may provoke symptoms
Reflex syncope	Gastrointestinal, genitourinary, or thoracic stimulation	Urination, defecation, cough, eating, swallowing, weightlifting
Neurocardiogenic (vasovagal)	Emotion, pain are common triggers; upright posture;gradual onset; rapid recovery once supine	Prodrome of light-headedness, graying or blurring of vision,nausea, sweats common
Hyperventilation	Emotion, pain; gradual onset; patient often unaware of rapid respirations	Perioral tingling, carpopedal spasms, extremity numbness
Narcolepsy	Often spontaneous	Known history
Basilar artery migraine	Specific triggers often known to patient	Visual prodrome often absent; more common in young women; vertigo and nausea common
Trigeminal or glossopharyngeal neuralgia	Sudden onset; specific triggers often known to patient	Lancinating pain in characteristic location
Subclavian steal	Moving affected arm	Thoracic outlet syndrome
Psychogenic	Variable	Anxiety or psychiatric history; diagnosis by examining symptom pattern and excluding organic cause
Breath-holding	Deliberate breath-holding	Usually toddlers or young children
Drop attack	Unpredictable	Not true syncope—no loss of consciousness; usually elderly;loss of tone, ataxia, vertigo

EMPIRICAL MANAGEMENT

Patients with significantly abnormal vital signs, recurrent syncope, or associated symptoms of a concerning nature such as chest pain, hypotension, abdominal or back pain, or shortness of breath should undergo rapid evaluation.

Patients with critical diagnoses are stabilized in the ED and admitted to the EICU or other appropriate inpatient unit.

Several scoring systems have been proposed as aids in the admission decision-making process, most notably the San Francisco Syncope Rule. In essence, this guideline suggests that in the absence of abnormal ECG findings, shortness of breath, hypotension (SBP <90 mm Hg), anemia (hematocrit <30%), or a history of HF the patient is at sufficiently low risk for outpatient disposition to be considered.

Hospitalization is required for patients with chest pain, unexplained shortness of breath, a history of significant CHF, or valvular disease. Patients with ECG evidence of ventricular dysrhythmias, ischemia, significantly prolonged QT interval, or new bundle branch block are also admitted. The clinician should consider monitoring patients with any of the following indications: age older than 45 yr, preexisting cardiovascular or congenital heart disease, family history of sudden death, serious comorbidities such as diabetes, or exertional syncope.

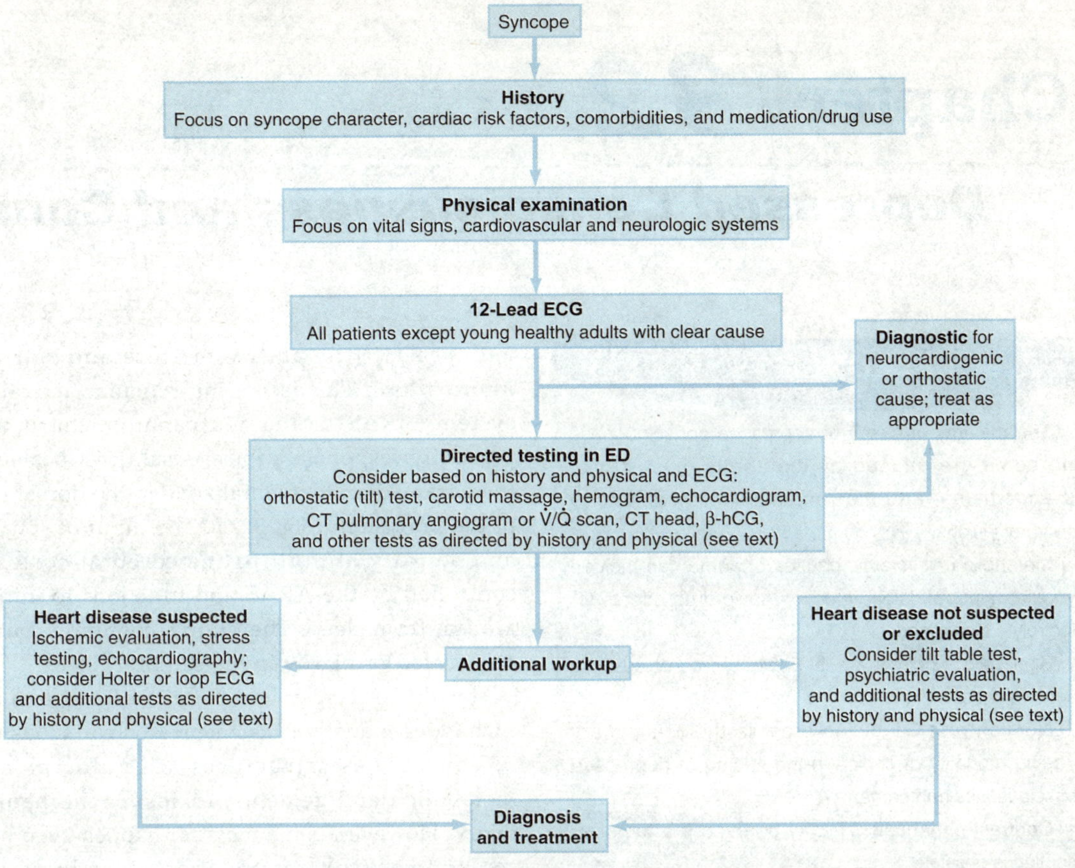

Fig. 31-2 Diagnosis algorithm for syncope.

(YANG Lishan)

Chapter 32

Depressed Consciousness and Coma

KEY CONCEPTS

The majority of cases of depressed consciousness and coma are caused by metabolic or systemic derangements, and the remainder are caused by structural lesions.

Metabolic or systemic causes of coma can include hypoxia, hypoperfusion, infection, toxic drug effects, or electrolyte disturbances.

Significant hypotension with depressed consciousness suggests shock.

Noncontrast CT of the brain is the preliminary imaging modality of choice in the setting of depressed consciousness and coma.

Contrast-enhanced CT may be used if a tumor or infection is possible.

Initial establishment of circulation, airway, and breathing (CAB) is of primary importance in stabilizing the patient with altered mental status.

PERSPECTIVE

Epidemiology

Depressed consciousness represents a spectrum of disease that ranges from sleepiness or decreased alertness to frank coma. The majority of cases of depressed consciousness and coma are caused by metabolic or systemic derangements, and the remainder are caused by structural lesions.

Pathophysiology

Consciousness includes the properties of *arousal* and cognition. *Cognition* is the combination of *orientation*, the accurate perception of what is experienced, *judgment*, the ability to process input data to generate more meaningful information, and *memory* (the ability to store and retrieve information). The ascending reticular activating system (ARAS) is the neuroanatomic structure primarily responsible for arousal. It is located in the paramedian tegmental zone in the dorsal part of the brainstem (Fig. 32-1). The input of somatic and sensory stimuli to the cerebral cortex is controlled by the ARAS and functions to initiate arousal from sleep. The brain's cognition centers are located primarily in the cerebral cortex.

Insults to the cerebral cortex or brainstem can each independently cause depressed consciousness or coma. These structures are vulnerable to metabolic derangements, toxins, or mechanical injury. However, coma may not happen even both cerebral hemispheres are affected, and this also depends on the size and speed of progression of the insult. Localized, unilateral lesions in the cerebral cortex usually do not induce depressed consciousness or coma. In contrast, small focal lesions in the brainstem can affect the ARAS. If the ARAS is impaired, the cerebral cortex cannot be aroused and depressed consciousness or coma occurs.

Potential causes of depressed consciousness can be broken down into a few general categories. Metabolic or systemic causes of coma can include hypoxia, hypoperfusion, infection, toxic drug effects, or electrolyte disturbances. Hypoxia can be the result of CHF, PE, carbon monoxide poisoning, or severe pulmonary compromise such as occurs in COPD, cystic fibrosis, and asthma. The various causes of shock can result in hypoperfusion states leading to depression of consciousness. These include anaphylactic, septic, hypovolemic, cardiogenic, and neurogenic origins of shock. Infection, both systemic (sepsis) and focal, can be another general cause of depressed consciousness. This is particularly true if CNS structures are involved as in meningitis,

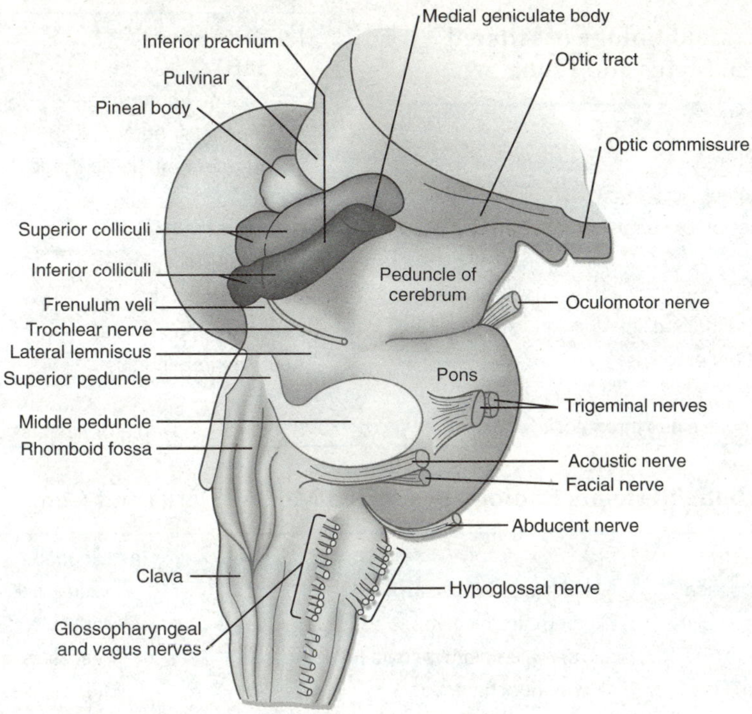

Fig. 32-1 Brainstem anatomy.

encephalitis, or CNS abscess. Toxic drug effects are imputed to the side effects of drugs (especially in overdose of drugs or in the elderly) are common causes of depressed consciousness in the ED. In addition, electrolyte and glucose abnormalities can be caused by multiple conditions, including diabetes, renal dysfunction, malignancy, and medication interactions or dosing errors.

Structural causes of coma and depressed consciousness are those most commonly arising from head trauma, stroke, tumor, or infection. Traumatic causes can include subdural and epidural hematomas, intraparenchymal or subarachnoid hemorrhage, or simply contusion or concussion. Strokes occur with embolic, thrombotic, or hemorrhagic mechanisms, but it is extremely unusual for ischemic (i.e., nonhemorrhagic) stroke to depress consciousness unless a massive insult to both hemispheres has occurred (e.g., diffuse, severe cerebral edema after a massive infarct). Depression of consciousness with CNS infections may be caused by mass effect and is common with severe bacterial meningitis, cerebral abscess or empyema, or parasitic mass. Malignancies, whether primary or metastatic, can cause depressed consciousness if their mass effect is sufficient or if surrounding edema devvelops rapidly.

Special consideration should be given to specific populations of patients. The elderly are susceptible to alterations in therapeutic medication dosage and drug-drug interactions. Even seemingly minor infections, such as urinary tract infections, upper respiratory infections, or viral gastroenteritis, may cause altered mental status, depressed consciousness, or coma. In addition, immunocompromised patients such as those with AIDS or those undergoing chemotherapy treatment for transplants, malignancy, or immunologic disease are vulnerable to a multitude of opportunistic infections not commonly seen in the general patient population.

CLINICAL EVALUATION

The differential diagnosis of depression of consciousness is extensive but can be greatly simplified by focusing attention on the distinguishing characteristics of the available patient history and physical examination (Boxes 32-1 and 32-2).

Box 32-1 Structural Etiology of Altered Mental Status and Coma

Trauma
- Subdural hematoma
- Epidural hematoma
- Cerebral concussion or contusion

Stroke Syndromes
- Embolism
  - Cardiac (Af, endocarditis)
  - Paradoxical (fat embolus)
- Thrombosis
  - Cerebral venous sinus thrombosis
- Hemorrhage
  - SAH
  - Pontine hemorrhage
  - Cerebellar hemorrhage
  - Intracerebral hemorrhage

Tumor
- Brainstem tumors
- Metastatic disease
- Angiomas
- Pituitary apoplexy
- Acute hydrocephalus

Infection
- Subdural empyema or abscess

Box 32-2 Metabolic/Systemic Etiology of Altered Mental Status and Coma

Hypoxia
- Severe pulmonary disease (hypoventilation)
- Severe anemia
- Environmental/toxin
  - Methemoglobinemia
  - Cyanide
  - Carbon monoxide
  - Decreased atmospheric oxygen (high altitude)
  - Near-drowning

Disorders of Glucose
- Hypoglycemia
  - Chronic alcohol abuse and liver disease
  - Excessive use of insulin or other hypoglycemic agents
  - Insulinoma
- Hyperglycemia
  - DKA
  - Nonketotic hyperosmolar coma

Decreased Cerebral Blood Flow
- Hypovolemic shock
- Cardiac
  - Vasovagal syncope
  - Arrhythmias
  - MI
  - Valvular disorders
  - CHF
  - Pericardial effusion/tamponade

Electrolyte/pH Disturbances
- Acidosis/alkalosis
- Hypernatremia/hyponatremia
- Hypercalcemia/hypocalcemia
- Hypophosphatemia
- Hypermagnesemia/hypomagnesemia

Endocrine Disorders
- Myxedema coma, thyrotoxicosis
- Hypopituitarism
- Addison's disease (primary or secondary)
- Cushing's disease
- Pheochromocytoma
- Hyperparathyroidism/hypoparathyroidism

Endogenous Toxins
- Hyperammonemia (liver failure)
- Uremia (renal disease)
- Carbon dioxide narcosis (pulmonary disease)
- Porphyria

Exogenous Toxins
- Alcohols
  - Ethanol, isopropyl alcohol, methanol, ethylene glycol
- Acid poisons
  - Salicylates
  - Paraldehyde
  - Ammonium chloride
- Antidepressant medications
  - Lithium
  - Tricyclic antidepressants (TCAs)
  - Selective serotonin reuptake inhibitors (SSRIs)
  - Monamine oxidase inhibitors(MAOIs)
- Stimulants
- Hallucinogens
  - Lysergic acid diethylamide (LSD)
  - Marijuana
  - Mescaline, peyote
  - Mushrooms
  - Phencyclidine (PCP)
- Herbs/plants
  - Aconite
  - Jimson weed
  - Morning glory
- Volatile substances
  - Hydrocarbons (gasoline, butane,toluene, benzene, choroform)
  - Nitrites
  - Anesthetic agents (nitrous oxide,ether)
- Other
  - γ-Hydroxybutyrate (GHB)
  - Ketamine
  - Penicillin
  - Cardiac glycosides
  - Anticonvulsants
  - Steroids
  - Heavy metals
  - Cimetidine
  - Organophosphates

Disorders of Temperature Regulation/Environmental
- Hypothermia
- Heat stroke
- Malignant hyperthermia
- Neuroleptic malignant syndrome
- HACE

Myocarditis
Infectious
Septic shock
Bacterial meningitis
Vascular/hematologic
Hypertensive encephalopathy
Pseudotumor cerebri
Hyperviscosity (sickle cell, polycythemia)
Hyperventilation
Cerebral lupus vasculitis
TTP
DIC

Metabolic Cofactor Deficiency

Thiamine (Wernicke-Korsakoff syndrome)
Pyridoxine (isoniazid overdose)
Folic acid (chonic alcohol abuse)
Cyanocobalamine
Niacin

Amphetamines/methamphetamines
Cocaine
Over-the-counter sympathomimetics
Narcotics/opiates
Morphine
Heroin
Codeine, oxycodone, meperidine, hydrocodone
Methadone
Fentanyl
Propoxyphene
Sedative-hypnotics
Benzodiazepines
Barbiturates
Rohypnol
Bromide

Dysbarism

Primary Glial or Neuronal Disorders

Adrenoleukodystrophy
Creutzfeldt-Jakob disease
Progressive multifocal leukoencephalopathy
Marchiava-Bignami disease
Gliomatosis cerebri
Central pontine myelinolysis

Other Disorders of Unknown Etiology

Seizures
Postictal states
Reye's syndrome
Intussusception

History

Family members, caregivers, or friends often can provide information that is unobtainable or unreliable from the patient who presents with depressed consciousness. They usually have some knowledge regarding the patient's past medical history, which may include diabetes, liver or renal disease, vascular disease such as hypertension, stroke or transient ischemic attacks, malignancy, seizures, immunocompromised states such as HIV, sickle cell disease or a history of organ transplant, or psychiatric illness. Symptoms in the hours to days preceding the occurrence of depressed consciousness are important. Specifically, the patient may have complained of headache, focal weakness or numbness, incoordination, or vision disturbances. The patient may have experienced nausea, vomiting, or fever. There may be a history of a traumatic fall or exposure to drugs or toxins. Family members may also be able to relay additional diagnostic clues such as rate of onset or waxing-waning characteristics of the patient's symptoms.

Causes of depression of consciousness vary with patient age (Box 32-3). The elderly are particularly vulnerable to infectious etiologies, medication changes, and alterations in their living environments. Young adults and adolescents are more likely to present after recreational drug use or trauma.

Box 32-3 Common Age-Related Etiology of Altered Mental Status

Adolescent/Young Adult

Toxic ingestion
Recreational drug use
Trauma

Elderly

Medication changes
Over-the-counter medications
Infection
Alterations in living environment
Stroke

Physical Examination

Level of consciousness is determined by the patient's ability to speak in full, coherent sentences and to respond appropriately to the examiner. A rapid, directed neurologic screening examination can determine whether the patient has a significant focal motor deficit. The presence of a distinctive odor on the breath, although uncommon, can cue the examiner to the presence of alcohol, ketones (diabetic/alcoholic ketoacidosis), or bitter almonds (cyanide toxicity). Undressing the patient promptly and completely permits evaluation for signs of trauma or skin lesions suggesting overwhelming infection.

Vital signs are paramount in the initial assessment of all patients. Significant hypotension with depressed consciousness suggests shock, and both diagnosis and therapy should be addressed immediately. Severe elevation in ICP can cause bradycardia and hypertension. Tachycardia and hypotension can be the result of primary cardiac, infectious, or toxic/metabolic causes. Both hypothermia and hyperthermia can result in altered mental status whether from infectious, structural, or toxic/metabolic causes. Hyperventilation, Kussmaul's or Cheyne-Stokes breathing, agonal breathing, apnea, or other alterations in respiratory patterns can suggest primary CNS abnormalities or toxic/metabolic derangements.

Immediately after an assessment of the patient's vital signs, a head-to-toe physical examination is performed.A methodical and complete head and neck examination is conducted, with particular emphasis on examination of the papillary reflexes and eye movements and any indications of head trauma (hemotympanum, scalp hematoma).

Examination of the neck should focus on evidence of infection, including nuchal rigidity, lymphadenopathy, or fluctuance. The cervical spine should be immobilized if there are signs of neck trauma, such as cervical spine tenderness, or evidence of blunt external trauma. Stridor indicates respiratory distress typically from infection, edema, or foreign body aspiration.

Chest examination focuses on pulmonary function, infection, CO, and the presence of injury. Potentially helpful abdominal findings include ascites, hepatosplenomegaly, ecchymosis, or striae. Gross blood, purulent drainage, or retained foreign bodies should be sought on genitourinary and rectal examination. In the absence or presence of signs of trauma, lesions on the skin such as rashes, signs of drug use (needle "tracks" or medication patches), or embolic phenomena can be differential clues.

A systematic neurologic examination, with particular attention paid to the eyes, is the most useful tool in differentiating a structural from a systemic or metabolic etiology of depressed consciousness or coma. A head-to-toe approach is a proven strategy. This should include evaluation of the patient's GCS (Box 32-4), level of alertness, cranial nerves, strength, reflexes, and cerebellar functions with emphasis on gait, pronator drift, finger-to-nose, heel-to-shin, rapid alternating movements, and Romberg testing. A change of two or more points in serial GCS testing represents a significant change in the patient's level of consciousness.

Box 32-4 Glasgow Coma Scale

		Score
Eye Opening	Spontaneous	4
	To voice	3
	To pain	2
	None	1
Verbal Response	Oriented	5
	Confused	4
	Inappropriate words	3
	Incomprehensible words	2
	None	1
Motor Response	Obeys commands	6
	Localizes pain	5
	Withdraws to pain	4
	Flexion to pain	3
	Extension to pain	2
	None	1

Discovery of a focal neurologic deficit is suggestive of a structural etiology. Particular attention should be paid to a focused eye examination. Unilateral dilatation of a pupil ("blown pupil") and loss of reactivity in a comatose patient are ominous signs of uncal herniation requiring immediate neurosurgical consultation and intervention. Papilledema in the setting of increased ICP or retinal hemorrhage associated with trauma can be found on funduscopic examination. The eye examination should also include testing of eye movements, which are coordinated by the medial longitudinal fasciculus located in the brainstem and ocular centers located in the cerebral cortex. Cranial nerves Ⅲ, Ⅳ, and Ⅵ are responsible for control of the extraocular muscles. Cranial nerve Ⅲ paralysis results in a persistently abducted eye, whereas a persistently adducted eye is caused by paralysis of cranial nerve Ⅵ. In the setting of trauma, a unilateralcranial nerve Ⅲ palsy suggests an ipsilateral compressive lesion such as seen with epidural hematoma. Cranial nerve Ⅵ palsies are often nonlocalizing as the nerve has a long intracranial course and compressive forces from intracranial mass effects (tumor, traumatic hematoma, increased ICP, etc.) may compromise cranial nerve function anywhere in its course. Horizontal disconjugate gaze is commonly seen in patients who are sedated, drowsy, or intoxicated, and vertical disconjugate gaze is usually more serious which suggests cerebellar or pontine dysfunction.

Oculocephalic (doll's eyes) and oculovestibular reflex testing are useful in looking at the functional integrity of the brainstem.

Oculocephalic testing is accomplished without contraindications (suspected cervical spine injury) by observing the patient's eye movements while the head is turned from side to side. The result is negtive if patients who exhibit a maintained forward gaze despite head turning, or positive if the eyes remain in a fixed position within the orbits. Oculovestibular or "cold water caloric" testing is a more sensitive test for brainstem involvement and cannot voluntarily be resisted (Fig. 32-2). Tympanic membrane perforation and cerumen impaction should be ruled out prior to performing this test. After elevation of the patient's head to 30° (this can be done in patients whose cervical spine is not cleared by placing the bed in the reverse Trendelenburg position), 10 to 30 mL of ice water is used to irrigate the external auditory canal. A negative response is a slow conjugate deviation of gaze toward the side of the cold water stimulus lasting 30 to 120 s. The reflex is short-lived and followed by corrective fast beats of nystagmus toward the midline. This corrective nystagmus is described by the mnemonic COWS, which stands for "cold-opposite, warm-same." A positive result means there is no response to the irrigation.

A negative result makes structural lesions in the brainstem very unlikely as the source of the patient's altered mental status, but a positive one means brainstem dysfunction.

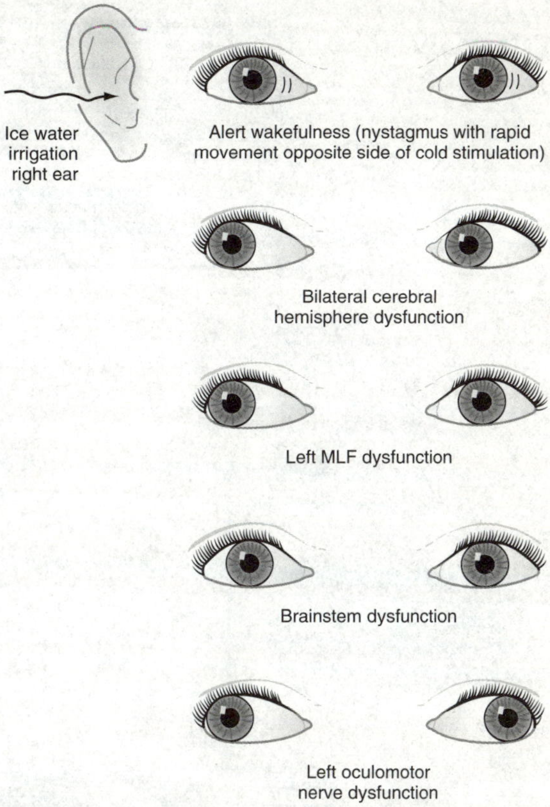

Fig. 32-2 Oculocephalogyric (caloric) responses to various central nervous system pathologic conditions. MLF, medial longitudinal fasciculus.

Diagnostic Algorithm

Information gathered from the history and physical examination of the patient with depressed consciousness must be used to direct the approach to diagnostic testing (Fig. 32-3). Most often, this information points toward a systemic or metabolic rather than a structural etiology. Neuroimaging studies are performed early in patients with suggested structural causes, but should not precede treatment of quickly reversible conditions such as possible opioid overdose or hypoglycema.

Systemic or metabolic causes of depressed consciousness and coma are most often found on analysis of laboratory studies. Bedside glucose testing definitively confirms or excludes hypoglycemia. Serum electrolytes identify derangements in sodium, CO_2, or AG. Changes in serum calcium can be a marker for metastatic disease. A urine dip test is a quick way to identify

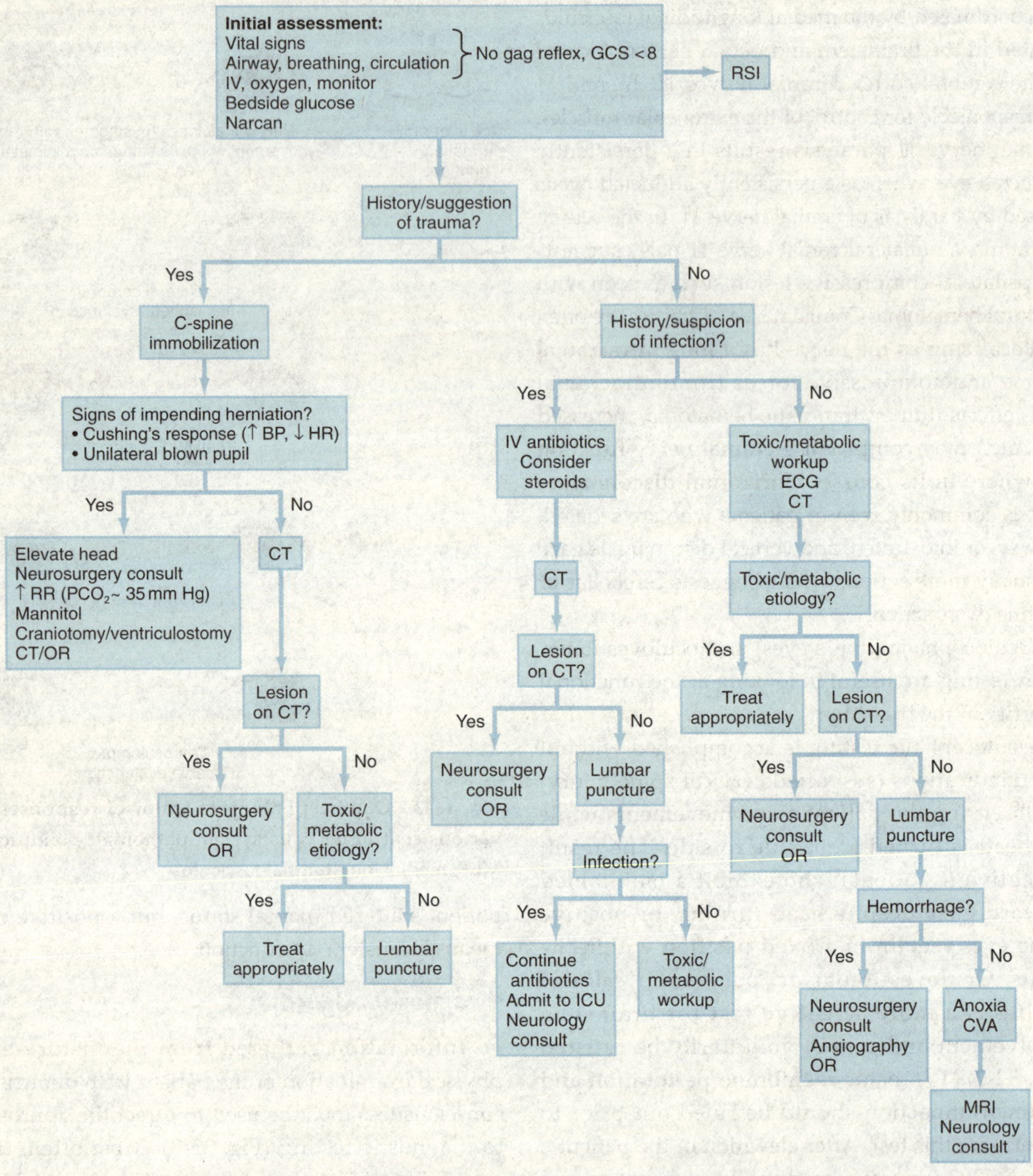

Fig. 32-3 Algorithm for diagnostic approach to altered mental status and coma.

infection, ketones, or spilling of glucose. Urinalysis itself provides valuable information regarding volume status (specific gravity and urine volume itself), infection, and the possible presence of calcium oxalate crystals in the setting of ethylene glycol ingestion. Urine drug testing may be helpful if another cause is not forthcoming.

Although an elevated white blood cell count can be a marker for infection, it is nonspecific and rarely helpful. An abnormally low WBC count suggests an immunocompromised state and should urgently direct clinical investigation toward an infectious etiology. Thrombocytopenia can be a marker for sepsis or intracranial hemorrhage and may sound a cautionary note against an invasive procedure such as obtaining central venous access or performing a LP. Elevated results from serum coagulation studies can be a marker for bleeding tendencies or liver disease. Serum ammonia levels are controversial and have not been shown to be a reliable marker in the setting of depressed consciousness. Thyroid function studies can reveal myxedema coma from hypothyroidism. When CNS pathology such as infection or hemorrhage is suggested but not seen on neuroimaging studies, cerebrospinal fluid analysis should be undertaken.

Noncontrast CT of the brain is the preliminary imaging modality of choice in the setting of depressed consciousness and coma. In the majority of ED settings, it is quickly available, making it more suitable for the patient with borderline stability. It is sufficiently sensitive to detect most intracranial hemorrhages that are large enough to cause coma. Contrast-enhanced CT may be used if a tumor or infection is possible. MRI is less feasible in most ED settings due to the patient's unstable condition and its limited availability as well as cost. Angiography may be available in the diagnosis or treatment of intracerebral aneurysms or arteriovenous malformations after initial identification of an intracranial hemorrhage on noncontrast CT.

Plain radiography may identify severe pneumonia or ARDS.

Electrocardiograms can point to certain ingestions (tricyclic antidepressants, etc.), electrolyte abnormalities (potassium, calcium, etc.), or hypothermia. If nonconvulsive status epilepticus is suggested, or if a patient with status epilepticus has required neuromuscular blockade, continuous electroencephalographic monitoring can provide key information about the patient's status and guide therapy.

EMPIRICAL MANAGEMENT

Initial establishment of circulation, airway, and breathing, CAB is of primary importance in stabilizing the patient with altered mental status. Initiation of IV access combined with the administration of oxygen and continuous telemetry monitoring should happen concomitantly within the first few minutes of the patient's arrival.In patients with a GCS score lower than 8, definitive airway control should be obtained unless the coma is readily reversible (e.g., hypoglycemia, opioid overdose). Patients with possible increased ICP should receive lidocaine prior to rapid sequence intubation. Trauma patients require spinal immobilization in addition to indicated fluid resuscitation.

Reversible causes of the patient's condition should be sought concomitantly with initial stabilization. Administration of the components of the "GI cocktail," which include dextrose, nalaxone, and thiamine, can quickly reverse the alterations in mental status caused by hypoglycemia, narcotic overdose, and thiamine deficiency, respectively. Specific attention should be given to identifying the focal neurologic abnormalities, including pupillary reflexes and pathologic eye movements that suggest mass effect or depressed brainstem function, prompting neuroimaging and evaluation by a neurosurgeon. Empirical administration of mannitol is indicated when there is evidence of transtentorial herniation in this setting. Ventriculostomy and ICP monitoring are commonly performed by the neurosurgeon in the ED. In trauma patients with suspected epidural hematoma who have evidence of brain herniation, the use of burr holes in the skull on the side of the dilated pupil may be a last resort. In patients with compromised brainstem function who lack evidence of herniation, a workup to investigate possible exposure to toxins or metabolic imbalances should proceed while supportive care is provided. Brain tissue is considered to be unsalvageable in patients who have not received sedative medications, are normothermic, and demonstrate lack of brainstem reflex activity.

In patients who demonstrate normal brainstem function, the workup proceeds as supportive care is provided. When an infectious cause is suggested, empirical administration of a broad-spectrum antibiotic should not be delayed for LP or other diagnostic tools. Lesions or masses found on brain imaging should prompt evaluation by a neurosurgeon and early operative intervention. In patients in whom a toxic ingestion is possible, specific toxin antidotes can be given. Early hemodialysis should also be considered in patients who have toxic or metabolic abnormalities amenable to this therapy.

The vast majority of patients who present with depressed consciousness or coma require admission to the hospital for further treatment and workup. Some patients who have returned to their baseline mental status after reversal of hypoglycemia or opioid overdose may be suitable for discharge directly from the ED or ED observation unit after a period of observation. Patients with alcohol or recreational drug intoxication and no other discernible cause of altered mental status can be discharged when they are clinically sober.

(TIAN Yingping)

Chapter 33

Seizure

KEY CONCEPTS

Seizures are episodes of abnormal neurologic functioning caused by pathologically excessive activation of neurons, either in the cerebral cortex or in the deep limbic system. *Epilepsy* is defined as recurrent unprovoked seizures due to a genetically determined or acquired brain disorder.

Seizures can be classified based on cause (primary or secondary),effect on mentation (generalized or focal), and motor activity (convulsive or nonconvulsive).

A generalized seizure is defined as abnormal neuronal activity in both cerebral hemispheres causing an alteration in the level of consciousness. Generalized seizures may be further divided into tonic-clonic, absence, atonic, and myoclonic.

Focal seizures usually involve one cerebral hemisphere, thereby preserving consciousness,though these seizures may progress and cause an altered sensorium.

Status epilepticus has been classically defined as at least 30 min of persistent seizures or a series of recurrent seizures without intervening return to full consciousness.

The first diagnostic task is to determine whether the patient actually experienced a seizure.

Hypoglycemia is the most common metabolic cause of seizure activity.

Bedside blood glucose levels should be measured early in every patient.

Seizures refractory to these initial treatments prompt an evaluation for nonepileptic causes of the convulsions.

PERSPECTIVE

Seizures are episodes of abnormal neurologic functioning caused by pathologically excessive activation of neurons, either in the cerebral cortex or in the deep limbic system. *Epilepsy* is defined as recurrent unprovoked seizures due to a genetically determined or acquired brain disorder; it is not an appropriate term for seizures that occur intermittently and predictably after a known insult, such as alcohol intoxication and withdrawal.

Presentation to the ED with a generalized convulsive seizure prompts immediate concern for airway protection and stabilization, followed by a focused search for the cause. Nonconvulsive seizures may be relatively obscure in their presentation, more diverse in their etiology, and are sometimes more difficult to recognize and control acutely.

Epidemiology and Classification

More than 10% of the United States population will experience at least one seizure during their lifetime;only 3% will be diagnosed with epilepsy. Alcohol and CNS pathologies (tumor, stroke, trauma, infection) are common causes in adults. Approximately 7% of patients who come to the ED with seizures are in status epilepticus.

Seizures can be classified based on cause (primary or secondary),effect on mentation (generalized or focal), and motor activity (convulsive or nonconvulsive). Primary seizures are unprovoked and not linked to an inciting event. Secondary seizures may be caused by trauma, illness, intoxications and poisonings, organ failure, other metabolic disturbances, cerebraltumors,preg nancy,and,paradoxically,supratherapeutic levels of some anticonvulsants.

A generalized seizure is defined as abnormal neuronal activity in both cerebral hemispheres causing an alteration in the level of consciousness. Generalized seizures may be further divided into tonic-clonic, absence, atonic, and myoclonic.Focal seizures usually involve one cerebral hemisphere, thereby preserving consciousness,though these seizures may progress and cause an altered sensorium. Some seizures are impossible to classify because of inadequate or inaccurate description of the ictal activity.

Convulsive seizures are characterized by uncontrolled, rhythmic motor movements and can affect part or all of the body.Nonconvulsive seizures do not result in abnormal motor activity;patients may display confusion, altered mental status, abnormal behavior, or coma.

Status epilepticus has been classically defined as at least 30 min of persistent seizures or a series of recurrent seizures without intervening return to full consciousness. The time criterion has been shortened to 5 min with recognition that the duration of seizure activity is related to outcome and that the likelihood of achieving seizure cessation with typical treatments decreases with ictal duration.Common causes of status epilepticus in adults are shown in Table 33-1.

Table 33-1 Etiology of Status Epilepticus in Adults

ETIOLOGY	PERCENTAGE OF CASES
AED noncompliance or withdrawal of AED	25-26
Alcohol related	15-24
Drug toxicity	2-10
Infection	8
Cerebral tumor	5-6
Trauma	3-5
Cerebrovascular disease or stroke	4-23
Metabolic abnormality	4-13
Hypoxia or cardiac arrest	4-12
Idiopathic	4-5

Pathophysiology

Seizures occur when the abnormal increased electrical activity of initiating neurons activates adjacent neurons and propagates until the thalamus and other subcortical structures are similarly stimulated.Given that the potassium current is the primary force behind repolarization of membranes, depolarization is prolonged in these patients, leading to an increase in neuronal hyperexcitability. Other studies have found that malformations of cortical development and glial cells may play a role in epileptogenesis.

Clinical seizure activity typically reflects the initiating focus. When the ictal discharge extends below the cortex to deeper structures, the reticular activating system in the brainstem may be affected, altering consciousness. In generalized seizures,the focus is often deep and midline, which explains the prompt loss of consciousness and bilateral involvement. Seizures are typically self-limited; at some point the hyperpolarization subsides and the bursts of electrical discharges from the focus terminate. This cessation may be related to reflex inhibition,neuronal exhaustion, or alteration of the local balance of neurotransmitters.

Focal seizures may represent a similar pathophysiologic process in which less recruitment occurs and the ictal activity does not cross the midline. Because of the more limited focus of abnormal activity, convulsive motor activity may not be the predominant clinical manifestation.

DIAGNOSTIC APPROACH

Differential Considerations

The first diagnostic task is to determine whether the patient actually experienced a seizure. Ictal activity can be irrefutably verified only by electroencephalography.Other abnormal movements and states of consciousness,including nonepileptic convulsions (pseudoseizures),can be confused with ictal activity. The differential diagnoses to consider when evaluating for seizure are listed in Table 33-2.

Table 33-2 Differential Considerations for the Diagnosis of Seizure

EPILEPTIC		NONEPILEPTIC	
Drugs of abuse	Alcohol	Cardiac	Vasovagal (neurocardiogenic) syncope
Intoxication or withdrawal	Stimulants LSD, PCP, NMDA Herbal products		Orthostatic syncope Cardiogenic syncope
Medications	Antibiotics Antiarrhythmic agents Pain medications Antidepressants Antipsychotics	Neurologic	Vertebrobasilar TIA, CVA Global transitory amnesia Migraine Movement disorders
Metabolic	Hypoglycemia or hyperglycemia Hyponatremia or hypernatremia Hypoxia Hypocalcemia Hypomagnesemia	Sleep disorders	Cataplex Periodic leg movements of sleep Arousal disorders Parasomnia associated with REM sleep
Infectious	Meningitis Cerebritis Encephalitis Cerebral abscess Non-CNS infections	Metabolic	Hypoglycemia or hyperglycemia Hyponatremia or hypernatremia Hyperthyroidism Pheochromocytoma
Structural lesions	Tumor Intracranial hemorrhage SAH Ischemic CVA	Psychogenic	Panic attacks Nonepileptic convulsion (pseudoseizure)
Systemic	Eclampsia Extreme fever Thyrotoxicosis	Toxic	Extrapyramidal symptoms of antipsychotics Delirium tremens Tetanus
Other	Trauma Posterior reversible encephalopathy syndrome		

Syncope can be confused with seizures by observers.In general, ictal tonic-clonic movements are more forceful and prolonged than the brief convulsive activity sometimes associated with fainting. In addition, most generalized seizures are characterized by a postictal state that syncope patients do not manifest. An important exception to this is an atonic seizure, or "drop attack," in which the patient experiences a sudden and complete loss of muscle tone associated with altered mentation; in this type of generalized seizure, motor activity is not displayed and a postictal state may not occur.

The cause of an unwitnessed, unprovoked loss of consciousness with a fall may be difficult to determine. Suggestions of seizure as the cause include retrograde amnesia, loss of continence (which also can occur with vasogenic and other forms of syncope), and evidence of oral trauma such as maceration of the buccal mucosa or bite lacerations of the tongue. Blood drawn soon after a true seizure may demonstrate a lactic acidosis.

Rapid Assessment and Stabilization

The patient who arrives with a history of possible seizure activity should be placed in a monitored area of the ED and prepared for prompt physician examination. An intravenous line or saline lock catheter should be placed in case anticonvulsants are emergently indicated. Blood glucose is checked at the bedside. Hypoglycemia is the most common metabolic cause of seizure activity. The only treatment may be administration of intravenous glucose.If the patient stopped seizing before arrival in the ED, the history, physical examination, and diagnostic course should focus on possible precipitants of the seizure. The patient should be protected from self-injury during this time.

If the patient is seizing in the ED, the first step is to confirm that a pulse is present and that the convulsions are not the result of cerebral hypoxia from lack of blood flow. After this, attention is paid to protecting and maintaining the airway. Nasopharyngeal airways and positioning the patient on the side generally are all that is required for airway management.Oxygen may be administered by nasal cannula if the saturation is below 90% or the patient appears cyanotic. Suction should be available but not used during seizure activity. Vascular access should be established, but benzodiazepine treatment can be initiated before placement of an intravenous line.

If the seizure persists after administration of anticonvulsant medication, preparation is made for endotracheal intubation.

Most seizures will terminate without intervention.If a patient begins to seize while under ED observation, it is prudent to administer low-dose benzodiazepines (approximately half of the doses for status epilepticus, Table 33-3). Patients who arrive at the ED with continued seizure activity,experience recurrent seizure without recovering from the postictal period, or experience witnessed convulsions lasting longer than 5 min are considered in status epilepticus and treated as indicated in Table 33-3.

Table 33-3 Medications and Dosages for Emergency Treatment of Prolonged Seizures and Status Epilepticus

MEDICATION	ADULT DOSE	PEDIATRIC DOSE	COMMENTS
Initial Therapy			
Diazepam	10 mg IV or 10-20 mg PR	0.15 mg/kg IV; 0.2-0.5 mg/kg PR (max 20 mg)	May repeat in 5-10 min; monitor respiratory status
Lorazepam	4 mg IV	<13 kg: 0.1 mg/kg IV (max 2 mg); 13-39 kg: 2 mg IV; >39 kg: 4 mg IV	Preferred IV benzodiazepine; may repeat in 10 min; monitor respiratory status
Midazolam	10 mg IV, IM, IN, buccal	0.2 mg/kg IV, IN (max 5 mg); 0.5 mg/kg buccal (max 5 mg); <13 kg:0.2 mg/kg IM (max 5 mg); 13-39 kg:5 mg IM; >39 kg: 10 mg IM	Preferred IM benzodiazepine; may repeat in 10 min; monitor respiratory status
Second-Tier Treatments			
Phenytoin	20 mg/kg IV infusion	20 mg/kg IV infusion	May cause hypotension and dysrhythmia
Fosphenytoin	20 mg PE/kg IV infusion or 20 mg PE/kg IM	20 mg PE/kg IV infusion	
Valproate sodium	20-40 mg/kg IV infusion		Max dose 60 mg/kg/d
Pentobarbital	5-15 mg/kg IV bolus then 0.5-5.0 mg/kg/hr		Titrate to EEG; intubation and hemodynamic support required
Phenobarbital	20-30 mg/kg IV infusion		Intubation likely required
Midazolam infusion	0.05-2 mg/kg/hr	0.5-2 mg/kg/hr	Monitor respiratory status
Propofol infusion	1-2 mg/kg IV bolus then 20-200 μg/kg/min infusion		Intubation required
Isoflurane inhalation			Titrate to EEG; intubation and hemodynamic support required

Continued

MEDICATION	ADULT DOSE	PEDIATRIC DOSE	COMMENTS
Special Situations			
Glucose	25 g IV (50 mL $D_{50}W$)	0-1 mo: 2 mL/kg IV $D_{10}W$ 1 mo-2 yr: 2 mL/kg IV $D_{25}W$ >2 yr: 2 mL/kg $D_{50}W$ (max 50 mL)	Titrate for blood glucose >100 mg/dL
Magnesium sulfate	6 g IV over 15 min, then 2 g/hr		First-line treatment for eclampsia; consider in women between 20 w-s' gestation and 6 w postpartum
Pyridoxine	Equal dosage of isoniazid ingestion (max 5 g) given 0.5 g/min IV until seizure stops, with remainder given over 4-6 hr	Max dose 70 mg/kg (up to 5 g)	
3% Hypertonic saline	100-200 mL over 1-2 hr	4-6 mL/kg over 1 hr (up to 100 mL)	Reserved for actively seizing and comatose hyponatremic patients; goal is to avoid raising serum sodium by > 12 mEq in 24 hr

Benzodiazepines are the optimal first-line agents for stopping seizure activity in patients of all ages. Available agents include lorazepam, diazepam, and midazolam. If intravenous access is established, lorazepam is the preferred first agent for the management of status epilepticus, particularly because of a long half-life, which decreases risk of seizure recurrence. For the patient without vascular access,immediate intramuscular midazolam is preferred over delayed intravenous lorazepam. Diazepam and midazolam can both be administered via alternate routes, and buccal midazolam is more effective than rectal diazepam in achieving seizure cessation. If repeated doses of benzodiazepines do not abort seizure activity,or if the patient's oxygen saturation remains persistently below 90%, emergent intubation is indicated. If possible,the patient should not receive long-acting neuromuscular blockade, so that recurrence or persistence of seizure activity can be monitored.

Medications for the treatment of status epilepticus are shown in Table 33-3.Most recommendations are supported by expert consensus.Moving quickly to a second-line agent is supported, and phenytoin is the most recommended second-line therapy for adults with persistent seizure activity. The prodrug, fosphenytoin, can be administered more quickly, can be given intramuscularly, and has less tendency to cause hypotension. Second-line therapy is phenobarbital for adults. Intravenous valproate sodium is safe and is an alternative for patients who are on chronic valproic therapy and whose levels are subtherapeutic.

Seizures refractory to these initial treatments prompt an evaluation for nonepileptic causes of the convulsions. Isoniazid overdose can cause prolonged seizures refractory to benzodiazepines.Pyridoxine is the only fully effective pharmacologic treatment for toxic isoniazid seizures, although benzodiazepines have been shown to suppress seizure activity in some cases. In seizing female patients of childbearing age, eclampsia may be the cause, and intravenous magnesium is the initial treatment. Eclamptic seizures refractory to magnesium may respond to benzodiazepines or barbiturates with or without phenytoin.

Patients who remain unresponsive to the third-level choice of pharmacologic intervention are by definition in *refractory* status epilepticus. Further choices for therapy are general anesthetic doses of midazolam or propofol, barbiturate coma,and isoflurane anesthesia; all of these treatments necessitate endotracheal intubation. A nondepolarizing neuromuscular blocking agent such as rocuronium or vecuronium is administered concomitantly to reduce the metabolic burden and potential hyperthermia that can ensue from prolonged status seizures; continuous electroencephalographic monitoring should be used.

Pivotal Findings

When the patient is stabilized with a secure airway and ictal activity is controlled, attention is turned to gathering more complete data.

History

History taking in the patient with seizure is directed by two main questions. First, "Was the incident truly a seizure?" This is important because of the broad differential diagnosis for seizures (Table 33-2). In general, ictal events have six properties:

1. Abrupt onset: Generalized seizures typically occur without an aura.
2. Brief duration: Seizures rarely last longer than 90 to 120 s.
3. Loss of consciousness: Present by definition, except for focal seizures.
4. Purposeless activity: For example, automatisms and undirected tonic-clonic movements.
5. Unprovoked: Especially with regard to emotional stimuli and substance withdrawal are notable exceptions.
6. Postictal state: An acute confusion state that typically occurs with all seizure types except focal and absence.

The second question to direct the history is, "Does this patient have a history of seizures?" If he or she does have a documented history of seizures, ED evaluation may be limited to a thorough history and consideration of measurement of anticonvulsant drug levels. Supratherapeutic and toxic levels of some anticonvulsants such as phenytoin and carbamazepine, may cause seizures. History should focus on intercurrent illness or trauma, drug or alcohol use, potential adverse drug-drug interactions with anticonvulsants, medication compliance, a recent change in anticonvulsant dosing regimens, or a change in ictal pattern or characteristics. Evaluation of injuries sustained during the seizure is also warranted.

If the patient does not have a history of seizures and the description of the event is truly consistent with a seizure, the history should focus on potential underlying medical, toxicologic, or neurologic causes.

Physical Examination

The physical manifestations of convulsive ictal activity include hypertension, tachycardia, and tachypnea from sympathetic stimulation.With more prolonged convulsions, skeletal muscle damage, lactic acidosis, and, rarely, frank rhabdomyolysis may ensue. Autonomic discharges and bulbar muscle involvement may result in urinary or fecal incontinence, vomiting, tongue biting, and airway impairment.

After the seizure activity has ceased, resting vital signs should be evaluated. Fever and underlying infection can cause seizures. Tachypnea, tachycardia, or an abnormal BP that persists beyond the immediate postictal period may indicate toxic exposure, hypoxia, or a central nervous system lesion. Pertinent physical findings may include nuchal rigidity, stigmata of substance abuse, lymphadenopathy suggestive of HIV disease or malignancy, dysmorphic features, or skin lesions. The examination should also focus on potential adverse sequelae of convulsive seizures, such as head trauma, tongue injury, posterior shoulder dislocation, or back pain.

Finally, a complete neurologic examination must be performed. A persistent focal deficit after a seizure (e.g., Todd's paralysis) often indicates the focal origin of the event. The patient should be carefully examined for papilledema; elevated intracranial pressure can both cause and result from ictal activity. Failure to note steady improvement of postictal depression of consciousness suggests the possibility of an underlying encephalopathy or nonconvulsive status epilepticus.

Ancillary Testing

Laboratory Bedside blood glucose levels should be measured early in every patient. Directed toxicologic screens should be obtained if substance abuse is possible. Serum sodium should be evaluated, particularly if mental status remains altered after apparent recovery from the postictal state. For medically ill adults and in patients with a first-time seizure or substantial change in seizure pattern,serum electrolytes are indicated. Liver function tests may be helpful if physical examination reveals liver disease or if there is history of liver infection or alcoholism. Eclampsia occurs late in pregnancy or in the early postpartum period, so pregnancy usually is clinically evident in such cases. Headache may be a feature of the patient's postictal state, but otherwise, presence of fever and headache or sudden onset of headache is an indication for CT scan, lumbar puncture, or both. Febrile patients are evaluated for the source of the fever. If there is *any* suggestion of central nervous system infection or subarachnoid hemorrhage, lumbar puncture should be performed.

Imaging Cranial CT is recommended for patients with new-onset seizures and is mandatory if neurologic examination identifies focal abnormalities postseizure. Box 33-1 lists the circumstances under which a head CT is recommended in the ED because of a higher likelihood of discovering an acute abnormality.

Box 33-1 Indications for Cranial CT in Patients with Seizure in the ED

- First seizure
- Acute intracranial process suspected
- History of acute head trauma
- History of malignancy
- Immunocompromised status
- Fever
- Persistent headache
- History of anticoagulation
- New focal neurologic examination
- Age older than 40 years without epilepsy history
- Focal onset before generalization
- Persistently altered mental status

EEG EEG is not consistently available in the ED and most appropriate for the follow-up evaluation of first-time seizures without clear cause after a complete ED evaluation.

MANAGEMENT

Usually, an acute seizure self-terminates or can be pharmacologically terminated before a need arises for active airway management. Rapidly reversible ictal insults (e.g., hypoglycemia, hypoxemia, Termination of pregnancy, isoniazid ingestion) should be considered. Identifying a new-onset seizure in the ED generates consideration for further management. The choice to initiate anticonvulsant therapy depends on the risk of seizure recurrence, any underlying predisposing disease, and the risk of initiating anticonvulsant therapy. Chronic anticonvulsant medication may be advisable, even in the short term, pending further outpatient evaluation, and the decision to initiate this should be made in consultation with the neurologist who will be following the patient after discharge from the ED. Prompt treatment of any apparent causative disorder discovered in the ED is appropriate.

DISPOSITION

Disposition plans are individualized according to the findings of the ED evaluation and the presence or absence of underlying disease.

(TIAN Yingping)

Chapter 34

Stroke

KEY CONCEPTS

Stroke can be defined as any vascular injury that reduces CBF to a specific region of the brain, causing neurologic impairment.

TIA is a "brief episode of neurologic dysfunction caused by a focal disturbance of brain or retinal ischemia, with clinical symptoms typically lasting less than 1 hr".

An emergent noncontrast cranial CT is the standard initial imaging technique for evaluating a patient with a potential stroke in the ED. It can quickly differentiate an ischemic stroke from ICH and other mass lesions.

Patients presenting with the signs and symptoms of an acute ischemic stroke within 3 hr of symptom onset should be evaluated for thrombolytic therapy.

Overly aggressive BP management should be avoided in patients with acute ischemic stroke.

The possibility of carotid or vertebral dissection should be considered in young patients with stroke and in patients with headaches and neck pain with acute stroke.

PERSPECTIVE

Background

Stroke is the third leading cause of death in the United States and a leading cause of long-term disability. It afflicts more than 700,000 patients per year, with an in-hospital mortality rate of 5% to 10% for ischemic stroke and 46% for ICH. Although 50% to 70% of stroke survivors will regain functional independence, 15% to 30% will be permanently disabled, and 20% will require institutional care at 3 months. In terms of emergency care, almost 2% of all 911 calls and 4% of hospital admissions from the ED are for patients with potential strokes.

Stroke can be defined as any vascular injury that reduces CBF to a specific region of the brain, causing neurologic impairment. The onset of symptoms may be sudden or stuttering, often with transient or permanent loss of neurologic function. Approximately 80% of all strokes are ischemic in origin, caused by the occlusion of a cerebral vessel. The rest are hemorrhagic strokes due to the rupture of a blood vessel into the parenchyma of the brain (ICH) or into the subarachnoid space (SAH). Only ischemic stroke and ICH are discussed in this chapter.

In the past, treatment for stroke consisted of stabilization, observation, and rehabilitation. In recent years, a better understanding of the pathophysiology of neuronal injury and the introduction of new therapies have led to a shift to early evaluation and treatment. Current interventional treatment regimens include BP management, anticoagulation, thrombolytic therapy, catheter-based interventions, and surgery. The key to success is early identification and treatment of patients with stroke before neurologic deficits become irreversible.

Epidemiology

Ischemic Stroke

An estimated 430,000 "first-ever" ischemic strokes occur each year in the United States, of which 10% to 15% are TIA. These may result either from in situ thrombosis or embolic obstruction from a more proximal source, usually the heart. In more than one third of these first-ever strokes, no cause is found.

Approximately one third of all ischemic strokes are thrombotic in nature. These can be due to either large- or small-vessel occlusions. The incidence of large-vessel occlusions is higher among men than among women and among whites than black Americans. Common areas for large-vessel occlusions are cerebral vessel branch points, especially in the distribution of the internal carotid artery. Thrombosis usually results from clot formation in the area of an ulcerated atherosclerotic plaque. A marked reduction in flow results when the stenosis occludes more than 90% of the blood vessel diameter. With further ulceration and thrombosis, platelets adhere to the region. A clot then either embolizes or occludes the artery.

Lacunae, or small-vessel strokes, involve small terminal sections of the vasculature and more commonly occur in black Americans and patients with diabetes and hypertension. A history of hypertension is present in 80% to 90% of patients who experience lacunar strokes. The subcortical areas of the cerebrum and brainstem often are involved. The infarcts range in size from a few millimeters to 2 cm and are seen most commonly in the basal ganglia, thalamus, pons, and internal capsule. They may be caused by small emboli or by a process termed *lipohyalinosis*, which occurs in patients with hypertensive cerebral vasculopathy. The most common of lacunar syndromes are pure motor strokes, pure sensory strokes, or ataxic hemiparesis, instead of cognitive impairment, aphasia, or simultaneous sensorimotor findings.

One fourth of all ischemic strokes are cardioembolic in nature. Embolization of a mural thrombus in patients with Af is the most common pathomechanism, and patients with Af have a four- to fivefold increased risk for development of a stroke. Almost 20% of stroke patients will have Af on their admission ECG. Strokes due to Af are more likely to involve large cerebral vessels, to be more severe, and to carry a higher mortality rate. Noncardiac sources of emboli may include diseased portions of extracranial arteries, resulting in an artery-to-artery embolus.

Approximately 12.2 ischemic strokes per 1000 nonfatal MI occur within 1 mo after the index event. Furthermore, 11.1 ischemic strokes per 1000 nonfatal MI occur during the patient's hospitalization. Independent predictors of stroke after AMI are advanced age, diabetes, HTN, history of previous stroke, anterior location of index MI, previous MI, Af, HF, and nonwhite race.

Approximately 3% to 4% of all strokes occur in patients between the ages of 15 and 45 yr. Although atherosclerosis is the most common cause in older patients, causative disorders and conditions in younger patients often are uncommon or are reversible. Pregnancy, the use of oral contraceptives, antiphospholipid antibodies (such as lupus anticoagulant and anticardiolipin antibodies), protein S and C deficiencies, and polycythemia all predispose patients to sludging or thrombosis, thereby increasing the risk of stroke. Fibromuscular dysplasia of the cerebral vasculature also may lead to stroke, and in rare instances, prolonged vasoconstriction from a migraine syndrome causes stroke. Recreational drugs such as cocaine, phenylpropanolamine, and amphetamines are potent vasoconstrictors that have been associated with both ischemic and hemorrhagic stroke.

Carotid and vertebral dissections often are associated with trauma but may follow such mild events as turning the head sharply. Carotid and vertebral dissections also are seen more frequently in people with underlying pathology of the vessel wall, such as in fibromuscular dysplasia and connective tissue disorders. Alteration in the vessel intima can lead to vessel stenosis, occlusion, or embolism. The patient may report a minor preceding event such as spinal manipulation, yoga, working overhead, coughing, or vomiting. This entity is considered a major cause of stroke in younger patients.

A TIA was historically defined as a neurologic deficit that has complete clinical resolution within 24 hr. A newer definition of TIA proposed by Albers is a "brief episode of neurologic dysfunction caused by a focal disturbance of brain or retinal ischemia, with clinical symptoms typically lasting less than 1 hr, and without evidence of infarction." This updated definition evolved as newer imaging techniques demonstrated infarction in up to 81% of patients with neurologic symptoms lasting less than 24 hr. TIA constitute an important warning sign for the future development of cerebral infarction. A majority of TIA last less than 5 min, but the course can be variable. Three or more TIA occurring within 72 hr are termed crescendo TIA.

Hemorrhagic Stroke

Spontaneous ICH causes 8% to 11% of all acute strokes and is twice as common as SAH. It carries a 30 d mortality rate of up to 50%, with one half of patients dying in the first 2 d. Among survivors, only 1 in 5 are living independently at 6 months. The incidence of ICH is higher in men than in women and in Asians than in whites, and it occurs more commonly in young and middle-aged black Americans than in whites of similar age.

ICH may occur in association with long-standing HTN (hypertensive hemorrhage), amyloid angiopathy in the elderly, or AVM. Two thirds of these bleeding episodes occur within the region of the basal ganglia. The most common sites for hypertensive hemorrhage are listed in Box 34-1. The hematoma that forms usually enlarges, causing local tissue injury and a subsequent increase in ICP.

Box 34-1 Most Common Sites for Hypertensive Intracranial Hemorrhage

Affected Area	Frequency(%)
Putamen	44
Thalamus	13
Cerebellum	9
Pons	9
Other cortical areas	25

ICH due to amyloid angiopathy tends to be lobar in nature and to occur more commonly in the elderly, with a higher incidence in whites than in black Americans. Sudden increases in BP that occur with such drugs as phenylpropanolamine and cocaine can cause ICH. Other causes include the use of anticoagulants, tumors, and AVM (especially in the young).

Bleeding from an arteriovenous malformation may be subarachnoid or intraparenchymal, or both.An arteriovenous malformation producing hemorrhage is more common in younger patients than hypertensive ICH. Such patients may have no history of hypertension.

PRINCIPLES OF DISEASE

Pathophysiology

The cerebral vasculature supplies the brain with a rich flow of blood that contains the critical supply of oxygen and glucose necessary for normal brain function. When a stroke occurs, there are immediate alterations in CBF and extensive changes in cellular homeostasis. A complete interruption of CBF, which is rare, results in loss of consciousness within approximately 10 s and death of vulnerable pyramidal cells of the hippocampus within minutes. In stroke, collateral circulation helps maintain some blood flow to the ischemic region. The normal CBF is 40 to 60 mL/100 g of brain per minute. When CBF drops below 15 to 18 mL/100 g of brain per minute,the brain loses electrical activity, becoming electrically "silent," although neuronal membrane integrity and function remain intact. Clinically, the areas of the brain maintaining electrical silence manifest a neurologic deficit, even though the brain cells are viable. When CBF is below 10 mL/100 g of brain per minute, membrane failure occurs, with a subsequent increase in the extracellular potassium and intracellular calcium and eventual cell death. The ischemic penumbra is the area of the brain surrounding the primary injury, which is preserved by a tenuous supply of blood from collateral vessels. As defined by CBF, the ischemic penumbra consists of brain tissue with blood flow of 10 to 18 mL/100 g of brain per minute in which electrical silence is present but irreversible damage has not yet occurred. In ischemic stroke, the duration of occlusion plays a critical role in neuronal survival.Increasing the duration of occlusion increases both the irreversibility of deficits and the amount of cerebral infarction.In patients with ICH, a complicated series of events including red blood cell lysis and increased blood-brain barrier permeability can lead to edema formation and secondary brain injury.

Anatomy and Physiology

Blood is supplied to the brain by the anterior and posterior circulations. The anterior circulation originates from the carotid system and perfuses 80% of the brain including the optic nerve, retina, and frontoparietal and anterior-temporal lobes. The first branch off the internal carotid artery is the ophthalmic artery, which supplies the optic nerve and retina. The internal carotid arteries terminate by branching into the anterior and middle cerebral arteries at the circle of Willis.

The anterior cerebral artery supplies the basal and medial aspects of the cerebral hemispheres and extends to the anterior two thirds of the parietal lobe. The middle cerebral artery feeds the lenticulostriate branches that supply the putamen, part of the anterior limb of the internal capsule, the lentiform nucleus, and the external capsule. Main cortical branches of the middle cerebral artery supply the lateral surfaces of the cerebral cortex from the anterior portion of the frontal lobe to the posterolateral occipital lobe.

Although the posterior circulation is smaller and supplies only 20% of the brain, it supplies the brainstem (which is critical for normal consciousness, movement, and sensation), cerebellum, thalamus, auditory and vestibular centers of the ear, medial temporal lobe, and the visual occipital cortex. The posterior circulation is derived from the two vertebral arteries that ascend through the transverse processes of the cervical vertebrae. They join to form the basilar artery, which branches to form the posterior cerebral arteries.

The extent of injury in either an anterior or a posterior stroke depends on both the vessel involved and the presence of collateral blood flow distal to the vessel occlusion.

CLINICAL FEATURES

Ischemic Stroke

The signs and symptoms of an ischemic stroke may appear suddenly and without warning or may have a stuttering, insidious onset. Ischemic strokes can be classified as anterior or posterior circulation strokes depending on the vasculature involved. The presence of neurologic deficits is highly dependent on collateral flow. A "stroke in evolution" is one in which focal neurologic deficits worsen over the course of minutes or hours. Approximately 20% of anterior circulation strokes and 40% of posterior circulation strokes will show evidence of progression. Anterior circulation strokes may progress within the first 24 hr, whereas posterior strokes may progress for up to 3 d.

With anterior circulation strokes (involving variously and primarily the carotid, anterior, and middle cerebral arteries), the clinical presentation rarely includes complete loss of consciousness. Occlusions in the anterior cerebral artery mainly affect frontal lobe function. The patient has altered mentation coupled with impaired judgment and insight, as well as the presence of primitive grasp and suck reflexes on physical exam. Bowel and bladder incontinence may be features. Paralysis and hypesthesia of the lower limb opposite the side of the lesion are characteristic. Leg weakness is more pronounced than arm weakness in anterior cerebral distribution stroke. Apraxia or clumsiness in the patient's gait also may be noted.

Marked motor and sensory disturbances are the hallmarks of occlusion of the middle cerebral artery. They occur on the side of the body contralateral to the side of the lesion and usually are worse in the arm and face than the leg. Such disturbances may involve only part of an extremity or the face but will almost always be accompanied by numbness in the same region as that of the motor loss. Hemianopsia, or blindness in one half of the visual field, occurs ipsilateral to the lesion. Agnosia, or the inability to recognize previously known subjects, is common, and aphasia may be present if the lesion occurs in the dominant hemisphere. Patients often have a gaze preference toward the affected hemisphere because of disruption of the cortical lateral gaze centers. The clinical aphorism is that a patient looks *at* a destructive lesion (stroke) but *away from* an irritative lesion (seizure focus).

Aphasia, a disorder of language in which the patient articulates clearly but uses language inappropriately or understands it poorly, also is common in dominant-hemisphere stroke. Aphasia may be expressive, receptive, or a combination of both. *Wernicke's aphasia* occurs when the patient is unable to process sensory input such as speech and thus fails to understand verbal communication (receptive aphasia). *Broca's aphasia* refers to the inability to communicate verbally in an effective way, even though understanding may be intact (expressive aphasia). Aphasia should be distinguished from dysarthria, which is a motor deficit of the mouth and speech muscles;

the dysarthric patient articulates poorly but understands words and word choices. Aphasia is important to recognize because it usually localizes a lesion to the dominant (usually left) cerebral cortex in the middle cerebral artery distribution. *Aphasia* and *dysphasia* are terms that are used interchangeably but must be distinguished from *dysphagia*, which is difficulty in swallowing.

Pathology in the vertebrobasilar system (i.e., posterior circulation strokes) can cause the widest variety of symptoms. The symptoms reflect cranial nerve deficits, cerebellar involvement, and involvement of neurosensory tracts. The brainstem also contains the reticular activating system, which is responsible for mediating consciousness, and the emesis centers. Patients with posterior circulation stroke can present with loss of consciousness and frequently have nausea and vomiting. The posterior cerebral artery supplies portions of the parietal and occipital lobes, so vision and thought processing are impaired. Visual agnosia, the inability to recognize seen objects, may be a feature, as may alexia, the inability to understand the written word. A third nerve palsy may occur, and the patient may experience homonymous hemianopsia. One of the more curious facets of this syndrome is that the patient may be unaware of any visual problem (visual neglect). Vertigo, diplopia, visual field defects, weakness, paralysis, dysarthria, dysphagia, syncope, spasticity, ataxia, or nystagmus may be associated with vertebrobasilar artery insufficiency. Posterior circulation strokes also demonstrate crossed deficits, such as motor deficits on one side of the body and sensory loss on the other. In anterior circulation strokes, by contrast, abnormalities are always limited to one side of the body.

A focused neurologic exam should assess level of consciousness, speech, cranial nerve function, motor and sensory function, and cerebellar function. Level of consciousness and fluency of speech can be rapidly assessed in a dialogue with the patient to determine the presence of dysarthria or aphasia. The head should be evaluated for signs of trauma. Pupillary size and reactivity and extraocular movements provide important information about brainstem function, particularly cranial nerves Ⅲ through Ⅵ; an abnormal third nerve function may be the first sign of tentorial herniation. Gaze preference suggests brainstem or cortical involvement. Central facial nerve weakness from a stroke should be distinguished from the peripheral causes of cranial nerves Ⅶ weakness. With a peripheral lesion, the patient is unable to wrinkle the forehead. Assessment of facial sensation, eyebrow elevation and squinting, smiling symmetry, gross auditory acuity, gag reflex, shoulder elevation, sternocleidomastoid strength, and tongue protrusion complete the cranial nerve evaluation.

Motor and sensory testing is performed next. Muscle tone can be assessed by moving a relaxed limb. Proximal and distal muscle group strength should be assessed against resistance. Pronator drift of the arm is a sensitive sign of motor weakness. Asymmetrical sensation to pain and light touch may be subtle and difficult to detect. Double simultaneous extinction evaluation tests for sensory neglect and can be easily performed by simultaneously touching the right and left limbs. Similarly, the ability to discern a number gently scratched on a forearm, graphesthesia, is another easily tested cortical parietal lobe function. These tests can help differentiate a pure motor deficit of a lacunar stroke from a sensorimotor middle cerebral artery deficit.

Cerebellar testing and the assessment of reflexes and gait complete the examination. Finger-to-nose and heel-to-shin evaluations are important tests of cerebellar functions. Asymmetry of the deep tendon reflexes or a unilateral Babinski's sign may be an early finding of corticospinal tract dysfunction.Observing routine ambulation and heel-to-toe walking can assess for subtle ataxia, weakness, or focal cerebellar lesions.

The National Institutes of Health Stroke Scale (NIHSS) is a useful and rapid tool for quantifying neurologic deficit in patients with stroke and can be used in determining treatment options (Box 34-2). The baseline NIHSS can identify patients who are appropriate candidates for fibrinolytic therapy as well as those at increased risk for hemorrhage. In addition, it has been used as a prognostic tool to predict outcome.

Box 34-2 NIH Stroke Scale Scoring Form

Item	Scoring Definitions	Score
1a. *Level of consciousness* (LOC)	0 = alert and responsive 1 = arousable to minor stimulation 2 = arousable only to painful stimulation 3 = reflex responses or unarousable	
1b. *LOC-related questions*: Ask patient's age and month, Must be exact.	0 = both correct 1 = one correct (or dysarthria, intubated, foreign language) 2 = neither correct	
1c. *Commands*: Open/close eyes, grip and release nonparetic hand. (Other one-step commands or mimic also acceptable.)	0 = both correct (acceptable if impaired by weakness) 1 = one correct 2 = neither correct	
2. *Best gaze*: Horizontal EOM by voluntary or doll's eye maneuver.	0 = normal 1 = partial gaze palsy; abnormal gaze in one or both eyes 2 = forced eye deviation or total paresis that cannot be overcome by doll's eye maneuver	
3. *Visual field*: Use visual threat if nec. If monocular, score field of good eye.	0 = no visual loss 1 = partial hemianopsia, quadrantanopia, extinction 2 = complete hemianopsia 3 = bilateral hemianopsia or blindness	
4. *Facial palsy*: If patient is stuporous, check symmetry of grimace to pain.	0 = normal 1 = minor paralysis, flat NLF, asymmetrical smile 2 = partial paralysis (lower face = UMN lesion) 3 = complete paralysis (upper and lower face)	
5. *Motor arm*: Arms outstretched 90 degrees (sitting) or 45 degrees (supine) for 10 s. Encourage best effort. Indicate paretic limb in score box.	0 = no drift for 10 s 1 = drift but doesn'ot hit bed 2 = some antigravity effort, but cann't sustain 3 = no antigravity effort, but even minimal mvt counts 4 = no movement at all X = unable to assess due to amputation, fusion, fracture, ect.	L or R
6. *Motor leg*: Raise leg to 30 degrees (from supine) for 5 s. Indicate paretic limb in score box.	0 = no drift for 5 s 1 = drift but doesn't hit bed 2 = some antigravity effort, but cann't sustain 3 = no antigravity effort, but even minimal mvtcounts 4 = no movement at all X = unable to assess owing to amputation, fusion, fracture, ect	L or R
7. *Limb ataxia*: Check finger-nose-finger, heel-shin position sense; and score only if out of proportion to paralysis.	0 = no ataxia (or aphasic, hemiplegic) 1 = ataxia in upper or lower extremity 2 = ataxia in upper and lower extremity X = unable to assess owing to amputation, fusion, fracture, ect	L or R

8. *Sensory*: Use safety pin. Check grimace or withdrawal if patient is stuporous. Score only stroke-related losses.	0 = normal 1 = mild-moderate unilateral loss but patient aware of touch (or aphasic, confused) 2 = total loss, patient unaware of touch; coma, bilateral loss
9. Best language: Describe cookie jar picture, name objects, read sentences. May use repeating, writing, stereognosis.	0 = normal 1 = mild-moderate aphasia (speech difficult to understand but partly comprehensible) 2 = severe aphasia (almost no information exchanged) 3 = mute, global aphasia, coma; no one-step commands
10. Dysarthria: Read list of words.	0 = normal 1 = mild-moderate; slurred but intelligible 2 = severe; unintelligible or mute X = intubation or mech barrier
11. Extinction/neglect: Simultaneously touch patient on both hands, show fingers in both visual fields, ask about deficit, left hand.	0 = normal, none detected (vis loss alone) 1 = neglects or extinguishes to double simultaneous stimulation in any modality (visual, auditory, sensation, spatial, body parts) 2 = profound neglect in more than one modality

Hemorrhagic Stroke

The classic presentation of ICH is the sudden onset of headache, vomiting, severely elevated BP, and focal neurologic deficits that progress over minutes. Similar to ischemic stroke, ICH often is associated with a motor and sensory deficit contralateral to the brain lesion. The patient may present with agitation and lethargy but may quickly deteriorate, with progression to stupor or coma. Almost 40% will demonstrate significant growth in hemorrhage volume within the first few hours. Although headache, vomiting, and coma are common, the clinical presentation may be similar to that of patients with ischemic stroke (Table 34-1).

Table 34-1 Clinical Findings Associated with Ischemic Strokes, ICH, and SAH

FINDING	ISCHEMIC STROKE	ICH	SAH
Headache	11%–17%	33%–41%	78%–87%
Vomiting	8%–11%	29%–46%	45%–48%
Decreased LOC	13%–15%	39%–57%	48%–68%
Seizure	0.3%–3%	6%–7%	7%

Ongoing assessment of airway and mental status is of paramount importance in patients with ICH. The respiratory pattern also may be affected in hemorrhagic stroke. Cheyne-Stokes respirations (increasing and decreasing depth of respirations with periods of apnea) may occur with a large ICH. Putaminal hemorrhages may cause deep, irregular respirations, whereas patients with cerebellar hemorrhage may have a normal respiratory pattern.

The pupillary examination can be extremely helpful in determining the location and extent of the insult. Pontine hemorrhage classically manifests with pinpoint pupils. Dilated pupils may result from bleeding into the putamen, whereas bleeding into the thalamus may manifest with anisocoria, miosis, or a sluggish pupillary response. Cranial nerve abnormalities may result from cerebellar hemorrhages. The parasympathetic fibers course along the outside of cranial nerves Ⅲ. As a result, compression of the nerve results in loss of pupillary reactivity before anisocoria.

Baseline NIHSS and GCS scores can be used to assess stroke severity, although the GCS score may be more feasible to follow for neurologic deterioration (Box 34-3).

As noted previously, the physical exam may be insufficient to distinguish an ischemic stroke from an ICH, and radiographic confirmation is required.

Box 34-3 Glasgow Coma Scale

Eye Opening (E)	Verbal Response (V)	Motor Response (M)
4 = Spontaneous	5 = Normal conversation	6 = Normal
3 = To voice	4 = Disoriented conversation	5 = Localizes to pain
2 = To pain	3 = Words, but not coherent	4 = Withdraws to pain
1 = None	2 = No words; only sounds	3 = Decorticate posture
	1 = None	2 = Decerebrate posture
		1 = None

Scoring

Total score = E + V + M

Poor prognostic indicators for patients with ICH include a decreased level of consciousness on arrival, intraventricular hemorrhage, and an ICH volume of greater than 40 cc, all of which can be assessed in the ED. The ABC/2 technique is a quick and accurate method of measuring ICH volume at the bedside (Fig. 34-1).

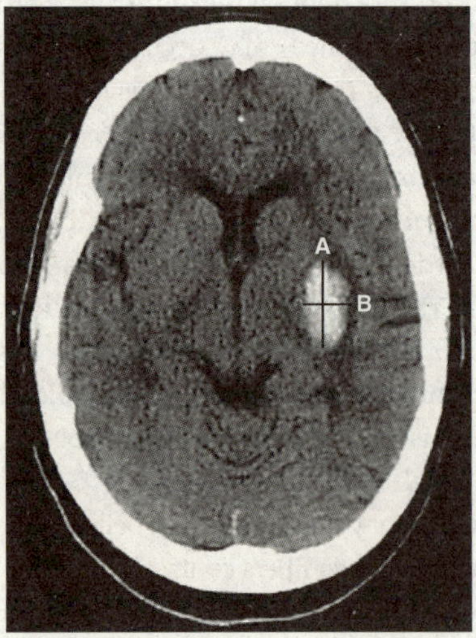

Fig. 34-1 The CT slice with the largest area of hemorrhage is identified. The largest diameter of the hemorrhage on this slice is measured in centimeters (A). The largest diameter 90 degrees to A on the same slice is measured (B). C is the approximate number of 10-mm slices on which the intracerebral hemorrhage was seen. The volume of the hemorrhage equals A multiplied by C, divided by 2 (ABC/2).

DIFFERENTIAL CONSIDERATIONS

Ischemic Stroke

Many diseases may all mimic stroke, so we should differentiate the followings: extra-axial collections of blood secondary to trauma such as epidural or subdural hematoma; Carotid dissection; brain tumors and abscesses; migraine, seizure, air embolism; metabolic abnormalities such as hypoglycemia or Wernicke's encephalopathy; Meniere's disease; any types of vasculitis, especially giant cell arteritis, et al. Compatible history and radiographic confirmation is required, such as CT or MRI scan, contrast angiography or MRA.

Venous sinus thrombosis is another cause of focal neurologic symptoms that most commonly affects the superior sagittal sinus and lateral sinuses. The diagnosis of cerebral venous thrombosis can be difficult because of the nonspecific nature of symptoms, as well as the variable time frame of symptom onset (from hours to a few weeks). Patients may present with generalized headaches, nausea, vomiting, paresis, visual disturbances, depressed level of consciousness, seizures or even symptoms generally ascribed to psychiatric disorders (such as depression).Depending on the location of the thrombus, physical examination of the patient may reveal papilledema, proptosis, or palsies of cranial nerves Ⅲ, Ⅳ, and Ⅵ, as well as other focal neurologic signs and symptoms.

The diagnosis of cerebral venous thrombosis sometimes can be made by CT. The so-called delta sign can be seen on a noncontrast CT scan as a dense triangle in the superior sagittal sinus. On a contrast-enhanced CT scan, this same area will lack demonstration of full contrast (the empty delta sign). At many institutions, MRI and MRV are the preferred modalities for the noninvasive detection of cerebral venous thrombosis.

The treatment of venous sinus thrombosis includes the use of heparin even in those patients with demonstrated hemorrhage.

The mortality rate from venous sinus thrombosis is approximately 10%. In women who are pregnant or have recently given birth, the possibility of venous sinus thrombosis should be a primary consideration in the setting of new-onset neurologic disorders.

Hemorrhagic Stroke

The differential diagnosis for ICH is similar to that for ischemic stroke; considerations include migraine, seizure, tumor, abscess, hypertensive encephalopathy, and trauma. Patients with hypertensive encephalopathy usually exhibit marked elevation in BP and other evidence of end-organ injury, including proteinuria, cardiomegaly, papilledema, and malignant hypertensive retinopathy. These patients usually improve significantly with treatment of their hypertension. Migraines frequently are associated with an aura, and the patient often has a history of similar headaches.

The differentiation between ICH and labyrinthitis can be especially difficult in the elderly. The abrupt onset of vertigo, vomiting, and nystagmus can represent a peripheral process such as labyrinthitis or a central process such as cerebellar or brainstem infarct or hemorrhage. Gross ataxia should be present with cerebellar stroke and absent with labyrinthine disease. A head CT scan should be strongly considered in patients older than 40, to assist in differentiating between labyrinthitis and cerebellar hemorrhage.

DIAGNOSTIC STRATEGIES

Ischemic Stroke

Although clinical data can help establish the diagnosis, cause, and location of the stroke, confirmatory diagnostic tests often are required to establish the final etiology or to eliminate other causes for the deficits. The immediate ED evaluation should include a blood glucose determination, cranial imaging (CT or MRI scan), and an ECG.

An emergent noncontrast cranial CT is the standard initial imaging technique for evaluating a patient with a potential stroke in the ED. It can quickly differentiate an ischemic stroke from ICH and other mass lesions. A CT scan can identify almost all parenchymal bleeds larger than 1 cm in diameter. In a majority of ischemic strokes, gross signs of infarction will not appear on routine CT scans for at least 6 to 12 hr, depending on the size of the infarct. However, subtle, early ischemic changes have been noted in up to 60% to 80% of noncontrast CT scans within the first 3 hr in patients with middle cerebral artery occlusions. These early ischemic changes include the hyperdense artery sign (acute thrombus in a vessel), sulcal effacement, loss of the insular ribbon, loss of gray-white interface, mass effect, and acute hypodensity (Fig. 34-2). Additionally,

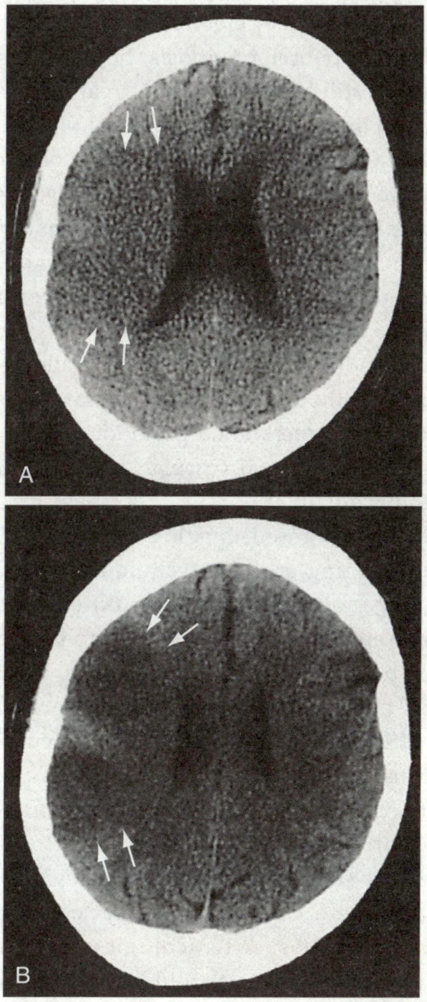

Fig. 34-2 A. CT scan taken 2 hr and 50 min after a large right middle cerebral artery occlusion. There are subtle, ultra-early ischemic changes, including loss of the gray-white interface *(arrows)* and subtle evidence of sulcal effacement. B. CT scan of same patient approximately 8 hr after symptom onset shows acute hypodensity *(arrows)* and more prominent sulcal effacement.

CTA can be used to identify the presence of intravascular thrombosis, vasculature dissection, or stenosis. In cases in which arterial dissection is suspected, imaging with MRA or CTA is indicated.

Only acute hypodensity and mass effect have been shown to be associated with an increased risk of ICH after fibrinolysis (over that in treated patients without these findings). Patients with a hyperdense artery sign and acute hypodensity of one third of the middle cerebral artery distribution tend to have a poorer prognosis; however, their outcomes are still better with t-PA treatment than without such treatment.

The role of MRI in the ED evaluation of stroke continues to evolve. MRI can visualize ischemic infarcts earlier and identify acute posterior circulation strokes more accurately than CT. However, availability, difficulty in accessing critically ill patients, and scan time limit its general use. Advances in MRA technology have allowed a noninvasive method of demonstrating large-vessel occlusions of the anterior and posterior circulation, though small intracranial vascular occlusions may not be readily apparent.

Diffusion-weighted imaging and perfusion-weighted imaging are MRI techniques that take minutes to perform and may allow differentiation between reversible and irreversible neuronal injury.

Other potential imaging modalities include CTA and perfusion scans.CTA and perfusion CT can differentiate reversible from irreversible ischemic insults.

An ECG should be obtained because Af and AMI are associated with up to 60% of all cardioembolic strokes. The hematologic evaluation should include a CBC with platelet count and coagulation studies. A toxicologic screen and cardiac isoenzyme assay should be considered if appropriate. Elevated blood viscosity even when hematocrit levels are not frankly polycythemic can affect blood flow and prognosis. A platelet count can identify thrombocytosis or thrombocytopenia, which may precipitate a thrombosis or hemorrhage. Coagulation studies are especially helpful to guide management for patients in whom anticoagulation is being considered or for patients with a hemorrhagic stroke. Cocaine or amphetamine ingestion should be considered with either an ischemic or hemorrhagic stroke in patients younger than 40 yr of age.

Other ancillary diagnostic tests to consider include an echocardiogram, carotid duplex scan, and angiogram. An echocardiogram can identify a mural thrombus, tumor, patent foramen ovale, or valvular vegetation in those patients in whom a cardioembolic stroke is suspected. An echocardiogram also should be considered in patients with no obvious cause for their stroke. Carotid duplex scanning may be helpful in patients with known or suspected high-grade carotid stenosis with worsening neurologic deficit or crescendo TIA.

Angiography is the definitive test to demonstrate stenosis or occlusion of both large and small blood vessels of the head and neck. It can detect subtle abnormalities, such as with dissection, that may not be demonstrated with other imaging techniques.

Hemorrhagic Stroke

The hematologic evaluation for the patient with hemorrhagic stroke should be performed in the same manner as for the patient with ischemic stroke. Particular attention should be directed to uncovering the presence of a coagulopathy. A drug screen should be obtained to evaluate for use of sympathomimetics if substance abuse is suspected. Increased sympathetic outflow secondary to the hemorrhage may lead to an increase in dysrhythmias. Dysrhythmias also may signal impending brainstem compression from an expanding hemorrhage.

As in ischemic stroke, the cranial CT scan is the diagnostic test of choice to evaluate for an ICH. Hemorrhages that are several days old may appear as isodense regions.

STROKE MANAGEMENT

Ischemic Stroke

With the recent focus on rapid recognition, evaluation, and treatment of stroke, EDs have attempted to streamline the care of these patients to meet recommended time goals (Table 34-2).

This has led to the development of various stroke protocols, critical pathways, and acute interventional stroke teams that often are deployed in the field before the patient even arrives to the ED.

Table 34-2 National Institute of Neurological Disorders and Stroke -Recommended Stroke Evaluation Targets for Potential Thrombolytic Candidates

MANAGEMENT COMPONENT	TARGET TIME FRAME
Door to doctor	10 min
Door to CT completion	25 min
Door to CT scan reading	45 min
Door to treatment	60 min
Access to neurologic expertise	15 min
Access to neurosurgical expertise	2 hr

In the prehospital setting, the focus should be on maintenance of the "ABC" (airway-breathing-circulation), rapid identification, early hospital notification, and rapid transport. Patients with intact protective airway reflexes should receive oxygen if they are hypoxic (oxygen saturation less than 95%), and a monitor and intravenous line established.

Overhydration should be avoided to prevent cerebral edema. By contrast, dehydration may lead to decreased cerebral perfusion, and saline infusion should be given if dehydration is suspected. Dextrose-containing solutions should be avoided in normoglycemic patients suspected of having had a stroke.Out-of-hospital personnel should attempt to rapidly ascertain the patient's blood sugar. Electrocardiographic monitoring is necessary because of the frequency of cardiac causes of ischemic stroke.

The circumstances surrounding the stroke as well as concomitant medical conditions should be ascertained. The initial out-of-hospital responders should document the exact time the patient was last seen to be neurologically normal and the level of neurologic functioning; reversible defects may completely resolve by the time the patient has arrived at the hospital. The level of consciousness, gross focal motor deficits, difficulty with speech, clumsiness, facial asymmetry, and any other focal deficits should be noted. Prehospital stroke scales have been developed to assist in differentiating patients who have had a stroke from those who have not and to identify potential candidates for fibrinolytic therapy.

In the ED setting, the ABCs should be reassessed on an ongoing basis, because patients may experience rapid deterioration, even with subacute stroke. They may be found at home 1 or 2 d after the event has occurred and may have concomitant illnesses, such as aspiration pneumonia, dehydration, hypothermia, rhabdomyolysis, or myocardial ischemia. Fever necessitates a thorough evaluation to identify the source of infection, followed by prompt institution of appropriate treatment.

Blood Pressure Management

The management of BP in patients with acute ischemic stroke and TIA is controversial.Current guidelines for the management of hypertension in patients with acute ischemic stroke recommend that antihypertensive treatment be reserved for those with markedly elevated BP, unless fibrinolytic therapy is planned or specific medical indications are present. These medical indications include (1) AMI, (2) aortic dissection, (3) true hypertensive encephalopathy, and (4) severe left ventricular failure.

Oral or parenteral agents should be withheld unless the patient's SBP is greater than 220 mm Hg or DBP is greater than 120 mm Hg or MAP is greater than 130 mm Hg (Table 34-3). If parenteral agents are used, labetalol or enalapril is favored because of ease of titration and limited effect on cerebral blood vessels. Sublingual nifedipine or sublingual nitroglycerin is not recommended because either agent can produce a precipitous drop in BP.

Table 34-3 Emergency Antihypertensive Therapy for Acute Ischemic Stroke

BLOOD PRESSURE	TREATMENT
Nonthrombolytic Candidates	
1. DBP >140 mm Hg	Sodium nitroprusside (0.5 μg/kg per minute). Aim for 10% to 20% reduction in DBP.
2. SBP >220, DBP >120, or MAP>130 mm Hg	10-20 mg labetalol IV push over 1-2 min. May repeat or double labetalol every 20 min to a maximum dose of 150 mg.

Continued

BLOOD PRESSURE	TREATMENT
3. SBP <220, DBP <120, or MAP<130 mm Hg	Emergency antihypertensive therapy is deferred in the absence of aortic dissection, AMI, severe congestive heart failure, or hypertensive encephalopathy.
Thrombolytic Candidates	
Pretreatment	
1. SBP >185 or DBP >110 mm Hg	1–2 inches of nitro paste or one to two doses of 10–20 mg labetalol IV push. If BP is not reduced and maintained at <185/110 mm Hg, the patient should not be treated with TPA.
During and after treatment	
1. Monitor BP	BP is monitored every 15 min for 2 hr, then every 30 min for 6 hr, and then hourly for 16 hr.
2. DBP >140 mm Hg	Sodium nitroprusside (0.5 μg/kg per minute)
3. SBP >230 or DBP 121–140 mm Hg	*Step 1*: Give 10 mg labetalol IV push over 1 to 2 min. May repeat or double labetalol every 10 min to a maximum dose of 150 mg, or give the initial labetalol bolus and then start a labetalol drip at 2–8 mg/min. *Step 2*: If BP is not controlled by labetalol, consider sodium nitroprusside.
4. SBP 180–230 or DBP 105–120 mm Hg	10 mg labetalol IVpush. May repeat or double labetalol every 10-20 min to a maximum dose of 150 mg or give initial labetalol bolus and then start a labetalol drip at 2-8 mg/min.

If fibrinolytic therapy is planned, stringent control of BP is indicated to reduce the potential for bleeding after the thrombolytic is administered (Table 34-3). Thrombolytic therapy is not recommended for patients whose SBP is consistently greater than 185 mm Hg or whose diastolic pressure is 110 mm Hg at the time of treatment. Simple measures can be used to try lowering BP below this level. Recommended approaches include the use of nitroglycerin paste and one or two doses of labetalol, 10 to 20 mg given intravenously. Once thrombolytic therapy has been initiated, BP must be monitored closely and hypertension treated aggressively.

Low BP can be quite detrimental to patients with ischemic stroke. Normally normotensive stroke patients with low BP or normally hypertensive stroke patients with low or even low-normal BP should be given a fluid bolus to try to increase cerebral perfusion. This is especially important in patients who present in a dehydrated state. If initial fluid challenge is ineffective, the patient may require vasopressor therapy (e.g., with dopamine) to gradually increase MAP and improve cerebral perfusion.

Acute Drug Therapy

To date, only the use of intravenous t-PA has been approved by the U.S. FDA for treatment of patients with acute ischemic stroke.The current recommendation for recombinant t-PA (rt-PA) is that it be administered intravenously at a dose of 0.9 mg/kg to a maximum of 90 mg (10% of the dose given as a bolus followed by an infusion lasting 60 min). Treatment must be initiated within 3 hr of the onset of ischemic symptoms in patients who meet strict inclusion and exclusion criteria (Box 34-4). Intravenous t-PA is not recommended when the time of stroke onset cannot be ascertained reliably, including strokes recognized on awakening. In addition, caution is warranted in treating patients with large strokes (NIHSS score of 20 or higher) or early CT changes from a recent major infarction (e.g., acute hypodensity or mass effect), because they are at increased risk for symptomatic hemorrhage.

Box 34-4 Fibrinolytic Therapy for Acute Ischemic Stroke: Inclusion and Exclusion Criteria

Inclusion Criteria

1. Age 18 yr or older
2. Clinical diagnosis of ischemic stroke causing a measurable neurologic deficit
3. Time of symptom onset well established to be less than 180 min before treatment would begin

Exclusion Criteria

1. Evidence of intracranial hemorrhage on noncontrast head CT
2. Only minor or rapidly resolving stroke symptoms
3. High clinical suspicion of subarachnoid hemorrhage even with normal CT findings
4. Active internal bleeding (e.g., gastrointestinal or urinary bleeding within last 21 d)

5. Known bleeding diathesis, including but not limited to:
- Platelet count <100,000/μL
- Patient has received heparin within 48 hr and had an elevated activated partial thromboplastin time (greater than upper limit of normal for laboratory)
- Recent use of anticoagulant (e.g., warfarin sodium) and elevated prothrombin time >15 s

6. Within 3 mo of intracranial surgery, serious head trauma, or previous stroke
7. Within 14 d of major surgery or serious trauma
8. Recent arterial puncture at noncompressible site
9. Lumbar puncture within 7 d
10. History of ICH, arteriovenous malformation, or aneurysm
11. Witnessed seizure at stroke onset
12. Recent AMI
13. On repeated measurements, SBP >185 mm Hg or DBP >110 mm Hg at time of treatment, requiring aggressive treatment to reduce BP to within these limits

Intra-arterial thrombolysis is an alternative treatment for eligible patients presenting beyond the 3 hr time window but within 6 hr of symptom onset.

A variety of mechanical clot retrieval devices are being investigated. The Mechanical Embolus Removal in Cerebral Ischemia (MERCI) retrieval device has demonstrated improved clinical outcomes.

Aspirin should not be given for the first 24 hr in patients who have received a fibrinolytic agent, because this has been associated with an increased risk of ICH and death.

The use of low-molecular-weight or unfractionated heparin is common in patients with acute ischemic stroke or TIA, but its value is unproved. However, heparin sometimes is considered in patients at high risk for stroke progression, including patients with crescendo TIA or TIA due to a cardioembolic source, patients with a high-grade carotid artery stenosis, patients with posterior circulation TIA, and patients with evolving strokes. Heparin is recommended for the treatment of carotid and vertebral artery dissection unless a contraindication such as intracranial extension is present. If a dissection is diagnosed and the patient has no symptoms of ischemia, treatment with antiplatelet therapy alone may be an option.Heparin therapy should not be initiated in patients with suspected endocarditis or in any patient until a CT scan has ruled out intracranial bleeding.

Other innovative approaches to stroke care, including mild to moderate hypothermia and early hemicraniectomy, are currently being investigated.

Management of Intracranial Hemorrhage

The patient with a potential ICH requires rapid assessment and transport to a care center with CT scanning capability and intensive care management facilities. Out-of-hospital management is similar to that for ischemic stroke.

Supportive care involving attention to airway management and perfusion is of the highest priority. Patients with hemorrhagic stroke are more likely to have an altered level of consciousness that may rapidly progress to unresponsiveness requiring emergent endotracheal intubation. Intravenous access should be established and cardiac monitoring should be initiated. Evaluation of blood glucose and appropriate dextrose and naloxone administration should be considered in any patient with altered mental status.

Considerable disagreement exists regarding optimal BP management in the patient with ICH. Hypertension may cause deterioration by increasing ICP and potentiating further bleeding from small arteries or arterioles. On the other hand, hypotension may decrease CBF, thereby worsening brain injury. In general, recommendations for treatment of hypertension in patients with ICH are more aggressive than those for patients with ischemic stroke. The current consensus regarding management of ICH is to recommend antihypertensive treatment with parenteral agents for SBP higher than 160 to 180 mm Hg or DBP higher than 105 mm Hg. Treatment for lower pressures remains controversial.Nitroprusside is the agent most commonly recommended. Nitroprusside provides a rapid onset, is titratable, and has no effect on mental status. Disadvantages include the need for careful monitoring and the theoretical risk of worsening the hemorrhage due to the vasodilatory effects of nitroprusside on cerebral vessels. Labetalol is another therapeutic option. More recently, nicardipine has been proposed as an optimal antihypertensive agent in the setting of cerebrovascular emergencies.

Hyperventilation and diuretics such as mannitol have been used when ICH is complicated by signs of progressively increasing ICP, clinical deterioration associated with mass effect, or impending uncal herniation. These interventions should not be used prophylactically.The effectiveness of mannitol in the setting of ICH is questionable. Hypertonic saline is being investigated as an alternative agent. Use of steroids in cerebral hemorrhage, once a common practice, appears to be harmful and is not recommended. Other experimental modalities include barbiturate coma and hypothermia.

Seizure activity can cause neuronal injury, elevations in ICH, and destabilization of an already critically ill patient. In addition, nonconvulsive seizure may contribute to coma in up to 10% of patients in a neuro-intensive care unit. Seizure prophylaxis (fosphenytoin 18 mg/kg) should be considered for patients with ICH, especially those with lobar hemorrhage.

Surgery is not beneficial in most cases of ICH. Selected patients with sizable lobar hemorrhage and progressive neurologic deterioration may benefit from surgical drainage. Surgery is more efficacious in patients with cerebellar hemorrhage.

DISPOSITION

Ischemic Stroke and Transient Ischemic Attacks

Patients with symptoms consistent with an acute stroke should be transported to ED capable of initiating fibrinolytic therapy within 1 hr of hospital arrival. At a minimum, this requires emergent CT capabilities, an institutional "acute stroke protocol," and availability of a physician versed in the use of thrombolytic therapy. Intensive care monitoring and neurosurgery capabilities should be available within 2 hr of drug initiation.

In most cases, once the diagnosis of an acute stroke or stroke syndrome is established and the patient is stabilized, hospitalization will be necessary for further evaluation and treatment. Patients may deteriorate over the first 24 hr and require close in-hospital monitoring. Most patients can be managed on a general medical or telemetry unit. Patients with large acute hemispheric strokes (associated with increased risk for herniation) or with significant posterior circulation-related changes and those treated with a fibrinolytic agent should be monitored in a step-down or ICU for at least 24 hr.

In select cases, patients with multiple previous strokes who have been thoroughly evaluated or those who experience mild new episodes or have a completed stroke days to weeks after the event may be treated in the ED and discharged home after discussion with their primary care physician or neurologist. Close follow-up should be arranged.

Patients with new-onset TIA should be hospitalized for evaluation and workup owing to the substantial short-term risk of stroke and other adverse events. Exception can be made for patients with only minimal anterior circulation symptoms, for whom an extensive ED evaluation constitutes appropriate management.

The ABCD (*a*ge,*BP*,clinical features,*d*uration of TIA symptoms) score has been validated as a good predictor of future stroke risk in patients with TIA treated in the ED. ABCD scores range from 0 to 6, with a higher score indicating a higher future stroke risk; this scoring system is based on the following criteria: age 60 yr or older = 1 point; SBP greater than 140 mm Hg and/or DBP greater than 90 mm Hg = 1 point; unilateral weakness = 2 points; speech disturbance without weakness = 1 point; symptom duration 10 to 59 min = 1 point; symptom duration 60 min or longer = 2 points. Patients with an ABCD score of 5 or 6 in the ED have a 30 d risk of stroke eight times that of patients with an ABCD score less than 5 (hazard ratio 8.01; 95% CI: 3.21 to 19.98).

Hemorrhagic Stroke

All patients with an acute hemorrhagic stroke in whom surgical intervention is a consideration should be admitted to EICU under the care of a neurologist or a neurosurgeon.

(TIAN Yingping)

SECTION 3

Surgical Emergencies

Chapter 35

Acute abdominal pain

KEY CONCEPTS

Pathology in the gastrointestinal and genitourinary tracts remains the most common source of pain perceived in the abdomen.

The location and severity of AAP may change over time.

AAP caused by ruptured abdominal aneurysm, or mesenteric ischemia may manifest atypically and be rapidly progressive in the elder patients.

The possibility of ectopic pregnancy in women of reproductive age greatly increases the risk of serious disease with a high potential for misdiagnosis.

Nonpregnant patients require evaluation for various ovarian and uterine pathologic states.

Ultrasound assessment should be part of the initial physical examination and can be invaluable in guiding treatment and disposition.

In the elderly population, CT results change management or disposition decisions in a significant proportion of patients.

PERSPECTIVE

Acute abdominal pain (AAP) is a common ED complaint. The nature and quality of AAP may be difficult for the patient to convey. Physical examination findings are variable and can be misleading. The location and severity of the pain may change over time. Initially benign symptoms and presentations may evolve into life-threatening conditions. Conversely, patients with severe symptoms may carry a relatively benign diagnosis. All of these factors make evaluation of patients with AAP challenging in the ED setting.

Epidemiology

AAP accounts for up to 10% of all ED visits. Some of the most common causes of AAP are listed in Table 35-1.Many patients have pain and other symptoms that are not typical of any specific disease process.

Elders with AAP are more likely to have a lifethreatening process as the cause of their pain. Conditions such as ruptured abdominal aneurysm, or mesenteric ischemia may manifest atypically and be rapidly progressive. Decreased diagnostic accuracy, coupled with increased probability of severe disease, results in increased mortality in elderly patients with AAP.

Increasingly, emergency physicians are seeing patients in immunocompromised states secondary to HIV and AIDS, uncontrolled diabetes, chronic liver disease, chemotherapy, and immunosuppressive drugs. Their clinical presentation can be misleading owing to atypical physical and laboratory findings, such as lack of fever.WBC count, which is unreliable in all cases of AAP, may be frankly misleading in such patients. With regard to infection, the scope of the differential diagnosis also should be broader than usual. Presentations in the immunocompromised patient may be highly variable.

The evaluation of AAP in women involves a differential diagnosis of considerable extent and often requires a more in-depth physical examination and further diagnostic testing. Pelvic organs may be the source of significant pathology in both the pregnant and the nonpregnant patient. The possibility of ectopic pregnancy in women of reproductive age greatly increases the risk of serious disease with a high potential for misdiagnosis. During pregnancy the uterus becomes an abdominal rather than a pelvic organ and may displace the normal intraperitoneal

Table 35-1 **Common Causes of AAP**

CAUSATIVE DISORDER OR CONDITION	EPIDEMIOLOGY	ETIOLOGY	PRESENTATION	PHYSICAL EXAMINATION	USEFUL TEST(S)
Gastric, esophageal, or duodenal inflammation	Occurs in all age groups.	Caused by gastric hypersecretion, breakdown of mucoprotective barriers, infection, or exogenous sources.	Epigastric radiating or localized, associated with certain foods. Pain may be burning. In some cases, exacerbation in supine position.	Epigastric tenderness without rebound or guarding. Perforation or bleeding leads to more severe clinical findings.	Uncomplicated cases are treated with antacids or histamine H_2 blockers before invasive studies are contemplated. Gastroduodenoscopy is valuable in diagnosis and biopsy. Testing for Helicobacter Pylori with blood or biopsy specimens. If perforation is suspected, an upright chest radiograph is obtained early to rule out free air. CT may be beneficial.
Acute appendicitis	Peak age in adolescence and young adulthood; less common in elders. Higher perforation rate in women and elders and in pregnancy.	Appendiceal lumen obstruction leads to swelling, ischemia, infection, and perforation.	Epigastric or periumbilical pain migrates to RLQ over 8-12 hr (50%-60%). Later presentations associated with higher perforation rates. Pain, low-grade fever (15%), and anorexia (80%) common; vomiting less common (50%-70%).	Mean temperature 38℃ (100.5°F). Higher temperature associated with perforation. RLQ tenderness (90%-95%) with rebound (40%-70%) in majority of cases. Rectal tenderness in 30%.	Leukocyte count usually elevated or may show left shift. Urinalysis may show sterile pyuria. CT is sensitive and specific. US may have use in women, pregnancy, and children with RLQ pain.
Biliary tract disease	Peak age 35-60 yr; rare in patients younger than 20. Female-tomale ratio of 3:1. Risk factors include multiparity, obesity, alcohol intake, and use of birth control pills.	Passage of gallstones causes biliary colic. Impaction of a stone in cystic duct or common duct causes cholecystitis or cholangitis.	Crampy RUQ pain radiates to right subscapular area. Prior history of pain is common. May have nausea or postprandial pain. Longer duration of pain favors diagnosis of cholecystitis or cholangitis.	Temperature normal in biliary colic, elevated in cholecystitis and cholangitis. RUQ tenderness, rebound, and jaundice (less common) may be present.	WBC count elevated in cholecystitis and cholangitis. Lipase and liver function tests may help differentiate this from gastritis or ulcer disease. US shows wall thickening, pericholecystic fluid, stones, or duct dilatation. Hepatobiliary scintigraphy diagnoses gallbladder function.

Continued

CAUSATIVE DISORDER OR CONDITION	EPIDEMIO LOGY	ETIOLOGY	PRESENTATION	PHYSICAL EXAMINATION	USEFUL TEST(S)
Ureteral colic	Average age 30-40 yr, primarily in men. Prior history or family history of stones is common.	Family history, gout, Proteus infection. Renal tubular acidosis and cystinuria lead to stone formation.	Acute onset of flank pain radiating to groin. Nausea, vomiting, and pallor are common. Patient usually writhing in pain.	Vital signs usually normal. Tenderness on CVA percussion with benign abdominal examination.	Urinalysis usually shows hematuria. Noncontrast CT is sensitive and specific. US with fluid bolus useful diagnostically.
Diverticulitis	Incidence increases with advancing age, affects males more often than females. Recurrences are common. Often called "left-sided" appendicitis.	Colonic diverticula may become infected or perforated or cause local colitis. Obstruction, peritonitis, abscesses, fistulae result from infection or swelling.	Change in stool frequency or consistency commonly reported. LLQ pain is common. Associated with fever, nausea and vomiting; rectal bleeding may be seen.	Fever usually of low grade. LLQ pain without rebound is common. Stool may be heme positive.	Results on most tests usually normal. Plain radiographs may show obstruction or mass effect. CT is often diagnostic.
Acute gastroent-eritis	Common diagnosis. Seasonal. Most common misdiagnosis of appendicitis. May be seen in multiple family members. History of travel or immunocompromise.	Usually viral. Consider invasive bacterial or parasitic cause in prolonged cases, in travelers, or immunocompromised patients.	Pain usually poorly localized, intermittent, crampy, and diffuse. Diarrhea is key element in diagnosis; usually large volume, watery. Nausea and vomiting usually begin before pain.	Abdominal examination usually nonspecific without peritoneal signs. Watery diarrhea or no stool noted on rectal examination. Fever is usually present.	Usually symptomatic care with antiemetics and volume repletion. Heme-positive stools may be a clue to invasive pathogens. Key is not using this as a "default" diagnosis and missing more serious disease.
Constipation and obstipation	More common in females, elders, the very young, and patients on narcotics.	Idiopathic or hypokinesis secondary to disease states (low motility) or exogenous sources (diet, medications).	AAP; change in bowel habits.	Variable, nonspecific without peritoneal signs. Rectal examination may reveal hard stool or impaction.	Radiographs may show large amounts of stool. This is a diagnosis of exclusion.
Nonspecific AAP	More common in persons of young and middle age, women of childbearing age, or persons of low socioeconomic status and patients with psychiatric disorders. Up to 10% of patients older than 50 yr of age will have intraabdominal cancer.	Unknown. Early or undiagnosed presentation of pathologic conditions.	Variable but tends to be chronic or recurrent.	Variable but no peritoneal signs. Rectal examination should be done to evaluate for subtle signs of pathology, including heme-positive stool, fistulae, and fissures.	Variable and often can be done on an outpatient basis.

RUQ: right upper quadrant; LLQ: left lower quadrant

contents, adding complexity to the evaluation of these patients. Nonpregnant patients require evaluation for various ovarian and uterine pathologic states.

Pathophysiology

Pathology in the gastrointestinal and genitourinary tracts remains the most common source of pain perceived in the abdomen. Also, pain can arise from a multitude of other intra-abdominal and extra-abdominal locations (Box 35-1).AAP is derived from one or more of three distinct pain pathways: visceral, somatic, and referred.

Box 35-1 Important Extra-abdominopelvic Causes of AAP

Thoracic
- AMI or UA
- Pneumonia
- PE
- Herniated thoracic disk (neuralgia)
- Pericarditis or myocarditis

Genitourinary
- Testicular torsion

Abdominal Wall
- Muscle spasm
- Muscle hematoma
- Herpes zoster

Infectious
- Streptococcal pharyngitis
- Rocky Mountain spotted fever
- Mononucleosis

Systemic
- DKA
- Alcoholic ketoacidosis
- Uremia
- Sickle cell disease
- Porphyria
- SLE
- Vasculitis
- Glaucoma
- Hyperthyroidism

Toxic
- Methanol poisoning
- Heavy metal toxicity
- Scorpion bite
- Snake bite
- Black widow spider bite

Visceral pain results from stimulation of autonomic nerves invested in the visceral peritoneum surrounding internal organs. Distention of hollow organs by fluid or gas and capsular stretching of solid organs from edema, blood, cysts, or abscesses are the most common stimuli. This discomfort is poorly characterized and difficult to localize. If the involved organ is affected by peristalsis, the pain often is described as intermittent, crampy, or colicky. In general, visceral pain is perceived from the abdominal region that correlates with the embryonic somatic segment, as follows:

- Foregut structures (stomach, duodenum, liver, and pancreas) are associated with upper AAP.
- Midgut derivatives (small bowel, proximal colon, and appendix) are associated with periumbilical pain.
- Hindgut structures (distal colon and genitourinary tract) are associated with lower AAP.

Visceral pain can be perceived in a location remote from the actual disease process. Localization occurs with the extension of the disease process beyond the viscera. A classic example is that of the early periumbilical pain of appendicitis (midgut). When the parietal peritoneum becomes involved, the pain localizes to the right lower quadrant of the abdomen, he usual location of the appendix.

Somatic pain occurs with irritation of the parietal peritoneum. This is usually caused by infection, chemical irritation, or another inflammatory process. Sensations are conducted by the peripheral nerves and are better localized than the visceral pain component. Fig. 35-1 illustrates some more typical pain locations corresponding to specific disease entities. Somatic pain is often described as intense and constant. As disease processes evolve to peritoneal irritation with inflammation, better localization of the pain to the area of pathology generally occurs.

Referred pain is defined as pain felt at a distance from its source because peripheral afferent nerve fibers from many internal organs enter the spinal cord through nerve roots that also carry nociceptive fibers from other locations, as illustrated in Fig. 35-2.This makes interpretation of the location of noxious stimuli difficult for the brain. Both visceral pain and

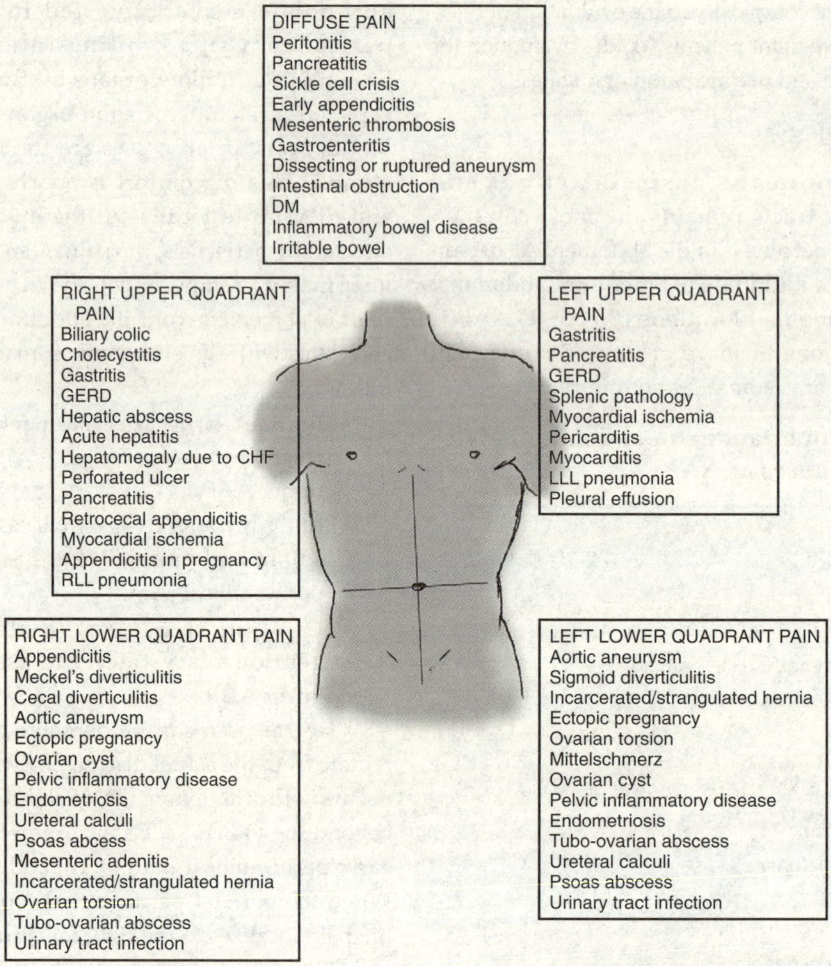

Fig. 35-1 Differential diagnosis of AAP. LLL, left lower lobe; RLL, right lower lobe.

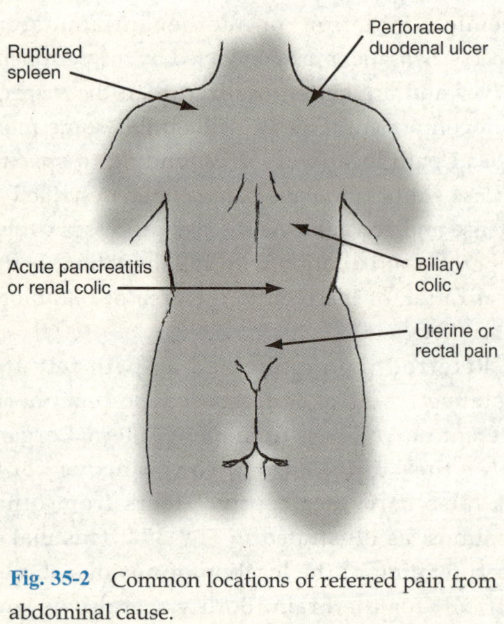

Fig. 35-2 Common locations of referred pain from abdominal cause.

somatic pain can manifest as referred pain. Two examples of referred pain are the epigastric pain associated with an inferior myocardial infarction and the shoulder pain associated with blood in the peritoneal cavity irritating the diaphragm. It is common for a patient to interpret pain originating from the hips as pelvic pain, especially in the very young or elderly. Lower lobe pneumonias can cause referred AAP secondary to diaphragmatic irritation. Finally, some metabolic disorders and toxidromes may manifest with AAP.

Notably, AAP in a female may represent referred pain from pelvic structures or an extension of a pelvic process, as in the case of perihepatic inflammation with pelvic inflammatory disease.

DIAGNOSTIC APPROACH

The clinical approach should focus on early stabilization, history, physical examination, and any ancillary tests collectively facilitating appropriate management and disposition plans.

Differential Considerations

Classically, potential diagnoses are divided into intraabdominopelvic (intraperitoneal, retroperitoneal, and pelvic) causes (e.g., appendicitis, cholecystitis, pancreatitis) and extraabdominopelvic processes (e.g., pneumonia, myocardial infarction, ketoacidosis, toxicologic).

Many disorders cause AAP, a few processes warrant careful consideration in the ED. Table 35-2

Table 35-2 Potentially Life-threatening Causes of AAP

CAUSE	EPIDEMIOLOGY	ETIOLOGY	PRESENTATION	PHYSICAL EXAMI-NATION	USEFUL TOOL(S)
Ruptured ectopic pregnancy	Occurs in females of childbearing age. No method of contraception prevents ectopic pregnancy. Approximately 1 in every 100 pregnancies.	Risk factors include nonwhite race, older age, history of STD or PID, infertility treatment, intrauterine contraceptive device placed within the past year, tubal sterilization, and previous ectopic pregnancy.	Severe, sharp constant pain localized to the affected side. More diffuse AAP with intraperitoneal hemorrhage. Signs of shock may be present. Midline pain tends not to be ectopic pregnancy.	Shock or evidence of peritonitis may be present. Lateralized abdominal tenderness. Localized adnexal tenderness or cervical motion tenderness increases the likelihood of ectopic pregnancy. Vaginal bleeding does not have to be present.	β-hCG testing necessary in all females of childbearing age (10-55 yr); combined with ultrasonography, preferably transvaginal in early pregnancy, usually is diagnostic. FAST examination is useful in evaluating for free fluid in patients with shock or peritonitis.
Ruptured or leaking abdominal aneurysm	Incidence increases with advancing age. More frequent in men. Risk factors include HTN, DM, smoking, COPD, and CAD.	Exact cause is undetermined. Contributing factors include atherosclerosis, genetic predisposition, HTN, connective tissue disease, trauma, and infection.	Patient often asymptomatic until rupture. Acute epigastric and back pain often associated with or followed by syncope or signs of shock. Pain may radiate to back, groin, or testes.	Vital signs may be normal (in 70%) to severely hypotensive. Palpation of a pulsatile mass is usually possible in aneurysms 5 cm or greater. The physical examination may be nonspecific. Bruits or inequality of femoral pulses may be evident.	Abdominal plain films abnormal in 80% of cases. Ultrasound can define diameter and length but can be limited by obesity and bowel gas. FAST examination can be helpful in evaluating for leak by looking for free fluid. Spiral CT test of choice in stable patients.
Mesenteric ischemia	Occurs most commonly in elders with CV disease, CHF, cardiac dysrhythmias, DM, sepsis, and dehydration. Responsible for 1 of 1000 hospital admissions. Mortality 70%. Mesenteric venous thrombosis associated with hypercoagulable states, hematologic	20%-30% of lesions are nonocclusive. The causes of ischemia are multifactorial, including transient hypotension in the presence of preexisting atherosclerotic lesion. The arterial occlusive causes (65%) are secondary to emboli (75%) or acute arterial	Severe pain, colicky, that starts in periumbilical region and then becomes diffuse. Often associated with vomiting and diarrhea. Sometimes postprandial. "Mes-enteric or abdominal angina."	Early examination results can be remarkably benign in the presence of severe ischemia. Bowel sounds often still present. Rectal examination important because mild bleeding with positive guaiac stools can be present.	Often a pronounced leukocytosis is present. Elevations of amylase and creatine kinase levels are seen. Metabolic acidosis caused by lactic acidemia is often seen with infarction. Plain radiographs of limited benefit. CT, MRI, and angiography are

Continued

CAUSE	EPIDEMIOLOGY	ETIOLOGY	PRESENTATION	PHYSICAL EXAMI-NATION	USEFUL TOOL(S)
	inflammation, and trauma.	thrombosis (25%).			accurate to varying degrees.
Intestinal obstruction	Peaks in infancy and elders. More common with history of previous abdominal surgery.	Adhesions, carcinoma, hernias, abscesses, volvulus, and infarction. Obstruction leads to vomiting, "third spacing" of fluid, or strangulation and necrosis of bowel.	Crampy diffuse AAP associated with vomiting.	Vital signs usually normal unless dehydration or bowel strangulation has occurred. Abdominal distention, hyperactive bowel sounds, and diffuse tenderness. Local peritoneal signs indicate strangulation.	Elevated WBC count suggests strangulation. Electrolytes may be abnormal if associated with vomiting or prolonged symptoms. Abdominal radiographs and CT are useful in diagnosis.
Perforated viscus	Incidence increases with advancing age. History of peptic ulcer disease or diverticular disease common.	More often a duodenal ulcer that erodes through the serosa. Colonic diverticula, large bowel, and gallbladder perforations are rare. Spillage of bowel contents causes peritonitis.	Acute onset of epigastric pain is common. Vomiting in 50%. Fever may develop later. Pain may localize with omental walling off of peritonitis. Shock may be present with bleeding or sepsis.	Fever, usually of low grade, is common; worsens over time. Tachycardia is common. Abdominal examination reveals diffuse guarding and rebound. "Boardlike" abdomen in later stages. Bowel sounds are decreased.	WBC count usually elevated owing to peritonitis. Amylase may be elevated; LFT results are variable. Upright radiographic view reveals free air in 70%-80% of cases with perforated ulcers.
Acute pancreatitis	Peak age in adulthood; rare in children and elders. Male preponderance. Alcohol abuse and biliary tract disease are risk factors.	Alcohol, gallstones, hyperlipidemia, hypercalcemia, or endoscopic retrograde pancreatography causing pancreatic damage, saponification, and necrosis. ARDS, sepsis, hemorrhage, and renal failure are secondary.	Acute onset of epigastric pain radiating to the back. Nausea and vomiting are common. Pain disproportionate to physical findings. Adequate volume repletion is important in the initial therapy.	Low-grade fever common. Patient may be hypotensive or tachypneic. Some epigastric tenderness usually present. Because pancreas is retroperitoneal organ, guarding or rebound not present unless condition is severe. Flank ecchymosis or periumbilical ecchymosis may be seen if process is hemorrhagic.	Lipase determination is test of choice. Ultrasound examination may show edema, pseudocyst, or biliary tract disease. CT scan may show abscesses, necrosis, hemorrhage, or pseudocysts. CT is ordered if severe acute pancreatitis is suspected. Rule out gallstones with ultrasound examination.

lists important potentially life-threatening nontraumatic causes of AAP.

Rapid Assessment and Stabilization

Most patients with AAP do not have hemodynamic instability. This percentage is higher in elders and immunocompromised patients.

Physiologically compromised patients should be brought to a treatment area immediately, and resuscitation initiated. Sepsis or protracted severe volume loss (emesis, diarrhea) can lead to shock; prompt resuscitation is required.

Extreme conditions, such as ruptured abdominal aortic aneurysm, massive gastrointestinal hemorrhage, ruptured ectopic pregnancy, ruptured spleen, and hemorrhagic pancreatitis, may necessitate blood or blood product replacement. Bedside ultrasonography can be used to quickly evaluate patients for free intraperitoneal fluid, volume status, and presence of aortic pathology. Ultrasound assessment should be part of the initial physical examination and can be invaluable in guiding treatment and disposition. Because any of the immediately life-threatening entities may necessitate surgical intervention or management, early surgical consultation is indicated.

Pivotal Findings

Symptoms

A careful and focused history is central to unlocking the puzzle of AAP. Box 35-2 lists some historical questions with high yields for serious pathology.

Box 35-2 High-Yield Historical Questions

1. *How old are you?* Advanced age means increased risk.
2. *Which came first—pain or vomiting?* Pain first is worse (i.e., more likely to be caused by surgical disease).
3. *How long have you had the pain?* Pain for less than 48 hr is worse.
4. *Have you ever had abdominal surgery?* Consider obstruction in patients who report previous abdominal surgery.
5. *Is the pain constant or intermittent?* Constant pain is worse.
6. *Have you ever had this before?* A report of no prior episodes is worse.
7. *Do you have a history of cancer, diverticulosis, pancreatitis, kidney failure, gallstones, or inflammatorybowel disease?* All are suggestive of more serious disease.
8. *Do you have HIV?* Consider occult infection or drug-related pancreatitis.
9. *How much alcohol do you drink per day?* Consider pancreatitis, hepatitis, or cirrhosis in patients with history or signs of significant intake.
10. *Are you pregnant?* Test for pregnancy—consider ectopic pregnancy.
11. *Are you taking antibiotics or steroids?* Effects of these drugs may mask infection.
12. *Did the pain start centrally and migrate to the right lower quadrant?* High specificity for appendicitis.
13. *Do you have a history of vascular or heart disease, HTN, or Af?* Consider mesenteric ischemia and abdominal aneurysm.

Abrupt onset often is indicative of a more serious cause; however, delayed presentations also may represent a surgical condition. Surgical causes of AAP are more likely to manifest with pain first, followed by nausea and vomiting, rather than with nausea and vomiting followed by pain, although in elder patients the progression may be reversed or pain may be absent entirely. Localization and pain migration also are helpful components of the pain history. Diffuse pain generally is nonsurgical, but it may represent the early visceral component of a surgical process. Colicky pain is indicative of hollow viscus distention, and duration and time of colic may give clues to the identity of the culprit organ, as displayed in Fig. 35-3, see color illustration.

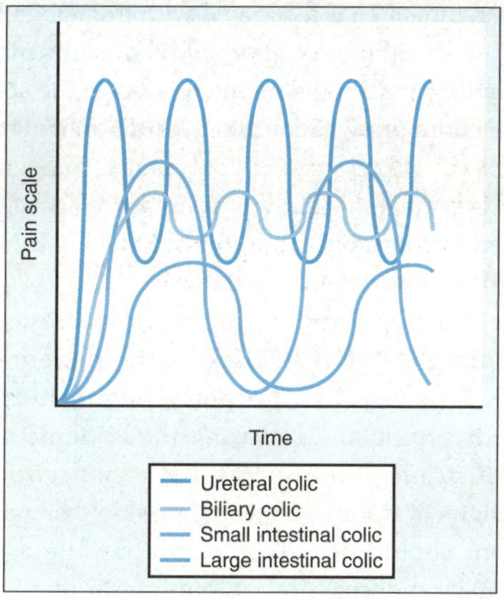

Fig. 35-3 The characteristics of colicky AAP.

The severity and descriptive nature of the pain are the most subjective aspects of the pain history, but a few classic descriptions are recognized, such as the following:

- The diffuse, severe, colicky pain of bowel obstruction
- The "pain out of proportion to examination" observed in patients with mesenteric ischemia
- The radiation of pain from the epigastrium straight through to the midback associated with pancreatitis, either related to primary organ inflammation or secondary to a penetrating ulcer
- The radiation of pain to the left shoulder

or independent pain in the left shoulder associated with splenic pathology, diaphragmatic irritation, or free intraperitoneal fluid
- The onset of pain associated with syncope seen in perforation of gastric or duodenal ulcer, ruptured aortic aneurysm, or ruptured ectopic pregnancy

A history of immunocompromised state or immunosuppressive medications may point to infection. A patient undergoing anticoagulation therapy or taking nonsteroidal anti-inflammatory medications may have gastrointestinal bleeding. Diabetics may be experiencing AAP as a feature of ketoacidosis. A patient undergoing chronic narcotic therapy may have constipation or even a bowel obstruction.

Signs

The objective evaluation begins with measurement of the vital signs. Significant tachycardia and hypotension are indicators that hypovolemia or sepsis may be present. Tachypnea may be an indication of metabolic acidosis from gangrenous viscera or sepsis, hypoxemia from pneumonia, or simply a catecholamine-induced reaction to pain. Elevated temperature often is associated with intra-abdominal infections. Although important, vital signs may be misleading and should be interpreted in the context of the entire presentation. Tachycardia may develop late for various reasons in hypovolemia. Temperature often is normal in elderly patients with laparotomy-proven intraperitoneal infections. Elders with sepsis also may demonstrate hypothermia.

A thorough abdominal examination is an essential part of evaluation of the patient with AAP. This requires properly positioning the patient supine and exposing the abdomen. The examination should begin with inspection for any signs of trauma, bruising, or skin lesions. The patient should be asked to localize the area of maximal tenderness by pointing with one finger. The abdomen can be divided into four quadrants: right upper, right lower, left upper, and left lower; each area is then examined individually. Tenderness in one quadrant often corresponds with the location of the diseased organ, which will direct the workup (Fig.35-1).Some disease processes may manifest with pain that is not exclusively within one specific quadrant, such as the suprapubic pain of a urinary tract infection or the midepigastic pain of a gastric ulcer. Although most patients with suspected appendicitis have right lower quadrant abdominal tenderness, a small percentage of patients with proven appendicitis do not.

Rectal examination may have limited use in the evaluation of AAP, except that associated with intraluminal gastrointestinal hemorrhage, prostatitis, or perirectal disease. The main utility of the rectal examination is in the detection of heme-positive stool, anal fissures or fistulae, or stool impaction. Rectal examination has not been shown to increase diagnostic accuracy for appendicitis when added to external physical examination of the abdomen.

The abdominal evaluation should include a pelvic examination in female patients with lower AAP and genital examination in male patients. The pelvic examination should be done early in the evaluation of the female patient with AAP to help differentiate an abdominal from a pelvic source. This information is helpful in choosing an imaging modality. Pelvic ultrasound examination is helpful in evaluating uterine and ovarian pathology, whereas CT is more beneficial in evaluation of suspected intra-abdominal pathology. Although the pelvic examination may guide the initial choice of imaging modality, overlap in examination findings is common. For example, a patient with right lower quadrant tenderness may have both right adnexal tenderness and tenderness over McBurney's point, necessitating exclusion of both appendicitis and ovarian torsion. The diagnosis highest on the differential list should be ruled out first through use of the corresponding imaging modality.

In the male patient with AAP, the urogenital examination is a routine and required part of the evaluation. Diseases such as prostatitis, orchitis, and epididymitis commonly cause AAP in males. Furthermore, inguinal hernias are more common in males, with the possibility of strangulation or incarceration in the inguinal canal, necessitating a thorough genitourinary examination.

Ancillary Testing

Urinalysis and testing for pregnancy are perhaps the most time-and cost-effective adjunctive laboratory tests available. Results often can be obtained quickly, so the former can lead to an early diagnosis and the latter may significantly affect further evaluation and management approaches. It is necessary to interpret urinalysis results within the context of the patient's clinical picture. Pyuria, with or without bacteriuria, often is present in a variety of conditions besides a simple urinary tract infection. For example, appendicitis may feature sterile pyuria. Similarly, hematuria usually is present with the relatively benign condition of nephrolithiasis but also may indicate a more severe pathology.

CBC frequently are ordered for patients with AAP, but findings seldom are contributory to a diagnosis. Despite the association of elevated WBC counts with many infectious and inflammatory processes, the WBC count is neither sufficiently sensitive nor sufficiently specific to be considered a discriminatory test to help establish or rule out a serious cause for the pain. Even serial WBC counts have failed to differentiate surgical from nonsurgical conditions. The WBC count is therefore not helpful for diagnosis, except when a low WBC indicates immunosuppression. Serum electrolytes, even in the presence of protracted emesis or diarrhea, are abnormal in less than 1% of patients. BUN concentrations can be elevated in gastrointestinal hemorrhage and dehydration, but such conditions are better detected and quantified by history and physical examination. Increased serum Cr usually is indicative of renal dysfunction. Blood glucose, AG, and serum ketone determinations are useful in DKA, one cause of AAP and tachypnea.

Liver enzymes and coagulation studies are helpful only in a small subset of patients with suspected liver disease. If pancreatitis is suspected, the most useful diagnostic result is serum lipase elevated to at least double the normal value, because it is more specific and more sensitive than serum amylase for this process. Measurement of serum amylase is of no value if a serum lipase level is available. Serum lactate levels are elevated late in bowel ischemia, and such determination may be useful if this entity is suspected, but serum lactate levels cannot be considered either sufficiently sensitive or specific enough to establish or exclude the diagnosis on their own.

Plain radiography of the abdomen has limited usefulness in the evaluation of AAP and should be performed only when bowel obstruction or radiopaque foreign body is suspected and there is no intent to obtain a CT scan. For suspected perforated hollow viscus, an upright chest radiograph is a better study than an abdominal film but is not indicated if the plan is to proceed to CT scan regardless of the findings on the plain film. CT of the abdomen has become the imaging modality of choice with nonobstetric, nonbiliary AAP. It allows visualization of both intraperitoneal and extraperitoneal structures and has a high degree of accuracy. CT is not indicated for biliary disease, however, for which ultrasound is a much better modality.

CT has increased diagnostic utility in elderly patients for several reasons. Older people with AAP are significantly more likely to require surgery and have a greatly increased mortality compared with younger adults. In the elderly population, CT results change management or disposition decisions in a significant proportion of patients. Table 35-3 lists the most common findings on CT scans in elders with AAP.

Table 35-3 Most Common Diagnostic CT Findings in older Patients in the ED with AAP

FINDING	PERCENT OF ABDOMINAL CT SCANS
Small bowel obstruction or ileus	18%
Diverticulitis	18%
Urolithiasis	10%
Cholelithiasis	10%
Abdominal mass or neoplasm	8%
Pyelonephritis	7%
Pancreatitis	6%

CT with IV contrast alone also has been shown to be sensitive and specific for the confirmation or exclusion of acute appendicitis. The exclusion of oral contrast in these patients significantly decreases ED time to disposition and improves patient satisfaction.

CT is an important adjunct in ED care, but the decision to scan is carefully weighed against the patient's history, physical examination findings, age, and gender. In particular, a patient with a history of chronic undifferentiated AAP, multiple previous CT scans, and alternative diagnoses may benefit from observation as opposed to another CT scan.

Bedside transabdominal and transvaginal ultrasonography have emerged as extremely useful adjuncts, decreasing time to diagnosis of life-threatening abdominopelvic conditions. Useful indications include the following:

- Identification of an intrauterine pregnancy
- Measurement of the cross-sectional diameter of the abdominal aorta to determine the presence of an abdominal aortic aneurysm
- Detection of free intraperitoneal fluid indicating hemorrhage, pus,or extrusion of gut contents
- Use as a diagnostic aid for detection of the following non–life-threatening conditions:
  - Gallstones or a dilated common bile duct, which may be a clue to the presence of choledocholithiasis
  - Pericholecystic fluid or gallbladder wall thickening, which may be indicative of cholecystitis
  - Free intraperitoneal fluid indicating ascites
  - Hydronephrosis indicating possible obstructive uropathy
  - Inferior vena cava distention or collapse as an indicator of volume status

The results of sonographic examinations are operator dependent, and misdiagnosis can occur because of failure to detect or identify pathology, incorrect identification of normal anatomy as pathologic, or overinterpretation of correctly identified findings (e.g., the mere presence of gallstones does not indicate that cholelithiasis is the cause of the pain).

DIFFERENTIAL DIAGNOSIS

The differential considerations with AAP include a significant number of potentially life- or organ-threatening entities, particularly in the setting of a hemodynamically unstable or toxic-appearing patient. Severely ill patients require timely resuscitation and expeditious evaluation for potentially life-threatening conditions. A focused history and examination should be conducted, and the patient should be placed in a monitored acute care area well equipped for airway control, quick intravenous access, and fluid administration. This approach is particularly important in dealing with elder or potentially pregnant patients (Tables 35-1 and 35-2).

Women of reproductive age with AAP should undergo pregnancy testing early, and a known pregnancy or a positive result on urine or serum pregnancy testing associated with AAP in the ED should be considered to represent an ectopic pregnancy until proved otherwise. If evidence of blood loss is present, early obstetric consultation and diagnostic ultrasonography should be promptly sought. Bedside transabdominal sonography may identify free intraperitoneal fluid during the evaluation of shock, which may be sufficient evidence to justify operative intervention in the context of a positive pregnancy test and appropriate history and physical examination findings. Despite the limitations already described, the approach to the differential diagnosis of AAP generally is based on the location of maximum tenderness. Fig. 35-1 shows locations of subjective pain and maximal tenderness on palpation related to various underlying causes. In women of childbearing age, a positive result on pregnancy testing may indicate ectopic pregnancy, but the entire spectrum of intra-abdominal conditions remains in the differential diagnosis, as for the nonpregnant patient. When the very broad differential list is compartmentalized by both history and physical examination, ancillary testing should proceed to either confirm or support the clinical suspicion.

Close to one half of the patients in the ED with AAP will have no conclusive diagnosis. It is incumbent on the clinician to reconsider the extra-abdominal causes of AAP (Box 35-1), with special consideration in elders and immunocompromised patients, before arriving at the diagnosis of "nonspecific AAP."

EMPIRICAL MANAGEMENT

The main therapeutic goals in managing AAP are physiologic stabilization, mitigation of symptoms and expeditious diagnosis, with consultation if required.

There is no evidence to support withholding analgesics from patients with AAP to preserve the accuracy of subsequent abdominal examinations. Pain relief may facilitate the diagnosis in patients ultimately requiring surgery. In the acute setting, analgesia usually is accomplished with intravenously titrated opioids. Meperidine (Demerol) has an unfavorable side effect profile and should be avoided. Intravenous ketorolac, the only parenteral nonsteroidal anti-inflammatory drug, is useful for both ureteral and biliary colic, as well as some gynecologic conditions, but is not indicated for general treatment of undifferentiated AAP. Ketorolac has been shown to cause increased bleeding times in healthy volunteers; it should be avoided in patients with gastrointestinal bleeding and potential surgical candidates.

Aside from analgesics, a variety of other medications may be helpful to patients with AAP. The burning pain caused by gastric acid may be relieved by antacids. Intestinal cramping may be diminished with oral anticholinergics, such as the combination agent atropine-scopolamine-hyoscyamine-phenobarbital (Donnatal).

Antiemetics such as promethazine, prochlorperazine, ondansetron, or droperidol can be useful for nausea and vomiting. Gastric emptying by nasogastric tube with suction is appropriate for suspected small bowel obstruction with intractable pain and vomiting.

If intra-abdominal infection is suspected, broad-spectrum antibiotic therapy should be initiated promptly. Abdominal infections are often polymicrobial, and coverage for enteric gram-negative, gram-positive, and anaerobic bacteria is included. In the choice of antibiotic or combination, the following should be considered:

- Unless local antibiotic resistance dictates otherwise, secondgeneration cephalosporins (e.g., cefamandole, cefotetan, cefoxitin) or quinolone (ciprofloxacin, levofloxacin) may be combined with metronidazole for the initial dose of antibiotics in the ED. Other noncephalosporin, β-lactam agents with β-lactamase antagonists (e.g.,ampicillin-sulbactam, piperacillin-tazobactam, ticarcillin-clavulanate) are alternatives.
- Many enteric gram-negative bacilli mutate rapidly to produce β-lactamases that are poorly antagonized by specific drug combinations containing clavulanate, sulbactam,or tazobactam. A carbapenem (e.g., imipenem, meropenem) or cefepime is an alternative for patients who may have recently received other antibiotics.

Whether to provide coverage for Enterococcus species is still a subject of debate, and the decision to treat for these bacteria specifically can be made after consultation. Immunocompromised patients may require antifungal agents.

DISPOSITION

Because up to 40% of patients with AAP receive the diagnosis of nonspecific AAP, decisions regarding disposition can be as difficult as the diagnosis in these patients. Categories for disposition may include surgical versus nonsurgical consultation and management, admission for observation, and discharge to home with follow-up evaluation. The decision to admit a patient to an observation unit or a hospital bed factors in the following:

- Information gained from the history, physical examination, and test results
- The likelihood of any suspected disease
- Any potential ramifications of progression of a known disease, or of incorrect diagnosis or management
- The likelihood of appropriate and timely follow-up after hospital discharge
- The ability of the patient to return if symptoms worsen Clinically stable patients may be discharged from the ED with appropriate follow-up care, possibly to include repeated physical examination or additional diagnostic imaging if indicated.

In the case of nonspecific AAP that is considered potentially worrisome, CT scan, observation, or follow-up reevaluation after 8 to 12 hr all are valid options. Follow-up evaluation can be done through a return visit to the ED, via an appointment with a primary care physician, or as part of an observation unit protocol.

Before discharge of a patient with an undiagnosed cause of nonspecific AAP, several conditions should be met. The abdominal examination findings should not indicate serious organ pathology or peritoneal irritation, and the patient should have normal or near-normal vital signs. Pain and nausea should be controlled, and the patient should be able to take fluids by mouth. If a patient is to be discharged home without a specific diagnosis, clear instructions are given and include the following information:

- What to do for relief of symptoms or to maximize chances of resolution of the condition (e.g., avoiding exacerbating food or activities, taking medications as prescribed)
- Under what circumstances, with whom, and in what time frame to seek follow-up evaluation, if all goes as desired on the basis of what is known when the patient is in the ED
- Under what conditions to seek more urgent care because of unexpected changes in the condition (such as with natural progression of the process before improvement, incorrect diagnosis made in the ED, or untoward reactions to medications).

(JIN Heng CUI Shuzhang)

Chapter 36

Abdominal Aortic Aneurysm

KEY CONCEPTS

AAA is a true aneurysm, meaning a localized dilation of the aorta (a diameter of 3 cm or more) caused by its weakening wall, and involving all three layers (intima, media, and adventitia) of the arterial wall.

A ruptured AAA should be considered in any patient older than 50 yr with otherwise unexplained abdominal or back pain. The complete triad of pain, hypotension, and a pulsatile mass is often absent.

An AAA can rupture into the gastrointestinal tract (aortoenteric fistula [AEF]) or IVC (aortocaval fistula).

Bedside ultrasonography can quickly confirm or exclude the presence of an aneurysm. A CT scan is appropriate only if it can be obtained very quickly without compromising the patient's care.

The hemodynamically unstable patient in whom a ruptured AAA has been diagnosed or is strongly suspected should be taken to the operating room as soon as possible.

PERSPECTIVE

AAA is a true aneurysm, meaning a localized dilation of the aorta caused by its weakening wall, and involving all three layers (intima, media, and adventitia) of the arterial wall (Fig. 36-1). A false aneurysm, or pseudoaneurysm, is a collection of flowing blood which communicates with the arterial lumen but is not enclosed by the normal vessel wall; it is contained only by the adventitia or surrounding soft tissue. Pseudoaneurysms can arise from a defect in the arterial wall or a leaking anastomosis after AAA repair.

AAA is distinct from aortic dissection, which

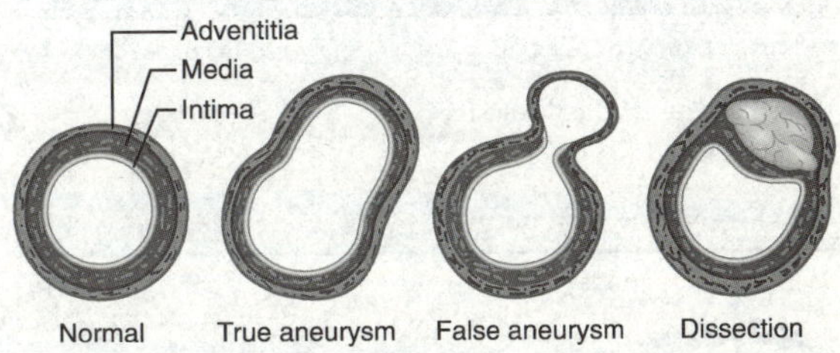

Fig. 36-1 Types of aortic aneurysms.

sometimes is incorrectly called a "dissecting aortic aneurysm". In aortic dissection, blood enters the media of the aorta and splits (dissects) the aortic wall.

An aneurysm can develop in any segment of the aorta, but most involves the aorta below the renal arteries. The diameter of the normal adult infrarenal aorta is approximately 2 cm, and a diameter of 3 cm or more defines an AAA.

Epidemiology

AAA is a disease of aging, and the prevalence of AAA is expected to increase as the population of elderly patients grows. AAA is rare before the age of 50 yr but is found in 2% to 5% of men older than 50.The average age at the time of diagnosis is 65 to 70, and men are affected much more often than women. The patient often has concomitant atherosclerotic occlusive disease of the coronary, carotid, or peripheral vessels, which may influence the clinical presentations, complications, and managements.

Several risk factors for the development of an AAA have been established. An AAA can be found in 5% to 10% of elderly men who are screened with ultrasonography and in an even higher percentage of patients with CAD or peripheral vascular disease. The presence or absence of risk factors should not strongly influence diagnostic considerations in any individual patient (Table 36-1). A family history of an AAA is a very strong risk factor; those with an affected first-degree relative have a markedly increased risk of developing an AAA. Smoking is also a significant risk factor for AAA. Although awareness of high-risk groups can speed the recognition of AAA, the consideration of AAA should not be restricted to patients in these groups.

Table 36-1 Prevalence of AAA in Selected Risk Groups

GROUP	INCIDENCE (%)
Men aged 65 yr or older	5-10
Patients with CAD or occlusive peripheral vascular disease	10-15
Brothers of patients with AAA	20-30

PRINCIPLES OF DISEASE

Pathophysiology

AAA have traditionally been attributed to atherosclerosis, but patients with advanced atherosclerosis have occlusive disease, not aneurysms. Recent data suggest that patients with AAA have biochemical abnormalities leading to the loss of elastin and collagen, the major structural components of the aortic wall. The propensity to form aneurysms may have a genetic basis, but the exact mode of inheritance is uncertain.

AAA may also have specific causes, such as infection, trauma, connective tissue diseases, and arteritis. However, such aneurysms are rare compared with nonspecific, degenerative aneurysms.

Natural History

AAA progressively enlarge, ultimately resulting in rupture of the aneurysm and fatal hemorrhage. Although other complications are possible, by far the most common and most critical is rupture.

The most important factor determining the risk of rupture is the size of the aneurysm. The risk increases dramatically with increased aneurysm size, and most ruptured AAAs have diameters greater than 5 cm. The growth rate of the AAA, in addition to other anatomic factors, may also be important in determining the risk of rupture. Although rupture of aneurysms smaller than 4 cm is rare, no aneurysm is completely "safe". Any aneurysm can rupture and cause the patient's ED presentation.

Rupture of an AAA usually occurs into the retroperitoneum, where hemorrhage may be temporarily limited by clot and tamponade at the rupture site, but 10% to 30% involve free intraperitoneal rupture, which is often rapidly fatal. Occasionally, rupture occurs into the gastrointestinal tract or the inferior vena cava.

Complications can also arise from an intact AAA. The walls of an AAA are often lined with clot and atheromatous material, which can embolize and occlude distal vessels. Aortic thrombosis may occur rarely. Patients can also have complications caused by impingement on adjacent structures.

In approximately 5% of AAA, a dense inflammatory and fibrotic reaction develops in the aneurysm wall and adjacent retroperitoneal tissue. In these "inflammatory" AAA, the periaortic fibrosis may incorporate and obstruct adjacent structures, such as the ureters or duodenum.

The overwhelming concern in the patient with an AAA is the potential for rupture of the aneurysm. The natural history of expansion and rupture can be interrupted only by timely repair.

CLINICAL FEATURES

Unruptured Aneurysms

Because most AAA cause no symptoms until they rupture, the prevalence of symptoms in patients with unruptured AAA is unknown. Patients may have symptoms that lead to the aneurysm's discovery and are therefore believed to be caused by the aneurysm, although true causation cannot be determined in most cases. These symptoms can include pain in the abdomen, back, or flank; an awareness of an abdominal mass or fullness; or a sensation of abdominal pulsations.

The pain associated with stable, intact aneurysms has a gradual onset and a vague, dull quality. It is usually constant but may be described as throbbing or colicky. Acute or severe pain is an ominous symptom that suggests imminent or actual aortic rupture.

In most cases, an AAA is asymptomatic and is discovered incidentally on physical examination, on a radiologic study done for other reasons, or by an ultrasonography aneurysm screening program. Symptoms usually do not develop until the aneurysm ruptures.

The most prominent physical finding is a pulsatile, expansile abdominal mass. The aortic bifurcation is at the level of the umbilicus, and an AAA can be palpated at or above this level. If the iliac arteries are also aneurysmal, the mass may extend below the umbilicus. The right border of an AAA may be palpable to the right of midline, whereas a normal or tortuous aorta is usually not. Most intact AAA are nontender; tenderness suggests aneurysm expansion or rupture.

Symptomatic aneurysms are usually fairly large and are often palpable. Likewise, the patient with an aneurysm large enough to warrant elective repair often has a palpable abdominal mass. However, an AAA may be difficult to palpate if the aneurysm is small or the patient is obese. There is virtually no risk of causing aneurysm rupture by abdominal palpation.

Physical examination may raise suspicion regarding an AAA even when the aorta is of normal size. A tortuous aorta may feel enlarged, and prominent aortic pulsations, especially in a thin patient, may simulate an aneurysm. Moreover, pulsations from a normal aorta may be transmitted to an adjacent abdominal mass. Nonetheless, clinical suspicion of AAA warrants further investigation.

Abdominal bruit is uncommon in patients with AAA. The presence of a bruit is also nonspecific, as bruits can originate in a stenotic renal, iliac, or mesenteric artery. A loud continuous bruit suggests the diagnosis of aortovenous fistula, a rare complication of AAA.

Perfusion distal to an AAA is usually well maintained, and most patients have normal femoral pulses. Diminished femoral pulses may result from iliofemoral occlusive disease or from hypotension in the patient with a ruptured aneurysm.

Thromboembolic complications can occur spontaneously or when atheromatous plaques are disrupted during invasive intravascular procedures. Large emboli can acutely occlude major vessels such as the iliac, femoral, or popliteal artery, causing acute painful lower extremity ischemia with absent distal pulses. Rarely, the aneurysm itself can thrombose, rendering both lower extremities acutely ischemic. More often, however, microemboli consisting of cholesterol crystals or clot obstruct small distal vessels, such as the digital arteries of the toes and arterioles and capillaries of the skin. These patients have livedo reticularis; one or more cool, painful, cyanotic toes; and palpable pedal pulses. This constellation of findings, often called the *blue toe syndrome*, is highly suggestive of a proximal source of emboli. When an AAA is the source, the aneurysm is often too small to palpate and may be discovered only after radiologic investigation.

Rarely, an intact AAA causes symptoms by compressing adjacent structures, with symptoms depending on the structures involved. Large, long-standing aneurysms can cause vertebral body erosion and severe back pain. Compression of the duodenum between the superior mesenteric artery and an AAA can cause duodenal obstruction, vomiting, and weight loss. Obstruction of the ureters in the patient with an inflammatory aneurysm can cause symptoms suggestive of ureteral colic.

Ruptured Aneurysms

Pain-Hypotension-Mass Triad

Although the classic triad of a ruptured AAA is pain, hypotension, and a pulsatile abdominal mass, many patients have only one or two components of this triad, and an occasional patient has none of the classic features.

Rupture is often the first manifestation of an AAA. Some patients, however, have a previously diagnosed AAA, and a decision not to operate electively may have been made because the aneurysm was small or the patient was considered too high risk. If such a patient has acute symptoms, the presumptive diagnosis is aneurysm rupture.

Most patients with a ruptured AAA experience pain in the abdomen, back, or flank. The pain is usually acute, severe, and constant and can radiate to the chest, thigh, inguinal area, or scrotum. If the patient's mental status is compromised by severe hypotension, the history of pain may be unobtainable.

In patients with a ruptured aneurysm, the duration of symptoms before presentation varies greatly. Some patients are seen shortly after severe pain and hypotension develop. In others, rupture is initially contained in the retroperitoneum, blood loss is small, and the presentation is delayed. Rare patients with a ruptured AAA may have symptoms for several days or even weeks before seeking medical attention; therefore a long duration of symptoms does not exclude the diagnosis of ruptured AAA.

Rupture of an AAA may be accompanied by nausea and vomiting, and sudden hemorrhage can cause syncope or near-syncope. Compensatory hemodynamic mechanisms may then return the BP and cerebral perfusion to normal. Transient improvement in symptoms is common but will be followed by hemodynamic deterioration if diagnosis and treatment are delayed.

Ruptured AAA are often large, and most patients have palpable abdominal masses. As with intact aneurysms, a ruptured AAA may not be palpable if the aneurysm is small or the patient is obese. The examination may be difficult if abdominal guarding is present or if an ileus causes significant distention. Aortic pulsations may not be prominent if the BP is low. When a mass is not palpable, the diagnosis may be delayed.

Hypotension is the least consistent part of the triad, occurring in approximately half of patients, and is often a late finding. When the initial blood loss is minor, vital signs are often normal. Patients with initially normal vital signs are more likely to be misdiagnosed and may quickly and unpredictably deteriorate and become hypotensive.

Occasionally, rupture into the retroperitoneum is sealed and contained for many weeks or months. When this occurs, patients develop abdominal or back pain, presumably at the time of aneurysm leakage, which subsequently diminishes or resolves completely. If the diagnosis is made, chronic rupture (organized hematoma) is found at surgery. These patients can have chronic pain and may progress to free rupture and massive hemorrhage at any time.

Aortoenteric Fistula

An AAA can rupture into the gastrointestinal tract (aortoenteric fistula [AEF]) or inferior vena cava (aortocaval fistula) . A primary AEF is formed when an unrepaired AAA erodes into the gastrointestinal tract, usually the third or fourth portion of the duodenum. A secondary AEF, a communication between the site of previous aortic surgery and the gastrointestinal tract, can occur as a late complication of AAA repair and should be considered as the leading diagnosis in any patient with a severe gastrointestinal bleed and a history of aortic graft placement.

Early in the formation of a primary AEF, the bowel wall is eroded from the outside by the adjacent AAA. This can lead to the leakage of intestinal contents, with local infection and sometimes abscess formation. Eventually, breakdown of the aortic wall leads to an AEF and gastrointestinal bleeding.

The patient with an AEF may have abdominal or back pain, fever and other signs of intra-abdominal infection, or gastrointestinal bleeding. Because most of these fistulaes are into the duodenum, hemorrhage usually manifests as hematemesis or melena. The initial bleeding results from erosion of vessels in the bowel wall and is often minor. Later, often after several days to a week or longer, massive bleeding results from rupture into the intestinal lumen.

Primary AEF, although rare, should be considered in any patients older than 50 yr with unexplained gastrointestinal bleeding. If an AAA is diagnosed by history, physical examination, or any other modality, the patient should be presumed to have an AEF until proven otherwise.

Aortovenous (Aortocaval) Fistula

An aortovenous (usually aortocaval) fistula arises when periaortic inflammation causes adherence of the aorta to an adjacent vein, with pressure on the vessel walls causing the development of an arteriovenous communication. If concomitant extravasation of blood into the retroperitoneum occurs, the clinical presentation is similar to that of other patients with ruptured AAA, often with hypovolemic shock. More commonly, however, the aneurysm ruptures into the vena cava without leaking externally, and the signs and symptoms of a large arteriovenous fistula dominate the clinical picture.

As in other patients with AAA, a patient with an aortovenous fistula may have abdominal or back pain. An aneurysm that becomes fistulous with the vena cava is usually large, and 80% to 90% are palpable. A continuous abdominal bruit can be auscultated in approximately 75% of patients with aortovenous fistulae, and 25% of patients have a palpable abdominal thrill.

Shunting of blood from the arterial to the venous system increases venous pressure, venous volume, and venous return to the heart. Signs and symptoms of high-output CHF (dyspnea, jugular venous distention, pulmonary edema) are often present. The increased venous volume and pressure can cause lower extremity edema or cyanosis, and dilated superficial veins can be seen on the legs or abdominal wall. Distention and rupture of veins in the bladder mucosa can cause gross or microscopic hematuria; rectal bleeding can occur for similar reasons. Because of shunting of arterial blood into the venous system, the lower extremities may be cool with diminished pulses.

The patient with an aortovenous fistula often has renal insufficiency caused by a decrease in renal perfusion as a result of high-output congestive heart failure and increased renal venous pressure. Such patients may exhibit hematuria, which is common when an aortovenous fistula is present but not in other patients with AAA. CTA can rule out aortovenous fistula formation.

DIAGNOSTIC STRATEGIES

Abdominal Radiography

Plain film radiography is not indicated in the evaluation of a patient for suspected AAA. A normal plain abdominal radiograph does not exclude the presence of an AAA and rarely identifies alternative pathology. Even if an aneurysm is identified on plain film because it is calcified, imaging with CT is required to identify whether the aneurysm is an incidental or culprit lesion in the patient's presentation (Fig. 36-2).

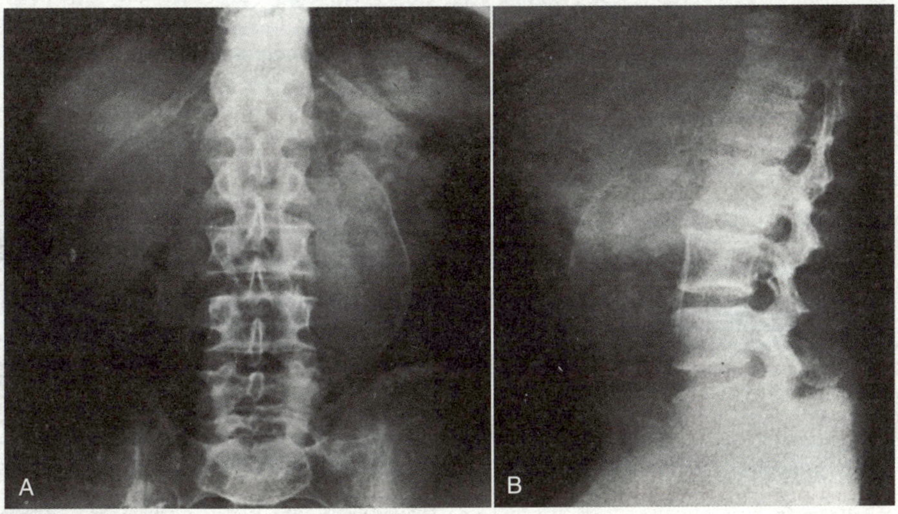

Fig. 36-2 Anteroposterior (A) and lateral (B) views of large abdominal aortic aneurysms with calcification of aortic wall.

Ultrasonography

Ultrasonography is virtually 100% sensitive in detecting AAA (Fig.36-3), when a technically adequate study can be obtained. Measurements of aortic diameter are very accurate and reproducible. Because it is relatively inexpensive and requires no contrast agents or radiation exposure, ultrasonography is used for nonemergency aneurysm diagnosis and to follow patients with known aneurysms.

Ultrasonography has distinct advantages in the emergency evaluation of a patient with a suspected ruptured AAA. It can be performed very rapidly at the patient's bedside, obviating the need to take a potentially unstable patient to the radiology suite. If an aorta with a normal diameter throughout its abdominal course is visualized, the patient does not have an AAA. In addition, ultrasonography sometimes provides alternative explanations for the patient's pain by revealing other conditions, such as acute cholecystitis.

However, ultrasonography has certain limitations. It is more operator-dependent than other diagnostic modalities and may be prone to technical or interpretive error. Even more than with elective

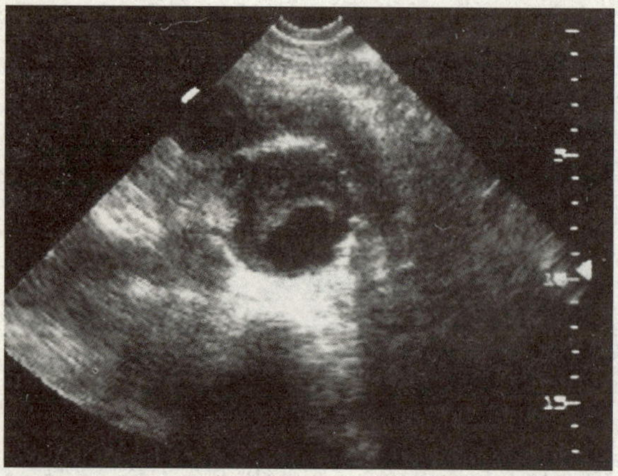

Fig. 36-3 Transverse sonogram of an abdominal aortic aneurysm. The central patent lumen is surrounded by an echogenic mural thrombus.

studies, in the emergency department the aorta may not be well visualized because of obesity or excess bowel gas. Ultrasonography is not immediately available in some EDs, requiring the patient to wait for the arrival of a technologist. Although ultrasonography is extremely sensitive in detecting an AAA, it cannot be relied on to reveal whether an AAA has ruptured.

Free intraperitoneal or retroperitoneal blood, seen in the presence of an AAA, confirms a rupture. However, the sensitivity of emergency ultrasonography in detecting extraluminal blood is very low. The purpose of the study is to confirm or exclude the presence of an aneurysm; clinical information (or a CT scan) must be used to determine the likelihood of rupture. Ultrasonography with the use of contrast agents may aid in the detection of leaking blood, but the clinical usefulness of this modality remains to be determined. If ultrasonography reveals an AAA in an unstable patient, aneurysm rupture is presumed, and the patient requires immediate aneurysm repair.

Computed Tomography

The abdominal CT scan is the diagnostic test of choice in the evaluation of a patient with suspected ruptured AAA and is virtually 100% accurate in determining the presence or absence of an AAA and the presence of bleeding.CT also provides detailed anatomic information about the aneurysm.

An intravenous contrast agent is desirable, but not essential, in emergency situations. With significant, prolonged hypotension or known renal disease, intravenous contrast should be avoided to prevent contrast-exacerbated nephropathy. Intravenous contrast will opacify the aortic lumen and distinguish the patent lumen from mural thrombus. It can also demonstrate periaortic fibrosis because the soft tissue surrounding an inflammatory AAA often enhances. However, intravenous contrast is not necessary to identify the aneurysm or acute hemorrhage.

CT is much more sensitive than ultrasonography in detecting retroperitoneal hemorrhage associated with aneurysm rupture. The reported sensitivity approaches 100% with the use of current generation scanning technology, with falsely negative studies sometimes occurring with very small ruptures. Blood is seen as a retroperitoneal fluid collection adjacent to the aneurysm, often tracking into the perinephric space or along the psoas muscle (Fig. 36-4).

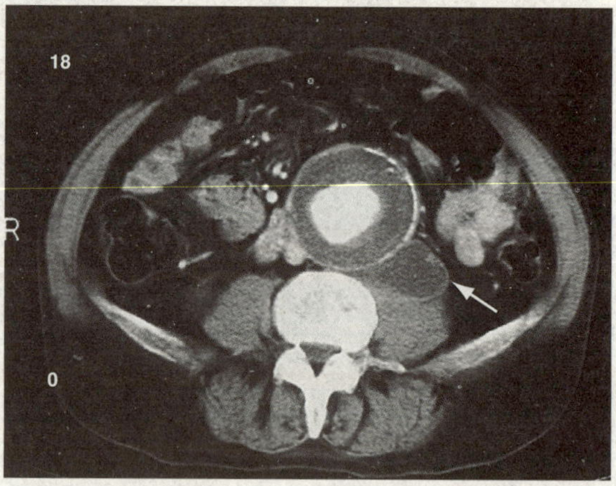

Fig. 36-4 CT scan of ruptured abdominal aortic aneurysm, with calcification of the aortic wall and intraluminal thrombus. The patent lumen enhances with the administration of contrast material, but the periaortic hematoma *(arrow)* does not.

Although a CT scan sometimes reveals signs of impending aneurysm rupture, it cannot reliably determine whether an AAA is the cause of the patient's pain or whether rupture of the aneurysm is imminent. Another cause of pain can be diagnosed only if the CT scan shows no aneurysm or shows an intact aneurysm and clearly demonstrates an alternative explanation for the patient's symptoms.

Other Diagnostic Modalities

Conventional angiography has no place in the emergency evaluation of the suspected ruptured AAA. Because contrast opacifies only the patent lumen and not mural thrombus, angiography often underestimates aneurysm size and can miss the aneurysm entirely. In addition, angiography is time-consuming and performed away from the ED. If detailed information is needed about the anatomy of the aneurysm or its relationship to nearby vessels, a CTA can provide the needed information.

MRI and MRA are very time-consuming, are logistically challenging, and provide no benefit over CT scan. Magnetic resonance scanning is not indicated in the evaluation of a patient with acute symptoms suspected to be related to AAA.

DIFFERENTIAL CONSIDERATIONS

Because the patient with a ruptured AAA usually has abdominal, back, or flank pain, with or without hypotension, common misdiagnoses are other disease processes that cause these symptoms (Box 36-1). The sudden onset of back pain often leads to the clinical suspicion of renal colic, with which AAA is often confused. Abdominal pain and tenderness can suggest pancreatitis, intestinal ischemia, or other intra-abdominal disorders. Musculoskeletal back pain is part of the differential diagnosis but should be confirmed by detailed history and physical examination, so that pain related to AAA is not mistakenly labeled as mechanical low back pain.

Box 36-1 Common Misdiagnoses in Patients with Ruptured Abdominal Aortic Aneurysms

Renal colic	Appendicitis
Acute abdomen	Perforated viscus
Pancreatitis	Bowel obstruction
Intestinal ischemia	Musculoskeletal back pain
Diverticulitis	AMI
Cholecystitis	

Presentation with epigastric pain and hypotension may lead to a presumptive diagnosis of acute myocardial infarction. Because the patient with a ruptured AAA often has coexistent CAD, blood loss from a ruptured aneurysm may diminish coronary perfusion and cause chest pain or electrocardiographic changes consistent with cardiac ischemia. These findings do not exclude the presence of a ruptured AAA.

Ruptured AAA should be considered in middle-aged or elderly patients with any part of the classic triad. The diagnosis of ruptured AAA should also be considered in making the diagnoses listed in Box 36-1, especially when the diagnosis is not clear-cut or the patient is at risk for an AAA.

MANAGEMENT

Ruptured Aneurysms

The patient with a ruptured AAA is unstable until the aorta is cross-clamped in the operating room or stabilized with endovascular techniques. No patient with a known or suspected aortic rupture should be considered stable, regardless of the initial vital signs or initial hemoglobin level. Patients taken to the operating room soon after ED arrival have a much higher survival rate than those in whom surgical care is delayed.

When the patient arrives at the ED, large-bore intravenous access should be established and blood sent for crossmatch. At least 6 units of blood should be made available initially, with notification to the blood bank of the potential need for significantly more, because patients with ruptured AAA often have large transfusion requirements. The surgical and anesthesia team should be notified immediately. Further management depends on the current hemodynamic condition and the level of diagnostic certainty.

The hemodynamically unstable patient in whom a ruptured AAA has been diagnosed or is strongly suspected should be taken to the operating room as soon as possible. Diagnostic testing should be kept to a minimum. The diagnosis can often be made from the clinical presentation and abdominal examination, and bedside ultrasonography can quickly confirm or exclude the presence of an aneurysm. A CT scan is appropriate only if it can be obtained very quickly without compromising the patient's care. Time-consuming tests inappropriately delay definitive therapy and increase the risk of exsanguination. Hypotensive patients may have to be taken to the operating room based on a strong clinical presumption of the diagnosis, without definitive diagnostic imaging. Some of these patients will not have ruptured aneurysms, but they usually have other acute abdominal conditions requiring laparotomy.

Attempts to resuscitate these patients fully and normalize the vital signs in the ED should be avoided. Hypotensive patients need to be taken to the operating room so that the aorta can be clamped, or occluded with a balloon, and hemorrhage stopped. Attempts to stabilize the patient in the ED are often fruitless and waste valuable time.

Fluid Resuscitation

The appropriate degree of preoperative volume resuscitation is controversial. Preoperative hypotension is the strongest predictor of mortality in the patient with a ruptured AAA. However, correction of the hypotension before the aorta is clamped may not improve mortality and may even be harmful.

It has been argued that hypotension slows bleeding in patients with AAA and allows local clot formation and tamponade of the rupture site. Raising the intravascular volume and BP before occluding the aorta may dislodge clots and cause further bleeding. Large volumes of crystalloid solution may contribute to bleeding by causing a dilutional coagulopathy. These concerns are similar to those in trauma patients with uncontrolled hemorrhage.

However, delaying resuscitation of hypotensive patients until they reach the operating room may also have deleterious effects. The patient with a ruptured AAA often survives the surgery but dies in the early postoperative period. These deaths are caused by complications of prolonged hypotension, such as myocardial infarction, respiratory failure, and renal failure. The patient with a ruptured AAA is usually elderly, often has coexisting conditions, and tolerates hypovolemia and hypotension poorly.

No prospective studies have compared different preoperative fluid regimens in hypotensive patients with ruptured AAAs, and the optimal resuscitation strategy has not been determined. The priority in these patients is expeditious transportation to the operating room for definitive control of aortic hemorrhage. In the prehospital setting and in the ED before the surgeon and the operating room are available, the BP should be raised with crystalloid or blood products to a level that maintains adequate cerebral and myocardial perfusion. The goal is to prevent irreversible end-organ damage. An arbitrary BP goal cannot be specified because the BP necessary for vital organ perfusion varies among patients, but a reasonable target is a SBP of 90 to 100 mmHg.

If blood products are to be administered in large amounts, FFP and PRBC are beneficial in patients with ruptured AAA. As with trauma patients, a PRBC: FFP ratio of less than 2 : 1 results in improved mortality.

Rarely, patients with ruptured AAA may be hypertensive on admission because of pain or underlying chronic hypertension. Unlike the situation with aortic dissection, no evidence exists that lowering the BP is beneficial in the patient with a ruptured AAA, and these patients are at risk of developing precipitous hypotension.

Diagnostic Confirmation

If an AAA can be diagnosed with bedside testing (abdominal examination or ultrasonography), the surgeon will often proceed immediately to the operating room with a clinical diagnosis of aneurysm rupture, as a delay in surgery places the patient with a ruptured AAA at risk for sudden and unpredictable hemodynamic deterioration. If the patient remains hemodynamically stable and an AAA can not be identified with bedside testing, or if anatomic detail is needed for endovascular repair, an abdominal CT scan can be obtained. This will confirm or exclude the presence of an aneurysm, define the aortic anatomy, and determine the patient's suitability for endovascular repair. The patient who is sent for a CT scan should be monitored closely and taken to the operating room immediately if hemodynamic deterioration occurs.

CT may provide confirmation of rupture, allowing the surgeon to avoid the complications of emergency surgery in a patient with an intact aneurysm. With emergency surgery, detailed anatomic evaluation and careful preoperative planning are often impossible, evaluation and optimization of the patient's cardiopulmonary and renal function may be precluded, and invasive hemodynamic monitoring may be unavailable. For these reasons, patients who are taken for emergency surgery and are found to have intact, symptomatic aneurysms have a higher mortality rate than patients undergoing elective aneurysm repair.

Surgery and Mortality

Ruptured AAA is uniformly fatal unless treated surgically. Thus once this diagnosis has been made, repair should be attempted in almost all patients. Attempts have been made to identify patients with a very low likelihood of survival, and it has been suggested that surgery can be withheld in patients with prehospital or ED cardiac arrest. However, no variables that can be assessed in the ED, including cardiac arrest, are universally predictive of a fatal outcome. Repair is indicated unless the patient's life expectancy is very short because of underlying illnesses or the patient's quality of life is so poor that repair is considered unreasonable. Hypotension is the most important factor predicting a poor outcome in patients undergoing surgery.

Although patients with ruptured AAA have a mortality of 30% to 40% with open repair, recent data suggest significantly lower mortality at centers experienced with the endovascular approach, with an operative mortality rate of 20% to 25%. Endovascular repair of ruptured aneurysms is becoming increasingly more common, even in unstable patients. If necessary, the surgeon can stabilize the patient by placing an aortic occlusion balloon above the aneurysm after rapidly accessing the femoral artery.

Not all patients with ruptured aneurysms will have an aorta that is anatomically suitable for endovascular repair. The method of repair will clearly be the surgeon's decision. Planning for the care of such patients should include the development of a well understood protocol that advises the ED staff about which services to mobilize and which diagnostic tests to perform for patients with ruptured AAA.

Unfortunately, even with the recent improvement in treatment outcomes, operative mortality rates significantly underestimate the true lethality of ruptured AAA. The patient with a ruptured AAA may die at home or may reach the hospital but die before surgery. When patients who do not reach the operating room are considered, the overall mortality rate may be as high as 80%.

Intact, Asymptomatic Aneurysms

An incidental diagnosis of AAA may be made in the ED. The decision to repair an asymptomatic aneurysm depends on the risk of aneurysm rupture, the patient's life expectancy and likelihood of dying from other causes, and the surgical risk. The last factors are determined by the patient's age and coexisting illnesses, whereas the risk of rupture is largely a function of aneurysm size.

Fewer small aneurysms are now repaired electively, potentially leaving a larger group of patients who may come to the ED with complications of an AAA. It is important to note that the "watchful waiting" approach is appropriate only for asymptomatic aneurysms, and rupture of the AAA should be strongly considered in the evaluation of any symptoms in these patients.

Traditional Repair

The conventional technique for repair of AAA is an open approach with a laparotomy. The aneurysm is opened longitudinally and repaired from within. A graft is inserted inside the aneurysm and anastomosed to uninvolved vessels above and below. If possible, a straight graft is used between the infrarenal and distal aorta, but if the aneurysm involves the aortic bifurcation or if iliac artery aneurysmal or occlusive disease is present, a bifurcation graft is used, with the distal anastomosis to the iliac or femoral arteries. The aneurysm wall is then closed around the graft to help separate it from adjacent structures.

Endovascular Repair

More than half of all AAA repairs are now performed without laparotomy, with use of endovascular techniques. A stent graft (a fabric graft supported by an internal wire frame) is placed into the femoral artery percutaneously or through a groin incision and is advanced under fluoroscopic guidance to a position that spans the aneurysm. The contralateral iliac limb is placed to form a bifurcated graft. Once in position, the graft is expanded to fit tightly against the walls of the aorta. Early straight (tube) grafts are now rarely used because of a high failure rate.

Endovascular surgery avoids the morbidity of a laparotomy and may allow the repair of AAAs in some high-risk patients who would not tolerate conventional surgery. Perioperative mortality is lower than that with open repair, but it is unclear whether this mortality benefit is sustained in the long-term. Endovascular repair requires more frequent reinterventions for graft-related complications. Because not all aneurysms are anatomically suitable for endovascular repair, detailed preoperative imaging and planning are required to make this determination. In addition, patients who have had endovascular aneurysm repair remain at risk for several complications, most importantly rupture of the aneurysm.

Survival

The operative mortality rate for elective AAA repair is approximately 1% to 2% for endovascular repair and 3% to 5% for open repair, in contrast to the much higher operative mortality with ruptured aneurysms. Patients who survive the operation have an excellent prognosis, with a long-term survival close to that of the general population. After repair of the aneurysm, long-term survival is primarily limited by associated cardiac disease.

LATE COMPLICATIONS OF REPAIR

Graft infection, AEF formation, and anastomotic aneurysm (pseudoaneurysm) formation can occur at any time from weeks to many years after the surgery. These complications often occur together, their clinical presentations overlap, and can be evaluated with angiography, CT scan, or ultrasonography. In addition, endovascular aneurysm repair has several unique complications, the most important of which is endoleak.

DISPOSITION

A patient with an acutely symptomatic AAA requires hospital admission and urgent or emergency repair. A patient whose aneurysm is asymptomatic and discovered incidentally should be referred for consideration of elective repair. The patient with an AAA should be referred for an outpatient workup only if it is clear that the symptoms prompting the ED visit are unrelated to the aneurysm. Although the incidental detection of AAA is common, such patients may suffer from poor subsequent follow-up and monitoring. If the patient is discharged, appropriate referral for follow-up is crucial, and instructions should be given to seek immediate medical attention if abdominal, back, or flank pain develops.

In the patient who has had an AAA repaired, unexplained fever, abdominal pain, or gastrointestinal bleeding suggests the presence of a graft-related complication and the need for inpatient evaluation.

(LI Lijun)

Chapter 37

Acute Disorders of the Small Intestine

KEY CONCEPTS

Postoperative adhesions are the most common cause of SBO, other common causes include neoplasms and hernias.

A closed loop obstruction can quickly lead to intestinal infarction and necrosis.

Only the CT finding of reduced intestinal wall enhancement, elevated WBC count, and guarding on physical examination were independent predictors of bowel strangulation.

AMEI should be considered in patients older than 50 yr with a history of cardiac disease who have acute abdominal pain, which may initially appear as severe pain that seems "out of proportion" to physical examination findings.

Within the diagnosis of AMEI are four distinct clinical entities with specific associated risk factors, clinical presentations, and treatments: mesenteric arterial embolism, mesenteric arterial thrombosis, nonocclusive mesenteric ischemia, and mesenteric venous thrombosis.

Recent advancements in multidetector CT angiographic scanning have made this modality a very sensitive and specific tool for the diagnosis of AMEI.

SMALL BOWEL OBSTRUCTION

Perspective

SBO is a relatively common problem encountered in the ED, accounting for an estimated 15% of all emergency admissions for abdominal pain.

There are several different types of SBO.The term mechanical obstruction implies the presence of a physical barrier to the movement of the intestinal contents. Obstructions of this type can be further subclassified according to the cause of the obstruction relative to the intestinal wall (Box 37-1). Lesions external to the intestinal tract can cause obstruction via compression from outside the gut. This is most commonly a result of postoperative adhesions, but hernias and intraperitoneal neoplasms are other causes. Lesions intrinsic to the intestinal wall itself can cause mechanical obstruction; such lesions include primary intestinal neoplasms, localized infection (i. e., intestinal wall TB), and trauma-related conditions (i. e., a hematoma of the intestinal wall). Lesions within the intestinal lumen itself can lead to obstruction. Bezoars, ingested foreign bodies, and gallstone ileus are all examples of the cause of this type of obstruction.

Box 37-1 Lesions Causing SBO Relative to the Intestinal Wall

External to Intestinal Wall
- Postoperative adhesions
- Hernias
- Volvulus
- Compressing masses (tumors, abscesses, hematomas)

Intrinsic to Intestinal Wall
- Primary neoplasms
- Inflammatory (e.g., Crohn's disease, radiation enteritis)
- Infectious causes (e.g., intestinal tuberculosis)
- Intussusception
- Traumatic (intestinal wall hematoma)

Intraluminal
- Bezoars
- Foreign bodies
- Gallstones
- *Ascaris* infestation

Another important distinction of SBO is whether

the obstruction is a simple or closed-loop obstruction. A simple obstruction occurs at a single point. On the other hand, in a closed-loop type obstruction the intestine is obstructed at two locations.This can occur when a twist develops in the mesentery or, in the case of an internal hernia, when a loop of bowel becomes entrapped in a defect in the mesentery (Fig. 37-1). If not promptly recognized and relieved, a closed loop obstruction can quickly lead to intestinal infarction and necrosis.

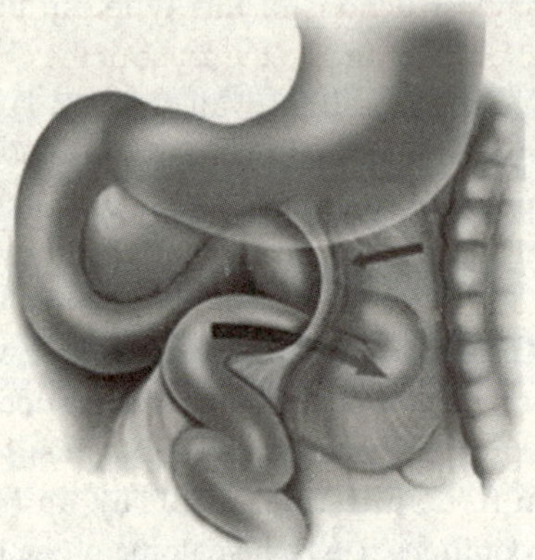

Fig. 37-1 Diagram of internal hernia. Note the formation of a "closed-loop," which creates a high risk for strangulation.

A neurogenic or functional obstruction occurs as a result of disruption of the normal coordinated peristaltic activity of the gastrointestinal tract in the absence of a physical blockage within the intestinal lumen. This is also commonly referred to as an adynamic ileus. The causes of adynamic ileus are listed in Box 37-2.

Box 37-2 Causes of Adynamic Ileus

- Metabolic disease (especially hypokalemia)
- Medications (e.g., narcotics)
- Infection (retroperitoneal, pelvic, intrathoracic)
- Abdominal trauma
- Laparotomy

Finally, the term pseudo-obstruction refers to a poorly understood and complex syndrome in which the signs and symptoms of a mechanical obstruction, including the appearance of dilated bowel on radiography, are present in the absence of a mechanical lesion.Pseudo-obstruction can arise from many causes, including degenerative neuropathies, autoimmune and paraneoplastic disease, and hereditary conditions.The symptoms of pseudo-obstruction are often chronic and respond poorly to treatment.

Principles of Disease

In the presence of a mechanical obstruction, the bowel proximal to the blockage first becomes mildly dilated by the accumulation of partially digested food and normal intestinal secretions.Increased intestinal dilation causes an increase in peristalsis throughout the intestines, which can trigger frequent and loose bowel movements early in the progression of the obstruction as well as episodes of nausea and vomiting. As the process continues, the bowel wall becomes edematous and the normal absorptive function of the intestinal wall decreases, leading to further accumulation of contents in the intestinal lumen proximal to the obstruction. Owing to the loss of normal intestinal motility, bacterial overgrowth begins to occur in the proximal small bowel. It is this overgrowth in a location of the intestines.As the obstruction continues, transudative fluid loss occurs into the peritoneal cavity, leading to worsening hypovolemia and dehydration. In addition, if the obstruction is proximal in location, continued bouts of emesis can lead to electrolyte abnormalities, metabolic alkalosis, and severe hypovolemia and shock.

In the presence of a closed-loop obstruction, the increase in the intraluminal pressure occurs much more rapidly because the intestinal contents cannot flow retrograde. Intestinal venous congestion and then arterial obstruction can also progress quickly to intestinal ischemia and infarction. This is referred to as a strangulation obstruction.

The second most common cause of SBO is tumors, which are responsible for roughly 20% of cases. This includes both malignancies, such as adenocarcinomas, carcinoid tumors, lymphomas, and sarcomas, and benign conditions, including adenomas, leiomyomas, and lipomas. In addition to these primary gastrointestinal tumors, gynecologic cancers, especially ovarian cancer, are a very common cause of SBO. There are also numerous case reports of metastatic disease leading to SBO, including metastatic breast, skin, and testicular cancers.

Hernias are the third most common cause of SBO. Similar to their relative frequency in general, ventral and inguinal hernias are most often encountered, but femoral hernia, parastomal hernia, lateral ventral hernia (also called spigelian hernia), and internal hernia may also lead to SBO.

Although rare in the general population, internal hernias (Fig. 37-1) are a recognized complication of bariatric surgery, especially when a Roux-en-Y type procedure has been performed.

Another rare type of hernia is the obturator hernia. This hernia is especially common in elderly women who have recently lost a significant amount of weight. The female pelvis is wider and the obturator canal is more oblique in women than in men. This often emaciated patients, predisposes to the development of an obturator hernia. Because an external mass is absent, the diagnosis can be especially challenging,it carries the highest mortality of any abdominal hernia, at nearly 70% when incarcerated.

Gallstone ileus is another rare but important cause of mechanical SBO (Fig. 37-2, see color illustration). It is most frequently seen in elder patients with significant underlying medical problems. The pathogenesis involves the entry of a gallstone into the intestinal tract through a biliary-enteric fistula. This results from the localized inflammation of cholecystitis, and in the majority of cases entry occurs via a cholecystoduodenal fistula.After entering the intestinal lumen, the gallstone migrates distally.Eventually, the gallstone becomes lodged,and the patient then develops symptoms of obstruction.

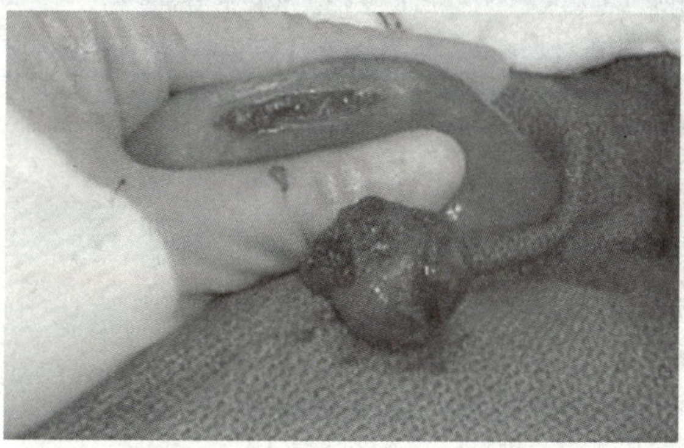

Fig. 37-2 Gallstone ileus of the small intestine at laparotomy.

Small bowel volvulus is a potentially catastrophic cause of SBO. Primary small bowel volvulus occurs in an otherwise normal abdominal cavity; secondary small bowel volvulus occurs when a congenital or acquired abnormality leads to the development of the volvulus.Diet is thought to play a role in some cases. Alterations in gut motility and increased small bowel length have also been suggested as possible predisposing factors. Secondary causes of small bowel volvulus include intestinal malrotation caused by the arrest of normal rotation of the embryonic gut or as a result of postoperative adhesions.

Intussusception describes the invagination or "telescoping" of a part of the small intestine into itself. This results in the development of venous and lymphatic congestion with consequent intestinal edema.A mechanical cause is found in more than 90% of adult cases. Tumors are discovered as the initiating cause in more than 65% of adult cases.

Clinical Features

History

Patients with SBO commonly report crampy abdominal pain, abdominal distention, nausea, vomiting, constipation, or the inability to pass flatus. The pain is often described as periumbilical in location and typically has a crescendo-decrescendo pattern. The recurrent waves of discomfort can last from seconds to minutes. In more proximal obstruction, symptoms of nausea and vomiting can be much more severe, and the onset of symptoms is often more abrupt. Distal obstructions typically cause symptoms over a slower period of 1 to 2 d and are frequently accompanied by greater abdominal distention. It is important to remember that the colon requires up to 24 hr to empty after the formation of SBO, and the associated small bowel distention stimulates peristalsis. Because of this, flatus and the passage of stool may continue even in the presence of a complete obstruction. A thorough past surgical history should be obtained, and any history of malignancy or inflammatory bowel disease should be determined.

Physical Examination

As with all patients in the ED, the physical examination should start with a careful evaluation of the patient's hemodynamic status, degree of distress, and general condition.Inspection of the patient should include a careful search for abdominal distention and hernias and should include a genital examination. Bowel sounds in SBO are frequently described as high pitched and "tinkling" in nature,they are also frequently decreased or absent in SBO.

The presence of peritoneal signs usually indicates late obstruction with complications, including strangulation. However, it should be noted that abdominal palpation in the setting of significant bowel dilation can give the false impression of peritonitis, because quick compression-decompression of dilated bowel may elicit a significant pain response for true peritonitis.

Complications

Persistent vomiting can lead to significant hypovolemia, metabolic alkalosis, and shock. If strangulation occurs, necrosis of the bowel can lead to perforation and leakage of contaminated bowel contents into the peritoneal space. This can cause peritonitis, intraabdominal abscess formation, and sepsis.There are also several potential complications related to surgical intervention for SBO, including wound infection and short bowel syndrome.For patients with SBO secondary to adhesions, the relative risk of recurrence increases with the number of prior episodes of obstruction.

Diagnostic Strategies

Although laboratory tests are not helpful in diagnosing the presence of SBO, they can be very useful in assessing the degree of dehydration and metabolic disruption resulting from the obstruction. These have included lactate and CPK.

Plain radiographic findings are estimated to be diagnostic in approximately 50% to 60% of cases of SBO, equivocal in 20% to 30%, and normal, nonspecific, or misleading in 10% to 20%.

Abdominal plain film radiographs should include both supine and upright or decubitus studies. An upright chest radiograph may also be obtained.Characteristic plain radiographic findings of SBO include distended loops of bowel, normally greater than 3 cm in diameter, seen centrally in the radiograph (Fig. 37-3).

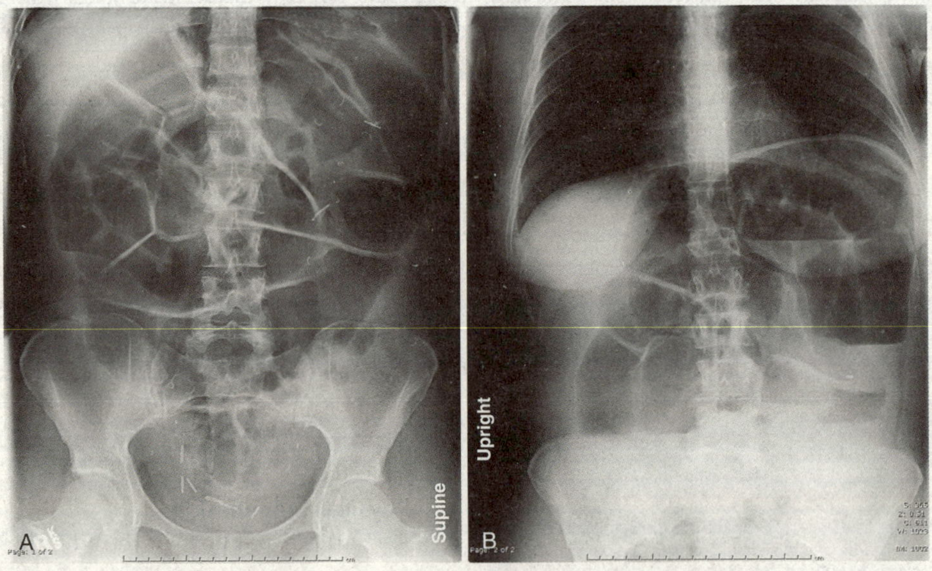

Fig. 37-3 A, Supine plain film radiograph showing dilated loops of small bowel in a patient with SBO. B, Upright abdominal plain radiograph revealing multiple air-fluid levels and small bowel dilation, consistent with a diagnosis of SBO.

If the obstructed small bowel contains more fluid than air, the classic radiographic findings may be absent.An adynamic ileus,tends to show extensive air-filled loops throughout the entire gastrointestinal system, and no small bowel dilation.

CT has been shown to detect SBO with a high degree of sensitivity and specificity. CT provides more information about the cause of obstruction, such as a tumor.

Finally,only the CT finding of reduced intestinal wall enhancement, elevated WBC count, and guarding on physical examination were independent predictors of bowel strangulation. Of these, the CT finding was by far the most specific at 96%, with a likelihood ratio of 9.3 for the presence of strangulation.

Differential Considerations

The diagnosis of SBO should be considered in any patient with abdominal pain and vomiting, especially if he or she has a history of prior abdominal surgery. It may be difficult to differentiate SBO from nonobstructive intestinal motility disorders such as adynamic ileus or intestinal pseudo-obstruction by history and physical examination alone.

The other conditions to consider in the differential diagnosis range widely from benign to potentially life-threatening. These include constipation, cholelithiasis or nephrolithiasis, ectopic pregnancy, pancreatitis, peptic ulcer disease, atypical MI, leaking AAA, and mesenteric ischemia.

Management and Disposition

Hemodynamically unstable patients should be aggressively resuscitated with crystalloid solution. In the era of modern antiemetics, if the patient's symptoms of nausea and vomiting can be controlled with medication, it may be reasonable to delay nasogastric tube insertion. However, if symptoms persist or if the patient has an altered level of consciousness that places him or her at risk for aspiration, a nasogastric tube should be promptly inserted.

All patients with SBO merit admission to the hospital.

Bacterial translocation is thought to result from simple SBO. However, there is no convincing evidence to recommend the empirical use of antibiotics in the nonoperative management of a simple SBO. In patients in whom surgical exploration is planned or perforation is suspected, antibiotics are recommended. The antibiotic used should provide coverage against the gram-negative and anaerobic organisms that colonize the intestinal tract (e.g., second-generation cephalosporins).

SBO in the presence of known malignancy is very common. Surgery should be the primary treatment for selected patients with malignant bowel obstruction.

Laparoscopy is a safe and effective surgical method in the treatment of SBO in adults, particularly those with obstructions caused by adhesions. The risk of recurrence seems to be similar to that of an open surgical approach.

ACUTE MESENTERIC ISCHEMIA

Perspective

The mortality rate of the patient with mesenteric vascular occlusion has remained as high as 60% to 80%, and the diagnosis and treatment of this vascular catastrophe have remained difficult.

Acute mesenteric ischemia (AMEI) involves the acute insufficiency of the blood supply to the small bowel and may also involve the right colon. The left colon has a much higher degree of collateral blood flow and is less prone to AMEI. When AMEI occurs, rapid intestinal injury results. This condition should be clearly differentiated from chronic mesenteric ischemia , which is often referred to as "intestinal angina" and often manifests as recurrent episodes of abdominal pain resulting from insufficient intestinal blood flow during periods of increased postprandial metabolic demand. Chronic mesenteric ischemia does not usually require emergent therapy; however, it is possible for AMEI to develop in these patients as well.

Overall AMEI is a rare clinical problem, accounting for 0.1% of hospital admissions. Within the diagnosis of AMEI there are four specific clinical categories that make up the overwhelming majority of causes. These categories include mesenteric arterial embolus, mesenteric arterial thrombosis, nonocclusive mesenteric ischemia, and mesenteric venous thrombosis.

Principles of Disease

The mesenteric vessels arise from the primitive ventral segmental arteries.There is a significant amount of person-to-person variability. These become the celiac trunk, superior mesenteric artery(SMA), and inferior mesenteric artery(IMA), respectively. The celiac trunk arises from the anterior aspect of the abdominal aorta and branches into the common hepatic, splenic, and left gastric arteries. These vessels supply the distal esophagus to the duodenum at the entrance of the bile duct. The SMA normally arises 1 cm below the celiac trunk and runs toward the cecum, terminating as the ileocolic artery. The SMA supplies the distal half of the duodenum to the proximal two thirds of the transverse colon. The IMA originates approximately 6 to 7 cm below the SMA and gives rise to the left colic artery, the sigmoid arteries, and the hemorrhoidal arteries. Anatomically, this vessel provides blood flow to the distal third of the transverse colon to the rectum.

The gut receives 20% of cardiac output at rest, and up to 35% after eating. Of this, up to 70% supplies the mucosa.

Intestinal blood flow is regulated by a complex combination of intrinsic and extrinsic mechanisms to match intestinal demands with blood supply. Intrinsic factors provide the moment-to-moment control of the intestinal circulation; they function independently from neural control. Smooth muscle relaxation can also be brought about directly by a decrease in the perfusion pressure in the arterioles themselves. These two mechanisms are referred to as the metabolic and myogenic pathways. Intestinal blood flow is also controlled extrinsically through neural and hormonal mechanisms. Hormonal influences include the direct action of angiotensin II released as a result of decreased extracellular volume, as well as vasopressin to cause mesenteric vasoconstriction.

Because of the high metabolic demands of the intestinal mucosa, within 15 min of absolute ischemia, structural damage to the intestinal villi can be observed histologically (Fig. 37-4, see color illustration). If not corrected, within 3 hr mucosal sloughing occurs. By 6 hr, transmural necrosis is complte.

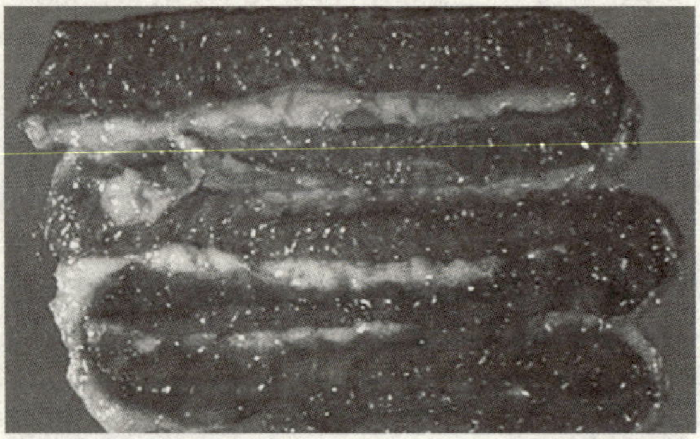

Fig. 37-4 Gross pathologic image of intestinal ischemia and infarction.

Mesenteric Arterial Embolism

Arterial emboli are the most common cause of AMEI.The median age of patients with mesenteric arterial emboli is 70 yr, and two thirds are women. Emboli are most often cardiac in origin and arise from left atrial or ventricular mural thrombi or valvular lesions. Risk factors for the development of such thrombi include myocardial ischemia or MI, cardiomyopathies, ventricular aneurysms, endocarditis, and Af.The SMA is most frequently affected.The embolus typically lodges 3 to 10 cm distal to the origin of the SMA (Fig. 37-5). The jejunum is most often involed.

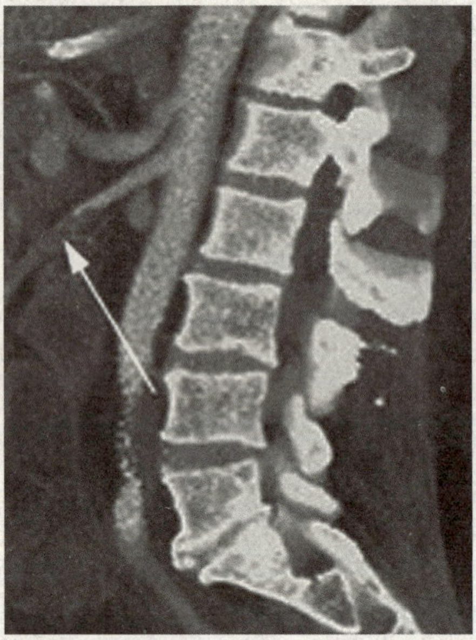

Fig. 37-5 Coronal abdominal CT angiogram with large superior mesenteric artery embolism *(arrow)*.

Mesenteric Arterial Thrombosis

Mesenteric arterial thrombosis results from the progression of atherosclerotic disease of the mesenteric vasculature. Risk factors for development include advanced age, hypertension, diabetes, and tobacco use. Affected patients frequently have a history suggestive of chronic mesenteric ischemia of several months' or years' duration.Thrombosis usually occurs in the proximal SMA at the origin of the vessel.

Nonocclusive Mesenteric Ischemia

Nonocclusive mesenteric ischemia occurs as a result of mesenteric vasospasm in the absence of a physical obstruction. This vasospasm is triggered by mesenteric hypoperfusion or excessive sympathetic nervous system activity. Mesenteric hypoperfusion can result from a wide variety of conditions, including sepsis, severe dehydration, pancreatitis, or hemorrhagic shock. Excessive sympathetic activity can result from CHF, or the use of medications and drugs such as vasopressors, cocaine, or digoxin. Once initiated, this vasospasm often persists even after correction of the underlying condition, and repeated episodes of ischemia and reperfusion occur.

Mesenteric Venous Thrombosis

Mesenteric venous thrombosis is the least common cause of AMEI. It most frequently involves the superior mesenteric vein and its branches. In the vast majority of cases (over 75%), an underlying inherited thrombotic disorder or an inherited or acquired hypercoagulable state can be identified. The most common cause is factor V Leiden mutation. Other inherited prothrombotic states implicated in the development of mesenteric venous thrombosis include deficiency in antithrombin Ⅲ, protein C, or protein S. Hematologic conditions predisposing to this condition include polycythemia vera and essential thrombocythemia. Oral-contraceptive use accounts for 9% to 18% of the episodes of mesenteric venous thrombosis in young women. Local intra-abdominal inflammation secondary to pancreatitis, malignancy, or inflammatory bowel disorders also increase the risk of mesenteric venous thrombosis. Finally, the venous stasis caused by portal hypertension is a recognized risk factor.

Box 37-3 summarizes causes of mesenteric venous thrombosis.

Unusual Causes of Mesenteric Ischemia

These include SMA dissection leading to occlusion, tumor emboli, retroperitoneal fibrosis, and various types of vasculitis, including Buerger's disease, polyarteritis nodosa, and Takayasu's arteritis.

Box 37-3 Factors Associated with Mesenteric Venous Thrombosis

- Hypercoagulable states
  - Polycythemia vera
  - Sickle cell disease
  - Antithrombin Ⅲ deficiency
  - Protein C or S deficiency
  - Malignancy
  - Myeloproliferative disorders
  - Estrogen therapy, oral contraceptive pills
  - Pregnancy
- Inflammatory conditions
  - Pancreatitis
  - Diverticulitis
  - Appendicitis
  - Cholangitis
- Trauma
  - Operative venous injury
  - Postsplenectomy
  - Blunt or abdominal trauma
  - Miscellaneous
  - CHF
  - Renal failure
  - Decompression sickness
  - Portal hypertension

Clinical Features

History

The traditional historical triad of AMEI is the sudden onset of poorly localized abdominal pain and gastric emptying (vomiting or diarrhea) in a patient with cardiac disease. This is especially true in cases of SMA embolism or thrombosis, in which symptoms and clinical deterioration can rapidly occur. In cases of mesenteric venous thrombosis the symptoms are slower in onset and often have been present for several days by the time the patients seeks medical attention. Approximately one third of patients with acute embolic mesenteric ischemia and one half of patients with acute mesenteric venous thrombosis have a personal history of an embolic event such as a PE, deep vein thrombosis, or ischemic stroke.

Physical Examination

The pain is classically described as being "out of proportion" to the physical examination findings. The patient may be writhing in pain but have a soft abdomen without guarding. As the parietal peritoneum becomes ischemic, the abdominal physical findings progress. If the ischemia progresses to infarction, peritonitis may be present. Heme-positive stools may also be noted. Hypotension, tachycardia, and tachypnea are all signs of severe ischemia and suggest a poor prognosis.

Complications

Secondary reperfusion injury is common, and bowel initially identified as viable may progress to necrosis. Other complications include wound infections, sepsis, and pneumonia. Given the population in which AMEI tends to occur, the physiologic stress of this disease process also places patients at high risk for MI, renal failure, and PE while in the hospital.

Diagnostic Strategies

The emergency physician should be especially vigilant in patients older than 50 yr with the complaint of the sudden onset of abdominal pain.

Initial laboratory results are often nonspecific and may include leukocytosis, an elevated hematocrit secondary to hemoconcentration, and metabolic acidosis.Early serum biomarkers of AMEI include lactate, D-dimer, IL-6, and serum ischemia-modified albumin levels.An elevated plasma lactate level was

100% sensitive for AMEI but only 42% specific.

Mesenteric angiography remains the "gold standard" in the radiographic evaluation for mesenteric ischemia.Plain radiographs in AMEI are most often nonspecific. Later in the disease course, plain radiograph findings may show so-called *thumbprinting*, in which multiple, round, smooth soft tissue densities project into the intestinal lumen . More specific but very late plain radiographic findings indicating infarction include pneumatosis intestinalis and portal venous gas.

CT has largely replaced conventional angiography (Fig.37-6).

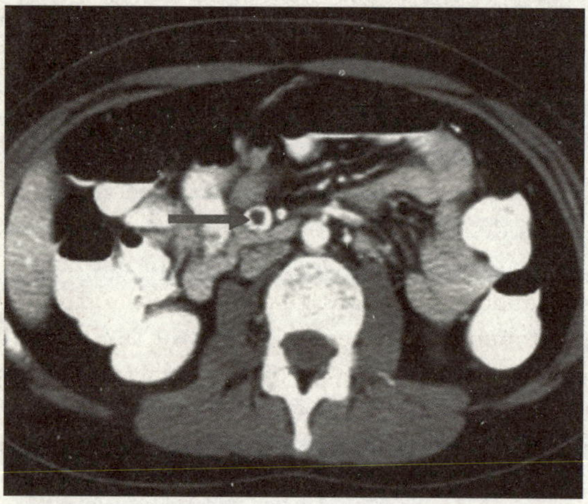

Fig. 37-6 Superior mesenteric venous thrombus (identified here by arrow) in a patient with nondescript abdominal pain. Hematologic workup revealed factor V Leiden thrombophilia.

Duplex sonography has also been evaluated as an imaging tool in the diagnosis of AMEI. It has been found to be very specific (92%-100%) for the detection of occlusions, but its sensitivity is decreased (70%-89%).

Differential Considerations

Other potentially devastating conditions to consider in the differential diagnosis of acute-onset severe abdominal pain include leaking AAA, perforated viscus, bowel obstruction, biliary disease, and atypical MI.

Management and Disposition

The goals of AMEI treatment are to restore mesenteric blood flow as rapidly as possible, manage underlying conditions, treat persistent mesenteric vasospasm if present, and mitigate the risk of further clot propagation. Initial interventions should focus on aggressive fluid resuscitation and hemodynamic stabilization.Invasive monitoring may be indicated. If vasopressors are required, dobutamine, low-dose dopamine, or milrinone is advised. Broad-spectrum antibiotics should be administered without delay, and a general or vascular surgeon should be immediately consulted.

Regardless of the cause, if signs of intestinal infarction or perforation with peritonitis are present, prompt emergent laparotomy is warranted.Numerous reports exist detailing the use of thrombolytic agents, angioplasty, embolectomy, or vascular stenting to restore mesenteric blood flow. In addition, the phosphodiesterase inhibitor papaverine may be continuously infused directly into the compromised vessel.A "second-look" laparotomy may be indicated, as bowel that initially appears viable may become gangrenous later.

Primary treatment of nonocclusive mesenteric ischemia involves aggressive interventions to reverse the underlying cause and consideration for papaverine infusion via angiographic catheter as well as intravenous heparin to prevent thrombosis in the vasospastic vessel. Papaverine infusion is often maintained for 24 hr. If peritoneal signs develop, laparotomy is indicated.

The treatment of mesenteric venous thrombosis is unique in that, in the absence of peritoneal findings, initial treatment with heparin infusion alone may be adequate. However, if peritoneal findings are present or develop later in the patient's hospital course, bowel necrosis is likely and prompt laparotomy. If the patient recovers, long-term anticoagulation with warfarin usually is provided to prevent recurrence. An appropriate workup for hypercoagulable conditions should be undertaken.

(WANG Xiujie)

Chapter 38

Wound Management Principles

KEY CONCEPTS

Risk factors for wound infection include prolonged time since injury; crush mechanism; deep penetrating wounds; high velocity missiles; and contamination with saliva, feces, soil, or other foreign matter.

The most effective intervention to decrease infection is thorough cleansing.

Soaking wounds in povidone-iodine (Betadine) is more toxic than beneficial to healthy tissue.

Antibiotics are indicated for through-and-through intraoral lacerations, cat bites, some dog bites, some human bites, puncture injuries to the foot in high-risk individuals, open fractures, and wounds involving exposed tendons or joints.

Tetanus immunization should be provided soon after injury but can be given days or weeks later. The usual incubation period for tetanus is 7 to 21 d (range, 3-56 d).

PERSPECTIVE

The goals of emergency wound treatment are to restore function, repair tissue integrity with strength and optimal cosmetic appearance, and minimize risk of infection. Risk of infection depends on the location, mechanism, host, and care. The risk for a clean facial wound produced by incision is less than 1%, whereas a dirty crush injury to the lower extremity may have more than a 20% risk.Wound infection generally results in delayed healing, decreased strength, and a poor cosmetic result.

Emergency physicians must also be aware of the medicolegal risk associated with soft tissue injuries. Including injuries to the hand, wound-related complaints are the fourth most common cause of malpractice claims against emergency physicians. Missed foreign body, wound infection, and missed tendon or nerve injury are the most common complications leading to these claims.

PRINCIPLES OF DISEASE

Anatomy of Skin and Fascia

The skin is a complex organ that protects the body against bacterial invasion and ensures thermoregulation. The skin also helps to regulate water content and register sensory stimuli.

The skin and fascia vary in thickness from 1 to 4 mm, depending on the part of the body. The epidermis, the outermost layer, is several cell layers thick. The most important parts of the epidermis are the stratum germinativum (basal layer), where new cells originate, and the stratum corneum, the outermost cell layer that gives the skin its cosmetic appearance. The layer of skin directly beneath the epidermis is the dermis. The much thicker dermis is primarily composed of connective tissue. The dermis is the key layer for the ultimate healing of skin wounds. Optimal healing and minimal scar formation depend on the removal of debris and devitalized tissue from the dermis.

The superficial fascia lies directly beneath the dermis and encloses the subcutaneous fat. This space must be irrigated and débrided to decrease the risk of infection. The deep fascia lies beneath the fat and is a strong, off-white sheath that covers and protects the underlying muscles and helps prevent superficial infection from spreading to deeper tissues. The deep fascia must be closed to maintain its protective and functional roles.

Wound Biology

Normal wound healing includes coagulation,

inflammation, collagen metabolism, wound contraction, and epithelialization. Maintaining the balance of these events is crucial for normal healing. Delaying any of the stages may result in a weak closure and dehiscence. Prolonging segments of the process may affect the ultimate scar appearance.

Soon after tissue integrity is altered, the process of coagulation begins. Platelet release factors initiate and enhance a response from inflammatory cells.Capillary permeability increases to allow WBC to migrate into the wound. Neutrophils and monocytes act as scavengers to rid the wound of debris and bacteria. Monocytes transform into macrophages, which seem to have a major role in subsequent healing phenomena. In addition to providing wound defense, macrophages release chemotactic substances, calling on other monocytes to stimulate fibroblast replication and trigger neovascularization.

Collagen is the principal structural protein of most tissues of the body. Normal tissue repair depends on collagen synthesis, deposition, and cross-linking. Fibroblasts synthesize and deposit collagen compounds 48 hr after injury. Immature collagen is highly disorganized because it has a gel-like consistency.

After a series of enzymatic processes, characteristic fibrils are produced. Subsequent intermolecular cross-links are responsible for a major portion of the strength of the collagen fibril. The entire process depends on tissue lactate and ascorbic acid and is directly related to tissue P_aCO_2. In the absence of vitamin C, prolyl and lysyl hydroxylase do not activate, and oxygen is not transferred to proline or lysine. Under hydroxylated collagen is produced, and characteristic collagen fibers are unable to form. Wound healing is poor, and capillaries are fragile. Without oxygen to hydroxylate proline and lysine, a local condition resembling scurvy tends to occur.

Under normal conditions, collagen synthesis peaks by day 7,coincident with rapid increases in tensile strength. The healing wound has the greatest mass at 3 w but remodels itself during the next 6 to 12 mo. However,the wound achieves less than 15% to 20% of its ultimate strength by 3 w and only 60% by 4 mo.

Wound contraction is the movement of whole-thickness skin toward the center of the skin defect. Immediately after injury, the wound edges retract and increase the size of the defect. Normal skin tension along the lines of minimal tension produces this retraction (Figs. 38-1 and 38-2). Wounds perpendicular to these lines are under greater tension and result in a larger scar.

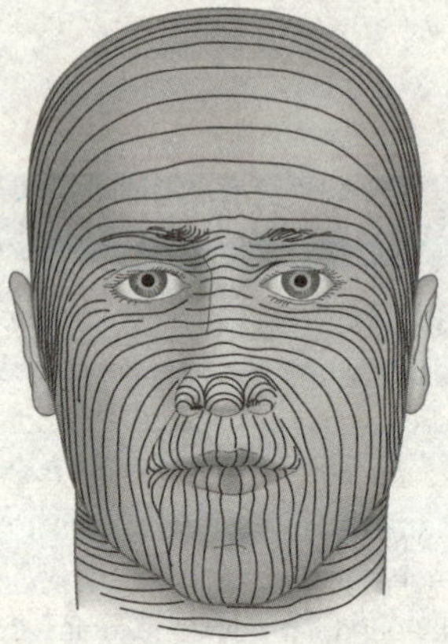

Fig. 38-1 Skin tension lines of the face.

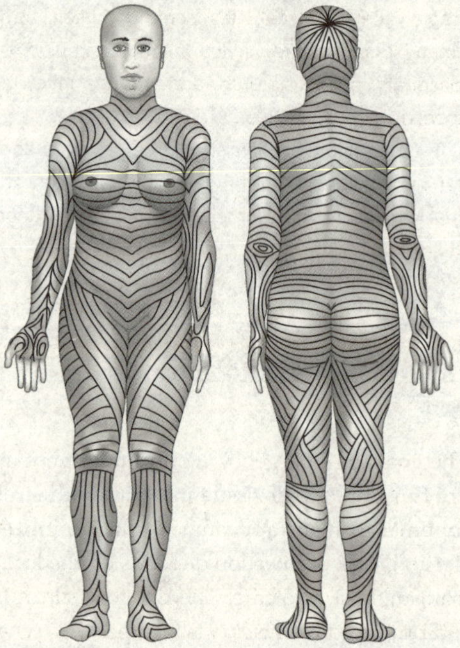

Fig. 38-2 Skin tension lines of the body surface.

During the next 3 or 4 d, the wound size shrinks as its edges move toward the center. This phenomenon is independent of epithelialization, and the presence of collagen is not necessary for it to occur. This process is considered beneficial to healing and should not be confused with contracture that results from scar shortening.

Contracture becomes more apparent when the normal healing process is prolonged. The effect is a disfiguring hypertrophic scar. Optimizing the duration of the inflammatory phase and minimizing wound tension help to produce a more "appealing" scar.

Epithelialization is a mechanism in the healing process whereby epithelial cells migrate across the wound. Mitosis appears at the wound edge near the basal cell layer within hours of injury. Eschar or other debris impedes this process. When a wound is properly cleansed and débrided and kept moist and protected, epithelialization proceeds at a maximum rate.

In a surgically repaired laceration, epithelialization bridges the defect by 48 hr. The new tissue proceeds to thicken and grow downward, beginning to resemble the layered structural characteristics of uninjured epidermis within 5 d. Simultaneously, keratin formation loosens the overlying scab.

Biomechanical Properties of Skin

Various forces (lines of tension) exist as a result of skin elasticity from collagen fibers. These static forces may vary more than fivefold with the respective area of body skin surface, but the static tension of a given area of skin remains constant. These static forces are shown clinically by the gaping of wounds after incision. The magnitude of static skin tension is directly related to ultimate scar width.

Uneven, jagged wounds have greater surface area than do linear lacerations. The skin tension is distributed over a greater area and is less per unit length of tissue. Meticulous reapproximation of the jagged edges results in a more appealing scar. Sharp débridement, converting a jagged wound to a linear laceration, is often unwise because it may cause too much tissue loss and produce a wider, more visible scar.

Skin forces produced by muscular contraction and movements of flexion and extension influence healing and scar size. These dynamic forces are greatest where skin elasticity is necessary for function.Lacerations parallel to skin folds, lines of expression, and joints do not impair function or produce unattractive scars. Wounds that traverse the skin lines heal with conspicuous scars and may impair function. Knowledge of these lines and forces is necessary for optimal wound repair.

CLINICAL FEATURES AND DIAGNOSTIC STRATEGIES

History

A detailed history should be obtained as part of routine wound evaluation. Serious complications can result when basic information is not obtained. If the patient has significant peripheral vascular disease, is immunocompromised, or has a high risk of a retained foreign body, wound care decisions may be changed. Essential historical information includes medical history, mechanism and setting of injury, and tetanus status.

Risk Factors

Risk factors for wound morbidity include prolonged time since injury; crush mechanism; deep wounds; age of the patient;high velocity missiles; and contamination with saliva, feces, soil, or other foreign matter (Box 38-1). Three hours after acute trauma, bacteria proliferate to a level that may result in infection. Standard wound care guidelines for the routine wound recommend closure within 8 to 12 hr of injury. Lacerations produced by fine cutting forces resist infection better than crush injuries. Reduction of blood flow to wound edges in the latter may increase the infective concentration of bacteria by 100-fold. High-velocity missile injuries produce damage remote from the missile tract. The extent of injury may not be apparent for several days. Clean, finely cut lacerations on the face may be safely closed in some patients 24 or more hours after injury, whereas blunt lacerations to the leg or thigh may be treated with delayed primary closure as early as 4 to 6 hr after injury. For sutured wounds, location appears to have the strongest association with infection. Lacerations repaired on the leg and thigh may have an infection rate greater than 20%, those on the torso and other extremities greater than 10%, and those on the face and scalp less than 4%.

Box 38-1 Risk Factors for Wound Infection

1. Injury more than 8-12 hr old
2. Location: leg and thigh, then arms, then feet, then chest, then back, then face, then scalp
3. Contamination with devitalized tissue, foreign matter, saliva,or stool
4. Blunt (crush) mechanism
5. Presence of subcutaneous sutures
6. Type of repair: risk greatest with sutures > staples > tape
7. Anesthesia with epinephrine
8. High-velocity missile injuries

Wounds contaminated by foreign matter are at high risk of infection. Saliva and feces are composed of a concentration of bacteria (approximately 10^{11} per gram wet weight) that greatly exceeds the numbers needed to produce infection ($\geqslant 10^6$ bacteria per gram tissue).

The presence of any foreign matter in the wound decreases resistance to infection. Soil fractions, which include organic components and inorganic clay particles, damage host defenses with adverse interactions between charged soil particles and WBC. The presence of these soil fractions greatly increases the infective potential of bacteria.

Wound closure decisions are individualized for each laceration. Sharp, clean lacerations of the face may be safe to close up to 24 hr after the time of injury, whereas highly contaminated blunt injuries to the feet should never be closed primarily. When the distal neurovascular evaluation is completed, the examination may proceed.There are three additional areas of concern: (1) immunocompetence of the host, (2) physical characteristics of the host (e.g., peripheral vascular disease), and (3) structural defects that invite bacterial seeding (e.g., damaged or prosthetic heart valves).

Physical Examination

When the injury occurs on an extremity,use of a sphygmomanometer may help to ensure a bloodless field. The blood pressure cuff is placed proximal to the injury, and the extremity is elevated above the heart for at least 1 min. Exsanguinating the extremity may be hastened by wrapping the limb tightly with an Ace bandage, beginning distally and ending at the base of the cuff.The sphygmomanometer is inflated to a pressure greater than the systolic pressure of the patient. A peripheral nerve block or Bier block should be used if inflation longer than several minutes is contemplated.

A thorough examination of the wound requires that the tissues be adequately anesthetized. Subcutaneous tissues quickly **reapproximate** after injury, giving the appearance of a shallow wound. In addition, significant subcutaneous swelling lends to this appearance and renders examination of the laceration more difficult, as in wounds of the scalp and face.Finger lacerations are rarely gaping, but crucial structures (e.g., tendons, nerves, and vessels) are often damaged. The examiner must pry the wound margins apart, ensure a blood-free field, and examine the tissues as the digit or extremity is placed through range of motion. The injured section of tendon may have been in a different state of tension and in a more proximal or distal location at the time of injury. Wounds that cannot be explored adequately and wounds with probable trauma to underlying tissues or with foreign matter require additional studies. It may be appropriate to extend the laceration to enable improved visualization of wound depth and extent.

Sterile gloves may not be a necessary part of wound closure. Clean nonsterile gloves should be worn to offer some protection for both the patient and the provider.

Foreign Body Assessment

No single method can guarantee the identification and removal of all foreign matter from wounds. Physical examination with wound exploration will discover about 78% of foreign bodies; plain radiography will detect glass foreign bodies in about 75% of cases, metal in 99%, and wood in 7%.

Attempts to visualize foreign matter by standard radiography are not as helpful as might be expected. The radiodensity of an object depends on the relative density of the matter and the adjacent tissue. Pieces of glass greater than 1 mm thick are visible when appropriate views are ordered. Many organic substances, such as wood, are not visible on plain films, but specifically requested soft tissue views may increase the yield.A radiolucent shadow may be seen on close inspection because the foreign substance displaces tissue in its path. Xerograms are better than plain radiography but still miss some plastics and organic matter. A CT scan is excellent for identifying all foreign substances but is expensive and results in significant exposure to radiation. Ultrasonography is a good technique, but the small size of many foreign bodies and pockets of air, edema, pus, and some calcifications may produce confusing echoes, limiting its clinical usefulness. When simpler, standard methods fail to locate a foreign body that is likely or definitely present, ultrasonography or a CT scan should be considered.

MANAGEMENT

Anesthesia

After an appropriate neurovascular examination is documented, the involved tissue should be anesthetized. Careful physical examination and thorough cleansing, irrigation, and debridement require that the patient be free of pain. Regional anesthesia may be preferable for wounds innervated by one superficial nerve. Injections at the wound site produce swelling and further distortion of landmarks. With a regional block, more than one laceration may be repaired in the same nerve distribution without additional anesthesia. Lacerations on the face, hands, fingers, feet, and toes and in the mouth are often well suited for regional anesthesia.

Anesthetic Agents

Lidocaine (Xylocaine) is the most common agent used for local and regional anesthesia. It is safe and fast acting. Onset of action for direct infiltration occurs within seconds, and effects last 20 to 60 min. When lidocaine is administered as a regional nerve block, onset occurs in 4 to 6 min and the effects generally last 75 min, although the block may remain effective for 120 min. A 1% lidocaine solution contains 10 mg/mL. It is safe to use 3 to 5 mg/kg, not exceeding 300 mg at a single injection. More volume can be added safely every 30 min. When epinephrine is added, the resulting vasoconstriction prolongs the effect for 2 to 6 hr, and the safe dose is increased to 5 to 7 mg/kg. However, the addition of epinephrine has been shown to delay healing and lower resistance to infection.Lidocaine with epinephrine should be avoided in wounds with higher risks of infection and when tissue viability is of concern. Traditional teaching has been to avoid epinephrine in the fingers and toes because of the risk of vasoconstriction in small arterioles. However, recent literature suggests that with careful screening epinephrine can be safely used in digital blocks. Digital artery vasospasm, accidentally induced by local injection of epinephrine, can be reversed successfully with a local injection of 0.5 to 2 mg of subcutaneous phentolamine or application of topical nitroglycerin.

Bupivacaine (Marcaine) provides anesthesia that is equal to that of lidocaine. Onset of action is slightly slower than that of lidocaine, but the duration of anesthesia is four to eight times longer. Bupivacaine is the preferred local anesthetic agent for the care of most wounds. In adults the maximal reported safe dose is approximately 2.5 mg/kg without epinephrine and 3.5 mg/kg with epinephrine. The dose can be repeated every 3 hr, not exceeding a total of more than 400 mg in a 24 hr period. The maximal intraoral dose is 90 mg.

Local injection of lidocaine with a 25-gauge needle is acceptable, but the more rapid injection can result in greater patient discomfort. The needle should be introduced through the cut margin to minimize the pain of the injection. The pain of injecting lidocaine can be ameliorated with the addition of bicarbonate to buffer the solution. Adding sodium bicarbonate in a 1:10 volume ratio to lidocaine (1 mL bicarbonate and 10 mL lidocaine) decreases the pain of injection without compromising the quality of anesthesia. A 1:100 volume ratio (0.1 mL of bicarbonate and 10 mL of bupivacaine) has been found to be effective. Warming the anesthetic solution is also an effective means of decreasing the pain of injection.

Topical anesthesia may be an effective painless alternative.A combination of tetracaine, adrenaline (epinephrine), and cocaine (TAC) (0.5% tetracaine, 1:2000 adrenaline, and 11.8% cocaine) can function effectively on skin lacerations. The solution is administered by soaking a cotton ball with 5 mL of the combined drugs (25 mg of tetracaine, 25 mg of adrenaline, and 590 mg of cocaine) and applying it to the wound for 10 to 20 min. TAC is similar to infiltrative lidocaine in all respects, including risk of complications. It is more effective on the face and scalp than on extremities. Half strength TAC solution is effective and may reduce the potential for toxicity. The tetracaine component may be superfluous and can be eliminated without compromising the quality of anesthesia. TAC increases the infection rate in contaminated wounds, this is not the case with routine wound care. The potential toxicity from TAC has been documented by measurable plasma cocaine levels. TAC should be avoided in the repair of highly contaminated wounds and in lacerations near mucous membranes.

The potential serious adverse effects of TAC have led to the increasing use of other topically applied anesthetic combinations. A mixture of lidocaine (1%-4%), epinephrine (1 : 1000 to 1 : 2000), and tetracaine (0.5%-2%) has been used successfully in place of TAC. This mixture avoids the untoward side effects of cocaine. Eutectic mixture of local anesthetics is a cream used to produce anesthesia of wounds. A newer technique that uses topical anesthesia in a progressively layered approach appears to be safe and effective.

Allergy

Allergy to local anesthetics is uncommon.The esters include procaine, tetracaine, and benzocaine. The second group, including lidocaine and bupivacaine, belong to the amide family. Allergy to the esters is uncommon.Good history taking is the best way to document a true allergic reaction. Many patients labeled as allergic have experienced uncomfortable drug effects or autonomic responses to the pain and the overall setting.

Apparent allergic reaction to lidocaine or bupivacaine may be a reaction to the methylparaben. Cardiac lidocaine does not contain preservatives, is a standard drug in ED, and can be used for wound anesthesia when there is concern about potential allergic reactions.

No cross-reactivity occurs between the amide and ester families, so an agent from a different group may be chosen. Single-dose vials of lidocaine or cardiac lidocaine are not mixed with methylparaben and may be used. A test dose of 0.1 mL may be administered intradermally before proceeding. The patient should be observed for 30 min. Aqueous diphenhydramine (1%) has also been shown to provide effective local anesthesia.

Skin Preparation

Disinfection of the skin may be accomplished with several different agents. The ideal agent is fast acting, has a broad spectrum of antimicrobial activity, and has a long shelf life. Povidone-iodine (Betadine) and chlorhexidine (Hibiclens) have all three characteristics. Although excellent as skin disinfectants, both products are toxic to wound defenses and may increase the incidence of wound infection. Povidone-iodine is effective against gram-positive and gram-negative bacteria, fungi, and viruses. Chlorhexidine is less effective against gram-negative bacteria. Care must be taken to avoid spilling these substances into the wound. Exposure of the eye to these agents can be disastrous. Chlorhexidine has been shown experimentally and in case reports to produce serious permanent corneal opacification.

Removal of the hair makes it easier for the patient to keep the area clean and ultimately facilitates accurate suture placement and removal. Exceptions are parts of the body where hairlines provide important landmarks for the accurate reapproximation of tissue margins, most notably the eyebrow.

Surgical studies show that hair removal with a razor is three to nine times more likely to result in a wound infection than is clipping the hair. The wounded follicle provides access for bacterial invasion and ultimately infection. For wounds considered to be at high risk of infection, clipping may be done with electronic shears or scissors.

Wound Preparation

Debridement

Debridement is the removal of foreign matter and devitalized tissue from the wound. With respect to ultimate wound healing and risk of infection, débridement is the most important consideration in wound care. The presence of any devitalized tissue in the wound delays healing and significantly increases the risk of infection. However, the benefits of débridement have to be weighed against the consequences of producing a larger tissue defect. The resultant closure is exposed to higher tension and may result in a wider scar. Skin edges that are clearly devitalized are debrided before wound closure. On the trunk, where there is little concern for specialized tissue, wide excision and débridement are feasible On the face and hands, where all tissue must be saved if possible, the process is more difficult. Meticulous sharp excision of small fragments of nonviable tissue should be performed only by experienced physicians. When the viability of large areas of skin or muscle is a significant concern, the wound should be prepared for delayed primary closure.

Wound Cleansing

An ideal wound cleanser has broad antimicrobial activity with a rapid onset.It is nontoxic to the tissue and does not reduce tissue resistance to infection, delay healing, or decrease the tensile strength of the healing wound.Many antiseptic solutions have been used clinically and studied in great detail (Table 38-1). Much debate exists regarding which agent comes closest to possessing these qualities.Povidone-iodine in various concentrations, saline, and, more recently, tap water have received the most attention.

Table 38-1 Antiseptic Solutions

AGENTS	ANTIMICROBIAL ACTIVITY	MECHANISMS OF ACTION	TISSUE TOXICITY	INDICATIONS AND CONTRAINDICATIONS
Povidone-iodine solution (iodine complexes) (Betadine)	Available as a 10% solution with polyvinylpyrrolidone (povidone) containing 1% free iodine with broadrapid-onset antimicrobial activity	Potent germicide in low concentrations	Decreases polymorphonuclear neutrophil leukocyte migration and life span at concentration >1% May cause systemic toxicity at higher concentrations; questionable toxicity at 1% concentration	Probably a safe and effective wound cleanser at a 1% concentration 10% solution is effective to prepare skin around the wound
Povidone-iodine surgical scrub	Same as the solution	Same	Toxic to open wounds	Best as a hand cleanser; never use in open wounds
Nonionic detergents Pluronic F-68 Shur-Clens	Ethylene oxide is 80% of their molecular weight No antimicrobial activity	Wound cleansers	No toxicity to open wounds, eyes, or intravenous solutions	Appear to be effective, safe wound cleansers
Hydrogen peroxide	3% solution in water has brief germicidal activity	Oxidizing agent that denatures protein	Toxic to open wounds	Should not be used on wounds after initial cleaning; may be used to clean intact skin
Hexachlorophene (polychlorinated bisphenol) (pHisoHex	Bacteriostatic (2%-5%) Greater activity against gram-positive organisms	Interruption of bacterial electron transport and disruption of membranebound enzymes	Little skin toxicity; the scrub form is damaging to open wounds	Never use scrub solution in open wounds Very good preoperative hand preparation
Alcohols	Low-potency antimicrobial most effective as a 70% ethyl and 70% isopropyl alcohol solution	Denatures protein	Kills irreversibly and functions as a fixative	No role in routine care
Phenols	Bacteriostatic >0.2% Bactericidal >1% Fungicidal 1.3%	Denatures protein	Extensive tissue necrosis and systemic toxicity	Never use >2% aqueous phenol or >4% phenol plus glycerol

Saline is the traditional wound-irrigating fluid of choice. However, tap water has consistently produced equivalent rates of infection and cosmetic outcomes. Tap-water irrigation allows a large volume of irrigation rapidly and inexpensively and is especially suited to upper extremity and scalp injuries.

Free iodine is too toxic to tissue and its defenses to have therapeutic value in the open wound. An iodophor is a complex of iodine with a carrier to increase its solubility and decrease the availability of free iodine. The most widely used iodophor is povidone-iodine. It is generally available in a 10% solution, which is 1% free iodine. The clinical benefit of this complex is a solution that maintains broad antimicrobial activity and eliminates most local and systemic toxicity.A 5% povidone-iodine solution is toxic to polymorphonuclear neutrophil leukocyte activity and may increase the infection rate. A 1% solution is safe and effective with little or no toxicity.Detergent containing cleansers, such as povidone-iodine scrub, may be excellent for skin preparation but are toxic to tissue defenses and should never be allowed to contaminate open wounds.

Tap-water irrigation soon may become the preferred method of irrigation because it is safe, is effective, requires no preparation, and is less expensive.

Irrigation

The quality of mechanical cleansing is one of the most important determinants of wound prognosis. The most effective form of wound cleansing is high-pressure irrigation. Irrigating with pressures greater than 7 pounds per square inch (psi) significantly decreases the number of bacteria and the incidence of infection. Although several commercial devices are available, attaching an 18-gauge needle to a 35 mL syringe yields a force of 7 or 8 psi. High pressures of 50 to 70 psi may be obtained with a commercial water pick. These pressures may cause some tissue damage, but the beneficial effect of ridding the wound of bacteria and debris outweighs this risk. Simply soaking the wound in an antiseptic solution is not beneficial and may be harmful. Scrubbing the wound with a sponge with large-pore cells inflicts tissue trauma and impairs the ability to resist infection. Tissue damage can be decreased by use of a sponge with a fine size of pore cell. Adding a surfactant further minimizes the mechanical trauma inflicted by the sponge. Flooding the wound under low pressure via a bulb syringe or gravity alone does not reduce the incidence of infection, regardless of the agent used.

Wound Closure

Decision-Making

The first determination required is whether the wound should be treated open or closed. Each wound, patient, and clinical circumstance must be handled individually. Certain lacerations, such as a fine linear laceration to the face, can be closed primarily 24 hr or more after injury. Other injuries may necessitate open management, regardless of the extent of delay. A large stellate laceration to the foot produced by blunt force and contaminated with dirt and grease should not be closed primarily; in addition, human and animal bites to the hand should not be closed primarily. Physician judgment is often the best method for deciding when it is safe to close a wound.

Three wound closure options are available. The wound may be (1) closed primarily in traditional fashion, (2) closed in 4 or 5 d (delayed primary closure), or (3) left open and allowed to heal on its own. Delayed primary closure is a safe alternative to traditional primary closure. Overall healing time is not affected, and the risk of infection is greatly decreased if proper technique is used. When a wound is slated for delayed primary closure, it is prepared, débrided, and irrigated in the same manner as for immediate closure. The wound should be packed to prevent it from closing on its own. If the wound is on an extremity, the injury should be splinted and dressed, and appropriate wound care instructions should be given. The patient should return for a wound check and packing change in 24 hr and should be instructed to follow up in another 72 hr for definitive repair, with wound closure undertaken 96 to 120 hr after injury. Prophylactic antibiotics offer no benefit.

Individuals who do not seek medical care after an injury select the option of leaving a wound open to heal on its own. The loosely closed wound approximates the tissue margins enough to allow the wound to seal itself completely within 48 hr. The infection risk when this method is used is the same as when the wound is closed traditionally.

Wound Tension

The goal of wound closure is optimal anatomic and functional reapproximation of tissue with minimal risk of complication. Consideration must be given to the wound's size, shape, location,depth, and degree of tension. Wounds with high static and dynamic tension that require meticulous closure cannot be closed with tape or staples. Delicate approximation of wound edges under tension can be accomplished only with suture.

Several techniques may be used to reduce wound tension. Deep sutures may be placed in subcutaneous tissue to help bring the wound margins closer together. In this manner, forces on the skin are reduced, and potential dead space can be closed. Care should be taken to avoid suturing adipose tissue because it may become necrotic, increasing the likelihood of infection. The number of dermal sutures depends on the characteristics of the wound. In general, the number should be kept to a minimum because suture material acts as foreign matter in the wound and can increase the risk of infection. Subcutaneous sutures should never be placed in the hand or foot because of the major structures that reside near the surface. Another method of ameliorating static tension from cut edges of the wound is to undermine at the lacerated margin. Undermining helps free the dermis from its deeper attachments, allowing the skin edges to be approximated with less force. Care must be taken to preserve the blood supply to the wound margins and not increase dead space in the process.

Suture Technique

Careful surgical technique is important to optimize the ultimate repair. If possible, pickups, hemostats, or forceps should not be used, especially on wound margins. Blind clamping in a wound can damage a nerve, artery, or tendon. Wound margins should be everted and the sutures tied just tightly enough to allow the edges to approximate lightly. The edges can be everted by ensuring that the needle enters and exits perpendicular to the skin. Wounds with opposing margins of different thickness can be difficult to close. If this difference is not considered and corrected, the ultimate scar has uneven margins that cast a shadow on the skin and is unsightly. In closing these wounds, the needle should be pulled through the cut margin of one side before entering the opposite edge. This method gives the emergency physician the best opportunity to take an equivalent amount of tissue on both sides of the wound. Viable edges of a jagged wound must be meticulously reapproximated. Because of the greater surface area and the ultimate contraction of the wound, preserving the jagged edges results in a more "natural"scar.

Most lacerations are closed with running or interrupted percutaneous suture. The running technique is appropriate for linear lacerations under minimal tension when there is a low risk of infection. This technique is more rapid, requires less suture material, and yields equivalent cosmetic results. Curvilinear or jagged wounds are best closed with interrupted sutures to distribute tension properly. Because tensile strength of interrupted sutures may be superior, wound edges subjected to higher levels of tension should be closed with interrupted sutures.

Basic and Advanced Techniques

Simple Sutures. Wound closure with simple interrupted sutures is the most common method of laceration repair in ED. The placement of simple sutures yields excellent cosmesis and a low infection rate.

Procedure. The needle is placed to one side of the laceration margin and enters the skin at approximately 90 degrees. To pass the needle through the tissue, the clinician supinates his or her wrist and guides the needle deep but parallel to the skin surface. Wrist supination is extended as the needle exits the skin on the opposite side perpendicular to the surface. Proper technique produces wound edges that are slightly everted and are lightly touching. The art of the process takes into consideration swelling while being careful not to secure the suture too tightly because necrosis of the wound margin tissue can seriously compromise healing.

Intradermal (Buried) Sutures. Placing cutaneous sutures in wounds under tension can lead to ischemia of the wound margin and an unsightly scar. Proper placement of buried intradermal sutures helps to approximate dermal margins and reduce wound edge tension. Buried sutures should not be used in contaminated wounds because they increase the risk of wound infection. Sutures through adipose tissue also increase infection and do not relieve skin tension.

Procedure. Placement of buried sutures differs from traditional suturing because of the need to bury the knot deep to the skin. Failure to do this can interfere with dermal healing and can leave a small lump under the surface of the skin. The needle is introduced deep in the wound in the subcutaneous tissue and emerges from the dermis below the skin surface. The needle is reintroduced in the dermis on the opposite wound margin and emerges from the subcutaneous tissue at the same level on the opposite side. The knot is secured and remains buried deep below the skin surface.

Scalp Laceration Repair. In contrast to small lacerations elsewhere on the body, most scalp lacerations require repair because of the propensity to bleed profusely. The dense connective tissue beneath the skin tends to hold vessels open and delay hemostasis. Frontal scalp lacerations in young men should be considered to be a cosmetically significant wound. Although the scalp laceration currently may be well hidden by hair, most men experience some balding. Care must be taken to explore the laceration thoroughly to look for a defect in the galea, an injury that requires repair with deep sutures. Staples may be ideal for the skin closure of simple linear scalp lacerations. Hair is less of a problem in placing staples, staples can be placed more quickly than traditional suture, and staples are easier to see and can be removed 1 to 3 d earlier than traditional sutures (Fig. 38-3). Staples may produce artifact on CT scans, but useful information may still be obtained if CT is necessary. Staples may move during MRI and should not be placed if this imaging modality is being considered. Lightweight stapling devices are available. Most devices come preloaded with five or more staples and are easy to use. Hair apposition may also be an option for the closure of many scalp wounds. The technique involves grabbing a bundle of hair on both sides of the wound and then twisting the hair bundles with a hemostat. A small dab of cyanoacrylate glue is applied to the twisted hair to prevent unraveling. Patient satisfaction is high with this approac.

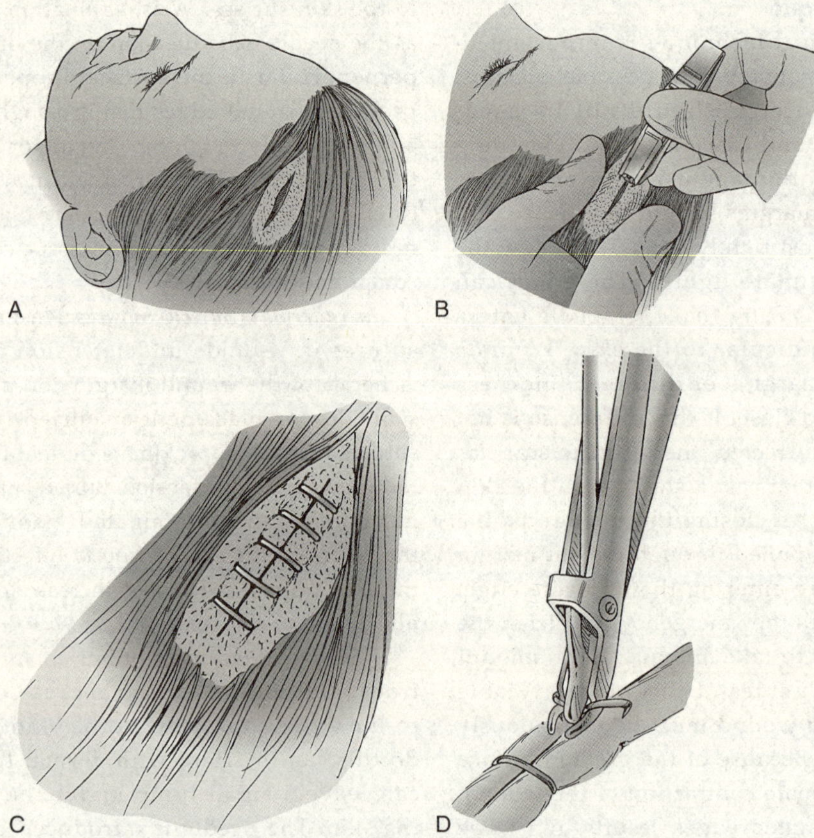

Fig. 38-3 Scalp laceration repair.

Traditional sutures are used to repair most scalp lacerations, usually with standard nylon suture. Absorbable chromic gut can be used in adults who may not return for suture removal.

Procedure. Anesthesia with epinephrine is recommended to help control bleeding. Hair removal is necessary only if the hair makes closure difficult. A defect in the galea is closed with 3-0 or 4-0 absorbable suture. Failure to repair the galea can lead to a cosmetic deformity related to frontalis muscle function. Linear superficial scalp lacerations that do not require deep sutures can be closed with staples or with monofilament nylon sutures applied with a simple interrupted or running technique. Jagged or macerated lacerations may require some débridement and horizontal mattress sutures. When one chooses to staple a scalp laceration, the adjacent skin margins are pinched together with forceps to evert wound margins. The "mouth" of the stapler is placed gently on the skin surface, taking care not to indent the skin. The handle of the stapler is squeezed carefully to eject the staple into the tissue. Ideally, the staple closely approximates the wound margins without indenting the surface of the skin. For release of the staple, the wrist is pulled back to disengage itself from the last staple.

Vigorously bleeding scalp lacerations often need temporizing measures to control bleeding while the patient is being evaluated and resuscitated. An anesthetic agent with epinephrine should be used and may be helpful to control some bleeding. Blindly clamping in an attempt to control bleeding is unwise and not likely to be successful. Raney scalp clips can be rapidly applied to the wound margins to quickly gain control of the bleeding. An applicator is used to apply and remove the clips so that they can be replaced with sutures once the patient has been stabilized. The clips are plastic and will not interfere with CT or magnetic resonance imaging.

Staple removal is simple, especially if the patient has kept the wound clean and free of dried secretions. The dual prongs on the disposable staple remover slide under the staple crossbar. As the handle is squeezed and the horizontal aspect of the staple is depressed, the sharp edges are eased out of the tissue for removal.

Skin Tears. Most commonly seen in the elderly and chronically ill, skin tears can be a treatment dilemma for emergency physicians. These tears are a result of shearing forces that separate the epidermis from the underlying dermal layer of the skin. Often the result of minor trauma, these injuries may be minor tears or as large gaping wounds with extensive loss of tissue. Approximating the wound margins by aligning thin fragile tissue can be very difficult. The use of Steri-Strips and or topical skin adhesives (cyanoacrylate-based derivatives) is currently the preferred option. Either material may be used alone; however, when tension exists, placing the Steri-Strips first, then the adhesive, may be the optimal approach. Care must be taken in deciding what type of dressing to use. Transparent films can cause fluid to collect and delay healing. Adhesives are difficult to remove and can cause additional tearing. If the wound must be covered, then hydrogel sheets, hydrocolloid dressings, or both are recommended.

Vertical Mattress Sutures. Vertical mattress sutures improve wound edge eversion. They are also used for the closure of gaping wounds and deep lacerations that may need more than simple sutures to close potential dead space. Areas of lax skin tension, generally where maximal skin mobility is needed such as over joint surfaces, may need assistance to ensure eversion of the wound margins. Vertical mattress sutures may be ideal to accomplish both tasks.

Procedure. A vertical mattress suture is a combination of deep and superficial components. The needle is introduced at a 90-degree angle approximately 1 cm from the wound margin. The needle courses through the depth of the wound and emerges on the opposite side, 1 cm from the laceration margin at a 90-degree angle. The needle is reintroduced 1 or 2 mm from the epidermal edge for final approximation of the wound.

Horizontal Mattress Sutures. Horizontal mattress sutures are useful to help disperse excess skin tension and to evert wound edges. The scalp is one area where gaping lacerations may benefit from this tension-reduction method. Horizontal mattress sutures may also be beneficial in thin, fragile skin of elderly people and for lacerations that have lost tissue from the injury or débridement.

Procedure. The initial step is to pass the needle as for a simple interrupted stitch (Fig. 38-4). On exiting the skin, however, the needle is reintroduced approximately 0.5 cm adjacent to the exit point. This second "bite" reemerges

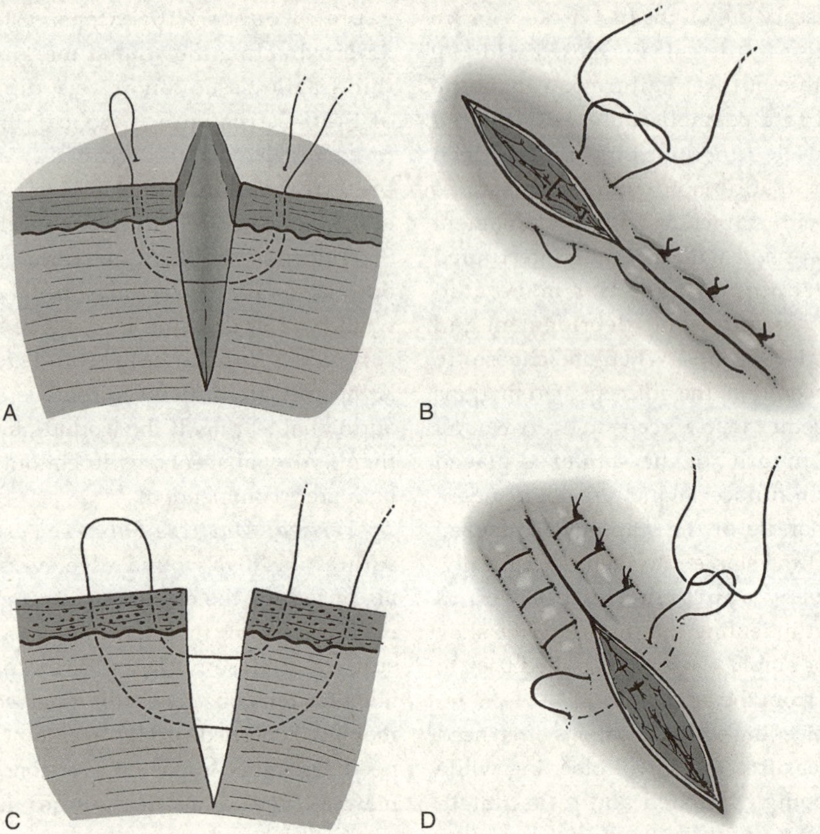

Fig. 38-4 Mattress suture.

0.5 cm adjacent to the initial insertion point and is tied. Unlike with vertical mattress sutures, each bite is always the same distance from the wound margin.

Dog-Ear Deformity Repair. Some redundant tissue may result on one side of the repair as the closure nears completion, especially in the closure of curvilinear lacerations. This redundant tissue generally can be avoided by placing the initial suture in the middle of a curvilinear wound. If the clinician has limited experience, excision and undermining of tissue are likely to result in complications and should not be attemped.

Procedure. The laceration repair begins in a traditional manner and continues to approximately the final 1 cm of the wound (Fig. 38-5). A short incision (approximately 1 cm) is made from the end of the laceration at a 45-degree angle. The angle is cut toward the side of the redundant, bunched tissue. In most cases the subcutaneous tissue from the start of the dog-ear defect to the newly created end of the wound must be gently undermined to mobilize the skin. The next step, the final step before suturing, is the most important. The work that has just been completed leaves a small triangular piece of excess tissue. The redundant piece is gently lifted with the tissue forceps and excised in a line parallel to the incision made above. The wound can now be closed with simple interrupted suture technique. Poor technique can result in a more unsightly repair. If too much tissue is undermined, the edge of the skin can lose its blood supply and necrse.

Corner Stitch (Half-Buried Horizontal Mattress Sutures). Jagged and triangular wounds create corners that can be difficult to repair. The clinician must avoid placing the suture directly in the tip of the flap. This practice may "stretch" the tissue and further compromise blood flow to the wound margin. The corner stitch allows optimal tissue approximation with minimal tension.

Procedure. The needle is introduced percutaneously through the nonlap side of the wound a few

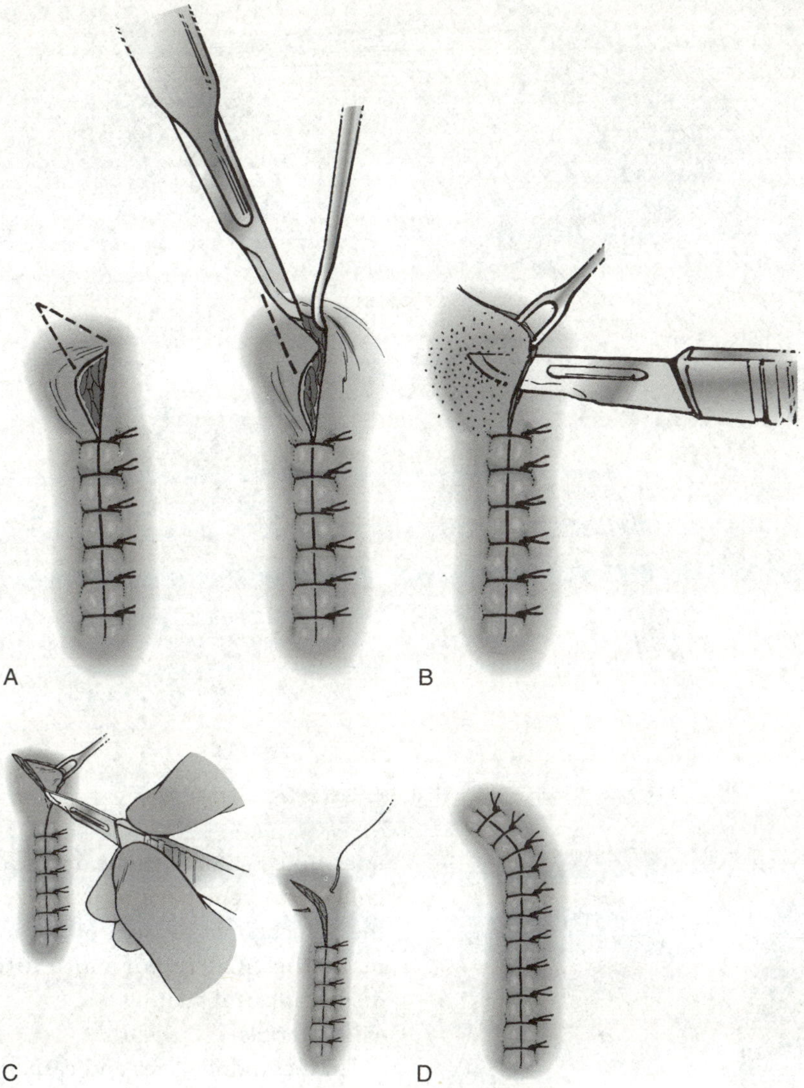

Fig. 38-5 Dog-ear repair.

millimeters from the corner of the wound (Fig. 38-6). The needle is passed horizontally through the dermis of the flap. The final step is to pass the needle into the dermis of the nonflap aspect of the wound a few millimeters from the opposite side of the corner. The suture is led out through the epidermis and tied. This technique can also be used to encompass multiple flaps either individually or simultaneously if the tips are adjacent to one another. The most difficult but important aspect of the corner stitch is to take bites of equal depth with each pass of the needle. Failure to take equal bites of tissue results in a wound with opposing sides that do not lie flat; this leads to a more obvious scar. When the corner has been repaired, the remaining two sides of the wound may be closed with simple interrupted or running suture techniue.

V-Y Wound Closure. The V-Y closure is indicated for the repair of V-shaped wounds with tissue loss or with nonviable margins that must be trimmed. The tissue loss is such that the adjacent mobile tissue is not sufficient to close the remaining defect.

Procedure. Nonviable tissue is trimmed with fine iris scissors (Fig. 38-7). The long V-shaped portion of the wound is sutured with simple interrupted percutaneous stitches. This first step brings the tip of the flap closer to the newly created corner of the wound. A corner stitch is used to secure the tip of the flap. The remaining limbs of the Y can be repaired with simple

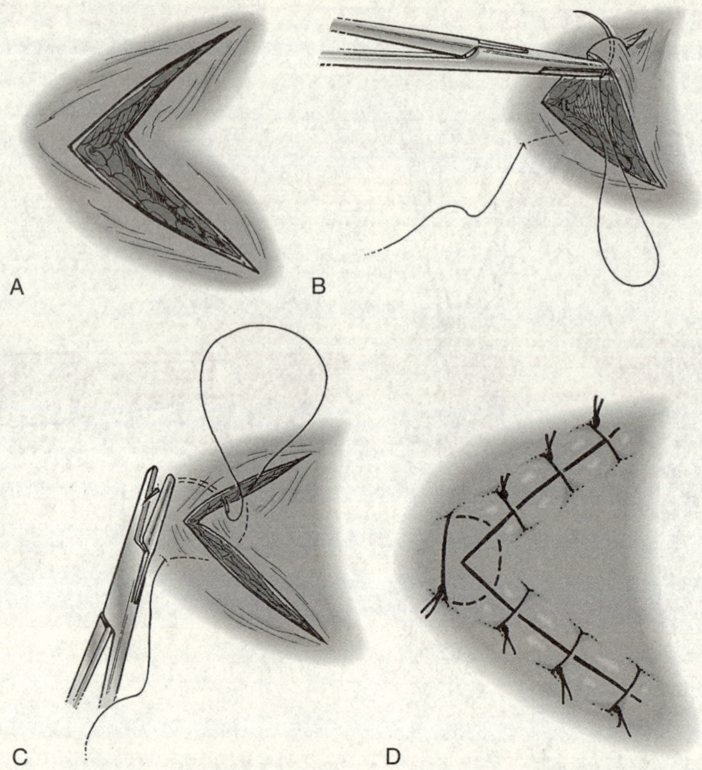

Fig. 38-6 Corner stitch (half-buried horizontal mattress).

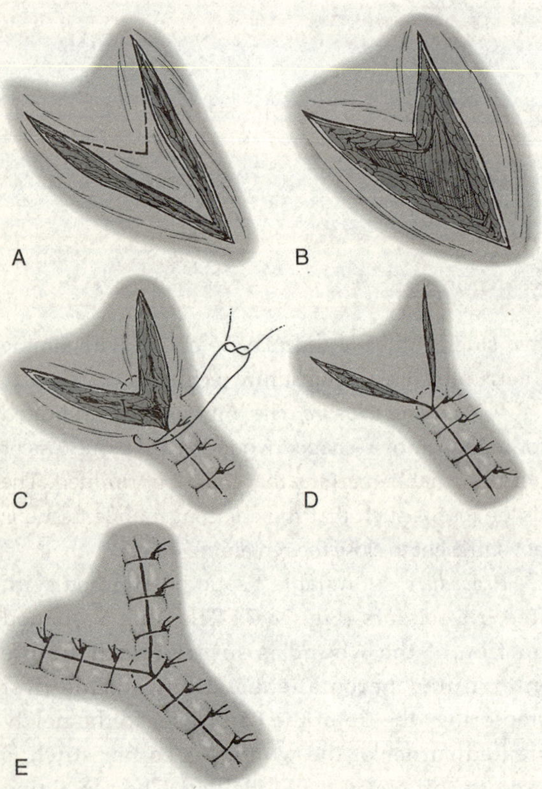

Fig. 38-7 V-Y closure.

interrupted stitches. Some degree of undermining is likely to be needed to mobilize tissue to close the defect. Débridement of too much tissue can make the final repair more difficult and can distort adjacent anatmy.

Materials

In the Middle Ages and earlier, materials used to close wounds included flax, hemp, fascia, hair, linen strips, pigs' bristles, reeds, grasses, and even the mouth parts of the pincher ant. In the early 1900s, natural organic protein products, including silk, cotton, and catgut, were the only available substances. Polyester (Dacron) and nylon were the first synthetic materials, available in the 1940s. Since then, a host of other synthetic materials have become available.

Suture. The ideal suture is inert to metabolism, is resistant to infection, has great tensile strength, does not tear tissue, is easy to work with and tie, and is available in convenient colors with a variety of cutting and noncutting needles (Table 38-2). A common classification of suture material relies on relative absorbability. In general, the materials that maintain their tensile strength for more than 60 d after implantation have been defined as nonabsorbable. Materials that undergo rapid degradation in tissue and lose their strength in less than 60 d are considered absorbable. A second classification considers the source and nature of the material. Biologic substances, which include catgut, collagen, silk, linen, and cotton, generally produce the greatest tissue reaction and have the lowest relative tensile strength but have good knot security. These characteristics are in contrast to synthetic materials, such as polyester (Dacron), polyamide (nylon), polypropylene (Prolene), polyglycolide and polylactide polymers (Dexon and Vicryl), polydioxanone (PDS), and steel, which usually have less tissue reactivity, greater strength, and less knot security.

Table 38-2 Suture Materials for Wound Closure

TYPE	DESCRIPTION	SECURITY	STRENGTH	REACTION	WORKABILITY	INFECTION	COMMENT
Nonabsorbables							
Silk		++++	+	++++	++++	++	Suitable around mouth, nose, or nipples, but too reactive and weak to be used universally
Mersilene	Braided synthetic	++++	++	+++	++++		Good tensile strength; some prefer for fascia repairs
Nylon	Monofilament	++	+++	++	++	+++	Good strength; decreased infection rate; knots tend to skip, especially the first "throw"
Polypropylene (Prolene)	Monofilament	+	++++	+	+	++++	Good resistance on infection; often difficult to work with; requires an extra throw
Ethibond	Braided coated polyester	+++	++++	++1/2	+++	+++	
Stainless steel wire	Monofilament	++++	++++	+	+	+	Difficult to use; painful to patient;some prefer for tendons
Absorbables							
Gut (plain)	From sheep intima	+	++	+++		+	Loses strength rapidly and is quickly absorbed; rarely used today
Chromic (gut)	Plain gut treated with chromic salts	++	++	+++		+	Similar to plain gut; can be used to close intraoral lacerations
Dexon	Braided copolymer of glycolic acid	++++	++++	+		++++	Braiding may cause it to "hang up"when knots are being tied
Vicryl	Braided polymer of lactide and glycolide	+++	++++	+		+++	Low reactivity with good strength; suitable for subcutaneous healing; good in mucous membranes
Polydioxanone	Monofilament	++++	++++	+	Excellent	Unavailable	First available monofilament synthetic absorbable sutures; appears to be excellent

Knotting properties and handling characteristics tend to vary inversely. Knot security is of particular importance in maintaining wound closure and the patient's confidence in the physician. Sutures with smooth or slippery surfaces produce little friction and glide effortlessly through tissue and are easy to tie. Smoother materials are more difficult to handle and more likely to untie spontaneously. Certain monofilament synthetic materials tend to return or spring back to their original shape. To overcome this suture memory, the first part of the tie should be a "double throw" pulled tightly enough to approximate the tissue, with care taken not to strangulate the margins. The second throw locks the tension of the first part into position. A third throw is used for added security. If this is done properly, additional knotting is not needed after the third throw.

The presence of any suture material in a wound increases the likelihood of infection. Subcutaneous sutures bear the greatest risk. The degree of risk depends on characteristics of the substances used. Braided multifilament materials, such as the polyesters, polyamides, polyglycolides, and silk, yield the highest infection rates, whereas monofilament synthetic substances have the lowest risk of infection. There are several nonabsorbable monofilament synthetic sutures and one absorbable monofilament (PDS). The degree of infectivity of PDS compares well with the low rates of infectivity of similar materials.

Consideration of patient comfort in suture selection is important. Although silk is highly reactive, it ties well, is easy to handle, and is comfortable for the patient. It is an excellent choice for use in and around the lips, where comfort is a major concern. PDS is a comfortable absorbable suture and can be left in intraoral mucosa to be absorbed, with apparently low risks of infection, or it can be removed in 5 to 7 d. Staples or metallic sutures are excellent when strength is needed, but they may be uncomfortable for the patient. Nylon and polypropylene, which are the most common sutures used on skin, produce little tissue reaction and offer good tensile strength. They tend to be stiff, produce discomfort near the lips, have poor knot security, and may be difficult to work with. A braided, coated polyester nonabsorbable material, such as Ethibond, is easier to work with and has better knot stability. Although Ethibond is more expensive than nylon, its characteristics and added patient comfort suggest that it may be preferable. Absorbable suture materials, such as polyglycolide and polylactide polymers (Dexon and Vicryl), have been used strictly for subcutaneous and mucosal closures. Their highly reactive nature allows them to be broken down and absorbed over weeks. Chromic catgut, another absorbable material, has been shown to be safe and effective for the closure of scalp wounds in children.

Needles. Surgical needles are available in a variety of sizes and shapes with myriad other characteristics. Cutting needles may be reverse cutting, conventional cutting, taper cut, or precision point. Most emergency wounds may be closed with a conventional cutting needle. In addition to its sharp point, it has two opposing cutting edges, with a third on the inside curve. Precision point needles are similarly shaped but are honed 24 extra times and maintain their added sharpness longer. These needles are used for delicate plastic or cosmetic surgery. Noncutting needles are reserved for organ repair and subcutaneous suturing. Cutting needles may also be used to repair subcutaneous tissue.

Tape. Tape closure may be superior to closure with sutures and staples if applied in the appropriate circumstances. In general, the laceration should be linear and subjected to weak static and dynamic forces. Tape is not considered for wounds requiring meticulous tissue approximation. Compared with other closure materials, tape is associated with lower risk of infection, less expense, and less physician time. In addition, a painful injection of local anesthetic is not needed.

The ideal wound closure tape allows water and gas exchange and possesses elasticity, strength, and optimal adhesiveness. For adhesive properties to be maximized, tincture of benzoin should be painted on the skin adjacent to the wound.

Staples. Staples offer several advantages over sutures. Monofilament stainless steel staples offer less risk of infection.The time necessary to accomplish closure may be significantly lessened. Acceptable wounds must be linear and subjected to weak skin forces. Wounds requiring accurate approximation of tissue are not candidates for staple closure.Staples are also uncomfortable while in situ and on removal. Stapled wounds gain tensile strength sooner, and the staples can be removed 1 to 3 d earlier than sutures. After removal, the staples should be replaced with wound closure tape for continued reinforcement.

Various stapling devices are available. The device must allow good visual access and flexible positioning for difficult angles. The angle of staple delivery is important. The device needs an ejector spring for smooth staple release and must be able to be handled without producing fatigue.

Tissue Adhesives. Tissue adhesives offer many advantages over traditional sutures. In addition, suture removal in 7 to 10 d is unnecessary because the adhesive sloughs off the skin in approximately the same amount of time. Evidence indicates that adhesives not only provide their own dressing but also have antibacterial properties and may decrease the rate of wound infections. Closing wounds with adhesives is less expensive than traditional suturing and carries no risk of needle-stick injuries.

Tissue adhesive may be applied in high-tension areas, but only if used in conjunction with subcutaneous or subcuticular sutures. If used alone, tissue adhesives are not recommended for lacerations longer than 4 cm or in areas of higher tension or frequent repetitive movements, such as joints or hands.

Other disadvantages of tissue adhesives include the inability to use antibacterial or other petroleum-based products on the wound; the recommendation not to swim, to limit forces that may prematurely remove the adhesive; and the greater risk of dehiscence. The tensile strength of tissue adhesives is significantly less than that of sutures. Tissue adhesives represent a tremendous advance in the management of routine uncomplicated lacerations in nontension areas.

Application of tissue adhesive begins with routine skin and wound preparation.The area must be dried and adequate hemostasis achieved before application of the adhesive. The wound margins are approximated as meticulously as possible, and care should be taken to prevent adhesive from getting between the wound margins. Applying tape (Steri-Strips) before application will facilitate wound margin approximation and make it easier to apply. Adhesive between the wound margins delays healing and increases the likelihood of wound dehiscence. The adhesive is applied to the entire length of the wound sufficient to cover 5 to 10 mm of skin adjacent to the margins. Three layers of adhesive are applied. A period of 30 to 45 s is allowed for the first layer to polymerize, and then the subsequent two layers are applied, with approximately 10 s allowed between applications. Special care is taken to ensure that the adhesive does not run off and disturb adjacent tissues.

Antibiotic Prophylaxis

Prophylactic antibiotics had no role in simple nonbite lacerations. Routine antibiotic use also has complications:Increasing resistance to antibiotics, gastrointestinal side effects, and allergic reactions are common.Prophylaxis must be tailored to each patient.

Contamination, Crush, and Host Factors

Antibiotic prophylaxis is often provided for patients with wounds with gross contamination, patients with severe crush injuries, and immunocompromised patients. Some authors recommend not closing these wounds. If circumstances require wound closure despite the infection risk, many emergency physicians recommend prophylaxis.

A patient with significant crush injury requires antibiotics. Crush injuries are high-risk wounds because they produce more devitalized tissue.

Patients with certain risk factors have increased wound infection rates. A prospective study of more than 23,000 surgical wounds showed an increased rate of wound infection in patients with diabetes, obesity, malnutrition, chronic renal failure, advanced age, and chronic steroid use. Because of higher rates of infection, some authors suggest the use of antibiotics in these patients, again based on individual circumstances.Some authors advocate prophylaxis for other host factors, such as prosthetic joints or risk for endocarditis.

Open Fractures, Joint Wounds, and Gunshot Wounds

Wounds that involve joints or open fractures necessitate use of prophylactic antibiotics. Indeed, the time to antibiotic administration in these wounds was found to be the most important factor in decreasing wound infection rates. Open fractures without evidence of significant soft tissue damage (avulsions and crushed or devitalized tissue) necessitate use of antibiotics for 24 hr. Open comminuted fractures or fractures with significant tissue damage necessitate 72 hr of antibiotics.For gunshot wounds, which are classified as a type of open fracture, the recommendations vary with the type of missile wound. Low-velocity missile wounds not treated with antibiotics.High-velocity wounds with fracture, on the other hand, are associated with an increased risk of infection, and antibiotic therapy should be initiated early and maintained for 48 to 72 hr.In addition, patients with shotgun wounds with fracture should receive prophylaxis as well.Appropriate antibiotic therapy would be a cephalosporin with or without an aminoglycoside plus penicillin (to cover Clostridia species).Use of cefazolin (Ancef) 1 g q8h and clindamycin 600 mg IV q8h may be considered. For the severely contaminated wounds, tobramycin 1 mg/kg q8h is added.

Bites and Puncture Wounds

Antibiotics are indicated for through-and-through intraoral lacerations, cat bites, some dog bites, some human bites, and some puncture injuries to the foot.

Cat Bites. Prophylaxis is required for patients with cat bites. These bites tend to be deep puncture wounds that are difficult to irrigate adequately.These wounds also tend to become infected at a much higher rate than other types of bites. Antibiotics seem to decrease the incidence of infection.

The organisms found in cat bites include Staphylococcus species, Streptococcus species, and, most often, Pasteurella multocida. P. multocida is usually found in infected cat bite wounds. P. multocida is sensitive to penicillin, but the infection is often polymicrobial. P. multocida is resistant to dicloxacillin, cephalexin, and clindamycin, and there are many erythromycin-resistant strains. Amoxicillin with clavulanate (875 mg bid for 7 d) is the current recommendation for antibiotic prophylaxis for cat bites.

Dog Bites. Antibiotic prophylaxis for dog bites is more controversial. Dog bites tend to involve more crush injuries with tearing and avulsions rather than puncture wounds. As such, dog bites are usually more amenable to irrigation and débridement. Dog bite wounds showed no benefit with antibiotics. It may be logical to limit the use of antibiotics to high-risk wounds, such as hand injuries, deep puncture wounds, and wounds in older or immunocompromised patients.

Hand Bites. In addition to the previous bite wound recommendations, antibiotic prophylaxis of injuries to the metacarpophalangeal joints is advised. These wounds are assumed to be human bites until proved otherwise. Also known as "fight bites," these wounds have a high incidence of infection. Patients without signs of infection may be managed as outpatients. Close inspection after anesthesia has been applied is necessary to thoroughly evaluate the area for tendon involvement and/or penetration of the joint. If the joint is involved,aggressive irrigation is required. In some institutions, all these patients are taken to the operating room for a thorough washout.Patients with early signs of infection are admitted for intravenous antibiotics and aggressive debridement and irrigation. The choice of antibiotics reflects the predominant organisms of hand bite infections. Streptococcus and Staphylococcus species are common, but Eikenella corrodens and Bacteroides species are also typical pathogens. Because Eikenella is often resistant to clindamycin,first-generation cephalosporins,and erythromycin, patients with early infection are treated with amoxicillin with clavulanate.Patients with later infection are treated with intravenous extended-spectrum antibiotics (e.g., ampicillin with sulbactam).

Intraoral Lacerations. Lacerations of the oral mucosa involve bacteria-rich oral secretions and may become infected slightly more often (6%-12%) than other wounds. Rates of infection for through-and-through lacerations may be twice the rates for simple mucosal lacerations. It may be reasonable to limit antibiotic use to high-risk patients with through-and-through wounds. Penicillin 500 mg bid for 5 d is an appropriate choice of antibiotic.

Puncture Wounds of the Foot. Puncture wounds of the foot are seen frequently in ED.These wounds are often caused by common nails, although other objects (e.g., glass, metal, and wood) must be considered.Despite their simple appearance, these wounds may produce significant morbidity. Most wounds occur on the plantar surface, from the neck of the metatarsal to the toes. Simple cellulitis accounts for half of these infections.More significant infections include septic arthritis, abscesses, and osteomyelitis. Pseudomonas organisms cause 90% of osteomyelitis cases from puncture wounds. No data suggest a benefit from prophylactic antibiotics, but given the high risk of infection and serious complications, their use may be considered in select puncture wounds. Consideration of Pseudomonas organisms when the puncture went through a rubber-soled shoe is essential.Patients with puncture wounds to the foot require early follow-up. Ciprofloxacin is the drug of choice to treat outpatients with suspected wound infection when Pseudomonas is of concern. Cephalexin (Keflex) or dicloxacillin is adequate for staphylococcal and streptococcal coverage unless methicillin-resistant Staphylococcus aureus(MRSA) is likely. In cases suspicious for MRSA, sulfamethoxazole-trimethoprim or doxycycline is recommended.

Drains, Dressings, and Immobilization

Drains

Drains probably have no role in ED wound care. In general, drains are placed when a collection of fluid exists or may develop. The presence of a drain reduces the wound's resistance to infection,regardless of the materials used in its construction, and the use of drains should be avoided. In wounds likely to collect fluid (e.g., around the elbow or knee), it is preferable to place the extremity at rest with a plaster splint or perform delayed primary closure.

Dressings

Various dressing materials are available. The microenvironment created by a dressing affects the biology of healing. The optimal wound climate must not interfere with the activity of fibroblasts and macrophages.The production of granulation tissue and migration of epithelial cells across the wound must be optimized.

Several factors should be considered in choosing the appropriate dressing.Dressings that prevent evaporation of water and keep tissues moist are helpful. A drying wound produces a thick, hardened scab that impedes the process of epithelialization. Excess fluid can lead to maceration of tissue and may be a potential culture medium for bacterial proliferation.Gaseous permeability is essential because epithelialization is accelerated greatly in the presence of oxygen. The wound-covering product should be impermeable to bacteria and other particulate matter that can contaminate the wound. It is important not to traumatize newly established tissue during dressing changes.The optimal dressing should have a nonadherent surface, be permeable to gases, and have a capacity to absorb some fluid but not allow desiccation.The outer barrier of the product should be impermeable to bacteria but permeable to water vapor. These products include films, hydrocolloids, foams, and hydrogels. The choice of dressing for ED wounds is primarily based on the amount of drainage that is expected.

Film dressings are thin membranes that are transparent, adhesive,and waterproof but are not absorptive. They are best reserved for wounds with low levels of drainage.Film dressings may be left in place for up to 7 d as long as they do not leak or separate from the wound bed. For wounds with a moderate amount of drainage, moderately absorptive hydrocolloid dressings may be indicated. These dressings are thicker than films, semiocclusive, waterproof, and very comfortable for the patient.Like films, they can be left on for up to 7 d. Foam dressings are more absorptive and made of a soft cushion spongelike material.Some may require a secondary dressing for adhesion and need to be removed every 3 d. Hydrogel dressings are moisture-donating water-based gels that are available in sheets attached to a semipermeable film. These dressings do not absorb fluids, so they must be used on relatively dry wounds. Patients often find these dressings to be the most comfortable, but they need to be changed every 1 to 3 d. These should be changed daily to prevent desiccation. Immobilization Wounds in proximity to joints must be immobilized as part of routine care. Splinting the injured body part places the injury at rest and hastens healing. Failure to splint appropriately exposes the healing tissue to the dynamic forces of muscular contractions, ultimately slowing the healing process and increasing scar size. In addition, immobilization decreases lymphatic flow and minimizes spread of microflora from the wound.

DISPOSITION

Wound Care Instructions

It is difficult for patients to identify and recognize the signs of infection (Box 38-2). Discharge instructions must be clear, understandable, and reasonably comprehensive.Instructions should include daily care, observation for signs of infection, suture removal dates, and a follow-up source. It should be recommended to the patient that injured extremities be elevated during the first 24 to 48 post-traumatic hr and explained that elevation lessens edema, hastens healing, and mollifies pain. The wound should be protected as described previously or cleaned daily to remove crust formations.It is safe for patients to bathe and get the wound wet 24 hr after injury. Daily swabbing with half-strength hydrogen peroxide rids the wound of debris and any blood clot that forms between the sutured edges. Hydrogen peroxide should not be used after separation of the scab because it is toxic to the epithelium and may produce bullae.

Box 38-2 Wound Care Instructions

A. Elevate the injured extremity above the level of the heart.Wear a sling when appropriate.
B. Cleanse daily in a gentle manner to remove debris and crusting that develops. Use dilute hydrogen peroxide.
C. Immobilization should be maintained at least until suture removal.
D. Signs of infection
  1. Redness
  2. Increasing pain
  3. Swelling
  4. Fever
  5. Red streaks progressing up an extremity
E. Wound check
  1. As needed to check signs of infection
  2. Routine at 48 hr for high-risk wounds
F. Suture removal (*Note*: Suture may be removed earlier if Steri-Strips reinforce the wound.)
  1. Face: 3-5 d (always replace with Steri-Strips)
  2. Scalp: 7-10 d
  3. Trunk: 7-10 d
  4. Arms and legs: 10-14 d
  5. Joints: 14 d

Wound infection is difficult for the untrained observer to distinguish from the inflammatory response of injury and subsequent healing. An injury classified as high risk must be reexamined 48 hr after the trauma, regardless of its appearance.

Suture removal times vary, but generally they are approximately 4 d for the face and 7 to 14 d for other body parts (Box 38-2). Considerations include cosmetics, dynamic forces in proximity to the injury, static skin tension, blood supply, and anticipated healing rates.

Tetanus Immunization

Immunization status needs to be considered in all patients with wounds, regardless of severity.

The usual incubation period for tetanus is 7 to 21 d (range, 3-56 d). Immunization is given as soon as possible but can be given days or weeks after the injury. The dose of tetanus toxoid (T) or diphtheria, pertussis, and tetanus toxoids (DTaP) is 0.5 mL intramuscularly, regardless of the patient's age. Inadequately immunized patients need a dose of DTaP and tetanus immune globulin (TIG). The TIG dose is 250 U for all ages 7 yr or older and 4 U/kg IM up to 250 U for ages younger than 7 yr (Table 38-3). A single injection of TIG provides protective levels of passive antibodies for at least 4 w. The immune globulin and toxoid may be given during the same visit but should be administered with a different syringe at separate sites.

Table 38-3 Tetanus Prophylaxis for All Patients with All Wounds

IMMUNIZATION HISTORY	DTAP (0.5 mL)	TIG (250 U)
Fully immunized, $<$10 yr since booster	No	No
Fully immunized, $>$10 yr since booster	Yes	No
Incomplete series ($<$3 injections)	Yes	Yes

SUMMARY

Box 38-3 summarizes the principles of wound care management.

Box 38-3 Summary of wound care

A. Stabilize patient
B. History (include tetanus immunization and allergies)
C. Physical examination
  1. Neurovascular examination
  2. Anesthesia: bupivacaine 0.5% without epinephrine,regional or local
  3. Bloodless field: tourniquet or sphygmomanometer for extremities

4. Sterile examination of anatomic structures, skin, nerves,tendons, blood vessels, bones, muscles, fascia, other (ducts, cartilage)
5. Consultation if indicated

D. X-ray films to detect injury to bone or the presence of foreign bodies (xeroradiograph or ultrasound)

E. Wound preparation
1. Cut—do not shave—surrounding hair
2. Prepare surrounding skin with povidone-iodine (Betadine)solution
3. Sharp debridement of foreign matter and devitalized tissue
4. High-pressure irrigation with saline, 1% Betadine, an antibiotic solution, or a nonionic solution

F. Wound closure
1. Tape, staples, or suture
2. Do not use subcutaneous sutures unless the wound is under high tension

G. Antibiotics
1. Apply topical antibiotics
2. No systemic antibiotics unless wound is very high risk

H. Dress and immobilize: Consider a transparent gas-permeable dressing

I. Wound care instructions (Box 38-2)
1. Signs of infection
2. Elevation
3. Wound check if necessary
4. Suture removal as soon as possible

(WANG Pei)

Chapter 39

Multiple Trauma

KEY CONSEPTS

The majority of life-threatening injuries that require intervention by out-of-hospital providers are related to airway, breathing, and circulation (ABC).

The goals of the secondary survey are to obtain pertinent historical data about the patient and injury as well as evaluate and treat injuries not found on the primary survey.

Care of the multiple trauma patient is complex and involves the coordination of multiple providers, including EMS personnel, emergency physicians, nurses, technicians, trauma surgeons, and subspecialists.

In the critically injured patient, imaging of the chest and pelvis and an eFAST exam should be obtained early in the evaluation.

All patients with potentially serious injuries should have blood type and screening done.

INTRODUCTION

The care of the injured patient remains one of the mainstays of emergency medicine practice. Emergency physicians play a vital role in the stabilization and diagnostic phases of trauma care. Management of these patients involves complex, time-dependent decision-making, leadership capability, and technical skill. Proper resuscitation can lead to functional outcomes, even in severely injured patients.

PRINCIPLES OF DISEASE

The emergency physician faces significant clinical uncertainty when a multiple trauma patient presents to the ED. Much of the diagnostic dilemma and subsequent evaluation can be directed based on knowledge of the mechanism of injury. Although mechanisms of injury alone are not good predictors of major trauma, common patterns of injuries can be anticipated and specifically assessed in ED patients. Table 39-1 outlines several blunt trauma mechanisms of injury with potential associated clinical findings.

MANAGEMENT

Out-of-Hospital

Management of the trauma patient frequently begins prior to arrival in the ED by first responders. The goals of out-of-hospital care include intervening in immediately life-threatening injuries, preventing additional injury, and rapid transport to trauma centers for definitive care.

The majority of life-threatening injuries that require intervention by out-of-hospital providers are related to airway, breathing, and circulation (ABC). Preventing aspiration of gastric contents and providing adequate tissue oxygenation are the primary goals of endotracheal intubation. Tension pneumothorax is the fundamental threat to adequate ventilation and requires immediate needle thoracostomy. Systemic hypotension with impaired end-organ perfusion mandates treatment in the trauma patient.

Preventing additional injury requires an awareness of not only clinically evident abnormalities but also potentially more serious injuries. Coordinated extrication and transport with rigid cervical immobilization, complete spinal precautions, intensive hemodynamic monitoring, and stabilization of fractures to prevent neurovascular compromise are examples of assuming the most serious injuries exist in multiple trauma patients.

Table 39-1 Blunt Trauma Mechanisms and Associated Injuries

MECHANISM OF INJURY	ADDITIONAL CONSIDERATIONS	POTENTIAL ASSOCIATED INJURIES
Motor vehicle collisions		
Head-on collision		Facial injuries Lower extremity injuries Aortic injuries
Rear-end collision		Hyperextension injuries of cervical spine Cervical spine fractures Central cord syndrome
Lateral (T-bone) collision		Thoracic injuries Abdominal injuries—spleen, liver Pelvic injuries Clavicle, humerus, rib fractures
Rollover	Greater chance of ejection Significant mechanism of injury	Crush injuries Compression fractures of spine
Ejected from vehicle	Likely unrestrained Significant mortality	Spinal injuries
Windshield damage	Likely unrestrained	Closed head injuries, coup and countercoup injuries Facial fractures Skull fractures Cervical spine fractures
Steering wheel damage	Likely unrestrained	Thoracic injuries Sternal and rib fractures, flail chest Cardiac contusion Aortic injuries Hemo/pneumothoraces
Dashboard involvement/damage		Pelvic and acetabular injuries Dislocated hip
Restraint/seat belt use		
Proper three-point restraint	Decreased morbidity	Sternal and rib fractures, pulmonary contusions
Lap belt only		Chance fractures, abdominal injuries, head and facial injuries/fractures
Shoulder belt only		Cervical spine injuries/fractures, "submarine" out of restraint devices (possible ejection)
Air bag deployment	Front-end collisions Less severe head/upper torso injuries Not effective for lateral impacts More severe injuries in children (improper front seat placement)	Upper extremity soft tissue injuries/fractures Lower extremity injuries/fractures
Pedestrian versus automobile		
Low speed (braking automobile)		Tibia and fibula fractures, knee injuries
High speed		Waddle's triad—tibia/fibula or femur fractures, truncal injuries, craniofacial injuries "Thrown" pedestrians at risk for multisystem injuries
Bicycle		
Automobile related		Closed head injuries "Handlebar" injuries Spleen/liver lacerations Additional intra-abdominal injuries Consider penetrating injuries

Continued

MECHANISM OF INJURY	ADDITIONAL CONSIDERATIONS	POTENTIAL ASSOCIATED INJURIES
Nonautomobile related		Extremity injuries "Handlebar" injuries
Falls	LD_{50} 36–60 ft	
Vertical impact		Calcaneal and lower extremity fractures Pelvic fractures Closed head injuries Cervical spine fractures Renal and renal vascular injuries
Horizontal impact		Craniofacial fractures Hand and wrist fractures Abdominal and thoracic visceral injuries Aortic injuries

Emergency Department

General Principles

Care of the multiple trauma patient is complex and involves the coordination of multiple providers, including EMS personnel, emergency physicians, nurses, technicians, trauma surgeons, and subspecialists. A systematic and comprehensive approach to these patients is necessary, incorporating providers from each discipline. Advanced Trauma Life Support(ATLS) guidelines delineate the use of defined trauma response teams, with providers performing assessments, diagnostics, and interventions simultaneously. With this approach, the physician team leader coordinates the management of the patient, considering the presence of life- or limb-threatening injuries in a sequential manner **(Table 39-2).**The priorities in the treatment of trauma patients are similar to those for any other life-threatening condition. Securing the airway, maintaining ventilation, controlling hemorrhage, and treating shock are first priorities because of their crucial importance for survival. The emergency physician should give consideration to the worst possible injury and act accordingly until the diagnosis is confirmed or excluded. The consequences of an overzealous evaluation are more acceptable than those of a missed injury. Based on ATLS, the phases of ED care are divided into the primary survey with interventions, initial diagnostics and imaging, the secondary survey, and disposition.

Table 39-2 American College of Surgeons Requirements for the Presence of a Surgeon in Major Resuscitations

A surgeon should be present in the emergency department on trauma patient arrival or within 15 min if any of the following major criteria are found:
Confirmed hypotension (systolic blood pressure 90 mm Hg)
Respiratory compromise requiring intubation
Penetrating gunshot wound to the neck, chest, abdomen, or pelvis
Glasgow Coma Scale score of < 8 attributed to trauma

Primary Survey

Airway and Breathing Proper assessment and management of airway, oxygenation, and ventilation in the trauma patient is of utmost importance but can be challenging. The goals of airway management are threefold: airway protection, adequate oxygenation, and adequate ventilation.

Airway protection is necessary in a variety of trauma patients. Airway obstruction mandates immediate intervention. Obstruction from debris, blood, or vomitus may be easily removed with suction. Neck or facial trauma may be more problematic. Swelling, distorted anatomy, and hematoma formation may all contribute to impending obstruction. Early airway control is safest because these conditions may rapidly worsen. Inability to adequately protect the airway, such as in patients with depressed levels of consciousness, is another indication for intervention. Airway control is recommended in patients with significant head injury (GCS < 9). Low GCS scores from intoxication, and not injury, may not necessitate intubation, as loss of airway reflexes cannot be predicted by GCS alone in this group.

As a general rule, all trauma patients should be placed on supplemental oxygen. Adequate oxygenation has a direct effect on outcome of many trauma patients. In head-injured patients, hypoxia in both out-of-hospital and hospital phases of resuscitation has been associated with poorer outcomes. Hypoxia may also worsen outcome in spinal cord injury. Maintenance of P_aO_2 greater than 60 mm Hg has been recommended. Inadequate ventilation, which may lead to respiratory acidosis, can be noted by the rate and quality of respirations. Signs of inadequate oxygenation may be more subtle and include agitation and restlessness. Assessment for injury that may compromise oxygenation, ventilation, or both requires careful inspection and auscultation of the chest. Signs of such compromising injury include increased work of breathing, tachypnea, penetrating wounds, flail segments, tracheal deviation, and distended neck veins. In determining the need for more aggressive airway management, these data are put into the context of the patient's overall presentation. Certain ventilatory problems, such as pneumothorax or hemothorax, may require tube thoracostomy in addition to intubation. Early intervention is preferable in the tenuous patient.

Once the decision to intubate the patient has been made, many considerations must be taken into account. If the patient's condition allows, a brief neurologic examination prior to paralytics can be helpful in determining the extent of injury. Also, cervical spine injury precautions should be considered for patients with blunt trauma and gunshot wounds to the neck. Rapid sequence induction and orotracheal intubation with in-line cervical stabilization provides a safe method. There are many approaches to airway control, and many alternative devices, such as the flexible fiberoptic scope, intubating laryngeal mask airway, and video-assisted laryngoscope, are now available to assist in intubation. The choice will be based on clinical scenario and physician comfort.

Surgical airways are indicated in cases of failure or contraindication to orotracheal or nasotracheal intubation. Cricothyrotomy is the preferred method. A variety of devices for percutaneous cricothyrotomy are available that show good success rates and are easy to use. If there is any question of the ability to identify the cricothyroid membrane, the traditional surgical approach with a vertical incision should be used.

Circulation Assessment of hemodynamics and circulatory status are of critical importance after the airway has been evaluated and controlled and adequate ventilation has been ensured.Clinical indicators of adequate perfusion include mental status, skin color and temperature, heart rate, blood pressure, and capillary refill. A normal finding of any single sign does not rule out shock. Mental status changes associated with hypoperfusion can include anxiety, agitation, or sedation. Cool, pale skin or extremities with delayed capillary refill suggest inadequate perfusion and shock. A normal HR and/or BP can be present despite significant hemorrhage. Conversely, tachycardia may be seen without evidence of significant volume loss.

Control of external hemorrhage is crucial. Traditionally, direct pressure to external bleeding sites has been advocated and the use of tourniquets has been discouraged. The use of direct pressure on bleeding remains first-line therapy.

Intravenous access is required early in the assessment of circulation. Two large-bore (14- or 16-gauge) intravenous catheters are recommended. Routine intravenous access may be difficult or unobtainable in certain cases. Intraosseous vascular access can be obtained rapidly and allows the safe infusion of large amounts of fluid or blood products.

Ultrasound-guided peripheral venous access should be considered in patients when blind peripheral attempts are unsuccessful. Central venous access may also be indicated in the appropriate clinical scenario. The use of ultrasound has been shown to increase successful vein cannulation and decrease complications in the placement of central venous lines.

The choice of fluids for resuscitation includes crystalloid, colloid, and blood products. Fluid replacement is generally based on a 3:1 ratio of fluids to blood loss. There are few clinically significant differences between lactated Ringer's and normal saline.No indisputable advantages of colloids have been demonstrated. Therefore, the less expensive and more readily available crystalloids are the routine mainstay as first line of therapy.Current ATLS guidelines standardize the ratio of replacement fluids to loss and recommend 2 L of crystalloid be infused in all patients in shock, followed by blood products. O-positive blood should be used except in women of childbearing age. Type-specific blood should be used when available, but emergent transfusion should not be delayed. The use of the antifibrinolytic agent tranexamic acid has been shown to decrease mortality in trauma patients at risk of major bleeding.

The concept of "permissive hypotension" is based on the concern that resuscitation to normal BP may increase bleeding from a site that is contained and not actively hemorrhaging. Clinically, restoration of normal blood pressure is delayed until active bleeding foci are ruled out. Permissive hypotension is contraindicated in the management of traumatic brain injury because of the risk of hypoperfusion.

The eFAST examination should be performed on all patients as an adjunct to the assessment of circulation. The presence or absence of free intra-abdominal, -thoracic, or -pelvic hemorrhage or pneumothorax diagnosed by ultrasound will direct the management of trauma patients. Pericardial effusions or tamponade can be readily identified. In addition, ultrasound evaluation of the inferior vena cava may be useful in the overall assessment of fluid status in resuscitation.

Disability. A rapid assessment of the patient's neurologic status is necessary early in the ED course. The GCS score is commonly employed.

Exposure. The final phase of the primary survey is completely undressing the patient in order to assess for inconspicuous injuries. Special attention to the axilla, perineum, and skin folds is needed. Preventing hypothermia is essential in this phase. Blankets, warming lights, and warm fluids may be used as indicated.

Secondary Survey

The goals of the secondary survey are to obtain pertinent historical data about the patient and injury as well as evaluate and treat injuries not found on the primary survey. An AMPLE (*a*llergies, *m*edications, *p*ast medical history, *l*ast meal, *e*nvironments and events) history should be obtained. Frequent reassessment of the ABC throughout the ED phase of management is necessary. If deterioration occurs, a complete reevaluation of the primary survey should be initiated. Features of the secondary survey and management are listed in Table 39-3.

Table 39-3 Secondary Survey

REGION/SYSTEM	ASSESSMENT/EXAMINATION
General	Level of consciousness GCS score Specific complaints
Head	Pupils (size, shape, reactivity, visual fields) Contusions Lacerations Evidence of skull fracture (hemotympanum, Battle's sign, raccoon eyes, palpable defects)
Face	Contusions Lacerations Midface instability Malocclusion
Neck (maintain Cervical immobilization)	Penetrating injury/lacerations Tracheal deviation Jugular venous distention Subcutaneous emphysema Hematoma Midline cervical tenderness
Chest	Respiratory effort/excursion Contusions Lacerations Focal tenderness/crepitus Subcutaneous emphysema Heart tones (muffled) Breath sounds (symmetrical)
Abdomen/flank	Contusions Penetrating injury/lacerations Tenderness Peritoneal signs
Pelvis/genitourinary	Contusions Lacerations Stability/symphyseal tenderness Blood (urethral meatus, vaginal bleeding,hematuria) Rectal examination
Neurologic/spinal cord	Midline bony spinal tenderness Mental status Paresthesias Sensory level Motor function, including sphincter tone
Extremities	Contusions Lacerations Deformity Focal tenderness Pulses Capillary refill Evaluation of compartments

Pitfalls

The goal of trauma management in the ED is to provide life-saving interventions and evaluate for injuries. The tenets of ATLS provide a structured approach to ensure a thorough assessment is performed. Because multiple trauma patients present with a variety of injuries from varying mechanisms, the initial focus is directed at defining the most serious pathology. The emergency physician must be aware of potential pitfalls. Head-injured, unconscious, and intubated patients frequently have injuries that are not identified early in their hospital course. More aggressive diagnostics may be indicated in this subset of patients when history and patient-specific complaints are not obtainable. When cervical radiography is indicated, it is essential that the imaging obtained is complete and adequate. Limited radiographic series and inadequate cervical spine imaging have been shown to result in missed or delayed diagnosis of injuries.

Radiographic Evaluation

In the critically injured patient, imaging of the chest and pelvis and an eFAST exam should be obtained early in the evaluation. These studies provide essential information on possible sources of hemorrhage in either the chest or abdomen or from a pelvic fracture.

Laboratory Evaluation

Laboratory evaluation of the trauma patient can provide an objective measure of the adequacy of resuscitation. It also provides much needed information for proper transfusion products and the onset of coagulopathy. Finally, it provides baseline information and values for follow-up studies (e.g., tracking hemoglobin values in a patient with a nonoperative splenic injury).Lactate and base deficit have both been used to measure adequacy of resuscitation in the trauma patient. New noninvasive devices, such as muscle tissue oxygenation and sublingual capnometry, have shown promise in assessing severity of shock and predicting multiorgan dysfunction and mortality. Using one of these objective markers can assist in ensuring proper resuscitation of these patients.

All patients with potentially serious injuries should have blood type and screening done. Cross-matched blood should be immediately ordered for those with apparent serious hemorrhage. As transfusion requirements increase, attention should be paid to the development of coagulopathy. international normalized ratio and fibrinogen should be followed in these patients. Routine electrolytes, BUN, Cr, CBC, and pregnancy testing (when appropriate) should be obtained as well.

DISPOSITION

The ED management of the multiple trauma patient is but one critical phase of the spectrum of care. The decision to admit the patient or transfer to a tertiary care facility should be coordinated based on available resources, consultation with the trauma surgeon, and consideration of institutional and regional guidelines.

(PENG Peng)

Chapter 40

Injury Prevention and Control

KEY CONSEPTS

Injury is the second most costly disease to society and the most serious disease of young people.

Through interdisciplinary research, a better understanding of the epidemiology and biomechanics of injury will lead to new control strategies.

Emergency physicians can incorporate injury control techniques into daily practice through clinical prevention services.

Increasingly, emergency physicians are leaders in addressing and preventing injuries and complex biosocial problems.

PERSPECTIVE

The science of injury control is based on the concept that trauma is like a disease rather than just the consequence of fate or random occurrences. Control of a disease as widespread and multifactorial as injury can occur only through broad interdisciplinary effort, including that of medicine, public health, policy makers, law enforcement, educated citizens, and others (Box 40-1).

Box 40-1 Multidisciplinary Team Approach to Injury Control: Prevention, Acute Care, and Rehabilitation

Prevention
Epidemiology
Biomechanics
Education
Public policy
Law enforcement
Engineering
Outcomes research
Emergency preparedness

Acute Care
Trauma system
EMS
ED care
Hospital care
Clinical guidelines
Clinical prevention services
Outcomes research

Rehabilitation
Physical therapy
Occupational therapy
Mental health providers

Emergency medicine plays a pivotal role in the care of injured patients and in injury control. Injury is the leading cause of death for many age groups. The emergency care system may be the patient's only interface with the health care system. In addition to providing state of the art acute care, emergency physicians should provide state of the art clinical preventive services for these injured patients, as well as work with surgeons, pediatricians, and other specialists to decrease injuries through clinical and policy-relevant research and education.

PRINCIPLES OF THE DISEASE OF INJURY

The major causes of injury include falls, car crashes, gunshots, drownings, and poisonings. Similar to other disease models, injury occurs from the interaction of agent and host through a vector and an environment that is conducive to exposure

(Fig. 40-1). *Injury* is a harmful event caused by the acute transfer of energy to a patient that results in tissue and/or organ damage. Energy is the agent that is delivered to the host (patient) by a vector in an environment with variable risk.

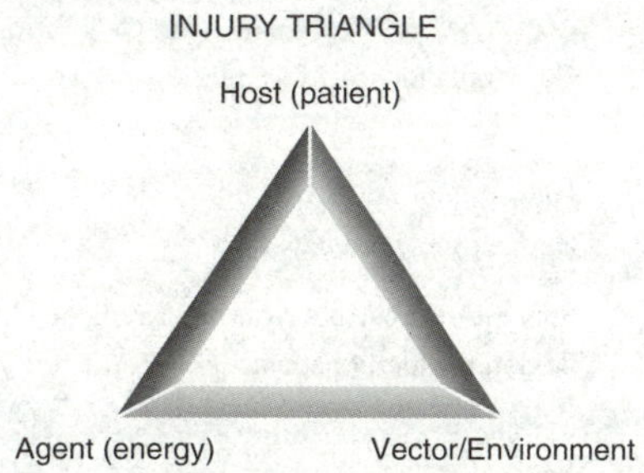

Fig. 40-1 The epidemiologic triad can be used as a framework for injury prevention.

The goal of injury control, similar to other forms of disease control, is to prevent or decrease the transfer of energy to the host by (1) separating the host from the agent through modification of the environment, (2) equipping the host with protection against the agent, or (3) eliminating or modifying the vector that transmits the energy.

Energy is transmitted to the host through a vector, such as motorized and nonmotorized vehicles (e.g., car, bicycle, and skateboard), firearms, piercing instruments (e.g., knife and arrow), explosives, and lit cigarettes. Modifying the vector (by elimination or modification of design) and separating the vector from the host are important methods to reduce injury.

When an injury occurs, host–agent interaction and energy transfer take place in an environment. This environment can be modified to decrease injury. If the environment does not permit energy transmission, the risk for injury, including intentional injuries to the host (patient), is eliminated. In contrast to altering host risk factors, most environmental modifications require no cooperation or action on the part of the host and are more effective when implemented.

William Haddon, the first physician administrator for the National Highway Traffic Safety Administration (NHTSA), first described using this type of approach in a landmark article on injury control in 1970. He laid out 10 methods for preventing injury (Table 40-1). Haddon later expanded these ideas to incorporate time and developed the Haddon matrix. The matrix recognizes that preventative interventions should be considered for the host, agent, vector, and environment prior to the event, during the event, and after the event. Any type or cluster of injuries can be prevented or reduced in severity using this matrix when the environment, vector, and population most at risk are identified and modified. An example of using this process to reduce car crash injuries is given in Table 40-2. The key to energy transfer reduction or prevention is understanding that (1) injuries are predictable, (2) they follow predictable patterns (e.g., by age or gender), and (3) reliance solely on human factors for prevention has significant limits. A fragile item sent through the mail arrives at its destination intact only if it is properly packaged to reduce the energy we anticipate being placed on the item during transport. Likewise, injuries to people can be prevented by using the cells of the Haddon matrix to mitigate the energy transfer of predictable events.

Table 40-1 Haddon's Strategies for Preventing the Transfer of Energy to the Host

TECHNIQUE	CAR CRASH	FALLS
1. Prevent the initial marshaling of energy	Manual task/Breathalyzer ignition interlocks Use of alternative transportation	Remove floor obstacles Prevent unnecessary climbing
2. Reduce the amount of energy marshaled	Speed reduction Vehicle mass restrictions	Climbing height restrictions
3. Prevent the release of energy	Breakaway light poles, roadway obstacle removal	Ambulation aids for elderly Worker safety harnesses
4. Modify the rate of spatial distribution of the release of energy from its source	Autobody crumple zones Safety belts, air bags Water barrel barriers	Land with a "roll" Use of safety nets

Continued

TECHNIQUE	CAR CRASH	FALLS
5. Separate the energy from the host in space or time	Reduce traffic density Homogeneous traffic flow Increase following distance Sidewalks for pedestrians	Safety zones at edge of raised work areas
6. Separate the energy from the host by barrier	Guardrails, concrete median barriers	Guardrails for scaffolds, raised work areas
7. Modify the surface or structure of impact	Collapsible steering columns, padded pillars and bolsters, safety glass	Padded flooring Helmets and hard hats
8. Strengthen the host receiving the energy	Detect and treat premorbid medical conditions	Prevent/treat osteoporosis and strengthen hip flexion in elderly patients
9. Rapidly detect and evaluate damage and counter its continuation and extension	911 and EMS availability Trauma system planning and implementations, and provision of state-of-the-art emergency care	911 and EMS availability Trauma system planning and implementation,and provision of state-of-the-art emergency care
10. Reparative and rehabilitative measures	Provision of state-of-the-art trauma care, rehabilitation, and aftercare	Provision of state-of-the-art trauma care,rehabilitation, and aftercare

Table 40-2 Typical Haddon Matrix (Constructed for Motor Vehicle Injury)

	HOST (DRIVER)	AGENT/VECTOR (CAR)	ENVIRONMENT
Pre-event (before the crash)	Alcohol use Fatigue Experience and judgment Vision	Brake condition Tire quality Center of gravity Load weight	Visibility of hazards Road curvature and gradient Surface coefficient of friction Shoulder height
Event (during the crash)	Medications Motor skills Cognitive function Age	Speed capacity Visual obstructions Speed at impact Vehicle size	Intersections, access control Weather Signalization Speed limits
Postevent (after the crash)	Age Physical condition Medications Social situation	Load containment Deformation zones Fuel system integrity	911 access EMS response Triage and transfer protocols Nearby level 1 trauma center

METHODS OF PREVENTION

The history of injury control began with the first injury. Pain from injury is a powerful stimulus for avoidance behaviors. Early prevention technology is seen in the instruments and garb of the earliest armies, shielding people from the harmful kinetic energy of weapons. Such technology included helmets, shields, and suits of armor. As the delivery of kinetic energy became more sophisticated, prevention technology did not keep pace. Firearms and automobiles represent new plateaus in harnessing kinetic energy as well as creating a new source of morbidity and mortality. The cultural belief was that individuals could avoid vehicular injury by safe driving, and if not, an "accident" occurred. It took more than 50 yr to acknowledge that behavior modification alone was insufficient to mitigate high-energy transmission to persons in a hazardous environment. Cars were not uniformly equipped with seat belts until the 1960s. It took another two decades before air bags became standard.

Implementation of effective injury control strategies depends on collaborative efforts with physicians, nurses, out-of-hospital care providers, epidemiologists, biomechanical engineers, public policy makers, law enforcement officers, and lawyers. A major challenge is the wide diversity of disciplines and interests involved in safety and injury control, many of which are isolated from one another. In the 1990s, important strides were made in community-based injury control programs that rely on coalitions of existing resources with the support of NHTSA, the CDC, and the State and Territorial Injury Prevention Directors Association. These community coalitions were created to garner existing resources and implement injury countermeasures using "the 3 E's" of public *e*ducation, *e*nforcement of laws, and *e*ngineering modification of hazardous devices and environmental conditions.

INJURY CONTROL IN MEDICAL PRACTICE

Traditionally, physicians have focused on treating the patient after the disease has occurred. As the causes of many diseases have become increasingly understood, education about risk assessment and clinically based prevention has been integrated into medical practice, particularly in areas such as infectious (immunizations) and cardiovascular (smoking cessation) disease. Emergency physicians are incorporating risk assessment, counseling, and referral of patients in high-risk groups for injury, such as with domestic violence patients. The Joint Commission has ED requirements for addressing abused patients. Emergency care providers are pivotal in the recording and accumulation of data about the injury event, which is useful for surveillance and epidemiologic analysis. Injury control techniques can be incorporated easily into emergency medicine practice as well. A rational approach to improve injury care in a community (Box 40-2) requires that emergency physicians, surgeons, pediatricians, and physiatrists assume specific roles and activities in promoting injury control. This role for emergency physicians in injury control has been advocated by the American College of Emergency Physicians. Documentation of injury information in the medical record, assessing risk factors in individual patients, counseling and referral, provision of systematized acute trauma care, and public health advocacy are all important.

Box 40-2 Injury Control in Emergency Medicine Practice

Clinical Preventive Services

Document injury information in the medical record

Ensure that medical records of injury cases contain E codes

Assess behavioral and comorbid risk factors for future injury

Provide risk screening, counseling, and referral

Assess biomechanical risk factors in individual patients

Use biomechanical risk factors for directed evaluation of injured patients

Provide systematized acute trauma care

Population Health, Research, and Policy

Participate in and advocate for inclusive trauma systems

Direct and advocate for rapid, competent emergency medical services response

Lead efforts in policy development, implementation, and evaluation

Lead efforts in educating high-risk groups

Lead efforts to address and modify the environment to reduce risk of injury

Collaborate in multidisciplinary research to reduce injury risk and to improve care

(PENG Peng)

SECTION 4

Enviroment Emergencies

Chapter 41

Heat Illness

KEY CONCEPTS

Heat syncope is a perplexing disorder and is characterized by temporary loss of consciousness.

Heat exhaustion (heat prostration) is a clinical syndrome characterized by volume depletion that occurs under conditions of heat stress.

Heatstroke results in elevation of body temperature to extreme levels, usually higher than 40.5°C (105°F), producing multisystem tissue damage and organ dysfunction.

Elderly patients, psychiatric patients, or those with chronic diseases are prone to classic heatstroke during periods of high ambient heat and humidity.

Immediate cooling is the cornerstone of treatment for heatstroke. Antipyretics are ineffective.

PERSPECTIVE

When environmental heat stress is maximal, strenuous exercise is not required to produce heat illness. While heat illness usually occurs in modern military organizations, athletes and the elderly and poor. In heat wave years in the United States, approximately 10 times as many deaths are reported as during non-heat wave years.It is also estimated that at least 10 times as many heat-aggravated illnesses occur because of MI, cerebrovascular accident, and other causes.

PRINCIPLES OF DISEASE

Physiology of Heat

Heat Production

Humans can be considered biochemical "furnaces" that burn food to fuel a complex array of metabolic functions. Water and carbon dioxide are produced and eliminated in large quantities, as are urea, sulfates, phosphates, and other chemical products. In the absence of cooling mechanisms, this baseline metabolic activity would result in a 1.1°C hourly rise in body temperature. Heat production can be increased up to 20-fold by strenuous exertion. Metabolic factors, such as hyperthyroidism and sympathomimetic drug ingestion, can dramatically increase heat production. Environmental heat not only adds to the heat load but also interferes with heat dissipation. The physics of heat transfer as it relates to human physiology involves four mechanisms: conduction, convection, radiation, and evaporation.

Conduction. Conduction is the transfer of heat energy from warmer to cooler objects by direct physical contact. Only approximately 2% of the body heat loss is by conduction. The thermal conductivity of water is at least 25 times that of air.

Convection. Heat loss to air and water vapor molecules circulating around the body is termed convection. Convective heat loss varies directly with wind velocity. Loose-fitting clothing maximizes convective heat loss.

Radiation. Radiation is heat transfer by electromagnetic waves. Radiation accounts for approximately 65% of heat loss in cool environments, it is a major source of heat gain in hot climates.

Evaporation. Evaporation is the conversion of a liquid to the gaseous phase. As ambient temperature rises, evaporation becomes the dominant mechanism of heat loss. In humans, the dominant mode of cooling in hot conditions is evaporation of sweat from the skin.

Heat Regulation

The regulation of body temperature involves

three distinct functions: thermosensors, a central integrative area, and thermoregulatory effectors.

Thermosensors. Temperature-sensitive structures are located both peripherally in the skin and centrally in the body. Skin temperature changes, however, correlate poorly with changes in the rate of heat loss.

Central Integrative Area. CNS interprets information received from the thermosensors to properly instruct thermoregulatory effectors. The concept of a central thermostat by which an alteration shifts effector thresholds in the same direction fits a variety of clinical situations.

Thermoregulatory Effectors. Sweating and peripheral vasodilation are the major mechanisms by which heat loss can be accelerated. In a warm environment, evaporation of sweat from the skin is the most important mechanism of heat dissipation. Each liter of completely evaporated sweat dissipates 580 kcal of heat. The ability of the environment to evaporate sweat is termed atmospheric cooling power and varies primarily with humidity but also with wind velocity. As humidity approaches 100%, evaporative heat loss ceases. Heat loss from the skin by convection and radiation is maximized by increased skin blood flow to facilitate sweating. The vascular response to heat stress is cutaneous vasodilation and compensatory vasoconstriction of splanchnic and renal beds.

For BP to be maintained, cardiac output increases dramatically.

Acclimatization

Acclimatization is defined as "a constellation of physiologic adaptations that appear in a normal person as the result of repeated exposures to heat stress." Daily exposure to work and heat for 100 min/d results in near-maximal acclimatization in 7 to 14 d. This is characterized by an earlier onset of sweating (at a lower core temperature), increased sweat volume, and lowered sweat electrolyte concentration.

As acclimatization proceeds, the sweat sodium concentration decreases while the volume increases.The cardiovascular system plays a major role in both acclimatization and endurance training, largely resulting from an expansion of plasma volume.Heart rate is lower and associated with a higher stroke volume.

Acclimatized individuals generate lower plasma levels of aldosterone during exercise heat stress.

For heat and exercise-induced adaptive responses to be maintained, heat exposure needs to continue intermittently at least on 4 d intervals. Plasma volume decreases considerably within 1 w in the absence of heat stress.

PATHOPHYSIOLOGY

Predisposing Factors for Heat Illness

Elderly patients, psychiatric patients, or those with chronic diseases who are taking medications predisposing to heat illness are prone to classic heatstroke during periods of high ambient heat and humidity.

Exertional heatstroke is most likely to occur in young, healthy people involved in strenuous physical activity, especially if they have not acclimatized to environmental factors.

Hydration can be monitored by measurement of body weight before and after training or athletic competition. A weight loss of 5% or 6% represents a moderately severe deficit and usually is associated with intense thirst, scanty urine, tachycardia, and increase in rectal temperature of approximately 2°C. A loss of 7% or more of body weight represents severe water depletion. Excessively high salt intake in relation to salt losses in sweat during initial heat exposure can impair acclimatization because of inhibition of aldosterone secretion. Excessive salt ingestion can also exacerbate potassium depletion. Evaporative cooling can be lost when clothing inhibits air convection and evaporation. Light-colored clothing reflects rather than absorbs light. The body's heat dissipation mechanisms are analogous to the cooling system of an automobile (Fig.41-1). Temperature is sensed by a thermostat (CNS), which alters coolant flow by a system of pipes, valves, and reservoirs (vasculature). Failure of any of these components can result in overheating.

Individuals with cardiac disease or those taking beta-adrenergic blocking agents or calcium channel blockers may be unable to

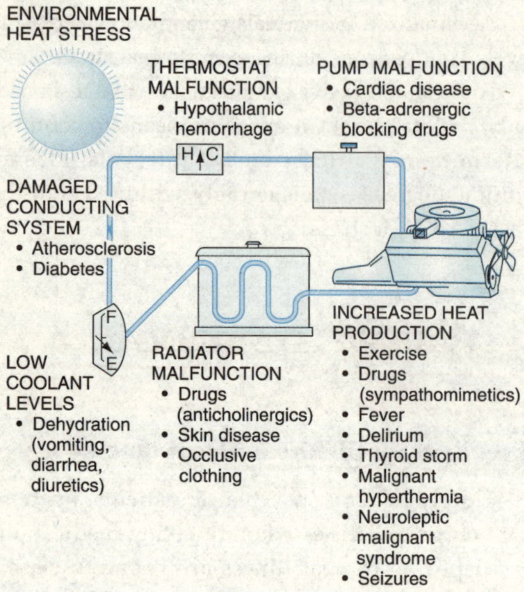

Fig. 41-1 Predisposing factors for heat illness.

increase their CO sufficiently to produce the necessary peripheral vasodilation to dissipate heat. Dehydration predisposes to heat illness. Dehydration alone increases body temperature at rest. Radiator function depends on the skin and sweat glands. Anticholinergic medications and some drugs of abuse interfere with sweating and produce heat illness.Various skin diseases, including miliaria, extensive burns, scleroderma, ectodermal dysplasia, and cystic fibrosis, are risk factors. Increased heat production causing heat illness most often accompanies exercise in hot, humid environments. Endogenous factors, such as hyperthyroidism and pheochromocytoma, can also drastically increase heat production. An overdose of sympathomimetics or stimulants, such as amphetamines, cocaine, and phencyclidine, can cause fatal hyperpyrexia. Certain patients undergoing general anesthesia rapidly experience severe hyperthermia, muscle rigidity, and acidosis. This syndrome, termed malignant hyperthermia, is the result of a genetically determined instability of skeletal muscle sarcoplasmic reticulum that allows inappropriate intracellular calcium release. Dantrolene is effective in the prevention and treatment of this syndrome. Neuroleptic malignant syndrome is induced by antipsychotic medications and is characterized by muscle rigidity, severe dyskinesia or akinesia, hyperthermia, tachycardia, dyspnea, dysphagia, and urinary incontinence. Some antipsychotics also cause suppression of thirst recognition. Other miscellaneous risk factors include obesity. Individuals with a history of heatstroke are at increased risk for a recurrence.

MINOR HEAT ILLNESS

Heat Cramps

Physiology

Heat cramps are brief, intermittent, and often severe muscle cramps occurring typically in muscles that are fatigued by heavywork. Heat cramps appear to be related to a salt deficiency.

Clinical Factors

Heat cramps tend to occur after exercise when the victim stops working and is relaxing (Box 41-1). Heat cramps are occasionally confused with hyperventilation tetany. Heat cramp victims exhibit hyponatremia, hypochloremia, and low serum sodium and chloride levels.

Management

Heat cramps are usually rapidly relieved by salt solutions. Mild cases without concurrent dehydration are treated orally with 0.1% or 0.2% salt solution. Severe cases respond rapidly to intravenous 0.9% NaCl.

Heat Syncope

Physiology and Clinical Features

Heat syncope is a perplexing disorder and is characterized by temporary loss of consciousness. Combined with volume loss and peripheral vasodilation, the dilation of cutaneous vessels can result in inadequate central venous return, a concomitant drop in cardiac output, and cerebral perfusion inadequate to maintain consciousness.

Management

The disorder is self-limited.Individuals at risk for heat syncope should be warned to move often,to flex leg muscles repeatedly when standing stationary,to avoid protracted standing in hot environments, and to assume a sitting or horizontal position when prodromal warning symptoms or signs occur. These include scintillating scotomas, tunnel vision, vertigo, nausea, diaphoresis, and weakness.

Box 41-1 Heat Cramps: Essentials of Diagnosis

Cramps of most worked muscles
Usually occur after exertion
Copious sweating during exertion
Copious hypotonic fluid replacement during exertion
Hyperventilation not present in cool environment

HEAT EXHAUSTION

Physiology

Heat exhaustion (heat prostration) is a clinical syndrome characterized by volume depletion that occurs under conditions of heat stress. Two types of heat exhaustion are classically described: water depletion and salt depletion.

Water depletion heat exhaustion results from inadequate fluid replacement by individuals working in a hot environment, usually laborers, athletes, military personnel, and incapacitated individuals without free access to water. Left untreated, water depletion heat exhaustion will progress to heatstroke. Salt depletion heat exhaustion takes longer to develop than the water depletion form. It occurs when large volumes of thermal sweat are replaced by water with too little salt. This syndrome is characterized by hyponatremia, hypochloremia, and low urinary sodium and chloride concentrations.

Clinical Features

The symptoms and signs associated with both types of heat exhaustion are variable and nonspecific and include weakness, fatigue, frontal headache, impaired judgment, vertigo, nausea and vomiting, and occasionally muscle cramps (Box 41-2). Orthostatic dizziness and syncope can occur.Sweating persists and may be profuse.The core temperature is only moderately elevated, usually below 40°C, and signs of severe CNS dysfunction are not present. Nevertheless, heat exhaustion should not be diagnosed in the presence of major CNS dysfunction (seizures and coma) or severe hyperthermia (40.5°C).If uncertainty exists, measurement of hepatic transaminases may prove helpful. Elevations to several thousand units can be seen in patients with heat exhaustion or in healthy runners after a marathon, whereas in patients with heatstroke, such levels are usually in the tens of thousands after 24 hr.

Box 41-2 Heat Exhaustion: Diagnosis

Vague malaise, fatigue, headache
Core temperature often normal; if elevated, below 40°C(104°F)
Mental function essentially intact; no coma or seizures
Tachycardia, orthostatic hypotension, clinical dehydration (may occur)
Other major illness ruled out
If in doubt, treat as heatstroke

Management

Heat exhaustion is primarily a volume depletion problem, and rapid recovery generally follows fluid administration.Decisions regarding the type of fluid and electrolyte replacements should be based on serum electrolyte measurements and the estimation of hydration status by clinical and laboratory parameters. Patients with significant volume depletion or electrolyte abnormalities require intravenous fluids. If the patient is orthostatic, normal saline should be administered. Free water deficits should be replaced slowly during 48 hr to avoid a decrease of serum osmolality more than 2 mOsm/hr. Overly rapid correction of hypernatremia is associated with seizures caused by cerebral edema.

Disposition

Young patients who respond rapidly to hydration do not require hospitalization. Older patients, particularly those with cardiovascular disease or other predisposing factors described in Fig 41-2, require more cautious inpatient fluid and electrolyte replacement and frequent reassessment (Box 41-3).

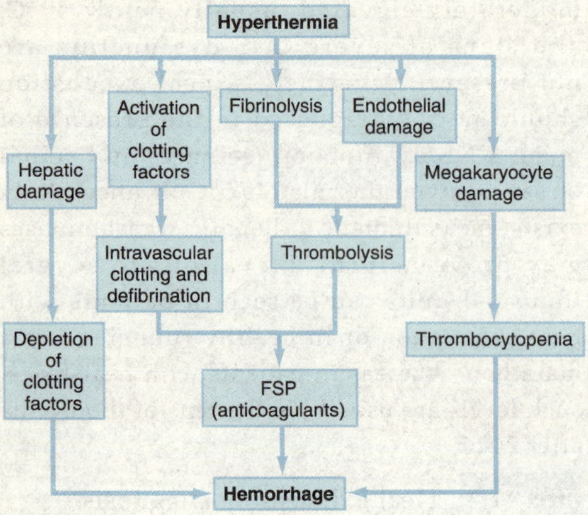

Fig. 41-2 Pathogenesis of hemorrhage. *FSP*, fibrin split products.

Box 41-3 Heat Exhaustion: Treatment

Rest
Cool environment
Assess volume status (orthostatic changes, blood urea nitrogen level, hematocrit, serum sodium concentration)
Fluid replacement: normal saline to replete volume if the patient is orthostatic; replace free water deficits slowly to avoid cerebral edema
Healthy young patients are usually treated as outpatients; consider admission if the patient is elderly, has significant electrolyte abnormalities, or would be at risk for recurrence if discharged

HEATSTROKE

Heatstroke is the catastrophic life-threatening emergency. This failure results in elevation of body temperature to extreme levels, usually higher than 40.5°C (105°F), producing multisystem tissue damage and organ dysfunction.

Clinical Features

Heatstroke versus Heat Exhaustion

The onset of heatstroke is sudden.Prodromal symptoms are nonspecific and may include weakness, dizziness, nausea, vomiting, anorexia, frontal headache, confusion, drowsiness, disorientation, muscle twitching, ataxia and signs of cerebellar dysfunction, and psychiatric symptoms ranging from anxiety and irritability to psychosis. Heat exhaustioncan progress to heatstroke if it is untreated. The usual manifestations of heatstroke include hyperpyrexia above 40.5°C,profound CNS dysfunction, and hot skin (Box 41-4). Persistent sweating can be observed in patients with rectal temperatures of 41.5 to 42.4°C with heatstroke.The cessation of sweating is not the cause of heatstroke, and continued sweating does not preclude the diagnosis.

Box 41-4 Heatstroke: Diagnosis

Exposure to heat stress, endogenous or exogenous
Signs of severe central nervous system dysfunction (coma,seizures, delirium)
Core temperature usually above 40.5°C (105°F), but may be lower
Hot skin common, and sweating may persist
Marked elevation of hepatic transaminases

Classic Heatstroke versus Exertional Heatstroke

The two forms of heatstroke have significantly different presentations and manifestations: classic heatstroke (CHS) and exertional heatstroke (EHS) (Table 41-1).CHS occurs during periods of sustained high ambient temperatures and humidity.Victims are often elderly and poor and live in underventilated dwellings without air conditioning. Victims of CHS commonly suffer from chronic diseases,alcoholism,or schizophrenia.Such patients are often prescribed medications (e.g., diuretics, antihypertensives, neuroleptics, and anticholinergics).Sweating ceases in the majority of CHS patients. Patients with EHS are usually young and healthy individuals. Rhabdomyolysis and acute renal failureare common in patients with EHS.Sweating is present in half the cases of EHS.Hypoglycemia may occur. Coagulopathy is common.Signs of profound CNS dysfunction dominate the early course of heatstroke.Delirium or coma is characteristic. Patients with heatstroke usually have hyperdynamic cardiovascular systems with low peripheral vascular resistance,tachycardia (up to 180 beats/min),and elevated cardiac index.Elevation of cardiac troponin I is common with CHS; but rarer in EHS. Most patients with CHS have respiratory alkalosis, those with EHS usually have a relatively pure lactic acidosis. Lactic acidosis is associated with a poor prognosis in cases of CHS but not necessarily in cases of EHS. Aberrations in coagulation are common in patients with severe heatstroke, and their presence is a poor prognostic sign.Abnormal hemostasis is manifested clinically by purpura, conjunctival hemorrhage, melena, bloody diarrhea, hemoptysis, hematuria, myocardial bleeding, or hemorrhage into the CNS.

Table 41-1 Usual Characteristics of Heatstroke

EXERTIONAL	CLASSIC
Healthy	Predisposing factors or medications
Younger	Older
Exercise	Sedentary
Sporadic	Heat wave occurrence
Diaphoresis	Anhidrosis
Hypoglycemia	Normoglycemia
DIC	Mild coagulopathy
Rhabdomyolysis	Mild CK elevation
Acute renal failure	Oliguria
Marked lactic acidosis	Mild acidosis
Hypocalcemia	Normocalcemia

Hepatic damage is so consistently featured in heatstroke. Jaundice typically appears 24 to 72 hr after the onset of severe heatstroke.Hypoglycemia is common in cases of EHS. Renal damage is also common. Microscopic examination reveals proteinuria with abundant granular casts and red blood cells.Acute oliguric renal failure complicates 25% to 30% of EHS cases and 5% of CHS cases. Pancreatitis is described with elevated serum amylase and lipase levels.

Diagnostic Strategies

Thermometry

Rectal thermometry is less variable but responds to changes in core temperature slowly. If, however, the temperature does not respond and the patient does not recover neurologically, other causes of fever and coma should be considered (Box 41-5). In patients with heatstroke, the spinal fluid should be crystal clear,with occasional lymphocytic pleocytosis and elevated protein levels. Cerebral falciparum malaria is seen in tropical areas where heat illness can also occur.In patients with thyroid storm,the clinical symptoms resemble those of heatstroke. Thyroid function test results are elevated.Drug-induced heat illness is an important consideration, particularly anticholinergic poisoning. Differentiation may be difficult because both heatstroke and anticholinergic poisoning produce hyperpyrexia,hot and dry skin,tachycardia,and abnormal mental status. Typhoid fever, typhus, delirium tremens, and hypothalamic hemorrhage all produce a symptom complex similar to that of heatstroke.Malignant hyperthermia and neuroleptic malignant syndrome are characterized by lead-pipe rigidity. Serotonin syndrome is classically a triad of mental status changes, autonomic hyperactivity,and neuromuscular abnormalities secondary to increased CNS serotonergic activity.

Box 41-5 Differential Diagnosis of Heatstroke

Central nervous system hemorrhage
Toxins, drugs
Seizures
Malignant hyperthermia
Neuroleptic malignant syndrome
Serotonin syndrome
Thyroid storm
High fever, sepsis
Encephalitis, meningitis

Management

Cooling

Immediate cooling is the cornerstone of treatment. Mortality correlates with the temperature, the number of dysfunctional organ systems and increases significantly when cooling is delayed. When the patient arrives at the hospital, clothes should be removed,a thermistor probe should be inserted, and the temperature should be continuously monitored. The ideal method of evaporative cooling uses a body cooling unit on which the patient lies suspended on a net surface while being sprayed with atomized 15°C water from above and below.Air warmed to 45 to 48°C is blown over the skin surface at 3 m/min.The unitmaximizes evaporative cooling by maintaining cutaneous vasodilation and avoiding heat generation caused by shivering. The combination of atomized tepid water at 40°C from a spray bottle and standing fans cools at rates comparable to both body cooling unit and immersion.Other evaporative techniques, including the use of downdraft from a helicopter, can be applied successfully.Immersion in ice water results in a rapid reduction of core temperature to below 39°C within 10 to 40 min but complicates the resuscitation.When the body temperature reaches 39°C,cooling measures should be discontinued.Continuous monitoring is necessary to maintain the core temperature at 37 to 38°C. Vasoconstriction from ice water immersion may be beneficial to hypotensive patients and may be better than evaporative cooling for victims in shock.Cooling modalities other than evaporation and immersion should be considered adjunctive treatments (Box 41-6).

Box 41-6 Cooling Modalities to Lower Body Temperature in Heatstroke

Preferred

Evaporative cooling with large circulating fans and skin wetting

Ice water immersion

Adjuncts

Ice packs to axillae and groin

Cooling blanket

Peritoneal lavage (unproven efficacy in humans)

Rectal lavage

Gastric lavage

Cardiopulmonary bypass

Resuscitation

Aspiration and seizures are common in patients with heatstroke, and airway control is essential. Hypoxemia may occur because of aspiration, pneumonitis and pulmonary infarction, hemorrhage, or edema.Circulatory fluid requirements are modest in some cases,averaging 1200 mL of isotonic crystalloid solution in the first 4 hr. The use of a CVP catheter to monitor fluid resuscitation may be deceptive. Hypotension is common in patients with heatstroke .Blood pressure usually rises with cooling. If the blood pressure rises,more fluids are given with careful monitoring of the CVP.Aggressive fluid replacement is continued until the blood pressure reaches 90/60 mm Hg or the CVP exceeds 12 mL H_2O. A variety of tachyarrhythmias commonly occur during heatstroke.These usually resolve with cooling, and electrical cardioversion should be avoided until the myocardium is cooled. Because the pathophysiologic processes of heatstroke and fever differ, antipyretics are not indicated and may be harmful for patient with heatstroke. If rhabdomyolysis is present, maintenance of urinary output of at least 2 mL/kg/hr is required.Urinary alkalinization higher than 6.5 should be considered early in patients with acidemia, dehydration, or underlying renal disease. After volume repletion, administration of mannitol may be considered to increase intravascular volume and to increase GFR. Mannitol should not be used in an oliguric patient. Persistent anuria, uremia, or hyperkalemia is an indication for consideration of hemodialysis. Hematologic evaluation should include arterial blood gas determination;complete blood cell count and platelet counts; electrolyte values and blood urea nitrogen,glucose,creatinine, aspartate transaminase,alanine transaminase,lactate dehydrogenase,creatine kinase,uric and lactic acid,and calcium levels;prothrombin and partial thromboplastin time;international normalized ratio;and fibrin degradation products and hepatic enzymes.Serum cardiac troponin I levels should be obtained. Acidosis is common, especially in patients with EHS. Lactate levels are usually elevated. Cooling modalities may induce violent shivering; this increases metabolic heat production and may impede cooling.Intravenous benzodiazepines are the treatment of choice for shivering. Neuroleptics, like chlorpromazine, have anticholinergic properties and should be avoided. Many patients are extremely agitated during the initial cooling period. Short-acting benzodiazepines can be used for sedation and to control seizures. Coagulopathies can occur during the first day of illness but are more common on the second and third days. Initial treatment after cooling should include replacement therapy with fresh frozen plasma and platelets.The clinician should monitor the laboratory signs of DIC.

(CHAI Yanfen)

Chapter 42

High-Altitude Medicine

KEY CONCEPTS

The symptoms of AMS can resemble a viral syndrome and include headache, nausea, anorexia, fatigue, and insomnia.

The management of altitude illness must include adherence to the principle that after the symptoms occur and until symptoms resolve, further ascent is contraindicated.

Dyspnea at rest is an early symptom of HAPE.

Altered consciousness and cerebellar ataxia must be recognized as early signs of HACE, and descent is mandatory.

Effective prophylaxis options for altitude illness include acetazolamide for AMS and nifedipine for HAPE.

EPIDEMIOLOGY

High-altitude illness is seen clinically in one of several forms that overlap and share a common pathophysiologic mechanism. Acute mountain sickness(AMS) is the relatively benign and self-limited presentation, whereas highaltitude pulmonary edema (HAPE) and high-altitude cerebral edema (HACE) represent the potentially life-threatening manifestations of high-altitude illness.

Mountain sports activities and tourism are attracting increasing numbers of participants each year. More than 1 million visitors travel annually to the remote high mountain ranges of Asia, Africa, and South America.Approximately 35 million visitors travel annually to high-altitude recreation areas in the western United States.

The incidence of high-altitude illness depends on many variables, including the rate of ascent, previous altitude exposure, and individual genetic susceptibility. Sleeping altitude, final altitude reached, and duration of stay at altitude are also risk factors for AMS development.AMS is common (67% incidence) among mountain climbers on Mt.The incidence of HAPE varies from 0.01% to 2% but has reached 15.5% among soldiers flown directly to 14,500 feet without a chance to acclimatize at a lower altitude. The incidence of HACE is lower. Both HAPE and HACE are more common with a longer duration of visit and higher sleeping altitude.

Age may be a relative risk factor.Younger individuals (<20 yr old) are more likely to have HAPE. Gender does not affect the incidence of AMS; however, women may have less risk for development of HAPE.No relationship appears to exist between AMS development and the menstrual cycle.The risk for AMS development in adults older than 50 yr may be less than in younger age groups.Pulmonary vital capacity decreases almost one third in elders ascending from sea level to 14,000 feet for 1w, producing a large decrease in both oxygen saturation and maximal oxygen uptake during exercise.

DEFINITIONS

High altitude is between 10,000 and 18,000 feet. Most serious altitude illness occurs at these levels. High-altitude illness is common with rapid ascent above 8000 feet, and individuals with underlying medical problems may be predisposed to development of altitude illness at lower levels. The pathophysiologic effects of high altitude begin when SaO_2 begins to fall below the 90% level.At an altitude of approximately 12,000 feet, the steep portion of the curve is encountered, and marked oxygen desaturation may occur with relatively small increases in altitude (Fig. 42-1).

At an altitude above 18,000 feet,complete acclimatization generally is not possible.

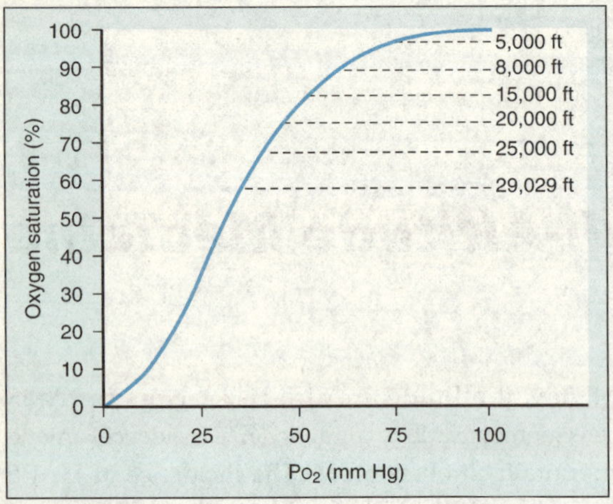

Fig. 42-1 Oxygen-hemoglobin dissociation curve.

ENVIRONMENTAL CONSIDERATIONS

Barometric pressure decreases logarithmically as the altitude rises.P_aO_2 in the atmosphere also decreases as altitude rises, but it remains a constant 20.93% of the barometric pressure.

Local weather can also have a significant effect on barometric pressure from day to day.

ACCLIMATIZATION

The term *acclimatization* refers to the series of integrated adaptations that take place at high altitude, which tend to restore the oxygen pressures within the tissues toward normal sea-level values despite the lowered PO_2 of the atmosphere. These processes occur gradually and involve multiple systems from protein synthesis to respiratory, cardiovascular, and hematologic adjustments. Gradual ascents made by mountaineers during several weeks have allowed the successful summiting of many of the world's highest peaks, including Mt.Rapid exposure to extreme altitude results in loss of consciousness, and death may occur in a matter of minutes.

Acclimatization begins at the altitude that causes the oxygen saturation of arterial blood to fall below sea-level values. The altitude at which this occurs depends on the rate of ascent, the duration of exposure, and the individual's physiology.People with preexisting conditions may have a decreased altitude tolerance. Of particular importance are both acute and chronic cardiac and respiratory illnesses.

The risk of high-altitude illness also depends on an individual's inherent ability to acclimatize. Previous successful acclimatization may be predictive of future responses for adults in similar conditions.

One of the most important physiologic changes that occurs during acclimatization is an increase in minute ventilation, causing a decrease in theP_ACO_2. The alveolar gas equation states that as the P_ACO_2 decreases, a corresponding increase in P_AO_2 occurs, thereby increasing arterial oxygenation (Box 42-1).

Box 42-1 Alveolar Gas Equation

$$P_AO_2 = P_IO_2\ (P_ACO_2/R)$$

P_AO_2	Partial pressure of oxygen in alveolus
P_IO_2	Partial pressure of oxygen in inspired air
P_ACO_2	Partial pressure of carbon dioxide in alveolus
R	Respiratory quotient

When a person arrives at high altitude, the peripheral chemoreceptors in the carotid bodies respond to a decrease in P_aO_2 and signal the respiratory control center in the medulla to increase ventilation. This increase in ventilation is known as the hypoxic ventilatory response (HVR), which may be inhibited or stimulated by numerous factors, including ethanol, sleep medications, caffeine, cocoa, prochlorperazine, and progesterone.

As ventilation increases, a respiratory alkalosis occurs. Within 24 to 48 hr of ascent, the kidneys excrete bicarbonate in an effort to compensate for the alkalosis. As the pH normalizes, ventilation rises slowly, reaching a maximum after 6 to 8 d. This process is enhanced by acetazolamide. The ability to achieve an adequate HVR varies and is related to the ability to acclimatize. A low HVR and relative hypoventilation are implicated in the pathogenesis of both AMS and HAPE.For the majority of people with intermediate HVR, however, ventilatory drive probably has no predictive value for AMS development.

The release of catecholamines on ascent is manifested by an elevation in heart rate, blood pressure, cardiac output, and venous tone.Except at extreme altitudes, acclimatization results in the gradual return of the resting heart rate to near sea-level values. Resting relative tachycardia is evidence of poor acclimatization.

The hematopoietic response to high-altitude acclimatization consists of an increase in both hemoglobin and the number of red blood cells.Long-term acclimatization leads to an increase in plasma volume and total blood volume. Erythropoietin is secreted in response to hypoxemia within hours of ascent, which in turn stimulates the production of red blood cells, leading to new circulatory red blood cells in 4 or 5 d. During the next 2 mo, red blood cell mass increases in proportion to the degree of hypoxemia.

Hypoxemia also results in an increase in 2,3-diphosphoglycerate, causing a rightward shift of the oxyhemoglobin dissociation curve, which favors a release of oxygen from the blood to the tissues.Some individuals with mutant hemoglobin and high oxygen-hemoglobin affinity are found to acclimatize more efficiently than their normal counterparts at moderate altitudes.

PATHOPHYSIOLOGY

AMS and HACE appear to represent differing manifestations of altitude illness on the same continuum, whereas HAPE appears to have a somewhat independent pathophysiologic mechanism.

The symptoms of AMS develop several hours after arrival at high altitude, whereas the development of HAPE and HACE generally requires several days of altitude exposure. Because hypobaric hypoxemia occurs within minutes of arrival, it cannot be the direct cause of high-altitude illness.The proposed mechanisms for the development of AMS, HAPE, and HACE are represented schematically in Fig 42-2.

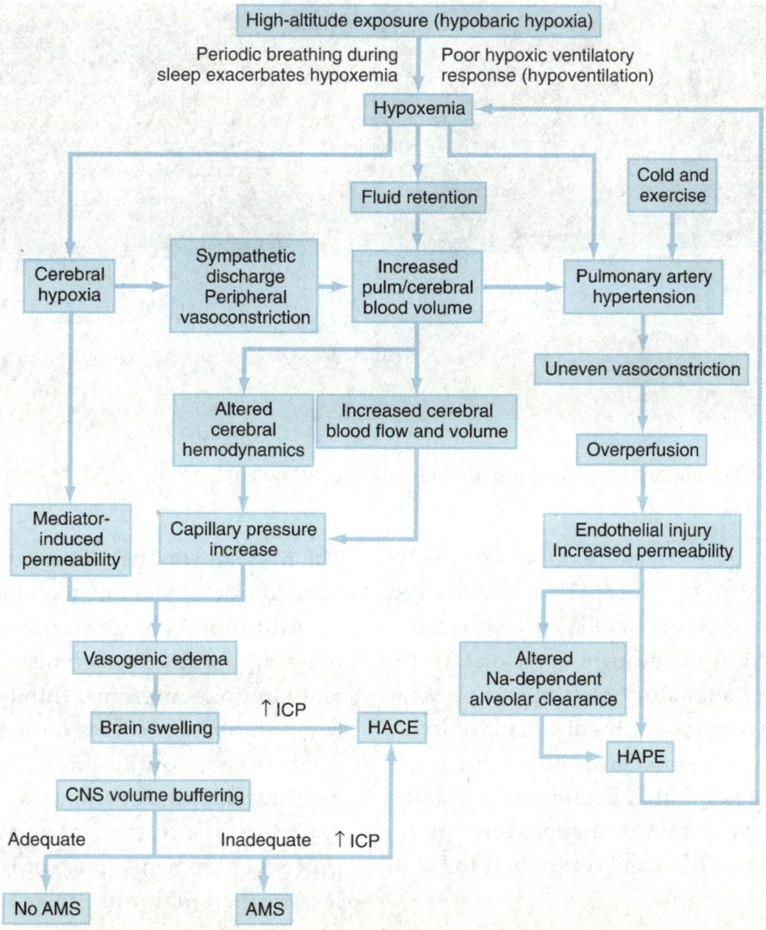

Fig. 42-2 Proposed mechanisms for the development of *AMS*, *HAPE*, and *HACE*. Significant hypoxemia initiates multiple systemic responses that involve the circulatory, pulmonary, endocrine, and CNS.

A poor HVR resulting in relative hypoventilation may be due to either the individual's genetic predisposition or extrinsic factors, such as medications, that decrease the ventilatory drive. Whenever the HVR is decreased, the protective effects of hyperventilation are lost and the hypoxemia of high-altitude exposure is exacerbated.

Hypoxemia alters fluid homeostasis, resulting in a generalized fluid retention followed by the shift of fluid into the intracellular spaces. This is manifested by peripheral edema, decreased urinary output, and increased body weight in patients with AMS. Several different mechanisms may account for these fluid shifts, including arginine vasopressin levels and sympathetic stimulation.Aldosterone, plasma renin, and atrial natriuretic levels are higher in people with AMS.

The hypoxemia play the cardinal role in the development of HAPE. Exercise and cold stress at altitude may increase hypoxemia and exacerbate pulmonary hypertension.Pulmonary blood volumes and pulmonary hypertension are increased by sympathetic nervous system stimulation and catecholamine release.In HAPE-susceptible individuals, pulmonary hypertension becomes severe, and an uneven distribution of pulmonary vasoconstriction results in overperfusion, increased capillary pressures, distention, and leakage in the remaining vessels. This explains the patchy nature of the infiltrate seen on a chest radiograph with HAPE (Fig. 42-3). These individuals deliver their entire cardiac output to one lung, predisposing them to overperfusion injury.

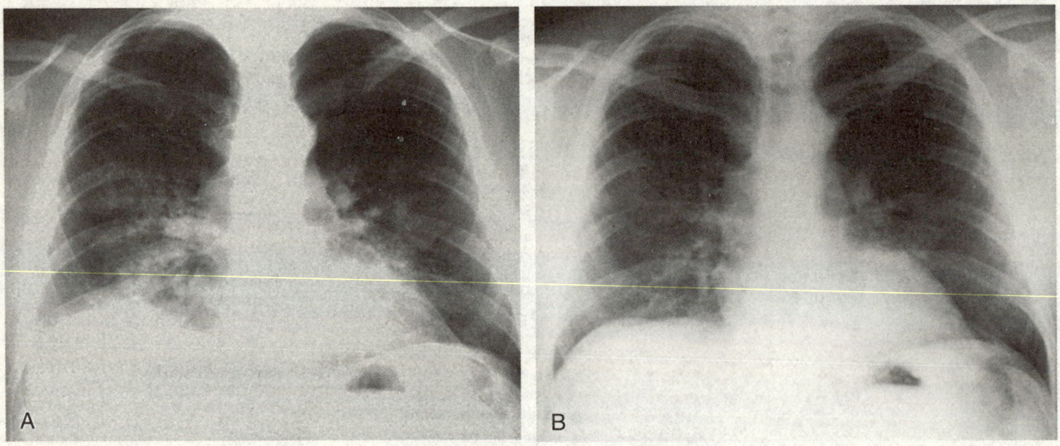

Fig. 42-3 Chest radiograph of a patient with high-altitude pulmonary edema. A, Before treatment. B, After treatment.

The importance of the excessive rise in pulmonary artery pressure in HAPE is emphasized. This implicates increased vascular pressure rather than inflammation as the primary cause of the vascular leak.Inflammatory mediators appear to be a secondary response to the mechanical injury caused by overperfusion.Once the vascular leak occurs and alveolar fluid accumulates, a defect in transepithelial sodium transport impairs the clearance of alveolar fluid and contributes to HAPE development.

Preexisting inflammation may also be a risk factor for HAPE. The clinical manifestations of AMS and HACE are the result of CNS dysfunction. The mechanistic theories involve altered cerebral hemodynamics and inflammatory mediators.

Additional circumstances, however, may be necessary for the development of vasogenic edema and clinical symptoms. Inflammatory mediators may contribute to edema formation.

As brain volume increases from increased cerebral blood volume, the volume-buffering capacity of the central nervous system may prevent an immediate rise of ICP.Individuals with less intracranial and intraspinal CSF buffering capacity have less compliance and become more symptomatic (i.e., develop AMS) from mild brain swelling.

ACUTE MOUNTAIN SICKNESS

Clinical Presentation

The symptoms of mild AMS are similar to those of a viral syndrome, an ethanol "hangover," or simple physical exhaustion.

For the diagnosis of AMS, a patient must be in the setting of a recent gain in altitude, be at the new altitude for at least several hours, and report a headache *plus* at least one of the following symptoms: gastrointestinal upset (anorexia, nausea, or vomiting), general weakness or fatigue, dizziness or lightheadedness, or difficulty in sleeping (Box 42-2).The symptoms of AMS develop within a few hours after arrival at high altitude and generally reach maximum severity between 24 and 48 hr, followed by a gradual resolution. Most individuals become symptom free by the third or fourth day.

Box 42-2 Acute Mountain Sickness

Incidence: 12% to 67%, varies with rate of ascent and individual susceptibility; rare below 8000 feet, most common with rapid ascent to altitudes above 10,000 feet

Symptoms and signs: Headache, anorexia, nausea, fatigue, dizziness, difficulty sleeping

Treatment: Mild cases are usually self-limited and do not require treatment; discontinue ascent, rest; for moderate case, administer acetazolamide; ibuprofen, aspirin, or acetaminophen for headache; prochlorperazine for nausea; supplemental oxygen if available; descend if persistent or severe; add dexamethasone in severe cases

Prevention: Gradual ascent to allow acclimatization; highcarbohydrate diet, avoidance of ethanol or smoking; acetazolamide if ascent is rapid or known history of recurrent acute mountain sickness

There are no diagnostic physical findings in cases of mild AMS.Dyspnea at rest is an early indication of HAPE. Similarly, any evidence of cerebellar dysfunction, such as mild ataxia or alteration in mentation, mandates descent because of early evidence of HACE.

Ultrasonography is emerging as an early, noninvasive diagnostic tool to assess ICP.Elevated ICP is associated with AMS and HACE.

Management

The management of AMS should include strict adherence to the principle that after the symptoms of altitude illness occur, further ascent to a higher sleeping altitude is contraindicated. The presence of neurologic abnormalities or evidence of severe pulmonary edema mandates immediate descent.

Most mild AMS is treated by stopping of further ascent and waiting for acclimatization. This may take 1 to 4 d.

Supplemental oxygen administration relieves AMS symptoms. Hyperbaric therapy is also effective.

Aspirin, ibuprofen, and acetaminophen are useful for the treatment of high-altitude headache. Narcotic analgesics should be avoided because of depression of the HVR and respiratory drive during sleep. For nausea and vomiting, prochlorperazine, stimulates the HVR.Periodic breathing causes insomnia, which is best treated with the respiratory stimulant acetazolamide. Doses of acetazolamide as low as 62.5 to 125 mg at bedtime may prevent periodic breathing and eradicate insomnia. Benzodiazepines and other sedativehypnotics should be avoided because of their tendency to decrease ventilation during sleep.low doses of benzodiazepines alone or in combination with acetazolamide are safe at high altitude.

Nonbenzodiazepine sleep agents (zolpidem and zaleplon) do not depress ventilation and may prove useful in AMS-related insomnia.

Acetazolamide accelerates acclimatization and rapidly resolves symptoms. Acetazolamide should be avoided in breast-feeding mothers and pregnant women.

Dexamethasone is an effective alternative treatment of AMS.

Prevention

Most of the symptoms of mild AMS are benign and well tolerated.

Slow ascent is the best method of prevention.

Mild to moderate exercise is thought to aid in acclimatization; however, overexertion can contribute to the development of AMS. Maintenance of adequate hydration is also recommended.Drinking of excessive amounts of free water may lead to hyponatremia and possibly complicate altitude illness.

The rate of ascent and prior history of altitude illness should be considered in the assessment of the risk for development of altitude illness (Table 42-1). Individuals who have a known susceptibility to the development of AMS should consider prophylactic medication in addition to gradual ascent.

Table 42-1 Risk Categories for Acute Mountain Sickness

RISK CATEGORY	DESCRIPTION
Low	Individuals with no prior history of altitude illness and ascending to ≤9200 ft Individuals taking ≥2 d to arrive at 8200-9800 ft with subsequent increases in sleeping elevation < 1600 ft/d
Moderate	Individuals with prior history of AMS and ascending to 8200-9200 ft in 1 d No history of AMS and ascending to >9200 ft in 1 d All individuals ascending >1600 ft/d (increase in sleeping elevation) at altitudes above 9800 ft
High	History of AMS and ascending to ≥9200 ft in 1 d All individuals with a prior history of HAPE or HACE All individuals ascending to >11,500 ft in 1 d All individuals ascending >1600 ft/d (increase in sleeping elevation) above> 11,500 ft Very rapid ascents (e.g., Mt. Kilimanjaro)

Acetazolamide for prevention of AMS in adults is effective.Acetazolamide(250 mg twice daily) starting 24 hr before ascent and continuing for the first 2 d at high altitude is effective.

Dexamethasone also prevents AMS.

Oxygen is an effective prophylactic modality for rescue personnel.

HIGH-ALTITUDE PULMONARY EDEMA

HAPE is the most common fatal manifestation of severe highaltitude illness (Box 42-3).HAPE can occur and even be fatal at altitudes as low as 8000 feet.

Box 42-3 High-Altitude Pulmonary Edema

Incidence: 0.01% to 15%, varies with rate of ascent; rare below 8000 feet and more common above 14,500 feet; usually occurs 2-4 d after arrival at high altitude

Symptoms and signs: Dyspnea at rest, cough, fatigue, headache, anorexia, cyanosis, rales, tachypnea, tachycardia

Treatment: Patients with mild cases may recover with bed rest; moderate cases can be treated with bed rest and supplemental oxygen if clinical monitoring is available; severe cases require oxygen and descent; use hyperbaric therapy if available; if oxygen or descent is unavailable, then nifedipine 30 mg slow-release every 12 hr; consider tadalafil 10 mg every 12 hr (unstudied)

Prevention: Gradual ascent and recognition of early AMS symptoms so that ascent is stopped before HAPE develops; with previous HAPE history, use nifedipine 30 mg slow-release every 12 hr during ascent, then continue for 3 d (monitor for hypotension)

Individuals who have been residents at high-altitude locations for extended periods may have pulmonary edema develop on reascent from a trip to low altitude. This phenomenon has been termed reentry HAPE.

Clinical Presentation

The initial symptoms of HAPE usually begin insidiously 2 to 4 d after arrival at high altitude. Most cases occur during the second night. Marked dyspnea on exertion, fatigue with minimal-to-moderate effort, and dry cough are early manifestations of the disease.

As the HAPE patient deteriorates, usually through the night, the dyspnea intensifies with effort and is unrelieved by rest. The cough becomes productive of copious amounts of clear, watery sputum, and hemoptysis may be seen in severe cases. As the condition intensifies, cerebral edema or simply severe hypoxemia causes CNS dysfunction. Coma may follow and precede death in a few hours if oxygen therapy or descent is not instituted.

The physical examination reveals a few rales in patients with mild HAPE, usually found in the region of the right middle lobe, progressing to unilateral or bilateral rales and then to diffuse bilateral rales. Cyanosis of the nail beds alone may progress to severe central cyanosis. Tachypnea and tachycardia become more pronounced as severity increases. Elevated temperatures are common, and a concurrent respiratory tract infection is occasionally seen.

Ancillary Tests

Chest radiographs can help elucidate the nature of the illness. The infiltrates seen in HAPE victims are alveolar and patchy in distribution, with areas of clearing between the patches. Unilateral infiltrates may be present in mild cases; however, bilateral infiltrates are seen in more advanced cases, with involvement of the right midlung field being most common (Fig. 42-3). Pleural effusion is rare. Of note, the radiographic findings of cardiomegaly,and Kerley B lines are absent in cases of HAPE.

Some mild HAPE may clear in 4 to 6 hr, and most clear by 24 hr. Radiographs of patients with severe HAPE may reveal infiltrates that persist for as long as 2 w, even though the clinical symptoms have resolved.

ECG reveals tachycardia and evidence of rightsided heart strain, including right axis deviation, P wave abnormalities, tall R waves in the precordial leads, and S waves in the lateral leads.

Ultrasonography to estimate pulmonary artery pressure is an emerging modality in the early detection and diagnosis of HAPE. Ultrasound lung comet tails, indicating extravascular water, may also be seen to support a HAPE diagnosis.

Differential Diagnosis

Pneumonia can be misdiagnosed in the setting of HAPE because the symptoms and signs of pneumonia are similar to those of HAPE.

High-altitude bronchitis and pharyngitis are common problems among climbers.Coughing spasms may be severe.

Death from pulmonary embolism at high altitude is described. The symptoms and signs of pulmonary embolism can mimic those of HAPE; however, embolic disease tends to have a more rapid onset, and pleuritic chest pain is a more prominent feature.

Management

Immediate descent is a lifesaving measure after diagnosis of HAPE. Descents of 3000 feet are generally adequate for a rapid recovery; however, descent should continue until symptoms resolve.

Warmth and rest are also important in HAPE therapy. Mild cases of HAPE can be treated without descent or oxygen with 1 or 2 d of bed rest.Moderate cases can be treated without descent if bed rest and adequate supplies of supplemental oxygen are available.

Oxygen administration (or hyperbaric therapy) can be a lifesaving measure.High-flow rates of oxygen (6-8 L/min) by mask should be delivered initially to victims with severe HAPE until improvement is seen.

Several portable, lightweight, fabric hyperbaric chambers are available and pressurized manually (Fig. 42-4, see color illustration). These devices can be lifesaving in patients with HAPE and HACE.

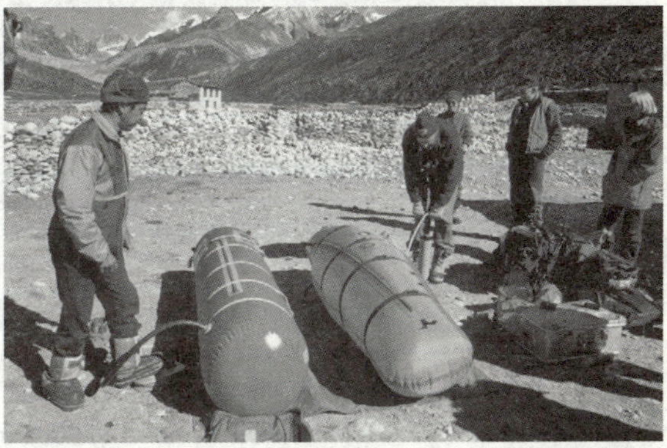

Fig. 42-4 Gamow bag *(left)* and Certec bag *(right)*: lightweight, portable hyperbaric chambers. Note the attached foot-operated pressure pump.

In treatment of HAPE, medications that lower pulmonary artery pressure, pulmonary blood volume, and pulmonary vascular resistance or enhance alveolar fluid clearance are useful.

Nifedipine is especially useful when oxygen is unavailable or descent is impossible.Patients should be monitored for the development of hypotension during nifedipine administration.

Inhaled beta-agonists have been used anecdotally for therapy of HAPE (salmeterol 125 μg inhaled twice daily).

The mainstay of treatment remains immediate oxygen if it is available and descent. Should these treatments not be available, nifedipine should be initiated.

Prevention

As with all forms of serious altitude illness, a gradual ascent that allows time to acclimatize and immediate cessation of further ascent at the onset of symptoms are the most effective means of prevention. Individuals with a prior history of HAPE should also avoid extreme exertion during the first 2 d at altitude. With a prior history of HAPE,the preferred medication is the nonspecific pulmonary vasodilator nifedipine, before ascent and continued at altitude for 3 d.

Sildenafil (40 mg every 8 hr) and tadalafil (10 mg every 12 hr) are effective in preventing HAPE. The phosphodiesterase type 5 inhibitors have the added benefit.Dexamethasone (8 mg every 12 hr) started 2 d before ascent also prevents HAPE. Acetazolamide aids in acclimatization and prevents HAPE, and it has utility in reduction of hypoxic pulmonary vasoconstriction.

HIGH-ALTITUDE CEREBRAL EDEMA

HACE is the least common but most severe form of high-altitude illness. Mild AMS can progress to severe HACE with coma in as few as 12 hr. Although the usual time course is 1 to 3 d for the development of severe symptoms, it may occur in 5 to 9 d (Box 42-4).

Box 42-4 High-Altitude Cerebral Edema

Incidence: Lower than 1% or 2%, uncommon as a pure entity; usually associated with the presence of severe AMS and HAPE

Symptoms and signs: Ataxia, severe headache, nausea and vomiting, altered mentation, seizures, coma

Treatment: Immediate evacuation to a lower altitude; oxygen, bed rest, dexamethasone, and hyperbaric therapy while awaiting descent

Clinical Presentation

HACE-specific signs include ataxia, generalized seizures, slurred speech, rarely focal neurologic deficits, and altered mentation, which can range from mild emotional lability or confusion to hallucinations and decreased levels of consciousness that may proceed to coma and death.MRI of patients with HACE reveals white matter changes consistent with vasogenic edema (Fig. 42-5).

Altered consciousness and cerebellar ataxia are the most sensitive signs for early recognition of HACE.The early appearance of ataxia reflects the particular sensitivity of the cerebellum to hypoxia. Retinal hemorrhages are common. Papilledema and occasionally cranial nerve palsy also occur.

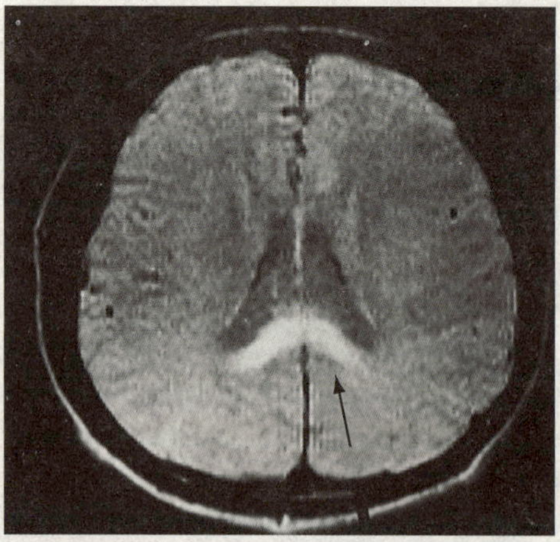

Fig. 42-5 Axial proton-weighted magnetic resonance image of a mountain climber with high-altitude cerebral edema. The arrow demonstrates the markedly increased signal (edema) in the splenium of the corpus callosum.

Management

Ataxia alone is an indication for immediate descent. High-flow oxygen should be administered. Steroid therapy is recommended and may result in recovery from HACE without neurologic deficits. The initial dose of dexamethasone is 8 mg parenterally or orally in mild cases, followed by 4 mg every 6 hr.

Patients with severely altered levels of consciousness require tracheal intubation. Hyperventilation, diuretics (e.g., furosemide), and hypertonic solutions (e.g., mannitol) may be used to manage severely elevated ICP. Caution is warranted; diuretic use could compromise adequate intravascular volume and reduce cerebral perfusion pressure.

Hyperbaric treatment of HACE is also effective and may result in temporary improvement.Early treatment of HACE generally results in good outcomes, but after coma is present, the mortality rate exceeds 60%.

HIGH-ALTITUDE RETINAL HEMORRHAGE

High-altitude retinal hemorrhage (HARH) is

common at altitudes above 17,500 feet.

Most patients with HARH are asymptomatic, noted only on retinoscopy.HARH is not generally related to the presence of mild AMS but does seem to be related to strenuous exercise at high altitude. At any altitude, in the setting of severe HAPE or HACE,retinal hemorrhages are commonly noted.

Hemorrhages usually spare the macula (Fig. 42-6, see color illustration). Retinal hemorrhages usually resolve without treatment in 2 or 3 w. HARH is more likely to occur among individuals with a previous history of these hemorrhages.

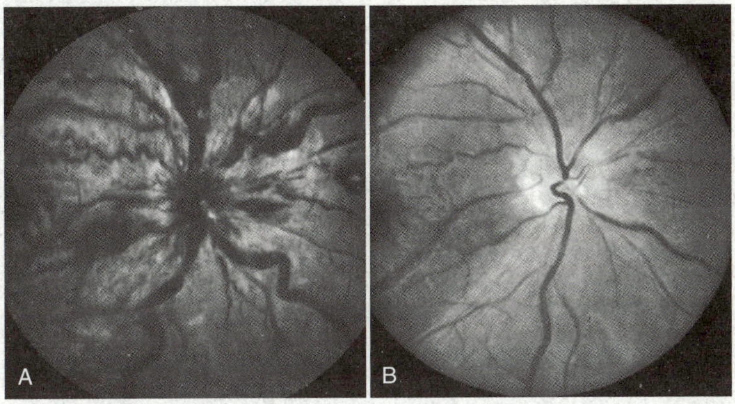

Fig. 42-6 High-altitude retinal hemorrhages. A. Acute; B. After 1 week of resolution.

ALTITUDE AND UNDERLYING MEDICAL CONDITIONS

Individuals with diseases such as moderate to severe COPD and CAD may have a more difficult time acclimatizing because these disease states are often aggravated by the hypoxic atmosphere at higher elevations. They may predispose these individuals to the development of high-altitude illness. Table 42-2 describes the risk associated with travel to altitude in individuals with a variety of underlying comorbidities.

Table 42-2 Risk Associated with Travel to Altitude in Individuals with a Variety of Underlying Comorbidities

ADVISABILITY OF EXPOSURE TO HIGH ALTITUDE FOR COMMON CONDITIONS (WITHOUT SUPPLEMENTAL OXYGEN)
Probably No Extra Risk
Young and old
Fit and unfit
Mild obesity
Diabetes
Previous coronary artery bypass grafting (without angina)
Mild COPD
Asthma
Low-risk pregnancy
Controlled hypertension
Controlled seizure disorder
Psychiatric disorders
Neoplastic diseases
Inflammatory conditions
Caution
Moderate COPD
Asymptomatic pulmonary hypertension
Compensated congestive heart failure
Morbid obesity
Sleep apnea syndromes
Troublesome arrhythmias
Stable angina or coronary artery disease
High-risk pregnancy
Sickle cell trait
Cerebrovascular diseases
Any cause of restricted pulmonary circulation
Seizure disorder (not taking medication)
Radial keratotomy
Contraindicated
Sickle cell anemia (with history of crises)
Severe COPD
Symptomatic pulmonary hypertension
Uncompensated congestive heart failure

Respiratory Illnesses

Travelers with COPD to moderate altitudes have underlying anatomic and physiologic changes that predispose them to development of hypoxemia, sleep apnea, pulmonary hypertension, and ventilation disorders. COPD is a risk factor for the development of AMS.High altitude increases hypoxic pulmonary vasoconstriction and may potentiate the development of cor pulmonale. Individuals with chronic COPD should be advised of the potential need for oxygen supplementation when traveling to moderate altitude. Use of a pulse oximeter can guide the need for increased oxygen supplementation.

Patients with asthma may have fewer problems at altitude . There are no descriptions of asthma exacerbations due to altitude.Even those with exercise-induced bronchospasm do not have worsening symptoms while exercising at 5000 feet.In addition, AMS incidence is not increased in asthmatics.People with asthma traveling to higher elevations should continue their usual medications and carry a rescue supply of bronchodilators and steroids.

Patients who ascend to high altitude with preexisting primary or secondary pulmonary hypertension should be considered HAPE susceptible, and those with primary pulmonary hypertension should be considered at increased risk for HAPE.Patients with known pulmonary hypertension should be advised against travel to higher elevations.Prophylactic nifedipine SR can prevent HAPE.Phosphodiesterase type 5 inhibitors and steroids may also be used.

Cardiovascular

In theory, People with diseased myocardium should be advised to avoid high altitude because of decreased environmental oxygen availability.To the contrary, long-term residents at high altitude may be protected from CAD by increased collateral vessel formation or a decrease in the development of atherosclerosis.

Many elderly people with known or suspected CAD have been safely exposed to acute hypoxia at altitude while breathing low oxygen mixtures or when being placed in a hypobaric chamber.

Patients with heart disease have increased sympathetic activity during the first 3 d at altitude. The resultant increases cardiac work and myocardial oxygen consumption, and this could increase dysrhythmias. Although both cardiac rhythm abnormalities and ST segment and T wave electrocardiographic changes are reported, none of these changes are associated with any clinical evidence of myocardial ischemia.

Travelers with heart disease do not appear to have an increased incidence of AMS.

Travelers with mild stable CAD should be advised to ascend gradually,and to continue antianginal and antihypertensive medications. Individuals who have more severe, symptomatic CAD or those in a high-risk group should avoid travel to high altitudes. Individuals with heart failure who travel to altitude may require increased use of diuretics to promote diuresis and acclimatization. Acetazolamide prophylaxis may be useful to speed acclimatization and to prevent AMS and its accompanying fluid retention.

Hypertension

High-altitude travel produces a mild increase in blood pressure and heart rate in healthy individuals.

People with severe hypertension should travel only to moderate altitudes. For individuals who have mild hypertension while traveling at altitude, treatment is not routinely necessary because the hypertension will rarely become dangerously high and will improve on descent.Patients with hypertension should be monitored frequently in the first few days at altitude and antihypertensive medications continued. For hypertensive patients with a rapid rise in blood pressure and who will be staying for several weeks, an alpha-blocker, nifedipine, or ACEI should be considered.

Seizures

Travel to altitude is implicated as a precipitant for seizure activity.Seizures attributable to high altitude are typically generalized tonic-clonic in nature.A focal seizure at altitude should prompt a thorough workup for a space-occupying lesion. Several pathophysiologic mechanisms include sleep deprivation from periodic breathing, hyperventilation, and the direct effect of hypobaric hypoxia.Seizures not responding to supportive care can be treated with benzodiazepines.Should an epileptic who is already taking seizure medicine experience a breakthrough seizure at altitude, standard seizure evaluation is warranted, and acetazolamide at 250 mg twice daily may be added. Acetazolamide itself has antiepileptic properties and may ameliorate the altituderelated metabolic derangements.

Pregnancy

Studies of permanent high-altitude residents in Colorado and Peru show an increased incidence of complications in maternal, fetal, and neonatal life.Infants born at high altitude have a lower birth weight compared with infants born at sea level because of a combination of factors, including altitude-related effects on fetal growth, changes in uterine blood flow, and increased premature births.

Pregnancy-induced hypertension, proteinuria, and peripheral edema (manifestations of toxemia and preeclampsia) are more common at high altitudes and may also be related to maternal and uterine hypoxemia.Although hypertension in pregnancy is more common at high altitudes, no evidence exists for an increase in spontaneous abortions, abruptio placentae, or placenta previa.

Travel by pregnant women to moderate altitudes appears to be safe, but caution is advised for lowland women with normal pregnancies who wish to travel above 13,000 feet, for pregnant women who wish to remain at high altitude for a prolonged period, and for women with complicated pregnancies.

(CHAI Yanfen)

Chapter 43

Drowning

KEY CONCEPTS

Drowning was defined as "the process of experiencing respiratory impairment from submersion/immersion in liquid."

Immersion syndrome refers specifically to syncope resulting from cardiac dysrhythmias on sudden contact with water that is at least 5℃ less than body temperature.

Aggressive pulmonary support is essential to optimizing the victim's chances for a favorable outcome.

In submersion incidents, the Heimlich maneuver is reserved for patients with a suspected airway occlusion by a foreign body.

The safest parameter is to continue resuscitative effort until the core temperature reaches at least 32 to 35℃.

Comatose patients who have been resuscitated after reasonable submersion time regardless of rhythm should not be rewarmed above 34℃.

PERSPECTIVE

Unintentional drowning is the sixth most common cause of accidental death, accounting for 4086 deaths (1.4 per 100,000) in the United States in 2007. Worldwide, it is estimated that 500,000 people die after drowning annually, which exceeds mortality due to war. Toddlers and older teenagers are at greatest risk of death by drowning, with annual incidences of 2.45 and 1.47 per 100,000, respectively. In china, drowning is the leading cause of death for children. Low and middle-income countries account for 97% of all drowning deaths.

Submersion injuries occur in domestic settings such as swimming pools, hot tubs, bathtubs, and large buckets and in all forms of natural bodies of water. Most (63%) deaths among older children occur in natural bodies of fresh water.

Drowning follows clear temporal patterns: Two thirds of pediatric deaths occur between May and August, and most submersion injuries occur on weekends between noon and 8:00 pm. Submersion victims older than 20 yr are most often participating in water sports or using watercraft.

Because of the recent natural disasters, the incidence of drowning injuries and fatalities is rising. In disasters such as floods and tsunamis, old populations are disproportionately affected.

PRINCIPLES OF DISEASE

Definitions

In the past, *drowning* referred to death within 24 hr of suffocation from submersion in a liquid, whereas *near-drowning* described victims who survived at least 24 hr past the initial event regardless of the outcome. In 2005, the World WHO published a new policy defining drowning. Drowning was defined as "the process of experiencing respiratory impairment from submersion/immersion in liquid." Furthermore, the WHO policy states that "drowning outcomes should be classified as: death, morbidity, and no morbidity. ... Use of the terms wet, dry, active, passive, silent, and secondary drowning should no longer be used." As such, the term near-drowning should not be used, and the association of the term drowning with a fatal outcome should be abandoned.

Immersion syndrome refers specifically to syncope resulting from cardiac dysrhythmias on sudden contact with water that is at least 5℃ less than body temperature. Proposed as mechanisms for the syndrome are vagal stimulation leading to asystole and Vf secondary to Q-T prolongation with a massive release of catecholamines on contact with cold water. The resultant loss of consciousness leads to secondary drowning. The risk of immersion syndrome is proportional to the difference between body and water temperature. Wetting the face and head before entering the water may prevent the inciting sequence of events.

Risk Factors

Age, gender affect the incidence of drowning. Toddlers and old teenagers are at greatest risk of death by drowning.

Ethanol consumption in proximity with water is also a major risk factor for submersion injury or death.

The relationship between swimming ability and the risk of drowning is unclear. Skilled swimmers have greater exposure to water and may be more prone to submersion incidents.

Numerous medical conditions confer an increased likelihood of drowning or submersion injury. Seizure disorders sharply increase the chance of drowning. Autism and other developmental and behavioral disorders increase risk in children as well. Prolonged Q-T syndrome is also a risk factor for drowning.

Pathophysiology

Unexpected submersion triggers breath-holding, panic, and a struggle to surface. Air hunger and hypoxia develop, and the victim begins to swallow water. As breath-holding is overcome, involuntary gasps result in aspiration. The quantity of fluid aspirated determines subsequent pulmonary derangement.

The historical emphasis on pathophysiologic differences between freshwater and salt water aspiration with respect to resultant electrolyte imbalance, hemolysis, and fluid compartment shifting was based on animal studies conducted in the early 20th century. Subsequent investigations have revealed that significant intravascular abnormalities do not occur until the amount of aspirated water exceeds 11 mL/kg of body weight, and autopsy studies show that most drowning victims aspirate less than 4 mL/kg. Aspiration of 1 to 3 mL/kg of either freshwater or salt water destroys the integrity of pulmonary surfactant, leading to alveolar collapse, atelectasis, noncardiogenic pulmonary edema, intrapulmonary shunting, and ventilation-perfusion mismatch. Profound hypoxia and metabolic and respiratory acidosis ensue, leading to cardiovascular collapse, neuronal injury, and, ultimately death.

The classic hypothesis was that 10% to 15% of drowning victims die without aspirating a significant amount of water. Death from such "dry" drowning putatively results from severe laryngospasm causing hypoxia, convulsion, and death without fluid entering the lungs. An exhaustive review of the literature failed to corroborate this hypothesis. Dry drownings more appropriately reflect deaths from causes other than simple submersion.

Many factors may influence the pathophysiologic sequence of events in submersion injury and affect the chance of survival, including age, water temperature, duration and degree of hypothermia, the diving reflex, and the effectiveness of resuscitative efforts. Hypothermia is generally a poor prognostic finding. Cold water immersion speeds the development of exhaustion, altered consciousness, and cardiac dysrhythmia. Activation of the diving reflex by fear or immersion of the face in cold water shunts blood centrally to the heart and brain. Apnea and bradycardia ensue, prolonging the duration of submersion tolerated without CNS damage.

CLINICAL FEATURES

Symptoms and Signs

Many submersion injuries are witnessed. The history of coughing, choking, or vomiting in a patient found near a body of water suggests the diagnosis. Signs of *pulmonary injury* may be obvious in a submersion victim who is hypoxic, cyanotic, and in obvious respiratory distress or arrest. More subtle clues, such as increased respiratory rate and audible rhonchi, rales, or wheezes, should alert the clinician to evolving respiratory compromise. Submersion victims swallow a significantly greater volume of water than is aspirated, and gastric distention from PPV during rescue is common. As a result, 60% of patients vomit after a submersion event. Aspiration of gastric contents greatly compounds the degree of pulmonary injury and increases the likelihood that

ARDS will ensue. In addition, aspiration of particulate contaminants such as mud, sewage, and bacteria may obstruct the smaller bronchi and bronchioles and greatly increase the risk of infection both bacterial and fungal in nature.

Victims with *CNS injury* may present with symptoms ranging from mild lethargy to coma with fixed and dilated pupils. CNS injury results from the initial hypoxic or ischemic insult and from the cascade of reperfusion injury that follows reestablishment of cerebral blood flow after an arrest.

Cardiac dysrhythmias may incite a submersion injury or develop as its consequence. Hypoxemia, acidosis, and, potentially, hypothermia are the primary factors responsible for dysrhythmias ranging from VT and Vf to bradycardia-asystole. Electrolyte disturbances are rarely significant enough to be dysrhythmogenic.

Other clinical sequelae of submersion injury may include *AKI*, present in approximately 50% of patients as the result of lactic acidosis; prolonged hypoperfusion; and, in some instances, rhabdomyolysis. *Coagulopathy* as a consequence of associated hypothermia or DIC may also occur.

Prognostic Factors

Hypoxia is the most important factor related to outcome and subsequent quality of life in drowning victims. Submersion victims who arrive in the ED alert with normal hemodynamics are unlikely to experience neurologic impairment. Circumstantial variables that portend a poor outcome include submersion for longer than 5 to 10 min, and initiation of CPR more than 10 min after rescue. Objective findings on ED arrival that are associated with an unfavorable prognosis include hypothermia, severe acidosis, unreactive pupils, a GCS score of 3, and asystole or the need for ongoing CPR.

DIFFERENTIAL CONSIDERATIONS

The precipitants of a submersion injury, such as drug or ethanol intoxication, cardiac arrest, hypoglycemia, seizure, and attempted suicide or homicide, should be considered in a patient who is found unresponsive in the water.

Potential head or cervical spine injury is an important consideration when a history of trauma is associated with the submersion.

DIAGNOSTIC STUDIES

Cardiac monitoring and an ECG must be obtained to determine the presence of significant dysrhythmias or Q-T prolongation. Pulse oximetry, capnography, and ABG should be monitored closely in all submersion victims for signs of hypoxemia, hypercarbia, and acidosis. Blood glucose, serum creatinine, and electrolytes should be obtained. Similarly, CBC is often normal with the exception of leukocytosis. Toxicologic screening may be appropriate. Subsequently, evidence of renal failure, hepatic dysfunction, and DIC may be noted on laboratory testing.

The initial chest radiograph may underestimate the severity of pulmonary injury, although infiltrates or pulmonary edema may be evident within hours. Cranial CT is rarely contributory initially unless significant trauma or other pertinent pathology is suspected. MRI of the brain may predict neurologic outcome after submersion injury.

MANAGEMENT

Resuscitation of pulseless and apneic patients should be attempted initially in most cases. The clinical presentation of severe hypothermia often mimics death, and case reports exist of functional recovery for individuals submerged for 66 min.

For a victim without vital signs, outcome depends on the interval preceding CPR. Mouth-to-mouth assisted ventilation should begin immediately, even before the victim is extricated from the water. Chest compressions should be initiated as soon as the individual is placed on a solid surface. Maneuvers such as those proposed by Heimlich and Patrick to remove fluid from the lungs are ineffective and dangerous in a victim at risk for aspiration and may delay ventilation. Use of such maneuvers is not recommended unless there is reason to suspect airway occlusion by a foreign body.

On arrival in ED, cardiac monitoring and continuous pulse oximetry should be established. A core temperature obtained for any unstable or lethargic patient. Rewarming a hypothermic patient may suffice for hemodynamic stabilization and improvement in mental status. Bedside blood glucose measurement and empirical naloxone administration are warranted. In a spontaneously breathing patient, monitoring for signs of developing pulmonary injury should be established. Initial chest radiographs are often unremarkable even in the setting of serious and evolving pathology. Frequent ABG measurements are indicated to monitor rapidly changing respiratory function.

The decision regarding tracheal intubation should be based on clinical impression and objective determination of the adequacy of oxygenation and ventilation. Apparent or developing respiratory distress, the absence of protective airway reflexes, and significant associated head or chest injuries are indications. A P_aCO_2 greater than 50 mm Hg mandates intubation and mechanical ventilation. Patients unable to maintain SaO_2 greater than 90% or a P_aO_2 greater than 60 mm Hg on high-flow oxygen require positive airway pressure to increase FRC, decrease intrapulmonary shunting, and reduce ventilation-perfusion mismatch. In an awake patient, this may be accomplished by face or nasal mask, but the risk of potential gastric distention, vomiting, and aspiration must be considered. Otherwise, tracheal intubation and mechanical ventilation with PEEP is necessary. The hemodynamic consequences of PEEP must be monitored carefully because increased intrathoracic pressure may compromise venous return and CO.

The safest parameter is to continue resuscitative effort until the core temperature reaches at least 32 to 35℃ because cerebral death cannot be diagnosed accurately in hypothermic patients with temperatures below this level.

The administration of corticosteroids in the setting of submersion injury and potential ARDS does not improve outcome. Barbiturate-induced coma, aggressive diuresis, neuromuscular blockade, and hyperventilation do not improve neurologic outcome and, particularly in the case of hyperventilation, may be harmful. Empirical antibiotics should be administered only to the rare patient who was submerged in grossly contaminated water or who shows signs of infection or sepsis.

Drowning victims in cardiac arrest are usually colder than 30℃ and require warming. Comatose patients who have been resuscitated after reasonable submersion time regardless of rhythm should not be rewarmed above 34℃.

DISPOSITION

Symptomatic patients must be admitted for treatment. Patients with a history of apnea, unconsciousness, or hypoxia and any patients who manifest dysrhythmia or an abnormal chest radiograph also require admission. Patients who are asymptomatic on presentation to ED, maintain a normal room air SaO_2, and have no chest radiograph or ABG abnormalities can be discharged safely after an observation period of 6 hr.

Preventive Efforts

An increased public awareness of preventive measures and an emphasis on public education with regard to CPR and the dangers of ethanol use in conjunction with water-related activities have contributed significantly to the reduction in fatalities.

Pool covers are inadequate and potentially dangerous as barriers.

Medical care providers are a vital resource for enhancing public awareness of the importance of these measures. Education in ED with regard to drowning prevention can have a positive impact on patient and family awareness of steps to lessen the likelihood of catastrophic drowning or submersion injury.

(LI Huiping)

Chapter 44

Electrical and Lightning Injuries

KEY CONCEPTS

High-voltage electrical injury causes significant tissue and organ damage along the path between the entrance and exit wounds.Injury assessment should be detailed.

Victims of lightning injury may appear to have significant injuries, but symptoms usually resolve with time.After spinal cord and intracranial injuries are excluded, observation is the mainstay of treatment.

Patients with low-voltage electrical injury may be discharged safely if they have a normal ECG and no urinary heme pigment.

With electrical injury, sensory findings may be patchy and not match motor levels of impairment.

PERSPECTIVE

Electrical Injury

Injuries from artificial electricity have been reported for almost 300 yr. The first recorded death caused by electrical current from an artificial source was reported in 1879 when a carpenter in Lyons, France, inadvertently contacted a 250-V alternating current generator.

In the United States, electrical burns account for 4% to 6.5% of all admissions to burn units and approximately 1000 fatalities per year. Occupational electrical incidents are uncommon but account for nearly 6% of all occupational fatalities annually. During adolescence, a more active exploration of the environment leads to more severe high-voltage injuries or death. At the time of presentation, documentation of injuries is important not only for the immediate resuscitation of the victim but also for medicolegal reasons. Many electrical injuries eventually involve litigation for negligence, product liability, or worker compensation.

Lightning Injury

The incidence of lightning-related deaths in the United States has declined to an average of 39 people annually. Lightning is fatal in 1 of 10 lightning strike victims. In typical years, lightning kills more people in the United States than any other natural disaster except floods, and it is consistently among the top four weather-related killers.In developing countries, particularly those in the tropics, lightning is a much bigger risk both because it is more common and because agricultural, mining, and construction continue to be labor-intensive, resulting in high exposure to the workers. The lack of safe housing and metal vehicles expose entire families and schools to injury whenever a thunderstorm occurs.

PRINCIPLES OF DISEASE

Physics of Injury

When an electrical current of high voltage passes through tissue, most of the injury seems to be thermal, and histologic studies reveal coagulation necrosis consistent with thermal injury. The theory of *electroporation* is that electrical charges insufficient to produce thermal damage cause protein configuration changes that threaten cell wall integrity and cellular function.

The nature and severity of electrical burn injury are directly proportional to the current strength, resistance, and duration of current flow (Box 44-1). *Current strength* is expressed in amperes and is a measure of the amount of energy flowing through an object. Current is determined by the voltage and resistance. Resistance is determined by the current's pathway through the body. The factors determining the severity of burn injury are summarized in Box 44-2. Unfortunately, none of these can be used to predict or to explain the damage that any individual may suffer.

Box 44-1 Electrothermal Heating Formulas

$$P = I^2Rt$$

and

$$I = V/R$$

where

P = thermal power (heat), in joules

I = current, in amperes (A)

R = resistance, in ohms (Ω)

t = time, in seconds

V = potential, in volts (V)

Box 44-2 Factors Determining Electrical Injury

Type of circuit
Duration
Resistance of tissues
Voltage
Amperage
Pathway of current

Type of Circuit

One of the factors affecting the nature and severity of electrical injury is the type of circuit involved, direct current or alternating current. High-voltage direct current contact tends to cause a single muscle spasm, often throwing the victim from the source. This results in a shorter duration of exposure but increases the likelihood of traumatic blunt injury. Brief contact with a direct current source can also result in disturbances in cardiac rhythm, depending on the phase of the cardiac cycle affected.

Alternating current exposure of the same voltage tends to be three times more dangerous than direct current. Continuous muscle contraction, or tetany, can occur when the muscle fibers are stimulated between 40 and 110 times per second. The standard frequency of electrical transmission in the United States is 60 Hz (cycles per second) versus 50 Hz in most other countries.

The terms *entry* and *exit* are commonly used to describe electrical injury patterns. The terms *source contact point* and *ground contact point* are more appropriate, however, when referring to alternating current injuries. The hand is the most common site of contact via a tool that is in contact with an alternating current electrical source. The flexors of the upper extremity are much stronger than the extensors, causing the hand grasping the current source to pull the source even closer to the body. Currents greater than the "let-go threshold" (6–9 mA) can prevent the victim from releasing the current source, which prolongs the duration of exposure to the electrical current.

Voltage

Voltage is a measure of the difference in electrical potential between two points and is determined by the electrical source. Electrical injuries are conventionally divided into low or high voltage using 500 or 1000 V as the most common dividing lines. Although both low or high voltage can cause significant morbidity and mortality, high voltage results in greater current flow and therefore has a greater potential for tissue destruction leading to major amputations and tissue loss.

No deaths are recorded from contact with the low voltages associated with long-distance communication lines (24 V) or telephone lines (65 V). Fatalities are reported, however, with exposure to 110 V household current, especially in special environmental circumstances such as bathtub-related electrocutions.

Resistance

Resistance is the tendency of a material to resist the flow of electrical current. It is specific for a given tissue, depending on its moisture content, temperature, and other physical properties. The higher the resistance of a tissue to the flow of current, the greater the potential for transformation of electrical energy to thermal energy. Nerves, designed to carry electrical signals, and muscle and blood vessels, because of their high electrolyte and water content, have a low resistance and are good conductors. Bone, tendon, and fat have a high resistance and tend to heat and coagulate rather than transmit current. The other tissues of the body are intermediate in resistance (Box 44-3).

Box 44-3 Resistance of Body Tissues

Least
Nerves
Blood
Mucous membranes
Muscle
Intermediate
Dry skin
Most
Tendon
Fat
Bone

Skin is the primary resistor to the flow of current into the body. Skin on the inside of the arm or back of the hand has a resistance of approximately 30,000 Ω/cm^2. Hardened skin can have 20 to 70 times greater resistance (Table 44-1).A surge of current internally can cause extensive deep tissue destruction. Moisture also lowers resistance. Sweating can decrease the skin's resistance to 2500 to 3000 Ω/cm^2, and immersion in water causes a further reduction to 1200 to 1500 Ω/cm^2.

Table 44-1 -- Skin Resistance

TISSUE	RESISTANCE (Ω/cm^2)
Mucous membranes	100
Vascular areas	
Volar arm, inner thigh	300-10,000
Wet skin	
Bathtub	1200-1500
Sweat	2500
Other skin	10,000-40,000
Sole of foot	100,000-200,000
Heavily calloused palm	1-2 million

Amperage

Current, expressed in amperes, is a measure of the amount of energy that flows through an object. As defined by Joule's law, the heat generated is proportional to the amperage squared. Amperage depends on the source voltage and the resistance of the conductor and must normally be estimated in human electric exposures. Although the voltage of the source is often known, the resistance varies according to the involved tissues.

The physical effects vary with different amperages at 50 to 60 Hz, which is the alternating current frequency used in European countries and the United States (Table 44-2). A very narrow range exists between the threshold of perception of current (0.2–0.4 mA) and *let-go current* (6–9 mA). Thoracic tetany also can occur at levels just above this let-go current and result in respiratory arrest owing to paralysis of the muscles of respiration. Vf is estimated to occur at an amperage of 60 to 120 mA.The 120 V household source usually causes minimal injury across dry skin, amperage delivered to the heart when the resistance of the skin is decreased by sweat or submersion in water can result in current sufficient to cause electrocution with cardiac arrest with no surface burns.

Table 44-2 Physical Effects of Different Amperage Levels at 50 to 60 Hz

PHYSICAL EFFECT	CURRENT (mA)
Tingling sensation	1–4
Let-go current	
Children	4
Women	7
Men	9
Freezing to circuit	10–20
Respiratory arrest from thoracic muscle tetany	20–50
Ventricular fibrillation	60–120

Duration of Contact

In general, the longer the duration of contact with high-voltage current, the greater the electrothermal heating and degree of tissue destruction. Once carbonization of tissue occurs, the resistance to current flow increases.

The physics differ with lightning. The extremely short duration and extraordinarily high voltage and amperage of lightning result in a short flow of current internally, with little, if any, skin damage and almost immediate flashover of current around the outside of the body.

Pathway

The pathway of low, high, or lightning voltages determines the tissues at risk, the type of injury, and the degree of conversion of electrical energy to heat. Current passing through the heart or thorax can cause dysrhythmias and direct myocardial damage. Cerebral current can result in respiratory arrest, seizures, and paralysis. Current with ocular proximity can cause cataracts.

Current density is the amount of current flow per area of tissue. As current density increases, its tendency to flow through the less resistant tissues is overcome. Eventually it flows through tissues indiscriminately, as if the body were a volume conductor, with the potential to destroy all tissues in the current's path. Because the current is often concentrated at the source and ground contact points, the greatest degree of damage is often observed there. Nevertheless, extensive deep destruction of the tissues may exist between these sites with high-voltage injuries, and the surface damage is often only "the tip of the iceberg." Damage to the internal structures of the body may be noncontiguous, with areas of normal-appearing tissue adjacent to burned tissue and with damage to structures at sites distant from the apparent contact points.

The most important difference between lightning and high-voltage electrical injuries is the duration of exposure to the current.

Lightning is neither a direct current nor an alternating current. At best, it is a unidirectional massive current impulse. The cloud-to-ground lightning impulse results from the breakdown of a large electrical field between a cloud and the ground that is measured in millions of volts.

After lightning meets the body, current is initially transmitted internally, after which skin breaks down, and ultimately external "flashover" occurs.

Lightning current seldom causes significant burns or tissue destruction. Thus burns and myoglobinuric renal failure are not common, whereas cardiac and respiratory arrest, vascular spasm, neurologic damage, and autonomic instability play a much greater role. Lightning tends to cause asystole rather than Vf.Other injuries caused by blunt trauma or ischemia from vascular spasms, such as myocardial infarction or spinal artery syndromes, also occur.

Mechanisms of Injury

Electrical Injury

The primary electrical injury is the burn. Secondary blunt trauma results from falls or being thrown from the electrical source by an intense muscular contraction or the explosive force that may occur with electric flashes from circuit box or transformer accidents. Electrical burns are classified into four different types (Box 44-4).

Box 44-4 Types of Electrical Burns

- Direct contact
- Electrothermal heating
- Indirect contact
- Arc
- Flame
- Flash

Heating of tissues secondary to current causes electrothermal burns. Usually, these burns are a result of a low-voltage shock with a limited affected area. Severe electrothermal burns can occur if a person grips a high-voltage conductor. The prolonged flow of current can result in significant burns anywhere along the current path. Typically, the skin lesions of electrothermal burns are well-demarcated, deep, partial-thickness to full-thickness burns.

The most destructive indirect injury occurs when a victim becomes part of an electrical arc. Because the temperature of an electrical arc is approximately 2500℃, it causes deep thermal burns at the point where it contacts the skin. With electrical arcs, burns may be caused by the heat of the arc, electrothermal heating due to current flow, or flames that result from the ignition of clothing.

Electrothermal heating is the main cause of muscle damage and is seen almost exclusively in high-voltage accidents with prolonged (seconds) contact and current flow.

The histologic change in muscle injury is coagulation necrosis.Similar to the muscle damage, serious vascular damage usually occurs only after a high-voltage accident.

The absence of a pulse may be a result of immediate arterial thrombosis or transient vascular spasm.

Damage to neural tissue also may occur via several mechanisms. An immediate decrease in neural conductivity occurs with coagulation necrosis . In addition, it may suffer indirect damage as its vascular supply or myelin sheath is injured or as progressive edema results in a compartment syndrome. Evidence of neural damage may develop immediately or be delayed hours to days.

The hands, feet, and skull are the most common contact points. Histologic studies of the brain reveal focal petechial hemorrhages in the brainstem, cerebral edema, and widespread chromatolysis .

Lightning Injury

Lightning injury may occur by electrical mechanisms and by secondary concussive or blunt trauma. Whereas direct strike is most commonly described as the mechanism of injury, it accounts for a very small proportion of injuries and deaths (Table 44-3)

Table 44-3 Distribution of Lightning Injury Mechanisms

MECHANISM	PERCENT
Direct strike	3%-5%
Contact injury	3%-5%
Side splash/flash	30%-35%
Ground current	50%-55%
Upward streamer	10%-15%
Blunt trauma	Unknown

Injury from contact occurs when the person is touching an object that is part of the pathway of lightning current, such as a tree, mental fence, indoor plumbing, or wiring. Side flash or splash occurs as lightning jumps from its primary strike object to a nearby person on its way to the ground. Step voltage, a difference in electrical potential between a person's feet, may occur as lightning current spreads radially through the ground. A person is a far better conductor of electricity than the earth.

Victims of lightning injury may also be exposed to low-current upward streamers or ball lightning.

Blunt injury from lightning can occur from two mechanisms. First, the person may be thrown a considerable distance by the sudden, massive contraction caused by current passing through the body. Second, an explosive or implosive force occurs as the lightning pathway is instantaneously superheated then rapidly cooled after the passage of the lightning. This concussive injury or barotrauma is associated with tympanic membrane rupture, contusions of various organs, and pneumothorax. Blunt or concussive injury can accompany electrical injury.

CLINICAL FEATURES

Patients with high-voltage injury commonly present with devastating burns. Patients with lightning injury and low-voltage injury may have little evidence of injury or may be in cardiopulmonary arrest.

Head and Neck

Electrical Injury

The head is a common point of contact for high-voltage injuries, and the patient may exhibit burns and neurologic damage. Cataracts more typically appear months after the injury. Visual acuity and funduscopic examination should be performed at presentation. Hearing loss is much less common.

Lightning Injury

Lightning strikes may cause skull fractures and cervical spine injury from associated blunt trauma. Tympanic membrane rupture is commonly found in lightning victims and may be secondary to the shock wave, a direct burn, or a basilar skull fracture. Although most patients recover without serious sequelae, disruption of the ossicles and mastoid, otorrhea, hemotympanum, perilymphatic fistulae, and permanent deafness may occur.

Ocular injuries include corneal lesions, uveitis, iridocyclitis, hyphema, vitreous hemorrhage, optic atrophy, retinal detachment, and choroidoretinitis. As a result, dilated, unreactive pupils are not a reliable indicator of death. As with electrical injuries, cataracts may develop later in some patients.

Cardiovascular System

Electrical Injury

Cardiac arrest, either from asystole or from Vf, is common in electrical accidents. Other electrocardiographic findings include sinus tachycardia, transient ST segment elevation, reversible Q-T segment prolongation, PVC, Af, and bundle branch block. AMI is relatively rare.

Lightning Injury

There are many proposed mechanisms of cardiac injury from lightning. Numerous dysrhythmias occur in the absence of cardiac arrest. Nonspecific ST-T wave segment changes and prolongation of the Q-T interval may occur, and serum levels of cardiac enzymes are often elevated. HTN is commonly present after lightning injury but usually resolves without treatment within a few hours.

Skin

Electrical Injury

Other than cardiac arrest, the most devastating injuries are burns, which are most severe at the source and ground contact points. The most common sites of contact with the source include the hands and the skull. The most common areas of ground contact are the heels. A patient may have multiple source and ground contact points. Burns in severe electrical accidents often appear as painless, depressed, yellow-gray, punctate areas with central necrosis, or the areas may be mummified. High-voltage current often flows internally and can create massive muscle damage. If contact is brief, however, minimal flow may have occurred, and the visible skin damage may represent nearly all of the damage.

A peculiar type of burn associated with electrical injury is the "kissing burn," which occurs at the flexor creases (Fig. 44-1, see color illustration).

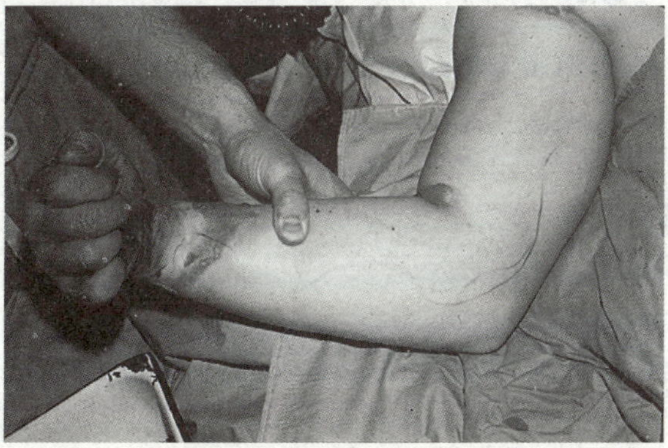

Fig. 44-1 Kissing burn.

Electrical flash burns are usually superficial partial-thickness burns, similar to other flash burns. Isolated thermal burns may also be seen when clothing ignites. The total body surface area affected by burns in electrical injury averages 10% to 25%. Severe burns to the skull and occasionally to the dura may occur.

Lightning Injury

Deep burns occur in fewer than 5% of lightning injuries. Patients may exhibit one or more of the following four types of superficial burns or skin changes: linear, punctate, feathering, or thermal burns.These transient lesions are pathognomonic for lightning injury and require no therapy (Fig. 44-2, see color illustration).

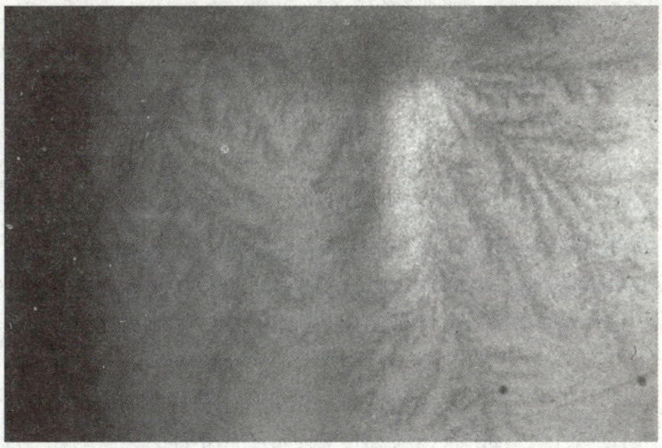

Fig. 44-2 Feathering burn.

Extremities

Electrical Injury

In high-voltage injuries, muscle necrosis can extend to sites distant from the observed skin injury, and compartment syndromes occur as a result of vascular ischemia and muscle edema.Massive release of myoglobin may lead to myoglobinuric renal failure.

Joint areas may exhibit more severe injury than the muscle along the long bone portions of an extremity. Burn injury becomes concentrated at joints.

Vascular damage from the electrical energy may become evident at any time.An extremity may initially appear edematous or ischemic. With severe injuries, the entire extremity may appear mummified when all tissue elements, including the arteries, experience coagulation necrosis.

Damage to the vessel wall at the time of injury may also result in delayed thrombosis and hemorrhage, especially in the small arteries to muscle. This ongoing vascular damage can cause a partial-thickness burn to progress into a full-thickness burn as the vascular supply diminishes to the area. Progressive loss of muscle because of vascular ischemia downstream from damaged vessels may mandate repeated deep débridements.

Lightning Injury

Lightning injury may cause transient vasospasm so severe that the extremities appear cold, blue, mottled, and pulseless. This condition usually resolves within a few hours and rarely requires vascular imaging or surgical intervention.

Skeletal System

As with electrical injury, numerous types of fractures, dislocations and soft tissue blunt trauma are reported with lightning injury. Fractures of the long bones are possible secondary to the trauma associated with electrical injury. Spinal fractures and ligamentous injury may occur.

Nervous System

Electrical Injury

In high-voltage injuries, loss of consciousness is usually transient, unless there is a significant concomitant head injury. Prolonged coma with eventual recovery also occurs. Patients may exhibit confusion, flat affect, and difficulty with short-term memory and concentration. Electrical injury to the CNS may cause a seizure. Neurologic symptoms may improve, but long-term disability is common. Even with low voltage, electrical injury may result in neurologic and psychological sequelae. In high-voltage exposures, spinal cord injury may result from fractures or ligamentous disruption of the cervical, thoracic, or lumbar spine. Patients with immediate damage have symptoms of weakness, and paresthesias develop within hours of the insult. Lower extremity findings are more common than upper extremity findings. Delayed neurologic damage may present days to years after the insult. Clinical presentations include ascending paralysis, or transverse myelitis. Motor findings predominate. Sensory findings are also common and may be patchy and not match motor levels of impairment. Significant autonomic system dysfunction may complicate the post injury recovery.

Lightning Injury

Whereas high-energy electrical injury is primarily a burn injury, lightning is primarily a nervous system injury. On initial presentation, two thirds of seriously injured lightning patients have *keraunoparalysis*, which is a unique temporary paralysis secondary to lightning strike. It is characterized by lower and sometimes upper extremities that are blue, mottled, cold, and pulseless. These findings are secondary to vascular spasm and sympathetic nervous system instability. Generally, this condition clears within a few hours.

Paraplegia, intracranial hemorrhages, seizures, and electroencephalographic changes occur after lightning injuries. Loss of consciousness for varying periods is common, and confusion and anterograde amnesia are almost universal findings. Peripheral nerve damage is also common, and recovery is usually poor. A lightning strike to the head can cause a visual cortex defect that results in complex visual hallucinations.A syndrome of delayed muscle atrophy caused by electrical injury of the nerves is described, even in the absence of cutaneous burns.

Other Viscera

Electrical Injury

Injury to the lungs is rare ,but damage to the pancreas, liver, small intestine, large intestine, bladder, and gallbladder is reported.

Lightning Injury

Pulmonary contusion, pneumothorax and hemorrhage are seen with lightning injury. Blunt abdominal injuries occur rarely.

Other Low-Voltage Injuries

Burns from low-voltage sources are usually less severe than burns from high-voltage sources, patients still may complain of paresthesias, experience cardiac dysrhythmias.

COMPLICATIONS

Electrical Injury

Cardiac arrest generally occurs only at the initial presentation . Many of the complications are similar to those of thermal burns and crush injuries, including myoglobinuria, infection, and clostridial myositis.

Neurologic complications, such as loss of consciousness, peripheral nerve damage, and delayed spinal cord syndromes, may occur.

Lightning Injury

Complications of lightning injury fall into three areas: (1) hearing loss from tympanic membrane rupture or paresthesias and paresis from neurologic damage; (2) long-term neurologic deficits and endocrine dysfunction; and (3) iatrogenic complications that are secondary to overaggressive management.

DIFFERENTIAL CONSIDERATIONS

Electrical Injury

Electrical injuries are usually self-evident. Alterations in consciousness or seizures can be caused by the electrical injury, associated traumatic brain injury.

Lightning Injury

The differential diagnosis of lightning injury includes many of the causes of unconsciousness, paralysis, or disorientation of unclear etiology. The presence of typical burn patterns, such as feathering, may be helpful.

MANAGEMENT

Out-of-Hospital

Securing the Scene

For high-voltage incidents, the power source must be turned off. Rescuers should ensure that the power is off before approaching the victim.

Triage Considerations

Cardiorespiratory arrest is the major cause of death in lightning injuries.The triage of lightning victims should concentrate on those who appear to be in cardiorespiratory arrest. CPR should be started on those who have no pulse or respirations. If the victim is adequately ventilated, perfusion may be maintained.

Initial Resuscitation

Electrical injury victims may require a combination of cardiac and trauma care. Spinal immobilization is indicated whenever associated spinal trauma is suspected. Fractures and dislocations should be splinted, and burns should be covered with clean, dry dressings.

Emergency Department

Assessment

Cardiac arrest and airway compromise, including burns, are the most serious initial complications. For patients suffering circumferential burns to the chest that limit chest excursion or to the extremities causing compartment syndromes, fasciotomy and escharotomy may be necessary.

The history obtained from bystanders and the nonhospital medical personnel regarding the type of electrical source, duration of contact, or environmental factors may be helpful. An electrical injury should be treated similarly to a crush injury, rather than a thermal burn. Standard crystalloid resuscitation in anticipation of myoglobinuria should be maintained. Cardiac monitoring is indicated for severely injured patients and for patients who have the indications listed in Box 44-5. All patients should have an ECG and cardiac biomarker determinations.

Box 44-5 Indications for Electrocardiographic Monitoring

- Cardiac arrest
- Documented loss of consciousness
- Abnormal electrocardiogram
- Dysrhythmia observed in out-of-hospital or emergency department setting
- History of cardiac disease
- Presence of significant risk factors for cardiac disease
- Concomitant injury severe enough to warrant admission
- Suspicion of conductive injury
- Hypoxia
- Chest pain

Most lightning victims behave as though they have had electroconvulsive therapy, with confusion and anterograde amnesia for several days. If any altered mentation or neurologic deterioration occurs after an electrical injury, a CT scan is indicated to assess for intracranial hemorrhage.

Lightning victims who do not experience cardiopulmonary arrest generally do well with supportive therapy. Patients who have cardiopulmonary arrest may have a poor prognosis, particularly if there is hypoxic brain damage.

Ancillary Tests

Electrical Injury

Patients should receive cardiac monitoring in the ED and an ECG . The following laboratory tests may be considered :CBC, electrolyte levels, serum myoglobin, BUN, serum creatinine, and urinalysis.

CK levels and isoenzyme analysis should be performed. Less specific cardiac biomarkers should be interpreted with care when diagnosing MI in the setting of electrical injury.Radiographs should be obtained if spinal injury is clinically suspected .CT or MRI may be useful in the evaluation of associated trauma.

Lightning Injury

In patients injured by lightning, an ECG should be obtained. Serum biomarkers for cardiac injury are indicated only in patients with chest pain, abnormal ECG, or altered mentation. The severity or nature of the injuries may require other laboratory studies.

Radiographic studies, particularly cranial CT or MRI evaluation, may be indicated, depending on the patient's level of consciousness at presentation and throughout the evaluation and treatment.

Specific Therapies

Rhabdomyolysis

Victims of electrical injury who have heme pigment in the urine usually have myoglobinuria. Alkalinization of the urine increases the solubility of myoglobin in the urine, increasing the rate of clearance. In an adult, urine output should be maintained at 1 to 1.5 mL/kg/hr until all traces of myoglobin have cleared from the urine, while the blood is maintained at a pH of at least 7.45 using sodium bicarbonate. Furosemide or mannitol may be used to cause further diuresis. In contrast to high-voltage injuries, rhabdomyolysis is rare with lightning injuries.

Burn Wound Care

Cutaneous burns should be dressed with antibiotic dressings, such as sulfadiazine silver. Electrical burns are especially prone to tetanus, and patients should receive tetanus toxoid and tetanus immune globulin on the basis of their immunization history.

Extremity Injuries

Management of electrical injuries of the extremities entails surgical management, including early fasciotomy, carpal tunnel release, or amputation of an obviously nonviable extremity.

DISPOSITION

Electrical Injuries

Admission

Indications for admission for electrocardiographic monitoring are listed in Box 44-5. In general, when corporeal conduction is suspected, the patient should be admitted for 12 to 24 hr of cardiac monitoring. Most patients with significant electrical burns should be stabilized and transferred to a regional burn center for burn care and extensive occupational and physical rehabilitation.

Outpatient Management

Asymptomatic patients with a normal physical examination after low-voltage exposure can be reassured and discharged without performing any ancillary tests. Patients with cutaneous burns or mild persistent symptoms can be discharged if they have a normal ECG and no urinary heme pigment.

Electrical injury during pregnancy from low-voltage sources may result in fetal demise.Obstetric consultation is advisable for all pregnant patients reporting electrical injury. Placental abruption, the most common cause of fetal death after blunt trauma, may result from even minor trauma, such as may be associated with electrical injuries. Patients in the latter half of pregnancy should receive fetal monitoring. First-trimester patients should be informed of the remote risk of spontaneous abortion and, if no other indications for admission exist, may be discharged with instructions for threatened miscarriage and close obstetric follow-up evaluation. The prognosis for fetal survival after lightning strike is most dependent on the extent of the mother’s injuries. Fetal demise occurs in 50% of cases.

Lightning Injuries

Most lightning survivors who appear well can be safely discharged. After spinal cord and intracranial processes are excluded, observation is the mainstay of treatment.

If there is a history of a loss of consciousness or if the patient exhibits confusion, hospital admission and observation are suggested. After evaluation, if the ECG is normal, asymptomatic patients may be discharged home.

(LI Huiping)

SECTION 5

Toxicology Emergencies

Chapter 45

General Approach to the Poisoned Patient

KEY CONCEPTS

A thorough history from many sources is the key to toxicologic diagnosis.

Patients who are contaminated with an agent require decontamination.

Gastric decontamination should not be undertaken routinely as it may result in morbidity, and patients often present too late for it to be effective.

Except for specific lifesaving antidotes against certain toxins, most poisoned patients require only supportive therapy for recovery.

A toxicology screen (usually urine, sometimes blood and urine) may identify the class of drugs ingested.

PERSPECTIVE

Most poisoned patients in ED are adults with acute oral drug overdoses. Other common clinical scenarios include accidental poisoning ; drug abuse through smoking, snorting, or injection; chronic poisoning from drug abuse or from environmental, industrial, and agricultural chemical exposure; medication reactions or interactions; and envenomation.

INITIAL APPROACH TO THE POISONED PATIENT

Patients who are contaminated with an agent require decontamination. Except for specific lifesaving antidotes against certain toxins, most poisoned patients require only supportive therapy for recovery.Hypoglycemia should be considered in a patient with altered mental status or seizures and should be evaluated by bedside glucose testing. Naloxone can be given to patients with suspected opioid overdose and respiratory depression while preparations are made to secure the airway because a positive response may obviate the need for intubation. Flumazenil use should be limited to confirmed acute benzodiazepine overdose in a patient who is not a chronic benzodiazepine user.The patient may have ingested tricyclic antidepressants or other drugs likely to cause seizures .The use of flumazenil can carry a substantial risk of seizures. Thiamine should be administered , alcoholic patients with altered mental status.A complete overdose history may be time-consuming but is important (Box 45-1).

Box 45-1 Obtaining an Overdose History

- Obtain all prescription bottles and other containers when possible. Perform a pill count. Be sure that the bottles contain the medications listed. Identify any unknown tablets.
- Contact the prescribing physician or the pharmacy as listed on the bottles to determine previous overdoses or other medications that the patient may have available. Identify underlying medical and psychiatric disorders and medication allergies. Review past medical records.
- Talk to the patient's family and friends in the emergency department. If necessary, call the patient's home to ask questions of others. The persons providing the important elements of the history should be identified in the chart.
- Search the patient's belongings for drugs or drug paraphernalia. A single pill hidden in a pocket, for example,may provide *the* most important clue to the diagnosis.

- Have family members (or the police) search the patient's home, including the medicine cabinet, clothes drawers,closets, and garage; such searches may also provide clues that make the diagnosis. This has the added benefit of involving the family in the patient's care.
- Look for track marks on the patient. Consider body packing or body stuffing.

Accurate vital signs, including pulse oximetry, are important in the diagnosis of poisoning and should be repeated as indicated. One measurement of temperature should be included. Respirations should be counted. A cardiac monitor or 12-lead ECG should be evaluated . The physical examination in a comatose patient should ensure that concomitant treatable conditions (e.g., trauma, intracranial hemorrhage, CNS infection) are not missed. Focal neurologic findings could be possible indicators of intracranial disease or severe head trauma.

The pupillary examination may give misleading information. Some opioid agonists, especially propoxyphene and pentazocine, may not produce the characteristic miosis of opioid intoxication. When multiple drugs are ingested, the expected pupillary findings related to any particular agent may be modified or absent.

Signs of infection (sepsis, abscess, endocarditis) should be investigated in patients suspected of injection drug abuse. Rectal, vaginal, and radiographic examination of the abdomen should be performed in these circumstances. Another important physical finding is evidence of aspiration or noncardiogenic pulmonary edema on chest auscultation. Bowel sounds may be increased or decreased if agents affecting the cholinergic nervous system have been ingested. A rectal examination to detect melena or hematochezia may also provide evidence of a coagulopathy.Skin examination may reveal evidence of skin popping, cyanosis (hypoxia or methemoglobinemia), or pressure marks if the patient has been unconscious.

Unusual odors of the patient's breath, skin, clothing, vomitus, or nasogastric aspirate may also provide useful diagnostic clues (Table 45-1).

Table 45-1 Odors in Overdose History

ODOR	POSSIBLE INTOXICANT
Bitter almonds	Cyanide
Carrots	Water hemlock (cicutoxin)
Fishy	Zinc or aluminum phosphide
Fruity	Ethanol, acetone, isopropyl alcohol, chlorinated hydrocarbons (e.g., chloroform)
Garlic	Arsenic, dimethyl sulfoxide (DMSO), organophosphates, yellow phosphorus, selenium, tellurium
Glue	Toluene, other solvents
Pears	Chloral hydrate, paraldehyde
Rotten eggs	Disulfiram, hydrogen sulfide, *N*-acetylcysteine, dimercaptosuccinic acid (DMSA)
Shoe polish	Nitrobenzene
Wintergreen	Methyl salicylate

TOXIC SYNDROMES AND ANTIDOTES

The most common toxidromes are the anticholinergic syndrome, sympathomimetic syndrome, opioid/sedative/ethanol syndrome, cholinergic syndrome, and serotonin syndrome (Table 45-2).

Table 45-2 Common Toxic Syndromes (Toxidromes)

Anticholinergic	
Common signs	Delirium with mumbling speech,tachycardia, dry flushed skin, dilated pupils, myoclonus, slightly elevated temperature, urinary retention, decreased bowel sounds. Seizures and dysrhythmias may occur in severe cases.
Common causes	Antihistamines, antiparkinsonians,atropine, scopolamine, amantadine,antipsychotics, antidepressants,antispasmodics, mydriatics, muscle relaxants, many plants (e.g., jimson weed,*Amanita muscaria*)
Sympathomimetic	
Common signs	Delusions, paranoia, tachycardia (or bradycardia with pure alpha-agonists),hypertension, hyperpyrexia, diaphoresis,piloerection, mydriasis, hyper-reflexia. Seizures, hypotension, and dysrhythmias may occur in severe cases.

Continued

Common causes	Cocaine, amphetamine,methamphetamine and its derivatives,over-the-counter decongestants (phenylpropanolamine, ephedrine,pseudoephedrine). In caffeine and theophylline overdoses, similar findings,except for the organic psychiatric signs,result from catecholamine release.
Opioid/Sedative/Ethanol	
Common signs	Coma, respiratory depression, miosis,hypotension, bradycardia, hypothermia,pulmonary edema, decreased bowel sounds, hyporeflexia, needle marks. Seizures may occur after overdoses of some narcotics (e.g., propoxyphene).
Common causes	Narcotics, barbiturates, benzodiazepines, ethchlorvynol, glutethimide ,methyprylon, methaqualone, meprobamate, ethanol, clonidine, guanabenz

The anticholinergic syndrome occurs frequently because many common medications and plants have anticholinergic properties. Anticholinergic CNS poisoning causes mild temperature elevation and acute delirium with mumbling speech and typical "picking movements" of the fingers. Suppression of cholinergic inhibition of the heart rate leads to tachycardia. Inhibition of the secretory functions of the integument causes dry mouth and skin, and the face is typically flushed. Unopposed sympathetic drive of the ciliary apparatus causes wide pupillary dilation.

The sympathomimetic syndrome is usually seen after acute or chronic abuse of cocaine, amphetamines, or decongestants (e.g., phenylephrine). Patients may be delusional; methamphetamine, in particular, may cause complicated, intricate, and paranoid delusions. Seizures may occur, and the postictal state can contribute to the altered mental status. Blood pressure is usually elevated, the pulse is rapid, the pupils are dilated, and piloerection may be seen. In massive overdoses of sympathomimetic agents, cardiovascular collapse can occur with the development of shock and wide-complex dysrhythmias. This clinical picture can mimic that of overdose of cardioactive drugs or cyclic antidepressants. In contrast to the dry skin seen with anticholinergic syndrome, diaphoresis would be expected with the sympathomimetic syndrome.

An extreme presentation of sympathomimetic excess can be excited delirium (Box 45-2). In this state, patients are agitated, hyperthermic, and violent and possess "superhuman strength." These individuals may have a severe metabolic acidosis and hyperkalemia.All sedative-hypnotic agents, when they are taken in sufficient dosage, cause general anesthesia with a complete loss of awareness and reflex activity. The CNS depressant (opioid/sedative/ethanol) syndrome is the most common toxic syndrome seen in ED, and a depressed sensorium is its hallmark. Mixing agents in this class (e.g., ethanol and benzodiazepines) is common.

Box 45-2 Toxins Causing Delirium

Alcohol and alcohol withdrawal	Muscle relaxants
Anticholinergics	Mushrooms with muscimol or ibotenic acid
Anticonvulsants	Opiates
Antidepressants	Phencyclidine
Antihypertensives	Salicylates
Antiparkinson medications	Sedative withdrawal
Antipsychotics	Solvents
Cardiac medications	Steroids
Cocaine	Sympathomimetics (cocaine, amphetamines)
Lithium	
Monoamine oxidase inhibitors	

Respiratory depression is particularly pronounced with opioid overdose, and the respiratory rate is often diminished before decreases in blood pressure or pulse occur. The diagnosis of opioid overdose is confirmed by the use of naloxone (Narcan) or nalmefene (Revex) in adequate doses. Comatose patients often present without a history and need to be managed aggressively, with securing of the airway when it is needed. These patients may need basic laboratory tests and a head computed tomography scan if their presentation or course is suggestive of stroke, infection, or head trauma while consideration is given to a drug overdose alone or in combination with one of these medical conditions. A serum or breath ethanol level that is not commensurate with the level of CNS depression raises suspicion of intracranial injury, hemorrhage, or infection.

The cholinergic syndrome is important to

recognize. Cholinergic syndrome causes the patient to be "wet," as opposed to the anticholinergic syndrome, which causes the patient to be "dry." The wetness is manifested by profuse sweating and excessive activity of virtually the entire exocrine system, often accompanied by vomiting, diarrhea, diaphoresis, and urinary incontinence. The mnemonic SLUDGE is used to recall the specific elements of the syndrome: salivation, lacrimation, urination, defecation, gastrointestinal cramping, and emesis. The CNS (e.g., confusion, coma, and seizures) and the skeletal muscles (e.g., weakness and fasciculations) can also be involved. The pupils are often miotic. Cholinergic syndrome is most frequently caused by organophosphate or carbamate pesticide exposure. Anticholinergic agents are also the foundation of "nerve agents" such as sarin.

Serotonin syndrome ensues when there is a drug interaction involving SSRI or an overdose of an SSRI.Fluoxetine (Prozac), sertraline (Zoloft), paroxetine (Paxil), fluvoxamine (Luvox), and citalopram (Celexa) are commonly used SSRI. Other drugs inhibit the reuptake of other neurotransmitters and are also SRI that can cause the syndrome. These drugs include venlafaxine (Effexor), nefazodone (Serzone), and mirtazapine (Remeron). Drug interactions between many drugs can cause the serotonin syndrome.These drugs include the SSRIs, SRIs, MAOI, tryptophan, sympathomimetics, tricyclic and other antidepressants, meperidine, dextromethorphan, and lithium. Serotonin syndrome is characterized by altered mental status, fever, agitation, tremor, myoclonus, hyper-reflexia, ataxia, incoordination, diaphoresis, shivering, and sometimes diarrhea.The diagnosis relies on the drug history, and it is difficult to distinguish serotonin syndrome from an overdose of cocaine, lithium, or MAOI and from the neuroleptic malignant syndrome or thyroid storm.As possible toxidromes are investigated, the use of specific antidotes should be considered (Table 45-3).

Table 45-3 Antidotes used in the Emergency Department

TOXIN USED FOR	ANTIDOTE	DOSE AND COMMENTS
Acetaminophen	*N*-Acetylcysteine	140 mg/kg PO, then 70 mg/kg q4h for up to 17 doses OR 150 mg/kg IV load during 1 hr with 50 mg/kg during 4 hr followed by 100 mg/kg during 16 hr
Anticholinergics	Physostigmine	1-2 mg IV in adults, 0.5 mg in children during 2 min for anticholinergic delirium, seizures, or dysrhythmias
Arsenic, lead, and mercury	BAL	3-5 mg/kg IM only
	d-Penicillamine	20-40 mg/kg/d; 500 mg tid in adults; may cross-react with penicillin in allergic patients
Benzodiazepines	Flumazenil	0.2 mg, then 0.3 mg, then 0.5 mg, up to 5 mg; not to be used if patient has signs of TCA toxicity; not approved for use in children but probably safe
Black widow spider bite	*Latrodectus* antivenin	One vial by slow IV infusion is usually curative; may cause anaphylaxis
Beta-blockers	Glucagon	5-10 mg in adults, then infusion of same dose per hr
	Insulin and glucose	1 unit/kg regular insulin IV push followed by 1-10 unit/kg/hr; blood glucose should be checked frequently; D10 at 100 mL/hr with boluses of D50 if hypoglycemia occurs
	Intralipid 20%	1.5 mL/kg during 2-3 min followed by infusion of 0.25 mL/kg/min Reported to be effective for highly protein bound drugs with large volumes of distribution,such as local anesthetics, beta-blockers, calcium channel blockers, and tricyclic antidepressants
Calcium channel blockers	Calcium	1 g calcium chloride IV in adults, 20-30 mg/kg/dose in children, during a few min with continuous monitoring; repeat as needed
	Glucagon	5-10 mg in adults, then infusion of same dose per hour
	Insulin and glucose	Same dose as for beta-blockers
Cyanide	Hydroxycobalamin	5 mg in 100 mL of NS during 15 min; repeat if necessary

Continued

TOXIN USED FOR	ANTIDOTE	DOSE AND COMMENTS
Cyanide, hydrogen sulfide	Sodium thiosulfate Sodium nitrite Hydroxycobalamin	50 mL of 25% (12.5 g; 1 ampule) in adults; 1.65 mL/kg IV in children 10 mL of 3% (300 mg; 1 ampule) in adults; 0.33 mL/kg slowly IV in children 5 g in 100 mL of NS given during 15 min
Digitalis glycosides	Digoxin-specific Fab	10-20 vials if patient is in Vf; otherwise dose fragments on the basis of serum digoxin concentration or amount ingested
Ethylene glycol	Fomepizole Pyridoxine Thiamine	15 mg/kg × 1, then 10 mg/kg q12h × 4, until ethylene glycol < 20 mg/dL; adjust dose during dialysis 100 mg IV daily, Thiamine 100 mg IV
Hydrofluoric acid	Calcium gluconate	3.5 g in 5 oz of KY jelly topical; apply liberally to affected skin
Iron	Deferoxamine	15 mg/kg/hr IV; higher doses reported to be safe
Isoniazid, hydrazine, and monomethylhydrazine	Pyridoxine	5 g in adults, 1 g in children, if ingested dose unknown; antidote may cause neuropathy in very large doses
Lead	DMSA (succimer) EDTA	Reported useful for arsenic and lead as well; one 100-mg capsule per 10-kg body weight tid for 1 week, then bid, with chelation breaks 75 mg/kg/d by continuous infusion; watch for nephrotoxicity, best done in hospital
Local anesthetics and others	Intralipid 20%	1.5 mL/kg during 2-3 min followed by infusion of 0.25 mL/kg/min Reported to be effective for highly protein bound drugs with large volumes of distribution, such as local anesthetics, beta-blockers, calcium channel blockers, tricyclic antidepressants, and others
MDMA-related hyperpyrexia	Dantrolene	2.5 mg/kg IV Lower doses have also been reported to be effective
Neuroleptics	Dantrolene	2.5 mg/kg IV for neuroleptic malignant syndrome
Methanol	Folate or leucovorin Ethanol Fomepizole	50 mg IV q4h in adults while patients have serious toxicity Loading dose, 10 mL/kg of 10%; maintenance dose, 0.15 mL/kg/hr of 10%; double rate during dialysis 15 mg/kg × 1, then 10 mg/kg q12h × 4, until methanol < 20 mg/dL; adjust dose during dialysis
Methemoglobin-forming agents	Methylene blue	1-2 mg/kg IV, one 10-mL dose of 10% solution (100 mg) is typical for an adult without anemia
Opioids	Nalmefene Naloxone	0.5-1 mg; much longer half-life than naloxone 2 mg; less to avoid narcotic withdrawal, more if inadequate response; same dose in children
Organophosphates and carbamates	Atropine Protopam	Test dose, 1-2 mg IV in adults, 0.03 mg/kg in children; titrate to drying of pulmonary secretions Loading dose, 1-2 g IV in adults, 25-50 mg/kg in children; adult maintenance, 500 mg/hr or 1-2 g q4-6h
Rattlesnake bite	CroFab antivenin	Five vials minimum dose by infusion in normal saline; increase is rate dependent on patient's tolerance; may cause anaphylaxis
Serotonin syndrome	Cyproheptadine	4 mg PO or by nasogastric tube as needed; no parenteral form available; antidote may cause anticholinergic effects
Sulfonylureas	Octreotide	50 μg SC q12h, 5-10 μg/kg/24 hr IV

Continued

TOXIN USED FOR	ANTIDOTE	DOSE AND COMMENTS
Tricyclic antidepressants	Bicarbonate	44-88 mEq in adults, 1-2 mEq/kg in children; best used by IV push and not by slow infusion
	Intralipid 20%	1.5 mL/kg during 2-3 min followed by infusion of 0.25 mL/kg/min Reported to be effective for highly protein bound drugs with large volumes of distribution,such as local anesthetics, beta-blockers, calcium channel blockers, and tricyclic antidepressants
Valproic acid	Carnitine	100 mg/kg IV or PO loading dose with 25 mg/kg q6h

A relatively new antidote, Intralipid, for the treatment of cardiotoxicity from local anesthetics has been reported. It has been successfully used for betablocker, calcium channel blocker, and tricyclic antidepressant poisoning and many other mostly lipophilic drugs.

TOXICOLOGY LABORATORY

A toxicology screen (usually urine, sometimes blood and urine) may identify the class of drugs ingested.The typical urine toxicology screen (U-tox) does not screen for many substances (Box 45-3). Some drugs, such as γ-hydroxybutyrate (GHB), are present relatively briefly in blood and urine, and therefore findings may be negative in samples collected even on the same day. Conversely, drugs found on screening may not be those currently responsible for the toxidrome, and drugs ingested therapeutically and not in overdose (e.g., Adderall containing amphetamine) and foods (e.g., poppy seeds containing morphine and codeine) can cause a misleading positive U-tox result.

A persistent, unexplained metabolic acidosis should prompt urine examination for oxalate crystals (suggestive of ethylene glycol poisoning), serum osmolality, serum salicylate level, and methanol and ethylene glycol levels. A normal ABG or electrolyte measurement does not rule out such ingestion because metabolic acidosis is delayed and does not appear until after metabolism of the acids from ethylene glycol and methanol or until after erratic and slow absorption of salicylate. Co-oximetry will confirm carboxyhemoglobin and methemoglobinemia, which will not be detected by pulse oximetry.

Rhabdomyolysis should be suspected when there is severe agitation or hyperthermia or if the patient is thought to have been unresponsive for a prolonged time (i.e., by history of presence or pressure sores). A urine dipstick test for blood (myoglobin) and determination of a serum creatine kinase concentration should be performed. Noncardiogenic pulmonary edema on a chest radiograph suggests opioid or salicylate overdose.

DECONTAMINATION

Gastric decontamination should not be undertaken routinely as it may result in morbidity, and patients often present too late for it to be effective.Gastric lavage is rarely if ever indicated.

Although activated charcoal may decrease drug absorption even if it is given hours after ingestion, it has not been proved to improve outcome.

Whole-bowel irrigation with a polyethylene glycol solution is sometimes recommended by poison centers for overdose of metals such as iron and lead. The scientific evidence that this procedure improves outcomes is lacking.

Exposure of the eye to caustic chemicals and irritants requires immediate irrigation with large amounts of water or readily available fluid.Exposure to a gas does not require decontamination.The exception is when the patient's skin or clothing is contaminated with a liquid that is evaporating. The most important intervention to limit dermal exposure is to remove all clothing as soon as possible. Skin should be irrigated with warm water, with special attention to skin folds and other areas that might be missed. This includes the axilla, beneath nails, behind the knees, the genitalia, and in the scalp. Ideally, skin decontamination occurs as soon as possible after exposure.

DISPOSITION AND CONSULTATION

Identification of an agent that causes a particular risk for the patient, especially cardiovascular instability, seizures, or respiratory depression, generally suggests admission to the hospital or to an observation unit in ED.For others, a 6-hour period of observation usually is sufficient to determine whether there is any significant toxicity. For extended-release preparations of toxic medications (e.g., beta-blockers), a longer observation period is warranted if drug effect is not subsiding by 6 hr. Patients with cardiac dysrhythmia, conduction disturbance, altered mental status requiring intubation, or the need for frequently titrated agents (e.g., pressors) should be admitted to a monitored bed or ICU. If the patient is acutely suicidal, a sitter or secure environment may be required.

Many drugs have been reported to cause QTc prolongation, a known risk factor for torsades de pointes.If the QTc is longer than 500 ms, even in a relatively asymptomatic drug overdose patient, monitoring is indicated until the QTc is decreasing.

Box 45-3 Drugs, Chemicals, and Groups Not Detected by a Comprehensive Toxicology Screen

Ammonia	Insect repellents
Anesthetic gases	Isoniazid
Antibiotics	Laxatives
Anticoagulants	Lithium
Beta-blockers	Metals
Borates	Monoamine oxidase inhibitors
Bromides	Most antihypertensives
Caustics and corrosives	Most cardiac medications
Colchicine	Muscle relaxants
Cyanide	Mushrooms
Digitalis glycosides	Newer antidepressants (e.g.,fluoxetine, sertraline,paroxetine, bupropion, buspirone)
Disulfiram	Nitrates and nitrites
Ergot alkaloids	Nonsteroidal antiinflammatory drugs
Ethylene glycol	Paraquat
Fentanyl and its derivatives	Pesticides
Fluorides	Phenol
H2 antagonists	Plants
Hallucinogens (e.g., LSD)	Solvents
Herbicides	Thyroid hormone
Household products	Vitamins
Hypoglycemics	

(CHAI Yanfen)

Chapter 46

Opioids

KEY CONCEPTS

Opioid is a term that applies to all natural, synthetic, and semisynthetic agents with morphine-like actions.

Diagnosis of opioid intoxication is based on history, physical examination, and response to naloxone.

The opioid toxidrome includes three prominent findings—CNS depression, respiratory depression, and miosis—but these may not be present in every patient.

Airway protection and management, ventilation, and early administration of naloxone are crucial to management of patients with opioid toxicity.

The duration of action of many opioids, especially after overdose, is significantly longer than that of naloxone.

Patients with known or suspected opioid withdrawal who also have altered cognition should be evaluated for another cause of the altered cognition.

PERSPECTIVE

Opioid is a term that applies to all natural, synthetic, and semisynthetic agents with morphine-like actions. It is more inclusive than the term opiate, which refers only to natural agents. Pharmacologic actions of opioids involve many organ systems, including the CNS, cardiovascular system, pulmonary system, and gastrointestinal system, and cause characteristic clinical effects. Globally, cannabis, amphetamine-type stimulant, and cocaine users outnumber opiate (heroin/opium) users, but opiates are associated with more harm with use. Mortality rate for dependent opiate users is between 6 and 20 times that expected for those in the general population of the same age and gender.

PRINCIPLES OF DISEASE

Anatomy and Physiology

The three established opioid receptors, mu/MOP (OPRM1 gene), kappa/KOP (OPRK1 gene), and delta/DOP (OPRD1 gene), are transmembrane, G protein–coupled receptors distributed throughout the CNS, concentrated in areas associated with nociception as well as in areas of euphoria and respiratory control. Systemically, opioid receptors are localized in sensory nerve endings, the gastrointestinal tract, cardiovascular endothelial cells, and immune cells.

Pathophysiology and Pharmacology

Toxicity

Opioids are well absorbed after gastrointestinal (oral and rectal) or parenteral administration but also through nasal, buccal, pulmonary, and transdermal routes, depending on the lipid solubility of the specific opioid. Heroin is usually abused through intravenous and subcutaneous routes, but it is also absorbed after nasal administration because it is lipid soluble. In general, opioid toxicity is less pronounced but more prolonged with ingestion than with parenteral administration. Absorption of opioids after ingestion occurs in the small intestine and with therapeutic doses is complete within 1 or 2 hr. However, because of delayed gastric emptying, absorption and clinical effects of toxicity may be prolonged after overdose.

Most opioids have a large volume of distribution. Clinical effects depend on lipid solubility, which affects the rate at which opioids and their metabolites cross the blood-brain barrier. All opioids undergo hepatic metabolism and renal elimination.The pharmacokinetics of the specific agent determine the clinical course of opioid toxicity. Heroin peaks in the serum within 1 min of intravenous injection, 3 to 5 min of intranasal administration, and 10 min of subcutaneous injection. Heroin's lipophilic nature allows rapid transport across the blood-brain barrier into the CNS. In the CNS and blood, heroin is rapidly hydrolyzed to 6-monoacetylmorphine and then morphine, which is less lipid soluble. In the liver, morphine undergoes conjugation with glucuronic acid to form more water-soluble compounds that are excreted by the kidneys. Morphine and heroin are not metabolized by cytochrome P_{450} enzymes and are not directly affected by P_{450} polymorphisms.

Withdrawal

Because the half-life of heroin is 30 min and the half-life of methadone is 15 to 40 hr, withdrawal symptoms occur 4 to 6 hr after discontinuation of heroin and 24 to 48 hr after discontinuation of methadone. Duration of symptoms is 7 to 10 d and 2 w, respectively.With chronic opioid exposure, cellular adaptation results in upregulation of cAMP. When the exposure is discontinued or an antagonist is administered, the result is a temporary elevation of cAMP levels and increased sympathetic activity .

CLINICAL FEATURES

Toxicity

The toxidrome of opioid toxicity is CNS depression, respiratory depression, and miosis..

Neurologic

Depression effects: Direct CNS depression and respiratory depression cause hypoxia and seizures.

Excitatory effects : Hypertonicity, myoclonus, and seizures have been reported with overdose of the synthetic opioids meperidine and propoxyphene. Dysphoria and acute psychosis may occur with an agonist-antagonist opioid.

Parkinsonian symptoms in injection drug abusers have been attributed to MPTP (1-methyl-4-phenyl-1,2,3,6-tetrahydropyridine), a side product during synthesis of a meperidine.MPTP metabolite accumulates in CNS cell mitochondria and is associated with focal lesions in the substantianigra and a syndrome clinically indistinguishable from idiopathic parkinsonism. The syndrome is irreversible in some patients.

Spongiform leukoencephalopathy, with psychomotor retardation, dysarthria, ataxia, tremor, and other neurologic abnormalities, is associated with "chasing the dragon," a practice of inhaling heroin heated typically on aluminum foil. This syndrome is thought to be related to a combination of mitochondrial injury and hypoxia from the heroin or, more likely, the method of preparation.

Serotonin syndrome is a clinical triad of mental status changes, autonomic instability, and neuromuscular changes and may be fatal. Most cases involve an interaction between a serotonergic agent and a second agent, usually a selective serotonin reuptake inhibitor or a monoamine oxidase inhibitor.

Respiratory

By suppressing the sensitivity of the medullary respiratory center to hypercapnia, opioids decrease respiratory rate and tidal volume in a dose-dependent manner.

Bronchospasm presented in patients with heroin use is rare, severe, prolonged, and refractory to beta-agonist therapy, it may require mechanical ventilation for several days. Acute lung injury occurs with therapeutic opioid use but is much more common after overdose. The capillary leak is likely to be from hypoxia rather than a direct drug effect.

Ophthalmologic

In opiate overdoses, stimulation of mu receptors in the Edinger- Westphal nuclei of the third nerve usually results in miosis.

Otologic

Sensorineural hearing loss has been reported with acute and chronic use of some opioids, including heroin, methadone, and hydrocodone, especially in combination with acetaminophen.

Cardiovascular

Opioids cause mild hypotension and relative bradycardia. Hypotension is from histamine release and can be blocked by antihistamines (H_1 antagonists). The hypotension is typically orthostatic and resolves with supine positioning. Cardiovascular toxicity included PR interval prolongation, QRS widening, and QT prolongation and QTc prolongation.

Gastrointestinal

Nausea and vomiting are common with therapeutic opioid use and overdose. Mechanisms include opioid-induced decreased gastrointestinal motility and delayed gastric emptying, direct stimulation of the chemoreceptor trigger zone, and vestibular stimulation. Severe cases may develop ileus. Antihistamines and dopamine antagonists (e.g., chlorpromazine) may be effective in treatment.

Urologic

Opioids can cause urinary retention from urethral sphincter spasm and decreased detrusor tone. Alpha-adrenergic antagonists may reverse this effect. Glomerulosclerosis and renal amyloidosis are seen in end-stage "heroin nephropathy" of chronic opioid addicts.

Dermatologic

Pruritus, flushing, and urticaria occur with certain opioids that release histamine and do not represent a true allergy. Pruritus and erythema are often localized to the area of injection. Symptoms are typically easily controlled with antihistamines.

Metabolic

Hypoglycemia and hypothermia occurs after opioid overdose, but the mechanism is unclear.

Withdrawal

Opioid withdrawal occurs in tolerant individuals when opioid use is discontinued or an antagonist is administered. Withdrawal is associated with the opposite symptoms of CNS excitation, tachypnea, and mydriasis. Pulse and BP are also increased.Opioid withdrawal is not life-threatening.

Neurologic manifestations are presented with restlessness, agitation, and anxiety are virtually universal, and rare seizures. Cognition and mental status are unaffected. Dysphoria and drug craving may be severe and prolonged.Nausea, vomiting, diarrhea, and abdominal cramps can be significant and lead to dehydration and electrolyte depletion. Other symptoms may also include diffuse myalgias and insomnia. Signs include piloerection, yawning, lacrimation, rhinorrhea, and diaphoresis but are frequently absent.

DIAGNOSTIC STRATEGIES

The diagnosis of opioid intoxication is usually based on history and physical examination. Other than hypoglycemia, specific laboratory abnormalities are not seen. Carbon dioxide and oxygen saturation monitoring is helpful for identification of respiratory depression and hypoxia. When the patient has hypoxemia and pulmonary rales, a chest radiograph can evaluate for acute lung injury. A 12-lead electrocardiogram can confirm a suspected dysrhythmia or evaluate for QRS widening or QT prolongation if propoxyphene or methadone overdose is suspected. An abdominal radiograph may identify packets of opioids or other illicit substances in a body packer. With ingestion of an unknown opioid preparation, acetaminophen and salicylate concentrations should be checked because many prescription opioids are available in combination products.

Opiates are detected on most qualitative antibody-based enzymatic immunoassay urine toxicology screens. Semisynthetic and synthetic opioids, such as fentanyl and its derivatives, are often missed on typical urine screens unless they are specifically included or the assay cross-reacts. A urine test result is positive for days after last use, depending on the half-life. Poppy seed ingestion leads to a positive opiate screen for morphine and codeine; however, detection of 6-monoacetylmorphine, a specific metabolite of heroin, can confirm heroin use.

As with opioid toxicity, no diagnostic test exists for opioid withdrawal.

DIFFERENTIAL CONSIDERATIONS

The diagnosis of opioid intoxication is usually based on history and physical examination. Other drugs that should be considered are clonidine, tramadol, valproic acid, γ-hydroxybutyrate, and sedative-hypnotic agents. The differential diagnosis encompasses all causes of depressed mental status, but the coexistence of miosis and respiratory depression greatly narrows the possibilities.

Opioid withdrawal is usually a straightforward diagnosis, and the patient typically reveals it as the chief complaint. Simultaneous intoxication with or withdrawal from other classes of agents, especially CNS depressants and stimulants such as cocaine in a "speed-ball," is common.

MANAGEMENT

Attention to the airway, oxygenation, and ventilation, including airway protection and ventilatory support, is of primary and vital importance.

Gastrointestinal Decontamination

Gastrointestinal decontamination is not routinely recommended,whole-bowel irrigation has been used to hasten passage of drug packets from body packers, body stuffers, or patients with ingestions involving opioid combination products or multidrug ingestions.

Antidote with Opioid Antagonist

Naloxone is the most useful antidote. It is ineffective after oral administration secondary to the first-pass effect, but intravenous, subcutaneous, intramuscular, inhalational, and endotracheal routes can be used. Naloxone competitively binds opioid receptors and can reverse all the receptor-mediated actions of opioids. Naloxone is indicated for patients with opioid intoxication who have significant CNS or respiratory depression. The initial intravenous dose is 0.4 to 2 mg for adults and children, but 10 mg (total initialdose) may be required to obtain a clinical response for synthetic opioids.Naloxone can precipitate acute withdrawal in chronic opioid users. In this population, naloxone should be started at 0.04 to 0.2 mg and then slowly titrated. The duration of action of naloxone is 1 or 2 hr. Consequently, either repeated doses or a continuous infusion may be required, starting at two thirds of the effective initial dose, given per hr. Naloxone has an excellent safety profile. Acute lung injury, hypertension, and dysrhythmia have been rarely associated with use of naloxone after general anesthesia and in patients with underlying cardiac or pulmonary disease. Complete clinical recovery in response to naloxone is strongly suggestive of opioid overdose. Naloxone has been given to overdoses with valproic acid, clonidine, tramadol, and captopril and ethanol intoxication because of a presentation similar to opioid intoxication.Some of these drugs may have activity at opioid receptors.

Nalmefene is an opioid antagonist with a long half-life (8-11 hr) and duration of clinical effect. Intravenous nalmefene has a rapid onset of action in reversal of opioid-induced CNS and respiratory depression. Alternative administration routes are oral, subcutaneous, and intramuscular. The initial intravenous dose is 0.5 to 1.5 mg. When a clinical response has been achieved with nalmefene, repeated doses or continuous infusions are generally not required; however, the duration of induced withdrawal symptoms may be longer with nalmefene. Naloxone remains the preferred antidote in patients at risk for withdrawal or other adverse effects and in patients with anticipated short duration of opioid toxicity.

Supportive Care

Patients with ALI may require oxygen and positive-pressure modalities. Circulatory support usually does not require more than a crystalloid infusion. Seizures associated with opioid toxicity resolve with correction of hypoxia, correction of hypoglycemia, or administration of benzodiazepines. Most opioids have a large volume of distribution and cannot be cleared by dialysis.

Withdrawal

Opioid withdrawal is not life-threatening, but supportive and symptomatic care can decrease the distress and avoid the associated complications. When withdrawal is produced by administration of naloxone, the symptoms are of short duration. Other patients with withdrawal can receive clonidine or symptomatic treatment (antiemetics, antidiarrheals, benzodiazepines) to alleviate symptoms in the ED. In addition, fluid and electrolyte replacement is important for patients with dehydration from gastrointestinal symptoms.

Methadone provides opioid replacement to treat or to prevent withdrawal in chronic heroin users admitted for other medical conditions but should not be used for patients in the ED with uncomplicated acute withdrawal. The onset of action of an initial dose of methadone of either 20 mg orally or 10 mg intramuscularly is 30 to 60 min. This initial dose typically controls significant symptoms.Some symptoms, particularly drug craving, may be ongoing and require a subsequent dose after several hours. Maintenance methadone therapy requires doses every 24 hr or may be tapered daily.

Clonidine is used for treatment of opioid withdrawal without opioid replacement. Clonidine controls symptoms by suppressing sympathetic hyperactivity. It may also shorten the duration of withdrawal. The initial dose is 0.1 mg orally. Repeated doses may be given every 30 to 60 min. Hypotension may limit the treatment but is not common in the setting of opioid withdrawal treatment. Patches for transdermal administration of clonidine are available, but onset of action is delayed 24 hr. Oral doses still must be given initially.

Buspirone is an azapirone compound used to treat ethanol and nicotine addiction.

DISPOSITION

Toxicity

Patients who receive naloxone should be observed for 2 hr to assess the extent of resedation, hypoxia, and pulmonary complications. Asymptomatic patients can be observed in the ED until 4 hr after an ingestion, at which time they can be discharged with appropriate psychiatric evaluation or drug abuse counseling. However, patients who have ingested an opioid with a longer half-life, active metabolite, or modified-release preparation, as well as patients with multiple drug ingestions involving an opioid, may require longer observation periods.

Asymptomatic patients who have a known or possible ingestion of diphenoxylate-atropine should be observed in a monitored unit.The metabolite of diphenoxylate, difenoxin, has a longer half-life and is five times more active than diphenoxylate, and it may cause delayed and prolonged toxicity.

Patients with a known or potential ingestion of packets of illicit opioid drugs, body packers and body stuffers, remain asymptomatic until one or more of the packets leak. Body packers are typically admitted until the packets are passed; body stuffers may be discharged after 6 hr.

Withdrawal

Patients with opioid withdrawal may be managed as outpatients. Clonidine may alleviate some of the symptoms of withdrawal but has a high incidence of postural hypotension. Patients with refractory complications (e.g., vomiting, dehydration, and electrolyte abnormalities) and patients with an uncertain diagnosis may require hospitalization. Some patients may need to be detoxified before entering chemical treatment programs. Substance abuse counseling and establishment of outpatient program referral should be completed before discharge.

(CHEN Xiaohui)

Chapter 47

Organophosphorus-poison

KEY CONCEPTS

Organophosphorus-poison is an acetylcholinesterase inhibitors. Inhibition of cholinesterase results in the accumulation and subsequent prolonged effect of acetylcholine at a variety of neurotransmitter receptors, including sympathetic and parasympathetic ganglionic nicotinic sites, postganglionic cholinergic sympathetic and parasympathetic muscarinic sites, skeletal muscle nicotinic sites, and CNS sites.

Morbidity in cholinesterase inhibitor exposure results from early airway compromise secondary to copious secretions, status epilepticus, and late respiratory failure.

Cholinesterase inhibitor exposure may include bradycardia or tachycardia, hypertension or hypotension, and miosis or mydriasis.

All patients exposed to cholinesterase inhibitors should have skin decontamination.

The clinical endpoint for atropine administration is drying of airway secretions.

Pralidoxime should be given to all organophosphorus-poisoned patients who require atropine regardless of time since exposure.

Intermediate syndrome occurs 24 to 96 hr after exposure and consists of proximal muscle weakness specifically of the respiratory muscles.

PERSPECTIVE

The first organophosphate insecticide, triethyl pyrophosphate, was synthesized in 1859 but did not replace nicotine as a pesticide until World War Ⅱ. After World War Ⅱ, these compounds were used as chemical warfare agents, as organophosphorus and carbamate insecticides, and as medicinal agents. With concern about the long half-life of the organochlorine dichlorodiphenyltrichloroethane (DDT), causing it to accumulate in the environment, the organophosphate insecticides became the most common pesticides for home and industrial use.

PRINCIPLES OF DISEASE

Organophosphorus insecticides are highly lipid soluble and are readily absorbed through dermal, gastrointestinal, and respiratory routes. This lipid solubility results in the buildup of organophos-phorus compounds in body fat, and toxic systemic levels often occur from repeated low-level exposures. The parent compound and its metabolites are acetylcholinesterase inhibitors, and because many parent organophosphorus compounds are less potent than their metabolites (e.g., parathion to paraoxon), delayed onset of clinical toxicity can occur.

Organophosphorus pesticides work by persistently inhibiting the enzyme acetylcholinesterase, the enzymatic deactivator of the ubiquitous neurotransmitter acetylcholine. Because of the global penetration of organophosphorus compounds, inhibition occurs at tissue sites (true acetylcholinesterase and represented by erythrocyte or RBC cholinesterase) and in plasma (circulating pseudocholinesterase). Inhibition of cholinesterase results in the accumulation and subsequent prolonged effect of acetylcholine at a variety of neurotransmitter receptors, including sympathetic and parasympathetic ganglionic nicotinic sites, postganglionic cholinergic sympathetic and parasympathetic muscarinic sites, skeletal muscle nicotinic sites, and CNS sites (Fig. 47-1).

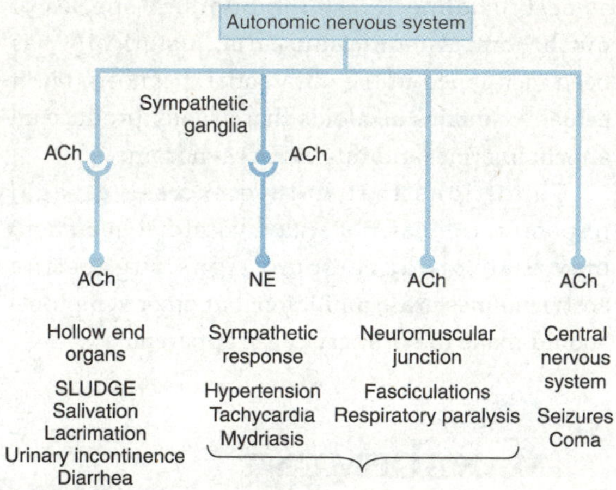

Fig. 47-1 The autonomic nervous system comprises the sympathetic and parasympathetic nervous systems. The sympathetic nervous system is also known as the thoracolumbar outflow; the cell body lies in the spinal cord, and the first synapse occurs in the sympathetic ganglia. The neurotransmitter in this first synapse is acetylcholine (ACh, preganglionic), and the neurotransmitter in the postganglionic neuron with the target organ is norepinephrine (NE). In the parasympathetic nervous system (craniosacral outflow), nerves from the medulla and sacrum use ACh as the neurotransmitter in preganglionic and postganglionic target organs. The autonomic nervous system is divided further into the muscarinic and nicotinic receptors; atropine can block the muscarinic receptors but not the nicotinic receptors. The neuromuscular junction uses ACh as the effector neurotransmitter. In the brain, ACh is just one of several active neurotransmitters.

CLINICAL FEATURES

Signs and Symptoms

The accumulation of acetylcholine results in the classic SLUDGE cholinergic syndrome, manifested by hyperactivity of cholinergic responses at the receptor sites indicated previously. The clinical syndrome of muscarinic acetylcholinesterase inhibition (Table 47-1) causes postganglionic acetylcholine-induced hollow end-organ general hypersecretion, resulting in miotic pupils, lacrimation, rhinorrhea, sialorrhea, bronchorrhea, vomiting, diarrhea, and urinary incontinence. Bradycardia is a classic sign of the cholinergic syndrome, but the increased release of norepinephrine from postganglionic sympathetic neurons precipitated by excess cholinergic activity at sympathetic ganglia may result in normal or even tachycardic HR (nicotinic effect). Sympathetic hyperactivity can cause diffuse diaphoresis. The most lethal components of acetylcholinesterase inhibition occur in the brain and neuromuscular junction. A combination of sympathetic stimulation, involvement of the N-methyl-Daspartate receptor, and enhanced acetylcholine concentrations can induce seizures. At the neuromuscular junction, excess acetylcholine causes hyperstimulation of the muscles with secondary paralysis, and when the diaphragm is affected, cholinesterase poisoning leads to respiratory arrest.

Table 47-1 SLUDGE Symptoms or DUMBELS

Salivation	Diarrhea/Diaphoresis
Lacrimation	Urination
Urinary incontinence	Miosis
Defecation	Bradycardia/Bronchorrhea/Bronc-hospasm
Gastrointestinal cramps	Emesis
Emesis	Lacrimation Salivation

Complications

Seizures, pulmonary hypersecretion (bronchorrhea), and bron- choconstriction are prominent mechanisms of early morbidity and mortality in cases of poisoning from acetylcholinesterase inhibitors. Bronchorrhea is often incorrectly called noncardiogenic pulmonary edema because the origin of the excessive pulmonary fluids is airway secretions, not transudation of fluid across the alveolar-capillary membrane. The obstruction of upper and lower airways, the potential intrusion of these bronchial secretions into alveolar sacs, and bronchoconstriction produce hypoxia, which is the primary concern in the initial stages of poisoning.

Nicotinic hyperstimulation of skeletal muscle leads to significant morbidity and mortality associated with acetylcholinesterase inhibitor toxicity. Signs of skeletal muscle hyperactivity include involuntary twitches, fasciculations, and hyperactive reflexes. Muscle hyperactivity eventually progresses to muscle fatigue and paralysis, including the respiratory musculature and particularly the diaphragm. Acetylcholinesterase inhibitors produce direct toxic effects on the CNS, leading to neurologic signs of confusion, combativeness, seizures, and coma.

A unique effect of organophosphorus insecticides results from "aging," the irreversible conformational change that occurs when the organophosphorus agent is bound to the cholinesterase enzyme for a prolonged time, causing clinical effects to persist for a prolonged time. On average, some aging for commercial organophosphorus agents will occur by 48 hr but may take longer. Once the enzyme has aged, an oxime antidote cannot regenerate the cholinesterase.

DIAGNOSTIC STRATEGIES

Any patient with a clinically apparent cholinergic syndrome should be treated empirically without waiting for laboratory confirmation of decreased cholinesterase activity. Known or suspected exposure to cholinesterase inhibitors can be evaluated by ordering of plasma and erythrocyte (RBC) cholinesterase levels.

After acute exposures, the plasma cholinesterase levels decrease first, followed by decreases in RBC cholinesterase levels. The RBC cholinesterase level correlates best with activity at the nerve terminal. Patients with chronic exposures may have a normal plasma cholinesterase level but have reduced RBC cholinesterase activity. The RBC cholinesterase level recovers at a rate of 1% per day in untreated patients and takes approximately 6 to 12 w to normalize, whereas plasma cholinesterase levels may recover in 4 to 6 w. Other laboratory studies should focus on the evaluation of pulmonary, cardiovascular, and renal function and fluid and electrolyte balance.

DIFFERENTIAL DIAGNOSIS

Few toxins or other clinical conditions produce the same constellation of symptoms as acetylcholinesterase inhibitors. A species of mushroom, Amanita muscaria, historically has been mentioned in the differential diagnosis, but it actually contains alkaloids that usually produce an anticholinergic (antimuscarinic) syndrome.

Conditions that induce excessive vagal responses (e.g., inferior wall myocardial infarction) may also produce some signs suggesting acetylcholinesterase inhibition, but other symptoms should make the primary cause apparent.

MANAGEMENT

Treatment is directed toward four goals: (1) decontamination, (2) supportive care, (3) reversal of acetylcholine excess at muscarinic sites, and (4) reversal of toxin binding at active sites on the cholinesterase molecule.

Decontamination should start in the out-of-hospital phase to prevent further absorption and subsequent toxicity and to protect care providers. Removal and destruction of clothing and thorough flushing of exposed skin may limit absorption and subsequent toxicity.In the case of ingestion, gastrointestinal decontamination procedures are of questionable benefit because of the rapid absorption of these compounds. Profuse vomiting and diarrhea are seen early in ingestion and may limit or negate any beneficial effect of additional gastrointestinal decontamination.

Because death is due to airway and respiratory failure, supportive care should be directed primarily toward airway management and include suctioning of secretions and vomitus, oxygenation, and ventilatory support.

The definitive treatment of acetylcholinesterase inhibition starts with atropine. A competitive inhibitor of acetylcholine at muscarinic receptor sites, atropine reverses the clinical effects of cholinergic excess at parasympathetic end-organs and sweat glands. Large doses of atropine may be required. The more rapid the atropinization, the faster control is obtained. Suggested dosing is 1 or 2 mg of atropine (0.02-0.05 mg/kg) intravenously, with doubling of each subsequent dose every 5 min until there is control of mucous membrane hypersecretion and the airway clears. If intravenous access is not immediately available, atropine may be administered intramuscularly. Patients may require 200 to 500 mg of atropine intravenously during the first hour, followed by prolonged continuous infusions of 5 to 100 mg/hr to maintain adequate secretion control. Tachycardia and mydriasis may occur at these doses, but they are not indications to stop atropine administration. The endpoint of atropinization is drying of respiratory secretions, easing of respiration, and MAP greater than 60 mm Hg. Atropine is not active at nicotinic sites and does not reverse the skeletal muscle effects (e.g., muscle fatigue and respiratory failure).

The second part of acetylcholinesterase inhibition treatment is the use of an oxime, such aspralidoxime (2-PAM, Protopam) or obidoxime (Toxogonin), to regenerate the organophosphate-acetylcholinesterase complex and to restore cholinesterase activity at muscarinic and nicotinic sites. TheWHO recommends an initial dose of pralidoxime is 30 mg/kg, followed by 8 mg/kg/hr continued for at least 24 hr or, if an infusion cannot be used, 30 mg/kg every 4 hr. The infusion may be continued for several days with no adverse effects attributable to the pralidoxime; however, rapid administration can lead to hypertension, vomiting, and a transient reversible neuromuscular blockade. The ideal dose of pralidoxime should be determined by monitoring of the clinical condition of the patient and serial cholinesterase levels; the patient may require higher doses of oxime than are recommended here. The WHO recommended infusion dose of obidoxime is 4 mg/kg, followed by 0.5 mg/kg/hr; alternatively, intermittent intravenous doses of 4 mg/kg, then 2 mg/kg, every 4 hr are given. Pralidoxime andobidoxime can be administered by intramuscular injection. Indications for oxime therapy include respiratory depression or apnea, fasciculations, seizures, arrhythmias, cardiovascular instability, and use of large amounts of atropine. Oxime therapy can be used whenever the patient requires more than a limited amount of atropine (2-4 mg) to completely reverse the signs and symptoms of intoxication or in any patient who requires repeated doses of atropine. Oxime therapy and atropine are synergistic.

In conjunction with atropine and the oximepralidoxime, patients with agitation, seizures, and coma should be treated with adequate doses of a benzodiazepine after the airway has been secured.

DISPOSITION

Because of the prolonged effects of acetylcholinesterase inhibition, most patients with significant exposures require hospital admission. Plasma cholinesterase levels may be useful for treatment and disposition decisions. Asymptomatic or minimally symptomatic patients with normal or minimally depressed levels may be discharged after 4 to 6 hr with close outpatient follow-up to ensure that progressive toxicity does not occur. Patients who arrive with known severely depressed levels require admission and close monitoring, usually in EICU. Patients may have rebound toxicity several days after apparently satisfactory response to initial treatment. Rebound toxicity may occur for many reasons, including persistent release of organophosphates from lipid stores.

A secondary syndrome, the intermediate syndrome, occurs 24 to 96 hr after exposure and consists of proximal muscle weakness specifically of the respiratory muscles. It is believed to be an abnormality at the neuromuscular junction. Patients with intermediate syndrome present with respiratory failure several days after the acute cholinergic symptoms have resolved and may require several weeks of ventilatory support. Finally, organophosphorus delayed neuropathy has been reported as a different entity. It affects an axonal enzyme, neurotoxic esterase, with a peripheral sensorimotor neuropathy 7 to 21 d after exposure.

(CHEN Xiaohui)

Chapter 48

Sedative Hypnotics Poisoning

KEY CONCEPTS

The life threat in severe barbiturate toxicity is respiratory depression.

Barbiturates have no specific antidote, the key to management of these patients is supportive care.

Serum barbiturate levels confirm the diagnosis but do not correlate with depth of coma or clinical outcome.A urine toxicology screen positive for barbiturates does not prove that the drug caused the patient's clinical condition.

Flumazenil is not needed in most benzodiazepine overdoses. Because it can precipitate seizures, it should not be used in patients who are regular benzodiazepine users.

BARBITURATES

Perspective

Although barbiturates are still useful for seizure disorders, they rarely are prescribed as sedatives, with the availability of safer alternatives, such as benzodiazepines.Barbiturates are addictive, producing physical dependence and a withdrawal syndrome that can be life-threatening.

Principles of Disease

Barbiturates depress the activity of all excitable cells, especially those in the CNS, by enhancing the activity of GABA, the major central inhibitor. In acute overdose, barbiturates decrease neural transmission in autonomic ganglia, the myocardium, and the gastrointestinal tract and also inhibit the response to acetylcholine at the neuromuscular junction.

The $GABA_A$ receptor is a protein complex found on postsynaptic membranes in the CNS. Structurally, it consists of several distinct receptor sites surrounding a chloride ion (Cl^-) channel (Fig. 48-1). GABA opens the chloride channel. The resulting flow of Cl^- into the cell increases the negative resting potential, hyperpolarizing and stabilizing the membrane. There are separate receptor sites for barbiturates and for benzodiazepines and a third site that binds GABA, ethanol, and meprobamate. Although barbiturates and ethanol can directly increase Cl^- conductance, benzodiazepines require the presence of GABA to affect Cl^- flow, which may account for the relative safety of benzodiazepines in comparison with barbiturates.

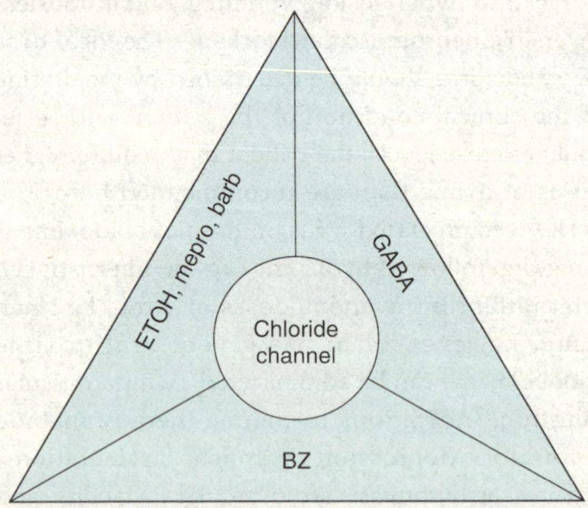

Fig. 48-1 The γ-aminobutyric acid (GABA receptor complex. BZ, benzodiazepine binding site; GABA, GABA binding site; ETOH, mepro, barb, binding sites for ethanol, meprobamate, and barbiturates, espectively.

Barbiturates produce dose-related depressive effects ranging from mild sedation to coma and fatal respiratory arrest. In the early stages of intoxication, some patients experience euphoria.

Barbiturates have no analgesic effect and can paradoxically increase the reaction to pain at low doses.

Barbiturates act directly on the medulla to produce respiratory depression. laryngospasm can occur at low doses.

Therapeutic oral doses of barbiturates produce only mild decreases in pulse and BP, similar to sleep. With toxic doses, more significant hypotension occurs from direct depression of the myocardium along with pooling of blood in a dilated venous system. Peripheral vascular resistance is usually normal or increased, but barbiturates interfere with autonomic reflexes, which then do not adequately compensate for the myocardial depression and decreased venous return. Barbiturates can precipitate severe hypotension in patients whose compensatory reflexes are already maximally stimulated, such as those with heart failure or hypovolemic shock. Barbiturates also decrease cerebral blood flow and intracerebral pressure. Higher doses can decrease gastrointestinal smooth muscle tone and peristaltic contractions and delay gastric emptying.

Barbiturates are classified according to their onset and duration of action (Box 48-1): ultra-short acting (onset immediate after intravenous dose, duration min), short acting (onset 10-15 min after oral dose, duration 6-8 hr), intermediate acting (onset 45-60 min, duration 10-12 hr), and long acting (onset 1 hr, duration 10-12 hr). Only long-acting preparations have anticonvulsant effects in doses that do not cause sedation. Short- and intermediate-acting preparations are almost completely metabolized to inactive metabolites in the liver, whereas 25% of a phenobarbital (long-acting) dose is excreted unchanged through the kidney. Because phenobarbital is a weak acid (pH 7.2), alkalinization of the urine will increase the amount of drug present in ionized form, minimizing tubular reabsorption and increasing drug clearance. Short- and intermediate-acting barbiturates are not significantly affected by pH changes in this range.

Box 48-1 Barbiturates

Ultrashort Acting

- Methohexital (Brevital)
- Thiopental (Pentothal)

Short and Intermediate Acting

- Pentobarbital (Nembutal)
- Secobarbital (Seconal)
- Amobarbital (Amytal)
- Aprobarbital (Alurate)
- Butabarbital (Butisol)
- Butalbital (Fiorinal)

Long Acting

- Phenobarbital (Solfoton, Luminal)
- Mephobarbital (Mebaral)

Clinical Features

Mild barbiturate toxicity is manifested with drowsiness, slurred speech, ataxia, unsteady gait, nystagmus, emotional lability, and impaired cognition.

In severe acute intoxication, CNS depression progresses from stupor to deep coma and respiratory arrest. Concomitant hypoxia can cause pupils to be fixed and dilated. Corneal and gag reflexes may be diminished or absent, muscle tone flaccid, and deep tendon reflexes diminished or absent. Flexor (decorticate) and extensor (decerebrate) posturing can occur in patients comatose from barbiturate intoxication. These neurologic signs are variable and do not always correlate with severity of intoxication or depth of coma. A fluctuating level of consciousness is commonly seen. High barbiturate levels depress gastrointestinal motility, delaying drug absorption. As the drug is metabolized and blood levels drop, peristalsis and drug absorption may increase, causing drug levels to rise.

The life threat in severe barbiturate toxicity is respiratory depression. Because respirations can be rapid but shallow, the degree of hypoventilation may not be apparent on clinical examination, and pulse oximetry or capnography may be needed to detect the ventilation compromise.

Hypotension is common in patients with severe intoxication, along with a normal or increased HR. Barbiturate overdose is associated with noncardiogenic pulmonary edema.Pneumonia may be delayed.

Barbiturate withdrawal syndrome includes tremors, hallucinations, seizures, and delirium. However, severe withdrawal occurs only after dependence on short- or intermediate-acting barbiturates (e.g., pentobarbital, secobarbital, amobarbital, or butalbital). Because these drugs are not commonly used, this syndrome is now very rare.

Diagnostic Strategies

The therapeutic level of phenobarbital is 15 to 40 μg/mL (65-172 μmol/L). A serum level greater than 50 μg/mL can be associated with coma, especially in a patient who is not a chronic user. Levels greater than 80 μg/mL are potentially fatal. Serial phenobarbital levels can monitor effectiveness of treatment. Other than phenobarbital, barbiturates have high volumes of distribution, so serum levels do not accurately reflect CNS concentrations or correlate with clinical severity. A positive urine screen establishes only exposure to a barbiturate but does not prove that the drug is present in toxic amounts and should not be relied on to explain decreased mental status.

Chest radiographs can detect noncardiogenic pulmonary edema or pneumonia. CT of the head may be helpful in comatose patients with evidence of trauma, focal neurologic signs, papilledema, or uncertain diagnosis to detect other causes of stupor and coma.

Management

Because barbiturates have no specific antidote, the key to management of these patients is supportive care, particularly with respect to the cardiovascular and respiratory systems.

Maintain stability

Severely intoxicated patients are unable to protect their airway and have decreased ventilatory drive. Supplemental oxygen may suffice for patients with mild to moderate overdose, but intubation is often required. Long-term induced paralysis is rarely necessary, and additional sedation usually is unnecessary for mechanical ventilation. Careful fluid replacement should maintain a SBP above 90 mmHg and adequate urine output. Patients should be monitored for fluid overload and pulmonary edema. Active warming should be initiated if the rectal temperature is below 30℃.

Gastrointestinal Decontamination and Enhanced Elimination

Gastric emptying by lavage is not indicated. For large overdoses, there is evidence that clearance of phenobarbital is markedly increased with multidose activated charcoal (MDAC). One dosage for MDAC is 25 g every 2 hr in an adult. If vomiting occurs, a smaller dose or antiemetics should be used. MDAC can also be administered slowly through a nasogastric tube. Contraindications to MDAC include an unprotected airway and gastrointestinal obstruction or perforation. Decreased peristalsis can result in constipation with MDAC and is a relative contraindication to MDAC. Although MDAC may shorten the duration of the intoxication, there is no evidence for improved outcome over supportive care.

There is no role for urine alkalinization in acute barbiturate poisoning.

Hemoperfusion was advocated over hemodialysis, because phenobarbital is 40% to 60% protein bound.

Disposition

An asymptomatic patient who arrives in the ED after ingesting barbiturates should be observed for 6 hr after ingestion for mental status changes, slurred speech, ataxia, hypotension, and respiratory depression. Symptoms generally occur within 1 hr of ingestion. Patients who remain asymptomatic and have no significant complicating coingestants or medical problems can be discharged. Patients who are still symptomatic after 6 hr should be admitted for observation and supportive care.

BENZODIAZEPINES

Perspective

Benzodiazepines emerged as the principal agents for the treatment of anxiety. Cardiac effects and fatalities from pure benzodiazepine overdose are rare, and respiratory depression is less than with barbiturates. In addition, drug-drug interactions involving benzodiazepines are uncommon.

Benzodiazepines remain among the most widely prescribed class of drugs (Table 48-1) and are the most common prescription drugs used in suicide attempts. Fortunately, most benzodiazepine overdoses follow a relatively benign clinical course.

Table 48-1 Benzodiazepines

NAME	USUAL DOSE	ORAL PEAK (hr)	HALF-LIFE (hr)	PARENT METABOLITE ACTIVITY
Alprazolam (Xanax)	0.25-0.5 mg	1-2	6-27	Inactive
Chlordiazepoxide(Librium)	5-25 mg	0.5-4	5-30	Active
Clonazepam (Klonopin)	0.25-0.5 mg	1-2	18-50	Inactive
Clorazepate (Tranxene)	7.5-15 mg	1-2	1-3	Active
Diazepam (Valium)	2-10 mg	0.5-1	20-50	Active
Estazolam (ProSom)	1-2 mg	2	8-28	Inactive
Flurazepam (Dalmane)	15-30 mg	0.5-1	2-3	Active
Halazepam (Paxipam)	20-40 mg	1-3	14	Active
Lorazepam (Ativan)	0.5-2 mg	2-4	10-20	Inactive
Midazolam (Versed)	0.025-0.1 mg/kg	1-2	1.5-3	Active
Oxazepam (Serax)	10-30mg	2-4	5-20	Inactive
Quazepam (Doral)	7.5-15 mg	2	39-41	Active
Temazepam (Restoril)	7.5-30 mg	1-2	3-19	Inactive
Triazolam (Halcion)	0.125-0.25 mg	1-2	1.5-5.5	Inactive

Principles of Disease

Benzodiazepines produce sedative, hypnotic, anxiolytic, and anticonvulsant effects by enhancing the inhibitory actions of GABA. Binding of a benzodiazepine to a specific benzodiazepine receptor potentiates GABA effects on the chloride channel at the $GABA_A$ receptor, increasing intracellular flux of chloride ions and hyperpolarizing the cell. The net effect is a diminished ability of the nerve cell to initiate an action potential, inhibiting neural transmission.

Three unique benzodiazepine receptors exist, distributed variably throughout the central and peripheral nervous systems. Classic benzodiazepines are nonselective, producing a broad range of clinical effects. Newer benzodiazepines interact selectively with a single receptor subtype to minimize unwanted effects.

Pharmacokinetics

Benzodiazepines are rapidly absorbed orally. Intramuscular use of chlordiazepoxide and diazepam is limited by erratic absorption, but lorazepam and midazolam are predictably absorbed after intramuscular injection. After absorption, benzodiazepines distribute readily and rapidly penetrate the blood-brain barrier. In plasma, benzodiazepines are highly protein bound.

All benzodiazepines are metabolized in the liver. Oxazepam, temazepam, and lorazepam are directly conjugated to an inactive, water-soluble glucuronide metabolite that is excreted by the kidney. Other benzodiazepines must first be converted by the hepatic cytochrome P450 system. Cytochrome P450 processes may be significantly impaired in elderly patients or those with liver disease, leading to prolonged elimination of some benzodiazepines. Coingestion of drugs that also undergo cytochrome P450 metabolism (e.g., cimetidine, ethanol) also prolongs the half-lives of these benzodiazepines.

Clinical Features

CNS depression is common in patients with benzodiazepine poisoning and ranges from mild drowsiness to coma. Respiratory depression is due mainly to upper airway obstruction and increased upper airway resistance from loss of muscle tone rather than central apnea. Significant respiratory depression can be seen with large oral overdoses or during intravenous conscious sedation, particularly when the benzodiazepine is combined with an opioid such as fentanyl. Hypotension is uncommon. Other potential complications include aspiration pneumonia and pressure necrosis of skin and muscles.

Prolonged or high-dose infusions of certain benzodiazepine preparations have been associated with the development of lactic acidosis. Patients with renal or hepatic insufficiency are at increased risk for this complication.

Diagnostic Strategies

Any patient with altered mental status should have a blood glucose level rapidly determined. Qualitative immunoassays for benzodiazepines in urine are available but do not aid management decisions. Serum drug concentrations are not routinely available and do not correlate with clinical severity. A lack of alcohol odor or a negative breathalyzer or blood ethanol test result suggests benzodiazepine or another sedative as a possible cause.

Differential Considerations

Benzodiazepine overdose is usually suspected or diagnosed because of the clinical presentation. Many patients are arousable and can provide supporting information. Atypical or focal findings suggest the presence of other conditions. Profound coma or cardiopulmonary instability is rare with pure benzodiazepine overdose and should prompt the search for a coingestant. Nontoxicologic causes of CNS depression should also be considered.

Management

General

Initial stabilization, including endotracheal intubation, should not be delayed by the administration of an antidote. Most benzodiazepine overdoses can be managed expectantly. Activated charcoal is generally not beneficial in overdose. MDAC, hemodialysis, and whole-bowel irrigation are not effective in benzodiazepine overdose.

Antidote

Flumazenil, a nonspecific competitive antagonist of the benzodiazepine receptor, can reverse benzodiazepine-induced sedation after general anesthesia, procedural sedation, and confirmed benzodiazepine overdose, but it is not recommended for the routine reversal of sedative overdose in the ED. Seizures and cardiac dysrhythmias can occur after flumazenil administration, and fatalities have been reported. Flumazenil use can precipitate acute withdrawal in patients who are dependent on benzodiazepines. Similarly, this antidote is hazardous when it is given to patients who have coingested seizure-causing drugs (such as cocaine or a tricyclic antidepressant) because of loss of the benzodiazepine's protective anticonvulsant properties. Coingestants that cause dysrhythmias, such as carbamazepine and chloral hydrate, may increase the likelihood of cardiac effects. The benzodiazepine antagonist flumazenil should not be routinely administered to patients with coma of unknown origin or suspected benzodiazepine overdose, either for diagnostic or for therapeutic purposes. Any possibility of concomitant tricyclic overdose contraindicates flumazenil use.

Other risk factors are summarized in Box 48-2.

Box 48-2 Use of Flumazenil

Indications

- Isolated benzodiazepine overdose in nonhabituated user (e.g.,accidental pediatric exposure)
- Reversal of conscious sedation

Absolute Contraindications

- Suspected coingestant that lowers seizure threshold (e.g.,tricyclic antidepressants, cocaine, lithium, methylxanthines,isoniazid, propoxyphene, monoamine oxidase inhibitors,bupropion, diphenhydramine, carbamazepine, cyclosporine, chloral hydrate)
- Patient taking benzodiazepine for control of a potentially life-threatening condition (e.g., seizures)
- Concurrent sedative-hypnotic withdrawal
- Seizure activity or myoclonus
- Hypersensitivity to flumazenil or benzodiazepines
- Patient with neuromuscular blockade

Relative Contraindications

- Chronic benzodiazepine use, not taken for control of life-threatening condition
- Known seizure disorder not treated with benzodiazepines
- Head injury
- Panic attacks
- Chronic alcoholism

The initial adult dose of flumazenil is 0.2 mg given intravenously during 30 sec. A second dose of 0.2 mg may be given, followed by 0.2-mg doses at 1-min intervals to a total of 1 mg. Because the duration of action of flumazenil is short (0.7-1.3 hr), resedation occurs in up to 65% of patients and requires either redosing or continuous infusion (0.25-1.0 mg/hr).

In summary, benzodiazepine overdose requires primarily supportive care (including intubation). Flumazenil may precipitate seizures or acute withdrawal and should be used only in highly selected cases, such as for accidental overdose of benzodiazepines during procedural sedation. When flumazenil is used, careful monitoring is necessary because of the risk for recurrent respiratory depression or resedation. Use of flumazenil has not consistently altered outcome, complication rate, number of costly procedures performed, or duration of hospital stay in ED patients.

Disposition

Patients remaining asymptomatic after 4 to 6 hr of ED observation may be medically cleared. For cases of deliberate overdose, appropriate psychiatric consultation should be obtained.

(CHEN Xiaohui)

Chapter 49

Toxic Alcohols

KEY CONCEPTS

A double-gap acidosis (anion gap and osmol gap) should suggest methanol or ethylene glycol toxicity.

Therapy should begin on the basis of clinical suspicion of exposure to ethylene glycol or methanol.

Three treatment goals exist for patients with methanol or ethylene glycol toxicity: (1) correction of metabolic acidosis with bicarbonate; (2) ADH enzyme blockade, which inhibits the metabolism of methanol and ethylene glycol to toxic metabolites; and (3) removal of the parent alcohol and its metabolites by hemodialysis.

METHANOL

Perspective

Methanol is a colorless, volatile, slightly sweet-tasting alcohol. Certain products found in the home may contain high concentrations of methanol. Illicit alcohol production remains a global source of methanol poisoning from products such as chang'aa (Kenya), raki (Turkey), and tuica (Romania). Although epidemic poisonings from methanol are reported occasionally, most exposures are sporadic. Treatment delay is associated with increased morbidity, making early recognition of clinical and laboratory clues crucial.

Principles of Disease

Pharmacology and Metabolism

Methanol is absorbed rapidly from the gastrointestinal tract, and blood levels peak 30 to 60 min after ingestion. Transdermal and respiratory tract absorption also has resulted in toxicity, especially in infants. Certain occupations, including painting, glazing, varnishing, lithography, and printing, are high risk for inhalational exposure to methanol. Inhalational abuse of methanol is a recent trend that can result in toxic serum levels.

At low serum concentrations, the elimination of methanol follows first-order kinetics; but at concentrations after overdose, zero-order kinetics predominate. This produces a prolonged half-life of 24 to 30 hr, which may be extended even further by the concurrent ingestion of ethanol. Small amounts of ingested methanol may be exceptionally toxic. In adults, the smallest lethal dose reported is 15 mL of 40% methanol, and 4 mL of pure methanol has led to blindness.

Methanol itself has little toxicity. Metabolites of the parent alcohol are extremely toxic, however. Although small amounts of methanol are eliminated by renal and pulmonary routes, 90% is metabolized in the liver. Methanol is oxidized by alcohol dehydrogenase(ADH) to formaldehyde, which is rapidly converted by aldehyde dehydrogenase to formic acid (Fig.49-1). Formic acid is the primary toxicant and accounts for much of the anion gap metabolic acidosis and ocular toxicity peculiar to methanol ingestion. Through a folate-dependent pathway, formic acid is degraded to

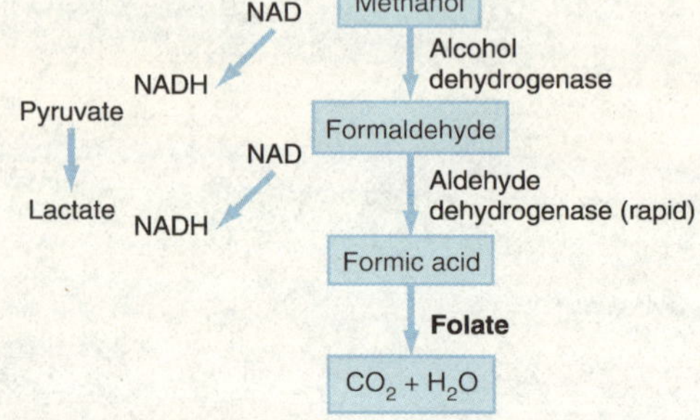

Fig. 49-1 Metabolism of methanol. NADH, reduced form of nicotinamide adenine dinucleotide.

carbon dioxide and water.

Pathophysiology

Optic neuropathy and putaminal necrosis are the two main complications of severe methanol poisoning. Long-term morbidity takes the form of visual impairment, including blindness, and parkinsonian motor dysfunction, characterized by hypokinesis and rigidity. Formic acid has a high affinity for iron and inhibits mitochondrial cytochrome oxidase, halting cellular respiration.

Methanol metabolism in the cytosol and mitochondria may account for a second mechanism of adenosine triphosphate depletion. Lactate accumulation resulting from hypotension or seizures further compounds the metabolic acidosis predominantly caused by formate. Other mechanisms of toxicity involve increased lipid peroxidation, free radical formation, and impaired protective antioxidant reactions. Severe dysfunction of subcellular metabolism from methanol also has been linked to significant disturbance in proteolytic-antiproteolytic balance.

The primary sites of ocular injury are the retrolaminar optic nerve and retina. Selective myelin damage to the retrolaminar optic nerve has been seen at autopsy after methanol toxicity. Müller cells, the principal glial cells of retinal neurons and photoreceptors, have been proposed as the initial target in methanolinduced visual toxicity. It seems that they alone harbor the enzymes necessary to metabolize methanol to formate. Histopathologic correlates suggest that retinal cells develop intra-axonal swelling, calcium influx, mitochondrial destruction, and microtubular disruption. Ultimately, this interferes with transport of essential proteins from the retinal neuron cell body to the nerve fiber axoplasm. Oligodendrocyte involvement causes myelin degeneration and leads to visual decrements. Acidosis may accelerate this process by enhancing nonionic diffusion of formic acid into neurons and further increasing lactate production. This self-perpetuating cycle of acidosis, termed *circulus hypoxicus*, underscores the need for aggressive correction of pH to accomplish ion trapping of formate outside the CNS.

Methanol adversely affects other areas of the CNS, specifically the basal ganglia. Bilateral, symmetrical putaminal hypodensities, hemorrhages, or cystic lesions are characteristic, occurring in 13.5% of patients. Necrosis is described in the subcortical white matter, spinal cord anterior horn cells, and cerebellum. Acute signs and symptoms may be lacking or may take several days to develop despite the presence of these radiographic findings. Quantitative neuropathologic studies conflict as to whether concentrations of formic acid within the putamen are higher than levels in the blood or other tissues. Massive edema adjacent to the putamen shown by MRI suggests a possible localized disruption of the blood-brain barrier. Other proposed mechanisms for the vulnerability of this region include the unique pattern of arterial blood supply and venous drainage and greater metabolic activity.

Clinical Features

With individual cases of methanol poisoning, the history may be unobtainable or unreliable. The diagnosis should be considered in patients with altered mental status, visual complaints, or metabolic acidosis and in patients with occupations that put them at high risk for exposure. Because methanol is a poor substrate for ADH, a latency period exists between the time of ingestion and metabolism to the formate that causes visual or metabolic disturbance. The typical 12 to 24 hr latency may be shorter when large amounts are consumed or longer when ethanol is coingested (range, 40 min to 72 hr). Formic acid accumulation may be ongoing, with risk for significant toxicity, in patients who present early despite being initially asymptomatic. When symptoms are manifested, they are primarily neurologic, gastrointestinal, or ocular.

Although methanol is less inebriating than ethanol, early symptoms of methanol poisoning include depressed mental status, confusion, and ataxia. Nonspecific complaints of weakness, dizziness, anorexia, headache, and nausea develop; in severe cases, coma and seizures may be seen. Although vomiting and abdominal pain commonly result from mucosal irritation, the absence of gastrointestinal complaints does not rule out a serious ingestion. Abdominal tenderness, however, may be so severe that it suggests an acute surgical abdomen. This may result from pancreatitis, and elevation of serum amylase is relatively common, but increased salivary amylase isoenzyme can occur without pancreatic inflammation.

Visual disturbances are seen in 50% of patients, and their development may precede or parallel that of other symptoms. Patients may complain of cloudy, blurred, indistinct, or misty vision or may note yellow spots or, rarely, photophobia. The most common acute field defect is a dense central scotoma. Some patients compare their visual symptoms with "stepping out into a snowstorm," a complaint unique to methanol ingestion. Patients can have a complete lack of light perception and total loss of vision. Visual acuity should be determined. On examination, optic disc hyperemia is seen at 18 to 48 hr after ingestion. Peripapillary retinal edema follows, is most striking in the nerve fiber layer along the vascular arcades, and only rarely involves the macula. Sluggishly reactive or fixed and dilated pupils indicate a poor prognosis. Pallor and cupping, indicative of optic atrophy, are late findings suggesting a poor prognosis for visual recovery. On occasion, the fundus may appear normal, even in patients with visualsymptoms.

Compensatory tachypnea heralds the onset of metabolic acidosis, which often may be severe, with reported serum bicarbonate concentrations of less than 5 mEq/L and an arterial pH less than 7.0. Early tachycardia has been noted, but in general, cardiovascular abnormalities are rare. Hypotension and bradycardia, when present, are preterminal findings. Historically, death is associated with a peculiar, abrupt cessation of respiration rather than with cardiovascular collapse. Multiple organ failure is rare.

Prognosis after methanol ingestion seems to correlate with the degree of acidosis, time to presentation, and initiation of treatment within 8 hours of exposure. Poor prognosis is associated with coma, seizures, or arterial pH less than 7.0. Patients surviving the acute phase of toxicity may be left with permanent blindness or neurologic deficits, such as parkinsonism, toxic encephalopathy, polyneuropathy, cognitive dysfunction, transverse myelitis, primitive reflexes, or seizures.

Diagnostic Strategies

A severe AG metabolic acidosis is the hallmark of methanol poisoning. In some cases, this sign may be the only diagnostic clue. Because the onset of acidosis may be delayed 12 to 24 hr, a normal AG does not rule out methanol exposure. Absence of high anion gap acidosis has been described in cases with concomitant ethanol, lithium, or bromide ingestion. In methanol toxicity, this AG is due primarily to the presence of formic acid, with a variable contribution from lactic acid. Another classic laboratory finding in methanol toxicity is an elevated osmol gap.

An osmol gap significantly greater than 10 mOsm/kg may be a useful aid in the diagnosis of toxic alcohol ingestion. In addition to methanol, ethylene glycol, and isopropanol, other low-molecular-weight solutes, such as ethanol, acetone, propylene glycol, mannitol, glycerol, and ethyl ether, may cause elevated osmol gaps. Caution should be taken, however, in ruling out toxic alcohol ingestion with a normal osmol gap for several reasons. First, calculated serum osmolality results may vary among laboratories and must be done by the freezing point depression method. Also, delayed presentation after toxic alcohol ingestion may be associated with prior metabolism of most of the parent alcohol. Because only the parent compound is osmotically active and because the charged metabolites are electrically balanced by sodium, there may be little or no osmol gap elevation in this setting. Finally, a toxic level of either methanol or ethylene glycol may be present with a gap of only 10 mOsm/kg. If there is clinical suspicion of toxic alcohol ingestion, direct measurement of the serum toxic alcohol level is necessary, and if it is not readily available, empirical treatment is warranted. Rhabdomyolysis,pancreatitis, and metabolic derangements, such as hypomagnesemia, hypokalemia, and hypophosphatemia, are alsodescribed with methanol poisoning.

CT may be indicated in an intoxicated patient with altered mental status. The characteristic finding of bilateral putaminal lesions suggests methanol poisoning, but this finding also may be seen with Leigh's syndrome, Wilson's disease, hypoxic-ischemic insult, encephalitis, and certain metabolic disorders. Ischemic necrosis, cerebral edema, or brain hemorrhages also may be noted. Follow-up scans may have prognostic value because parkinsonian features are unlikely to develop in patients whose putaminal lesions resolve within a short time frame. MRI may also detect putaminal aberrations or optic neuropathy from methanol intoxication.

Differential Considerations

Methanol and ethylene glycol cause inebriation and are ingested as ethanol substitutes. The differential diagnosis of a patient with altered mental status includes hypoglycemia, head trauma, postictal state, carbon dioxide narcosis, hypoxia, infection, hepatic encephalopathy, other metabolic disorders, thiamine deficiency, endocrinopathy, drug abuse, and other poisoning. For patients who present with severe abdominal pain and altered mental status, the differential diagnosis could include a long list of intraabdominal entities. When an AG acidosis is identified, however, the differential diagnosis should be tapered toward entities that cause this, and a primary decision should be made as to whether the acidosis is a result of an ingested toxin or some other cause (e.g., mesenteric ischemia, diabetic ketoacidosis). Toxic alcohol ingestion should be included in the differential diagnosis for patients with depressed mental status of unknown cause. Causes of an elevated anion gap in patients without evidence of renal failure, hypotension, hypoxemia, diabetes, seizures, or alcoholism include methanol, ethylene glycol, paraldehyde, isoniazid,iron, salicylates, toluene, and lactic acidosis from myriad toxicants, including metformin, carbon monoxide, cyanide, and cocaine. Isopropanol does not cause an increased anion gap. Ethylene glycol and methanol may cause a "double gap" (i.e., an osmol gap in addition to the anion gap). Other substances that contribute to an elevated osmol gap include isopropyl alcohol, ethanol, propylene glycol, mannitol, glycerol, and ethyl ether. Other situations in which double-gap acidosis may be encountered include diabetic ketoacidosis; alcoholic ketoacidosis; acetonitrile, methanol, ethylene glycol, and propylene glycol toxicity; multiple organ failure; chronic renal failure; and critical illness. Hyperlipidemia and hyperproteinemia, by decreasing the measured sodium concentration, can increase the osmolal gap.

Certain unique characteristics of methanol and ethylene glycol intoxication may lead to the specific diagnosis. The presence of ocular complaints unique to methanol poisoning is a valuable clue. Ethylene glycol ingestion often is associated with calcium oxalate crystalluria, which is not seen in methanol ingestion. Ultimately, a definitive diagnosis requires the documented presence of the parent alcohol through laboratory tests that may not be routinely available. It is often necessary to start treatment on the basis of clinical suggestion alone. Because the initial treatment for methanol and ethylene glycol is almost identical, identification of the specific toxic alcohol is not crucial to the initiation of therapy.

Management and Disposition

See the discussion on management in the following section on ethylene glycol.

ETHYLENE GLYCOL

Perspective

Ethylene glycol is a viscous, colorless, odorless, slightly sweettasting liquid. Because it lowers the freezing point of water, its primary utility is as a commercial antifreeze or coolant. If it is treated early and aggressively, ethylene glycol poisoning is unlikely to result in death. Conversely, failure to treat ethylene glycol ingestion may result in multiorgan failure and death within 24 to 36 hr.

Principles of Disease

Pharmacology and Metabolism

Absorption of ethylene glycol is rapid after ingestion. Peak blood levels are reached within 1 to 4 hr after ingestion. In contrast to methanol and isopropanol, ethylene glycol is nonvolatile at room temperature, so absorption by inhalation is unlikely. Reported half-lives range from 3 to 8.6 hr. When metabolism is blocked by fomepizole or ethanol, the half-life increases to 11 to 15 hr or 17 hr, respectively. The toxic and lethal doses of 100% ethylene glycol have been reported as 0.2 mL/kg and 1.4 mL/kg. Twenty-seven percent of ethylene glycol is excreted unchanged by the kidneys. The remainder is oxidized through hepatic ADH and other oxidative enzymes to various toxic organic aldehydes and acids (Fig. 49-2).

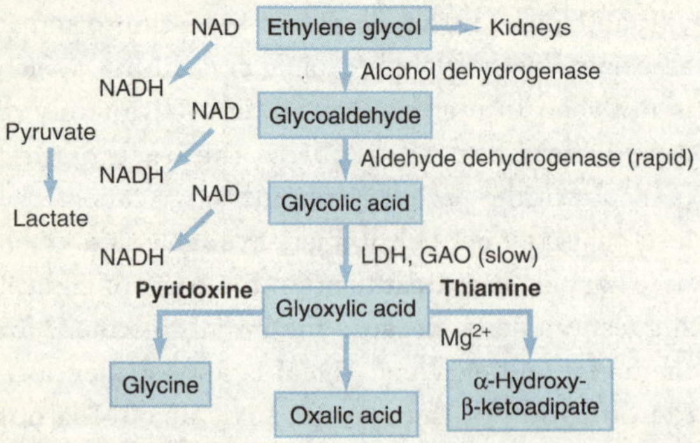

Fig. 49-2 Metabolism of ethylene glycol. *NADH*, reduced form of nicotinamide adenine dinucleotide.

Pathophysiology

Unmetabolized ethylene glycol has limited toxicity, yet all metabolites are toxic. In humans, 2.3% of a dose of ethylene glycol ultimately is converted to oxalic acid, most of which is excreted in the urine. A fraction of oxalic acid combines with calcium to form calcium oxalate crystals, which precipitate in renal tubules, brain, and other tissues. Because the intermediate metabolite, glyoxylic acid, theoretically can be shunted toward pyridoxine-dependent or thiamine-dependent pathways to generate the nontoxic products glycine and α-hydroxy-β-ketoadipate (Fig. 49-2), both pyridoxine and thiamine are routinely used in therapy.

On histologic examination, proximal renal tubular dilation with hydropic change and vacuolar degeneration, intratubular crystal deposition, and edema of the interstitium are seen. Relative sparing of the glomeruli is typical, although glomerular interloop space crystal deposition may occur. Glomerular function is preserved, but tubular dysfunction manifesting as protein leak is noted. Neuropathologic changes induced by ethylene glycol include diffuse calcium oxalate deposition with petechial hemorrhages in the retina, brain, vessel walls, and perivascular spaces, with evidence of cerebral edema and chemical meningoencephalitis. Similar changes also have been noted in the liver, spleen, pancreas, pleura, lungs, pericardium, and blood vessel walls throughout the body. Myonecrosis occurs in skeletal and myocardial muscle, and rhabdomyolysis and myocardial dilation occur. Fatty liver with focal necrosis has been noted.

The metabolism of ethylene glycol results in a profound anion gap metabolic acidosis, caused mainly by glycolic acid. Elevated lactate, triggered by the altered redox potential within cells and inhibition of the citric acid cycle by products of glyoxylate metabolism, is a minor contributing factor to the severe acidosis.

Clinical Features

The clinical syndrome with ethylene glycol ingestion is divided into four stages: (1) acute neurologic stage, (2) cardiopulmonary stage, (3) renal stage, and (4) delayed neurologic sequelae stage. The severity of illness in each stage and the progression through stages may vary. Stages may be skipped and patients may die in any stage of ethylene glycol poisoning. Poor prognostic factors include hyperkalemia, severe acidosis, seizures, and coma. Metabolic acidosis and symptoms typically occur within 4 to 8 hr but may be delayed for 12 hr or longer if ethanol has been coingested.

Stage Ⅰ, the acute neurologic stage, occurs 30 min to 12 hr after ingestion. The parent alcohol causes approximately the same degree of inebriation as ethanol does, with CNS depression, slurred speech, nystagmus, ataxia, and vomiting. With large ingestions, more dramatic neurologic findings, such as hallucinations, seizures, and coma, may be present during the early phase of intoxication. Ocular findings including decreased pupillary reflexes, decreased visual acuity, optic disc blurring, papilledema, and loss of color discrimination have been reported, but methanol exposure was not ruled out in most of these case reports.

Stage Ⅱ, the cardiopulmonary stage, occurs 12 to 24 hr after ingestion. Often, the patient exhibits mild hypertension and tachycardia. Tachypnea may reflect the underlying profound metabolic acidosis or may herald the onset of cardiogenic or noncardiogenic pulmonary edema. The mechanism of ARDS is unclear but may be related to the toxicity of glycolic and glyoxylic acids and to the deposition of calcium oxalate crystals within the lungs. Pulmonary infiltrates are described during this phase. Circulatory collapse may occur as a result of myocardial depression. Hypocalcemia, rarely associated with tetany or cardiac dysrhythmia, occurs in 30% of patients as a result of systemic chelation of calcium by oxalate.

Myositis with muscle tenderness and CK elevation results from skeletal muscle inflammation and necrosis.

Stage Ⅲ, the renal stage, occurs 24 to 72 hr after ingestion. Awake patients may complain of flank pain or have costophrenic angle tenderness. Calcium oxalate monohydrate or dihydrate crystalluria is seen in only 50% of cases. Hematuria and proteinuria are common, however, as with other causes of acute tubular necrosis, oliguria is not always present, but it may develop 12 hr after ingestion and may progress to frank anuria. Prolonged hemodialysis may be necessary, although recovery of renal function has been reported. Delayed onset of ARDS has been reported to occur during this stage, but it is more typically seen in stage Ⅱ. The degree of acidosis, delay in presentation, and glycolate levels correlate better than ethylene glycol levels with the development of renal failure.

Stage Ⅳ, the delayed neurologic sequelae stage, occurs 6 to 12 d after ingestion and typically is manifested as cranial neuropathy. All cases have been associated with renal failure. Facial diplegia, occasionally with deafness, is most frequently encountered. Other reported findings include dysarthria, dysphagia, tongue deviation, visual deterioration, and internal ophthalmoplegia. Delayed and persistent cognitive and motor deficits, such as ataxia, chorea, coma, and late personality changes, are also reported. Total paralysis from severe axonal peripheral polyneuropathic degeneration with oxalate deposition and polyradiculopathy from nerve root (not distal) disease are also reported. Although some improvement in neurologic status has been noted at follow-up, most patients are left with residual neurologic deficits.

Diagnostic Strategies

Useful laboratory tests for evaluation of a patient with potential ethylene glycol toxicity include serum electrolyte values; calcium, BUN, creatinine, and serum glucose concentrations; serum osmolality; blood ethanol level; arterial blood gas analysis; ethylene glycol level; electrocardiogram; and urinalysis. Although crystalluria is considered the hallmark of ethylene glycol ingestion, its absence does not rule out the diagnosis because less than half of patients have this finding. Crystalluria may take the form of envelope-shaped calcium oxalate dihydrate crystals or needle-shaped calcium oxalate monohydrate crystals. Other crystal shapes and composites have been noted so that in the setting of combined anion and osmolal gap elevation, the presence of any type of crystalluria warrants a search for ethylene glycol. Monohydrate crystals are thought to be more specific for ethylene glycol poisoning. Irrigating the urinary bladder with 50 to 100 mL of saline, centrifuging the irrigant, and examining the sediment for crystals may yield the diagnosis in patients who are already anuric. Other findings reflecting tubular dysfunction include decreased specific gravity, proteinuria, microscopic hematuria, pyuria, and cylindruria. Falsely elevated ethylene glycol levels may be seen in the face of elevated lactate or lactate dehydrogenase with certain enzymatic assays.

Freshly voided urine can be examined for fluorescence with Wood's lamp. Sodium fluorescein is added to antifreeze to aid in the detection of radiator leaks. Urinary fluorescence may be seen 6 hr after ingestion of fluorescein-containing antifreeze. The lack of fluorescence does not rule out ethylene glycol ingestion, however, because examiner sensitivity, specificity, and inter-rater reliability are low.

Leukocytosis may be seen in ethylene glycol poisoning, with a typical white blood cell count of 10,000 to 40,000/μL, but it is neither a sensitive nor a specific finding and is not of diagnostic value. The hematocrit and platelet counts are normal. One third of patients have hypocalcemia, which is most likely caused by calcium precipitation with oxalate. QT prolongation on the electrocardiogram leads to the early diagnosis of hypocalcemia. Rarely, profound hypocalcemia resulting in seizures and tetany may occur. The CK level can be elevated as a result of toxic effects of ethylene glycol metabolites on muscle tissue.

Similar to methanol, ethylene glycol often causes a profound anion gap metabolic acidosis when the metabolites glycolic acid and glyoxylic acid (and, to some extent, lactic acid) accumulate. False elevations of lactic acid levels may occur in the presence of glycolate with certain analyzers. Similar to methanol toxicity, an elevated osmolal gap as measured by freezing point depression can be a clue, but lethal concentrations can be associated with a normal or only slightly elevated osmolal gap. The cerebrospinal fluid may be normal or have a cloudy or bloody appearance, with increased protein or a polymorphonuclear pleocytosis.

Imaging studies show cerebral edema with decreased attenuation in the mediobasilar portions of the brain, typically with a return to isodensity within 1 week; this does not correspond to the clinical picture. MRI in one patient with delayed cranial neuropathy showed gadolinium enhancement of cranial nerve V bilaterally, possibly secondary to calcium oxalate deposition. Electroencephalographic findings have been nonspecific.

Differential Considerations

Classically, patients who ingest ethylene glycol appear intoxicated without the odor of ethanol and have an anion gap metabolic acidosis, increased osmolal gap, and calcium oxalate crystalluria. Without evidence of alcoholic ketoacidosis or diabetic ketoacidosis, the differential diagnosis of the double gap should include methanol and ethylene glycol. The hallmark finding with late presentation is renal toxicity. Toxicant-induced acute renal failure is extensively reviewed elsewhere; substances commonly implicated include antimicrobials, NSAIDs, acetaminophen, halogenated hydrocarbons, radiocontrast media, metals, antineoplastic agents, and myoglobin. Hypocalcemia and a prolonged QT interval are important diagnostic clues.

Toxicant-induced hypocalcemia is unusual and may be related to aminoglycosides, calcitonin, cisplatin, loop diuretics, interferon alfa, mithramycin, pentamidine, and phosphate infusions. Healthy individuals with dietary excesses of vitamin C or foods rich in oxalate, such as tomatoes, garlic, spinach, rhubarb, cocoa, and tea, may exhibit calcium oxalate crystalluria.

Management

Methanol and ethylene glycol ingestions are treated essentially in the same manner, and the following recommendations apply to both. As in any overdose, resuscitation and stabilization are paramount, including naloxone, bedside glucose determination, and thiamine, if indicated. Specific blood levels that confirm the presence of these substances may not be readily available, and a delay in therapy can lead to irreversible organ damage or death. For any significant history of exposure, treatment should be initiated pending a confirmatory toxic alcohol blood level.

Methanol and ethylene glycol are absorbed rapidly from the gastrointestinal tract; because gastric emptying has not been shown to alter clinical course or outcome and may be associated with complications, its use is restricted to possible nasogastric suction for patients who have ingested more than a swallow and arrive in the emergency department within 30 to 60 min of ingestion. Even in these cases, it is of unproven value. Forced diuresis is of no value and may cause pulmonary edema and ARDS. Early intubation may be indicated to protect the airway against aspiration and in anticipation of further deterioration in mental status.

Three treatment goals exist for patients with methanol or ethylene glycol toxicity: (1) correction of metabolic acidosis with bicarbonate; (2) ADH enzyme blockade, which inhibits the metabolism of methanol and ethylene glycol to toxic metabolites; and (3) removal of the parent alcohol and its metabolites by hemodialysis. The acidic metabolites of methanol and ethylene glycol can cause a profound bicarbonate-resistant metabolic acidosis, with several hundred milliequivalents of excess acid produced per hour. In contrast to lactic acid, these acids are not metabolized to bicarbonate, and massive amounts of bicarbonate may be necessary merely for partial correction of the acidosis. Early correction of metabolic acidosis may be beneficial in reversing methanol-induced visual impairment, most likely related to the induction of a larger fraction of dissociated formic acid, which should decrease the amount of formic acid entering the CNS. Depending on the severity of the patient's acidosis, bicarbonate can be administered intravenously by intermittent boluses, by an initial bolus followed by an infusion, or by infusion alone. Boluses of 1 to 2 mEq/kg to attain a target serum pH of 7.45 to 7.50 followed by an infusion of 150 mEq/L of sodium bicarbonate in 5% dextrose at 1.5 to 2 times the maintenance fluid rate are suggested.With ethylene glycol, the potential for worsened hypocalcemia during the administration of large amounts of sodium bicarbonate should be considered.

To prevent further production of the toxic and acidic metabolites of methanol and ethylene glycol, metabolism of the parent compounds by the enzyme ADH must be blocked by either ethanol or fomepizole (Antizol). As experience has been gained with fomepizole, it is generally thought to be more advantageous than ethanol from a safety and convenience perspective. ADH blockade should be carried out in any adult or child with symptoms or with methanol or ethylene glycol levels greater than 20 mg/dL, even if the patient is asymptomatic. If ethanol is used to block ADH, the goal is to maintain the blood ethanol level between 100 and 150 mg/dL, which completely saturates ADH. The affinity of ADH for ethanol is 10 to 20 times greater than for methanol and 100 times greater than for ethylene glycol. When the metabolism of methanol and ethylene glycol is blocked by ethanol, their half-lives increase to more than 30 hr and 17 hr, respectively. Prevention of methanol and ethylene glycol metabolism by ethanol explains the delayed toxicity seen in patients who ingest ethanol in combination with either of these substances. In dosing of ethanol, it also is important to measure the patient's initial blood ethanol level. If it is greater than 100 mg/dL, a loading dose is unnecessary, and a maintenance infusion can be started (Table 49-1). The required maintenance dose of ethanol may nearly triple during hemodialysis because ethanol also is efficiently removed. Ethanol may be given orally or intravenously. Potential side effects of intravenous administration include CNS and respiratory depression, hypotension, vomiting, hypoglycemia, and thrombophlebitis, although even in children, adverse effects are limited. Oral ethanol loading may be associated with gastritis. Initial close monitoring of serum ethanol and glucose levels every 1 to 2 hr is essential until a steady-state level of 100 to 150 mg/dL is achieved. Levels should be checked every 2 to 4 hr thereafter. Monitoring of ethanol therapy ideally is accomplished in ICU.

Table 49-1 Standard Range of Therapeutic Doses of Ethanol Based on Average Pharmacokinetic Values

	AMOUNT ABSOLUTE ETHANOL	VOLUME (43% ORAL SOLUTION)	VOLUME (10% IV SOLUTION)
Loading dose	600 mg/kg	1.8 mL/kg	7.6 mL/kg
Standard maintenance dose (nondrinker)	66 mg/kg/hr	0.2 mL/kg/hr	0.83 mL/kg/hr
Standard maintenance dose (chronic drinker)	154 mg/kg/hr	0.46 mL/kg/hr	1.96 mL/kg/hr
Maintenance dose during dialysis (nondrinker)	169 mg/kg/hr	0.5 mL/kg/hr	2.13 mL/kg/hr
Maintenance dose during dialysis (chronic drinker)	257 mg/kg/hr	0.77 mL/kg/hr	3.26 mL/kg/hr

Similar to ethanol, fomepizole blocks the metabolism of methanol and ethylene glycol by ADH and prevents the formation of toxic metabolites. When the metabolism of methanol and ethylene glycol is blocked by fomepizole, their half-lives increase to an average of 52 hr and 17 hr, respectively. Advantages of fomepizole over ethanol include ease of administration, predictable pharmacokinetics, improved patient safety profile, standardized and less complicated dosing regimen that does not require direct observation or frequent blood monitoring, longer duration of action, and lack of CNS depression. Nonetheless, simply blocking toxic alcohol metabolism does not alter the toxicity of preformed metabolites. The use of neither fomepizole nor ethanol supplants the need for hemodialysis. The main disadvantage of the use of fomepizole is its cost. The dosing regimen for adults and pediatric patients is 15 mg/kg, followed by 10 mg/kg every 12 hr for four doses. After five doses, the dose increases to 15 mg/kg every 12 hr until the ethylene glycol concentration is undetectable or less than 20 mg/dL and the patient is asymptomatic with a normal arterial pH. Dosing changes are required during hemodialysis. Side effects of fomepizole include headache, nausea, dizziness, inflammation at the site of infusion, rash, eosinophilia, and mild reversible transaminase elevation. A single case of hypotension and bradycardia related to the rapid infusion has been described. However, a 10-year review of adverse events in patients showed fomepizole to be safer than ethanol.

Rapid removal of the methanol or ethylene glycol through hemodialysis before it has been metabolized remains the cornerstone of therapy. In addition, hemodialysis, preferably with use of a dialysate high in bicarbonate, corrects acidosis and uremia, aids in fluid management and cardiovascular stabilization, and removes the toxic metabolites in late presenters. Hemodialysis decreases the half-life of methanol and ethylene glycol to 2.5 to 3.5 hr. Peritoneal dialysis and hemoperfusion are much less effective.

In general, hemodialysis is indicated for patients who have metabolic acidosis, renal insufficiency, deterioration despite intensive care, electrolyte disturbance, or visual disturbances with methanol. In addition, a blood level of either substance greater than 50 mg/dL usually calls for dialysis, but in patients with normal kidneys, prolonged fomepizole treatment alone has been used without hemodialysis. For ethylene glycol, a glycolic acid level greater than 8 mmol/L, an anion gap greater than 20 mmol/L, or an initial pH less than 7. predicts renal failure and the need for hemodialysis. Methanol and ethylene glycol levels should be interpreted in the context of the clinical status and the time after ingestion. An acidotic patient with a low blood level after a delayed presentation requires more aggressive treatment than an asymptomatic patient with a high level.

The endpoint for hemodialysis is an undetectable serum ethylene glycol or methanol concentration and the disappearance of acid-base abnormalities and signs of systemic toxicity. Resolution of the anion gap also may serve as an endpoint for hemodialysis in situations in which levels are not available or reliable (i.e., in patients with delayed presentation).

In methanol poisoning, the rate of the final degradation reaction of formic acid to carbon dioxide and water depends on the cofactor folate in primates (Fig. 49-1), so 50 mg of leucovorin (folinic acid) should be given intravenous every 4 hr to adults with methanol toxicity. Likewise, the cofactors thiamine and pyridoxine have theoretic benefit on the basis of their use in humans with primary hyperoxaluria, although no clinical trials have studied their efficacy in the treatment of ethylene glycol toxicity. Adequate cofactor levels minimize oxalic acid production by favoring the production of other, less toxic metabolites (Fig.49-2). The recommended adult doses are thiamine, 100 mg intravenous every 6 hr, and pyridoxine, 50 mg every 6 hr for 2 d. With symptomatic hypocalcemia, intravenous calcium should be supplemented,albeit cautiously, to avoid further precipitation of calcium oxalate crystals in tissues. Asymptomatic hypercalcemia need not be treated. Magnesium is a cofactor along with thiamine for the detoxification of glycolic acid and should be replaced in patients who are deficient.

Disposition

Admission is generally necessary for patients undergoing treatment for ethylene glycol or methanol exposure. In addition, all patients with clinical or laboratory findings consistent with these ingestions should be admitted, even when the history is lacking or unavailable. Early consultation with a nephrologist for possible hemodialysis is necessary in the management of suggested toxic alcohol ingestion. If such services are not available, the patient should be given an ADH inhibitor and transferred to a setting where dialysis is available. A regional poison center or medical toxicologist may be contacted to guide management. An ophthalmologist can evaluate visual injury fully in patients with methanol poisoning. Neurologic consultation and follow-up monitoring of patients with either methanol or ethylene glycol toxicity are prudent given the potential for delayed or persistent neurologic sequelae.

Prevention

The bittering agent denatonium benzoate (Bitrex) has been added to consumer automotive products containing 10% or more ethylene glycol or 4% or more methanol, but the effect of this effort has not yet decreased the frequency or severity of pediatric antifreeze poisoning. Another opportunity for prevention is the substitution of less toxic glycols, such as propylene glycol, into commercial antifreezes.

ISOPROPYL ALCOHOL

Perspective

Isopropyl alcohol (isopropanol) is a clear,

colorless liquid with a slightly bitter taste. It is the second most commonly ingested alcohol after ethanol. Isopropanol and its major metabolite acetone cause twice the CNS depression of ethanol, so intentional ingestion as an alcohol substitute is encountered frequently in adults. Isopropanol is not associated with the toxicity of ethylene glycol or methanol poisoning, and death after exposure is rare. The typical fatality involves a chronic, older alcoholic with mixed ethanol-isopropanol intoxication after a drinking binge.

Principles of Disease

Pharmacology and Metabolism

Absorption of isopropanol is rapid and complete; 80% of a dose is absorbed within 30 min of ingestion. The kidneys excrete 20% as unchanged isopropanol. A small portion is re-secreted into the stomach and saliva; the remaining 80% is metabolized in the liver to acetone by ADH (Fig. 49-3). Acetone is excreted primarily by the kidneys, with small amounts expired through the lungs.

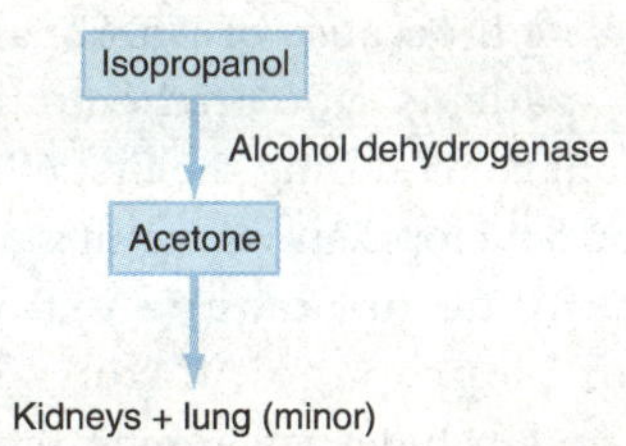

Fig. 49-3 Metabolism of isopropanol.

Isopropanol blood levels peak 30 min to 3 hr after ingestion, and elimination follows first-order kinetics, with a half-life of 3 to 7 hr. Acetone is eliminated more slowly, with a half-life of 22 hr. The rate of elimination of isopropanol may be increased by chronic ethanol abuse and decreased by hepatic damage. A potentially lethal dose in adults is 150 to 240 mL (2-4 mL/kg).

Pathophysiology

Isopropanol is a potent CNS depressant, but the mechanism of action is unclear. Acetone is also a CNS depressant, and it has been suggested that coma may be prolonged by the extended elimination of this metabolite. The extent to which acetone contributes to coma is brought into question by the report of a patient who was awake and conversant with acetone levels of 200 mg/dL. In large doses, isopropanol causes hypotension from peripheral vasodilation and direct myocardial depression. Topical effects include corneal de-epithelialization and dermal burns, described in premature infants as a result of skin de-esterification. Acetone does not seem to be shunted into the formation of acetoacetate or β-hydroxybutyrate; the finding of ketosis without acidosis is characteristic of isopropyl ingestion. Pulmonary congestion at autopsy is nonspecific and typical of deaths involving druginduced CNS depression.

Clinical Findings

Gastrointestinal and CNS complaints predominate clinically. Intoxication may be suggested by apparent inebriation with the odor of acetone rather than of ethanol detected on the breath. The patient may have headache or dizziness and may exhibit neuromuscular incoordination, confusion, and nystagmus. Severe ingestions may result in deep coma, which is prolonged compared with ethanol. Respiratory depression or failure may occur. Patients may have a loss of deep tendon, corneal, or protective airway reflexes and have an extensor response to plantar reflex testing. Pupillary size varies, but miosis is most common. Because isopropanol is a gastrointestinal irritant, the patient may complain of abdominal pain, nausea, and vomiting. Gastritis can occur with dermal and oral exposure. Hematemesis and upper gastrointestinal bleeding stem from gastritis but are rare.Hypotension, although rare, signifies severe poisoning, with a mortality rate of 45%. One case series found mortality only when coma and hypotension were present. Sinus tachycardia is common, but other atrial and ventricular dysrhythmias are rare and generally found only with confounding hypoxia, acidosis, or shock. Hypothermia is frequent. Rarely, myoglobinuria, acute tubular necrosis, hepatic dysfunction, and hemolytic anemia have been reported. A distinguishing feature is that metabolic acidosis is not present with isopropanol intoxication unless it is accompanied by hypotension, gastrointestinal bleeding, or coingestants. Hyperglycemia may be noted, but hypoglycemia has not previously been described.

Diagnostic Strategies

Most of these patients do not need any laboratory testing unless they are severely ill. Peak isopropanol levels occur soon after ingestion, whereas acetone levels peak later at 4 hr after ingestion. The most common laboratory abnormality is ketosis with little or no acidosis and normal blood glucose levels. The ketosis is from the metabolite acetone, which can be detected in the blood 15 min after ingestion and in the urine 3 hr after ingestion. Acetone is uncharged, so it does not elevate the anion gap. Isopropanol and acetone contribute to the increased osmol gap.

One early laboratory clue to the diagnosis of isopropanol ingestion is "pseudo-renal failure," or isolated false elevation of creatinine with a normal BUN concentration. This condition results from interference of acetone and acetoacetate by the colorimetric method of creatinine determination. Creatinine is expected to increase 1 mg/dL for every 100 mg/dL of acetone. A CK level may detect coma-induced myoglobinuria and rhabdomyolysis.

Differential Considerations

The differential diagnosis includes all of the causes of altered mental status in an alcoholic patient.The presence of ketosis warrants a search for DKA, alcoholic ketoacidosis, salicylism, cyanide, or starvation ketosis. A distinguishing feature of isopropanol ingestion is the presence of ketosis without acidosis.In the setting of a high or rising creatinine concentration and normal BUN concentration, acute rhabdomyolysis also should be considered. Other substances that falsely elevate creatinine are cimetidine, nitroethane, and nitromethane, often mixed with methanol in formulating radio-controlled vehicle fuel. Detection of isopropanol in acetonemic patients not exposed to isopropanol is well described.

Management and Disposition

Neither gastric emptying nor activated charcoal administration is warranted. Intubation is indicated if the patient is unable to protect the airway; it may also be indicated on the basis of coingestants or if the patient's mental status is poor and deteriorating. In contrast to methanol and ethylene glycol ingestion, ADH blockade with ethanol or fomepizole is not indicated. Hypotension should be managed with fluids and vasopressors as needed. If the patient remains hypotensive or has further vital sign deterioration despite these measures, dialysis is indicated. Some authors also recommend dialysis for isopropanol serum levels greater than 400 mg/dL. Coma itself is not an indication for dialysis but may necessitate mechanical ventilation. Peritoneal dialysis and hemodialysis have been successful, but hemodialysis is much more effective and is preferred. Because of isopropanol's rapid absorption, patients who are hemodynamically stable without coma during the first 6 hours are at low risk for development of significant sequelae and generally do not require extracorporeal removal of isopropanol. Care is otherwise supportive and includes rewarming, evaluation for hypoglycemia, and monitoring for gastrointestinal bleeding.

(ZHANG Jianfeng)

SECTION 6

Toxinlogy Emergency

Chapter 50

Venomous Snake Bite

KEY CONCEPTS

Snake venom causes neurotoxicity and hematotoxicity depending on the species of snake.

The initial 6 to 8 period after a snakebite is critical. During this time, medical therapy can help prevent the morbidity associated with severe envenomation.

ED care of a snakebite focuses on supportive care and rapid treatment with the appropriate antivenin.

The amount of crotalid antivenin given depends on the grade of envenomation, from 0 (minimal or no sign of envenomation) to IV (severe envenomation).

PERSPECTIVE

Epidemiology

Of the 3000 species of snakes, approximately 10% to 15% are venomous. Of the 14 families of snakes, four contain venomous species. Snakes are distributed throughout most of the earth's surface, including fresh and salt water. The major exceptions are the Arctic and Antarctic zones, New Zealand, Malagasy, and many small islands. Most snakebites occur in tropical and subtropical climates, especially in agricultural settings where the inhabitants go barefoot. Sea snakes are found only in the Pacific and Indian Oceans. Snakes are poikilotherms, which accounts for their distribution and activity. Their inability to raise their body temperature above ambient levels restricts their activity to a fairly narrow temperature range, approximately 25 to 35℃.All snakes are carnivorous, and their venom apparatus evolved for the purpose of obtaining food.

Snakes alone are estimated to inflict 2.5 million venomous bites annually,with approximately 125,000 deaths.

Approximately 45,000 snakebites occur annually in the United States;7000 to 8000 are inflicted by venomous snakes, and 5 to 10 result in death.

The American Association of Poison Control Centrol Centers began collecting data in 1983 on deaths caused by venomous snakes injuries(Table 50-1).

The number of exposures and deaths from exotic snakes seems to be increasing, possibly because of interest in collecting so-called "hot" or venomous varieties such as cobras, mambas, and vipers. Most exposures occur from April to October, when snakes are most active and potential victims are outdoors and involved in activities that might increase their risk for envenomation. Most deaths seem to occur in very young, elderly, or inappropriately treated patients.

Table 50-1 Venomous Snakes Injuries and Deaths, 1983-2009

ANIMAL	ENVENOMATIONS	DEATHS
Copperheads	14,580	1
Rattlesnakes	21,122	28
Coral snakes	1,337	0
Exotic snakes 2,196 3	2,196	3
Nonvenomous snakes	37,001	0
Unknown snakes	41,758	4

The incidence of reported venomous snakebites in the United States is greatest in the South. States having the highest death rates are North Carolina, Arkansas, Texas, and Georgia. Of all snakebites, 97% occur on the extremities, with two thirds on the upper extremities and one third on the lower extremities. Bites that occur accidentally are considered "legitimate," whereas bites that occur during attempts to handle or disturb a snake are considered "illegitimate." Men are bitten nine times more frequently than women.

Venom Delivery

Snakes that have developed specific venom glands and venom delivery systems can be found. The toxin and toxic apparatus vary from class to class. Snakes can be considered poisonous because of various toxins distributed in their tissues.

Classification and Characteristics

The four venomous families of snakes are the Colubridae, Elapidae, Viperidae, and Atractaspididae. The Colubridae, although representing 70% of all species of snakes, have very few venomous members dangerous to humans; these include the boomslang and bird snake. They are rear-fanged snakes, and although many possess venom, they generally do not envenomate humans. The Elapidae are more common and include the cobras,kraits, mambas, and coral snakes. The Hydrophiidae are sea snakes and a subfamily of the Elapidae. The Viperidae, or true vipers, are represented by Russell's viper, the puff adder, the Gaboon viper, the saw-scaled viper, and the European viper. The Crotalidae, or pit vipers, are sometimes considered a separate family and sometimes a subfamily (Crotalinae) of the Viperidae. The Atractaspididae are the mole vipers, which have sidepositioned fangs; they rarely envenomate humans and are found only in Africa and the Middle East.

Pit vipers are classified into three main groups: true rattlesnakes (genus Crotalus), copperheads and water moccasins (genus Agkistrodon), and pygmy or Massasauga rattlesnakes (genus Sistrurus).

The Colubridae and Hydrophiidae have few venomous encounters with humans and are responsible for even fewer injuries.

Identification

There are two key principles for identifying venomous snakes:Only experts should handle live snakes, and even dead snakes can envenomate careless handlers. It is not difficult to differentiate between pit vipers and harmless snakes found in the United States (Fig. 50-1). Pit vipers, as their name implies, have a characteristic pit midway between the eye and the nostril on both sides of the head. This pit is a heat-sensitive organ that enables the snake to locate warm-blooded prey. Pit vipers may be identified through other methods, but this characteristic is 100% consistent. The triangular shape of the head, the presence of an elliptical pupil, the tail structure, and the presence of fangs are useful characteristics but are inconsistent. The arrangement of subcaudal plates may be used for Crotalinae if the head has been damaged or is unavailable. An individual specimen may not fit the classic description,depending on the age of the snake, the time of the year, and the condition of the tail and mouthparts. Neither color nor skin pattern is a reliable method of identifying pit vipers (Fig. 50-2). Size is not an important factor in identifying various reptiles. Venomous snakes range in length from several inches to several feet. Although a 6-foot eastern diamondback rattlesnake is much more dangerous than a 10-inch copperhead, all venomous snakes are able to envenomate from birth and should be treated as

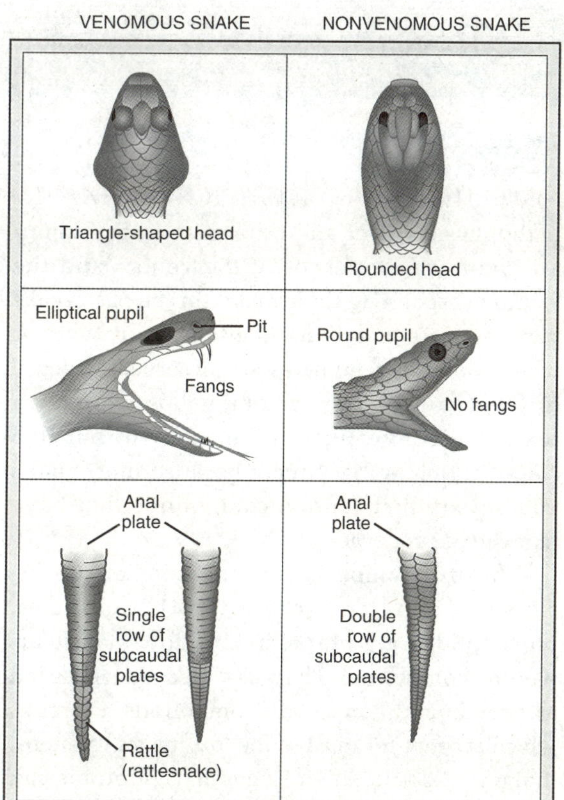

Fig. 50-1 Identification of venomous and nonvenomous North American snkes.

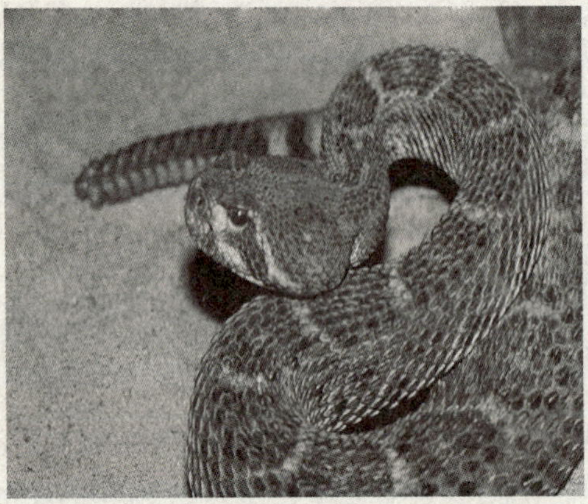

Fig. 50-2 Western diamondback rattlesnake.

though they are dangeous.

Exotic snakes that are not pit vipers are not as easily identified. If possible, they should be safely transported to an expert for positive identification. Local zoos, herpetology groups, and colleges often have individuals who can identify unknown snakes.

PRINCIPLES OF DISEASE

Toxins

The two main factors influencing the pathophysiology of any venomous animal injury are the toxic properties of the venom and the victim's response to these toxins. In the past, snake venoms were classified as either neurotoxic or hematotoxic, depending on the observed response of the victim to the various venoms. Modern toxicologic investigation has shown that this classification is inadequate because most snake venoms studied contain compounds that have many toxic properties.

The toxic components of snake venom can be classified into four broad categories: enzymes, polypeptides, glycoproteins, and low-molecular-weight compounds.They can also be classified as protein and nonprotein compounds. Proteins, which account for most of the toxic manifestations, make up 90% to 95% of venom. Symptoms can generally be classified as local or systemic. Local effects are usually caused by enzymatic action on the various cellular and noncellular structures in the victim's tissues. These enzymes can cause coagulation, anticoagulation, cell lysis, hemorrhage, hemolysis, and the destruction of nucleic acid, mitochondria, and other organelles.

Polypeptides are structurally smaller and more rapidly absorbed than proteins and may account for the venom's effects on presynaptic and postsynaptic membranes and other organ systems.

Phospholipase A can inhibit electron transfer at the level of cytochrome c and render mitochondrial-bound enzymes soluble. It can hydrolyze phospholipids in nerve axons, break down acetylcholine vesicles at the myoneural junction, cause myonecrosis, and induce lysis of red cell membranes. This single enzyme has been identified in all venoms of Hydrophiidae, Elapidae, Viperidae, and Crotalinae thus far investigated.

Elapidae and Hydrophiidae venoms have predominantly systemic effects, whereas Colubridae, Viperidae, and Crotalinae venoms have mainly local effects.

Venom Delivery

The mechanism for delivering venom is fairly standard among snakes. It consists of two venom glands, hollow or grooved fangs, and ducts connecting the glands to the fangs. The glands, which evolved from salivary glands, are located on each side of the head above the maxillae and behind the eyes. Each gland has an individual muscle and a separate nerve supply that allow the snake to vary the amount of venom injected. The venom duct leads from the anterior portion of the gland along the maxilla to the fangs. Pit vipers have fangs that are large anterior maxillary teeth. These teeth are hollow and rotate outward from a resting position to a striking position. The coral snake has fixed, hollow maxillary teeth that are much smaller than those of pit vipers. The fangs in most snakes are shed and replaced regularly, and it is not unusual to see a snake with double fangs on one or both sides of its mouth.

The snake can control the amount of venom injected. In biting a human, a prey much too large to swallow, the snake may inject little or no venom (a "dry" bite), especially if injured or surprised However, the snake may inject more than 90% of the contents of the gland for the same reasons.

CLINICAL FEATURES

The signs and symptoms of a venomous snakebite vary considerably and depend on many factors. From 30% to 50% of venomous snakebites result in little or no envenomation. A person with impaired cardiovascular, renal, or pulmonary function is less able to cope with even a moderately severe envenomation. Because of these multiple variables, the individual clinical response is the only way to judge the severity of a venomous snakebite. Factors that influence the effects of a snakebite are the age, health, and size of the snake; the relative toxicity of the venom; the condition of the fangs; whether the snake has recently fed or is injured; the size, age, and medical problems of the victim; and the anatomic location of the bite.

Local envenomation, if left untreated, can cause serious systemic problems (e.g., DIC, pulmonary edema, and shock) as the toxic products are absorbed. The victim's autopharmacologic response to the envenomation must also be taken into account. An gE-mediated anaphylactic-type reaction may develop in victims of a previous snakebite when reexposed to the venom. Many venoms contain enzymes that trigger the release of bradykinin, histamine, and serotonin from the patient's cells, which may cause fatal anaphylactoid reactions. A wave of effects ranging from minimal pain to multisystem failure and death can occur over a period of several days.

Infection

Although snakebite envenomation has been stressed here, any bite or puncture wound carries a risk for bacterial contamination. Gram-negative organisms predominate when snake venom and mouthparts are cultured. Prophylactic antibiotics are not indicated for snakebite, tetanus, osteomyelitis, cellulitis, or gas gangrene may occur in cases of snakebite with or without envenomation. This is especially true when a large amount of local tissue destruction has occurred, treatment has been delayed, or inappropriate first aid was attempted.

MANAGEMENT

Out-of-Hospital Care

All snakebites are considered an emergency, and any victim should be medically evaluated. The initial 6 to 8 hr period after a snakebite is critical. During this time, medical therapy can help prevent the morbidity associated with severe envenomation. Effective out-of-hospital care can be important.

Out-of-hospital care is relatively simple if guided by four basic concepts. First, the estimated time until arrival at a medical facility, as well as the skill of the on-scene assistants, must be considered when first aid is instituted. Separate the victim from the snake if possible to prevent further bites. A stick, pole, or other object longer than the snake can be used to move the snake away from the victim or, if necessary, to kill the snake by striking it behind the head. Rapid transportation to a medical facility is the best first aid for a snakebite. Any constricting jewelry or clothing should be removed from an extremity to prevent a tourniquet effect proximal to the swelling.

Second, spread of the venom should be slowed if possible;several methods are known. The patient's excitement and physical activity, movement of the bitten area, alcohol consumption, and greater depth of the bite may increase the spread of venom. Except for the last factor, these issues can be addressed by calming the victim, immobilizing the bitten area with a sling or splint, and not giving anything by mouth. A method of first aid for venomous snakebites that was developed in Australia—the immobilization and compression technique (also called the Commonwealth Serum Laboratory technique)—slows uptake of Elapidae venom and mock venom in humans. The bitten extremity is either wrapped in an elastic bandage or placed in an air splint. In another technique from Australia called the Monash method, a thick pad and bandage are placed over the bite wound and extremity. Both these techniques have similar postulated mechanisms of action: The lymphatic vessels and superficial veins are collapsed, and the proximal spread of venom is slowed. If less than 30 minutes has elapsed since the bite, a constricting band applied tightly enough to impede superficial venous and lymph flow, but not arterial blood flow, may be used. The band is applied loosely enough to admit a finger between the band and the skin after application. It is used with caution to prevent the development of a tourniquet effect under swollen tissue, which may cause more destruction than the snakebite. Incision of bite wounds has no proven efficacy and poses potential danger to underlying structures and therefore is not recommended. The use of ice is not helpful in slowing the spread of venom, but an ice bag wrapped in a towel and applied to the bite area helps relieve pain. Ice water immersion and packing of the extremity in ice are dangerous and only contribute to tissue destruction. The use of suction devices has not been shown to be beneficial.

Third, when feasible, the snake should be identified or brought to the treating facility with the victim, though this should not delay transport of the patient to definitive medical care. Identification of the snake must be done safely—usually only by someone expert in handling snakes. A photo may be useful in identifying the snake if a close-up of the head and tail are included. Care should be taken to not touch the head of the snake because envenomation can occur even after death.

Fourth, additional medical interventions, if available, should be initiated, including cardiac monitoring, intravenous fluids, and analgesics.

Emergency Department Care

Many snakes do not envenomate the victim when they bite, which has provided false support for the historical use of whiskey, clam juice, or split chickens in the treatment of snakebite. The only proven therapy is antivenin. ED care of a snakebite focuses on supportive care and rapid treatment with the appropriate antivenin. Rapid decision-making is required to determine the optimal type, amount, and route of administration of the antivenin. By the time the emergency physician examines a snakebite victim, the venom may have already caused much damage, both locally and systemically. In this case, the emergency physician must be prepared to support the victim's cardiovascular and respiratory systems.

Patient History

Specific historical information includes time elapsed since the bite, the number of bites, whether first aid was administered and what type, location of the bite, and symptoms (e.g., pain, numbness, nausea, tingling around the mouth, metallic taste in the mouth, muscle cramps, dyspnea, and dizziness). A brief medical history includes the last tetanus immunization, medications, and cardiovascular, hematologic, renal, and respiratory problems. An allergy history with emphasis on symptoms after exposure to horse or sheep products, previous injection of horse or sheep serum, and a history of asthma, hay fever, urticaria, or allergy to wool, papain, chymopapain, papaya. Or pineapple should be obtained if antivenin treatment is being considered.

Patient Examination

The bite area is examined for signs of fang marks or scratches and local envenomation (e.g., edema, petechiae, ecchymosis, and bullae). The area distal to the bite is checked for pulses. A general physical examination is performed, with emphasis on the cardiorespiratory system and the neurologic examination, especially if a Mojave rattlesnake, coral snake, or exotic snake is suspected. If the bite involves an extremity, the circumference of the extremity at the site of the bite and approximately 5 inches proximal to the bite should be measured and recorded. These data aid in objectively estimating both spread of the venom and the effect of antienin (Fig. 50-3, see color illustration).

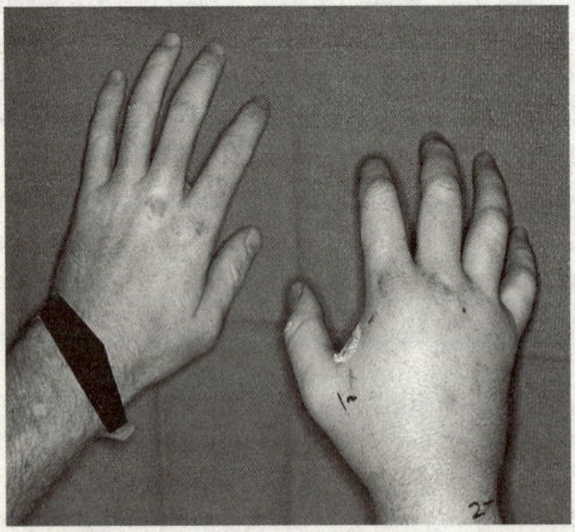

Fig. 50-3 Northern copperhead (Agkistrodon contortrix mokasen) bite on right hand with normal left hand for comparison.

Initial Medical Care

If the bite occurred less than 30 min before arrival in ED, first-aid measures can be instituted, including a constricting band until antivenin, can be obtained. Snakebite victims with clinical evidence of envenomation should have an intravenous line with normal saline placed in an unaffected extremity. An ECG, CBC, urinalysis, protime, and levels of fibrinogen, fibrin split products, electrolytes, blood urea nitrogen, and creatinine are recommended; blood should be typed and crossmatched for 4 U of packed red blood cells.

The patient's vital signs are monitored closely. Snakebite victims may be hypotensive because of third-space losses and hemorrhage. In an edematous extremity, the distal pulse may have to be examined with a Doppler instrument. If a compartment syndrome is suspected, insert a pressure monitor and obtain surgical consultation. If signs and symptoms of compartment syndrome are present, pressure greater than 30 mmHg may necessitate fasciotomy, although there is evidence that administration of antivenin may lower compartment pressures.

Once stabilization is initiated, the severity of the bite must be determined and a decision made regarding whether to administer antivenin. The more distal the bite on the extremity, the less toxicity associated with the bite. Intravenous bites may be rapidly fatal. Bites occurring on the trunk, neck, and face have increased risk because of rapid transit of the venom.

Antivenin

The emergency physician must determine the type of antivenin to administer, how much, and over what period. If the bite is from a pit viper, the problem is not too difficult. Bites from copperheads usually cause a moderate amount of edema but generally do not require antivenin, although it may be indicated in selected cases. Envenomation may be classified according to severity into five grades, from grade 0 (no sign of envenomation) to grade Ⅳ (very severe envenomation). The amount of antivenin to be given is correlated with the grade of envenomation:

- Grade 0 (minimal). There is no evidence of envenomation,but snakebite is suspected. A fang wound may be present.Pain is minimal, with less than 1 inch of surrounding edema and erythema. No systemic manifestations are present during the first 12 hr after the bite. No laboratory changes occur.
- Grade Ⅰ (minimal). There is minimal envenomation, and snakebite is suspected. A fang wound is usually present. Pain is moderate or throbbing and localized to the fang wound, surrounded by 1 to 5 inches of edema and erythema. No evidence of systemic involvement is present after 12 hr of observation. No laboratory changes occur.
- Grade Ⅱ (moderate). There is moderate envenomation, mores evere and widely distributed pain, edema spreading toward the trunk, and petechiae and ecchymoses limited to the area of edema. Nausea, vomiting, and a mild elevation in temperature are usually present.
- Grade Ⅲ (severe). The envenomation is severe. The case may initially resemble a grade Ⅰ or Ⅱ envenomation, but the course is rapidly progressive. Within 12 hr, edema spreads up the extremity and may involve part of the trunk. Petechiae and ecchymoses may be generalized. Systemic manifestations may include tachycardia and hypotension. Laboratory abnormalities may include an elevated WBC count, CPK, prothrombin time, and partial thromboplastin time, as well as elevated fibrin degradation products and D-dimer. Decreased platelets and fibrinogen are common. Hematuria, myoglobinuria, increased bleeding time, and renal or hepatic abnormalities may also occur.
- Grade Ⅳ (very severe). The envenomation is very severe and is seen most frequently after the bite of a large rattlesnake. It is characterized by sudden pain, rapidly progressive swelling that may reach and involve the trunk within a few hours, ecchymoses, bleb formation, and necrosis. Systemic manifestations, often commencing within 15 min of the bite, usually include weakness, nausea, vomiting, vertigo, and numbness or tingling of the lips or face. Muscle fasciculations, painful muscular cramping, pallor, sweating, cold and clammy skin, rapid and weak pulse, incontinence, convulsions, and coma may also be observed. An intravenous bite may result in cardiopulmonary arrest soon after the bite.

Dart and colleagues have advocated slightly different grading systems and higher doses of antivenin: Grades 0 and Ⅰ correspond to minimal envenomation, grade Ⅱ represents moderate envenomation, and grades Ⅲ and Ⅳ correspond to severe envenomation.Either system can be used interchangeably.

Onset of symptoms after a pit viper bite may be delayed andmay involve a variety of neurologic symptoms, including weakness, ptosis, stupor, bulbar paralysis, and other cranial nerve dysfunction, as well as nausea, abdominal pain, and headache.

Administration of Antivenin. Any victim of a venomous snakebite with moderate or severe envenomation is a candidate for antivenin. The choice of antivenin depends on the species of snake, and the antivenin may be horse serum- or sheep-derived Fab fragments. Wyeth Laboratories, producer of the polyvalent horse serum–derived antivenin for Western Hemisphere pit vipers, no longer manufactures that antivenin. Many zoos and hospitals still maintain vials of this antivenin until it can be replaced with the ovine-derived Fab antivenin (FabAV). This antivenin is derived from four species of U.S. pit vipers and has not been clinically studied with regard to bites from Mexican, Central American, or South American pit vipers.

Most antivenin for exotic snakes and the eastern coral snake is derived from horse serum. A recent polyvalent Fab(2) antivenin derived form horse serum and produced in Mexico has been shown to be effective against both North and South American crotalid species. Skin testing was commonly performed before administration of horse serum–derived antivenin, but it is not medically indicated because of the inaccuracy of the test.Moreover, testing with normal horse serum may precipitate an allergic reaction, and even a positive test result may not preclude treatment if a patient has sustained severe envenomation. The incidence of allergic reactions with Fab antivenins has been much less than previously seen with whole IgG. The incidence of allergic reactions was 17% for early reactions and 12% for late reactions in postmarketing analysis. This was thought to be a result of incomplete purification of one lot contaminated by Fc fragments. Most of these reactions were minor and did not require stopping the infusion of the antivenin. The true incidence is unknown.

Dosage and Precautions. Current treatment of pit viper envenomation in the United States is to use a FabAV polyvalent antivenin rather than the horse serum product. This is designed to limit the allergic reactions associated with horse serum antivenin by use of antigen-binding fragments (Fabs) of sheep (ovine) immunized against four species of venomous snake found in the United States. CroFab has been shown to be as effective as the Wyeth antivenin, with fewer allergic reactions. Because of more rapid clearance of smaller Fab fragments by the kidney, however, a repeat-dose regimen must be used to prevent the recurrence of coagulopathy. The duration of action of the venom may be longer than the therapeutic effect of the antivenin. Initial studies have shown promise for a new affinity-purified, mixed monospecific ovine Fab antivenin that has been tested with favorable results in humans after minimal to moderate crotalid envenomation. Its efficacy in pit vipers from South America or Asia has not been proved. Purification of antivenin by separation of active fractions may lead to safer administration of horse serum–derived antivenin. An algorithm has been developed that can aid in decisionmaking after a crotalid bite (Table 50-2 and Fig. 50-4). In the next decade, snakebite management will probably change radically throughout the world. Phytotherapy (botanical therapy) and other nonantivenin drug therapies for snakebite have shown promise in experimental animal studies, and some centers have successfully treated snakebite with medical support only. Hyperbaric oxygen therapy has also been used as an adjunct to antivenin in the treatment of venomous snakebite.

Table 50-2 Antivenin Dosage for Pit Viper Envenomation

ENVENOMATION	*FabAV*	
	INITIAL DOSE TOTAL	MAINTENANCE DOSE
Moderate	4-6 vials	2 vials
Severe	8-12 vials	2-4 vials
Very severe	12-18 vials	4-10 vials

The following are general guidelines to maximize patient care when antivenin is used:

1. Because anaphylaxis may occur whenever antivenin is administered, appropriate therapeutic agents (e.g., oxygen supply, airway support, epinephrine, and other pressors) must be ready for immediate use. Any patient requiring antivenin should have two intravenous lines

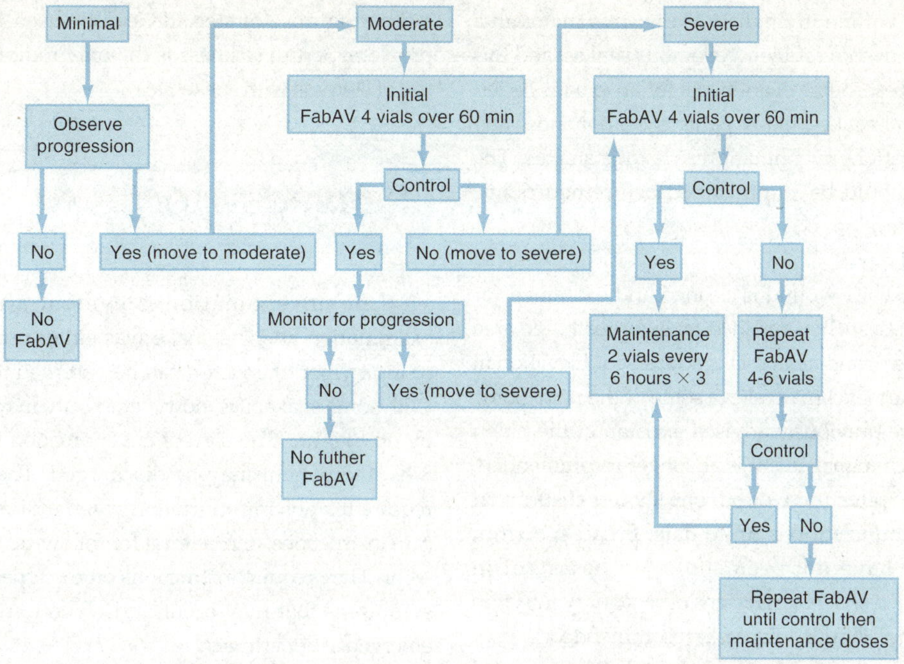

Fig. 50-4 Algorithm for use of FabAV (antivenin).

inserted. If an allergic reaction occurs, the line with the antivenin can be clamped and the other line used for resuscitation. Administration of 0.3 mg of 1 : 1000 epinephrine subcutaneously before administration of antivenin may prevent allergic reactions to horse serum–derived antivenin and, if not contraindicated, should be used. If an allergic reaction occurs, then the epinephrine can be given intramuscularly as needed.

2. The initial dose of antivenin is prepared. The smaller the body of the patient, the larger the relative initial dose that may be required. All antivenin is administered intravenously.
3. Pregnancy is not a contraindication to antivenin therapy.
4. Administration of antivenin at or around the site of the bite is not recommended.
5. The need for subsequent doses is based on the patient's clinical response. The patient is monitored closely after the initial dose, and local and systemic symptoms, as well as laboratory findings, are determinants of the need for further antivenin. Additional injections of one to five vials of antivenin are administered every 1 or 2 hr if symptoms progress. Most pharmacies do not stock large amounts of antivenin, and the pharmacy should be notified to obtain additional antivenin for treating a severe bite.
6. Even with a history or signs of allergy, patients with severe envenomation are treated with a dilute form of antivenin and epinephrine to maximize antivenin administration but minimize allergic symptoms.

Coral and Exotic Snakes. It is recommended that all victims of bites by the eastern coral snake (Micrurus fulvius) be given antivenin even before any symptoms develop. Unfortunately, this antivenin is no longer manufactured by Wyeth, and existing stocks are slowly being depleted. The toxicity of this venom has a rapid onset, and once symptoms develop, it may be too late to reverse the effects with antivenin. The recommended dose is three to five vials in 300 to 500 mL of normal saline. Antivenin is given based on the clinical response. If no antivenin is available, management is based on meticulous supportive care emphasizing the respiratory and neurologic status.

The problems with bites of exotic snakes are threefold: Positive identification of the specimen is sometimes difficult, even for experts; specific antivenin is not always readily available; and even if the antivenin is available, the instructions for reconstitution and dosage may not be written in English. Many zoos maintain a supply of antivenin for their venomous snakes, and this may be the best source of antivenin for an exotic species. As with coral snakes, many patients do not show any early signs after envenomation by exotic snakes. The antivenin should be administered before neurologic symptoms develop.

Wound Care

The snakebite wound is cleaned and examined for foreign bodies, such as retained fangs or teeth, the area is immobilized, and analgesia is addressed. Elevation at or above heart level may relieve some of the pain. Some authors have previously advised excision of the bitten area, but such management is no longer recommended. As with any puncture wound, one should ensure that tetanus immunization is up-to-date. Broad-spectrum antibiotics have not been shown to be useful in uncomplicated snakebites.If signs of secondary infection develop, ampicillin clavulanate is recommended.

Patients admitted to the hospital require serial determinations of platelets, fibrinogen, prothrombin time, and urinalysis every 4 hr to check for myoglobin and hemoglobin. Blood products, including packed red blood cells, fresh frozen plasma, and other coagulation factors, are administered as needed. Usually, it is best to wait until antivenin therapy has been started, or the use of the blood products may be futile. Awake patients who have no nausea or abdominal pain can be given oral fluids. Local wound care includes daily cleansing with soap and water and the application of a sterile dressing to open wounds.

Surgical consultation is recommended for débridement or skin grafting. Débridement should probably not be performed earlier than 3 d after the bite, until the coagulopathy has resolved. Surgical exploration of the bite wound is not necessary and may be harmful. Skin grafts are occasionally necessary after bites by pit vipers that produce large necrotic areas. Fasciotomy is not usually indicated unless compartment pressures are elevated above 30 mm Hg and signs of compartment syndrome are present. Physical therapy is often needed and should begin soon after the acute phase of the envenomation is complete.

Serum Sickness

In most patients who receive more than 10 vials of horse serum–derived antivenin and in approximately 15% of those who receive FabAV, serum sickness develops up to a week later. The administration of diphenhydramine plus cimetidine, and in severe cases a tapering dose of steroids, can be used to treat this problem. Serum sickness is the only indication for the use of steroids with snakebite.

DISPOSITION

If no envenomation is evident after clinical examination and the snake was either nonvenomous or a pit viper, the victim can be observed for 6 to 8 hr. With some snakebites, however,toxicity may be delayed by up to 8 hr. If no sign of envenomation is seen after 8 hs, the patient may be discharged. These patients require tetanus immunization when indicated, wound care instructions, and referral for follow-up within 24 to 48 hr. They require instructions on the types of delayed symptoms that may occur and when to return to the emergency department.

If only local pain and minimal edema have occurred, the patient is closely watched for 12 hr in the emergency department. If the pain and swelling decrease and no systemic symptoms or laboratory abnormalities develop, the patient may be treated with the same precautions as a patient with no signs of envenomation. Any patient with moderate or severe envenomation should be admitted to an intensive care unit for monitoring during antivenin therapy. Depending on the severity of the bite, blood products, vasopressors, and invasive monitoring may be necessary.

Any patient bitten by a coral snake, a Mojave rattlesnake, or an exotic snake is at risk for severe neurologic sequelae that may not become evident for many hours. As a result, these patients require hospital admission, preferably to an intensive care unit where they can be monitored closely. Arrangements should be made to have a ventilator, invasive monitoring, and dialysis equipment available if necessary. Appropriate antivenin should be obtained and treatment initiated at the earliest onset of symptoms. Some experienced clinicians may wait until symptoms develop before administering antivenin. All patients receiving antivenin require close monitoring for recurrence of coagulopathy, which may occur several days after initial envenomation.

(ZHANG Jianfeng)

SECTION 7

Other Emergencies

Chapter 51

Shock Syndrome

KEY CONCEPTS

Shock has been classified into four broad categories based on Blalock's 1934 description: hematologic, neurologic, vasogenic, and cardiogenic.

The three common causes of shock are Hemorrhagic shock, septic shock and cardiogenic shock.

Circulatory shock can occur with normal arterial BP, and not all patients with arterial hypotension have circulatory shock.

Urine output is a reliable index of vital organ perfusion in patients with suspected shock.

Lactate concentration greater than 4.0 mM or a base deficit more negative than −4 mEq/L predicts the presence of circulatory insufficiency severe enough to cause subsequent multiple organ failure.

Ill patients with tachycardia, a worsening base deficit, and low urine output should be diagnosed with circulatory shock.

Patients should be resuscitated within the first 6 hours of care to achieve normalization of markers of preload (CVP) and perfusion (MBP) and adequate oxygen delivery ($ScvO_2$ 70% or lactate clearance 10%).

PERSPECTIVE

Whether shock results from hemorrhage, sepsis, or cardiac failure, mortality rates exceed 20%. When the clinical impression and the quantitative data suggest widespread organ hypoperfusion, emergent resuscitation is used to restore normal tissue oxygenation and substrate delivery to prevent deterioration into systemic inflammation, organ dysfunction, and death.

Classification

Shock has been classified into four broad categories based on Blalock's 1934 description: hematologic, neurologic,vasogenic, and cardiogenic.Box 51-1 outlines five categories of shock that generally have specific mechanisms and treatments.

Box 51-1 Categories of Shock According to Primary Treatment

Causes That Require Primarily the Infusion of Volume

- Hemorrhagic shock
  - Traumatic
  - Gastrointestinal
  - Body cavity
- Hypovolemia
  - Gastrointestinal losses
  - Dehydration from insensible losses
  - Third-space sequestration from inflammation

Causes That Require Improvement in Pump Function

- Myocardial ischemia
  - Coronary artery thrombosis
  - Arterial hypotension with hypoxemia
- Cardiomyopathy
  - Acute myocarditis
  - Chronic diseases of heart muscle (ischemic, diabetic,infiltrative, endocrinologic, congenital)
- Cardiac rhythm disturbances
  - Atrial fibrillation with rapid ventricular response
  - Ventricular tachycardia
  - Supraventricular tachycardia
- Septic shock with myocardial failure ("hypodynamic shock")
- Overdose of negative inotropic drug
  - Beta-blocker
  - Calcium channel antagonist
- Structural cardiac damage
  - Traumatic (e.g., flail mitral valve)
  - Ventriculoseptal rupture
  - Papillary muscle rupture

Causes That Require Volume Support and Vasopressor Support
- Septic shock
- Anaphylactic shock
- Central neurogenic shock
- Drug overdose

Problems That Require Immediate Relief from Obstruction to CO
- Pulmonary embolism
- Cardiac tamponade
- Pneumothorax
- Valvular dysfunction
  - Acute thrombosis of prosthetic valve
  - Critical aortic stenosis
- Congenital heart defects in newborn (e.g., closure of patent ductus arteriosus with critical aortic coarctation)
- Critical idiopathic subaortic stenosis (hypertrophic obstructive cardiomyopathy)

Cellular Poisons That Require Specific Antidotes
- Carbon monoxide
- Methemoglobinemia
- Hydrogen sulfide
- Cyanide

Specific Causes

Hemorrhagic Shock

Hemorrhagic shock results from a rapid reduction in blood volume.Responses of HR and BP are notoriously variable in hemorrhage.Blood loss causes the pulse pressure to narrow. As blood loss continues, ventricular filling decreases and cardiac output drops,followed by a reduction in SBP. Consequently, acidemia will often precede any significant decrease in cardiac output with hemorrhage.A normal base deficit is more positive than −2 mEq/L. Accordingly, the arterial and venous blood base deficit can become more negative early in hemorrhage even while blood pH and BP remain in the normal range. The base deficit, therefore, crudely represents the physiologic endpoint that distinguishes trivial blood loss from clinically significant hemorrhage.After approximately one third of the total blood volume has been acutely lost, cardiovascular reflexes can no longer sustain adequate filling of the arterial circuit and frank hypotension supervenes. Hemorrhagic shock causes an activation of the hypothalamic-pituitary-adrenomedullary axis, with release of stress hormones that cause glycogenolysis, lipolysis, and mild hypokalemia.Patients who have sustained traumatic hemorrhage generally have an arterial lactate concentration greater than 4.0 mmol/L, a P_aCO_2 less than 35 mm Hg, and mild hyperglycemia (150-170 mg/dL) and hypokalemia (3.5-3.7 mEq/L).

The second phase of organ injury from hemorrhagic shock occurs during resuscitation. During resuscitation, neutrophils become most aggressive, binding to the lung endothelium and causing capillary leaks that characterize ARDS. Inflammatory cytokines are liberated during resuscitation, and membrane injury occurs in many cells.During resuscitation from hemorrhagic shock, the normal balance of vasodilation by NO versus vasoconstriction by endothelins becomes distorted, producing patchy centrilobular ischemic damage in the liver, which may produce an immediate rise in blood transaminase levels.Depending on the degree of hypotensive insult, the kidney may manifest acute spasm of the preglomerular arterioles, causing acute tubular necrosis. Systemic metabolic changes can impair fuel delivery to the heart and brain, secondary to depressed hepatic glucose output, impaired hepatic ketone production, and inhibited peripheral lipolysis.

Septic Shock

Septic shock can be produced by infection with any microbe.Infusion of lipopolysaccharide into humans or animals will produce cardiovascular, immunologic, and inflammatory changes.Two lines of reasoning suggest that gram-positive sepsis in hospitalized patients will continue to increase in prevalence:

1. More patients are being treated at home for chronic immunocompromising diseases with indwelling catheters.
2. The frequency of community-acquired infections caused by antibiotic-resistant gram-positive organisms has greatly increased in recent years, including infections caused by S. aureus, Streptococcus pneumoniae, and Streptococcus pyogenes.

Septic shock often causes three major effects that must be addressed during resuscitation: relative hypovolemia, cardiovascular depression, and induction of systemic inflammation. Septic shock produces relative hypovolemia from increased venous capacitance.Septic shock often causes absolute hypovolemia from gastrointestinal volume losses, tachypnea, sweating, and decreased ability to drink during development of the illness. Sepsis also induces capillary leak, which leads to relative loss of intravascular volume into third spaces.Septic shock causes myocardial depression simultaneously with vasodepression and capillary leak. Multiple mechanisms may explain depressed heart function in sepsis,including actions of specific cytokines,overproduction of NO, and possibly impairment in mitochondrial oxidative phosphorylation coincident with reduced mechanical efficiency. Evidence indicates that circulating mediators, myocardial cellular injury from inflammation, and deranged metabolism interact synergistically to injure the heart during septic shock. Systemic inflammation causes capillary leak in the lung, which may cause alveolar infiltration characteristic of ARDS early in the treatment of septic shock.With the potential for early development of ARDS, more profound ventilation-perfusion ($\dot{V}/\dot{Q}$) mismatching, and pneumonia or pulmonary aspiration, hypoxemia is more severe with septic shock than hemorrhagic shock.

Cardiogenic Shock

Cardiogenic shock results when more than 40% of the myocardium undergoes necrosis from ischemia, inflammation, toxins, or immune destruction.Patients with severe dysfunction are far more likely to have a cardiogenic cause of shock.

CLINICAL FEATURES

In general, patients with shock exhibit a stress response: they are ill appearing, asthenic, pale, often sweating, and usually tachypneic or grunting, and often have a weak and rapid pulse (Box 51-2).BP initially can be normal because of adrenergic reflexes. A single systolic BP less than 100 mm Hg in the ED is associated with a threefold increase in in-hospital mortality and a tenfold increase in sudden and unexpected death.The HR/SBP ratio may provide a better marker of shock than either measurement alone; a normal ratio is less than 0.8. Urine output provides an excellent indicator of organ perfusion.

lactate concentration greater than 4.0 mM or a base deficit more negative than −4 mEq/L predicts the presence of circulatory insufficiency severe enough to cause subsequent multiple organ failure. Fig. 51-1 shows a potential sequence of decisions to help arrive at a diagnosis in a patient with undifferentiated shock.

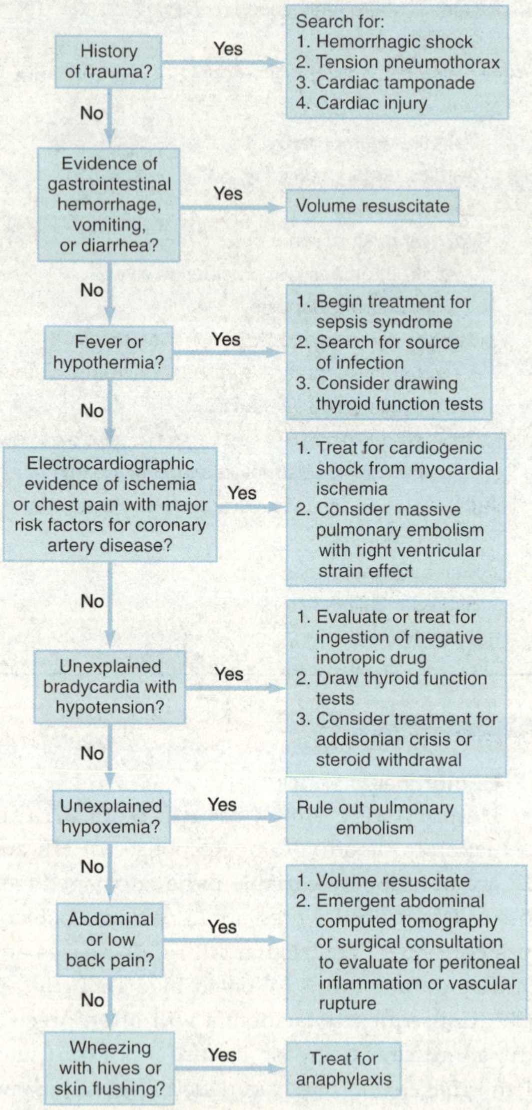

Fig. 51-1 Flow diagram to classify undifferentiated shock.

Box 51-2 Empirical Criteria for Diagnosis of Circulatory Shock

- Ill appearance or altered mental status
- Heart rate >100 beats/min
- Respiratory rate >20 breaths/min or P_aCO_2 <32 mm Hg
- Arterial base deficit <−4 mEq/L or lactate >4 mM/L
- Urine output <0.5 mL/kg/hr
- Arterial hypotension >30 continuous minutes duration

On physical examination, dry mucous membranes suggest dehydration,whereas distended jugular veins suggest cardiac failure or obstruction from PE or cardiac tamponade. Muffed heart sounds suggest cardiac tamponade, whereas a loud machine-like systolic murmur indicates acute rupture of a papillary muscle or rupture of the interventricular septum. Bilateral pulmonary rales in a patient with a normal rectal temperature help to define presence of primary left ventricular failure. Wheezing suggests bronchospasm from anaphylaxis. Abdominal tenderness may indicate peritoneal infammation or occult trauma. Rectal examination may disclose occult gastrointestinal hemorrhage. Rectal temperature is the preferred method for measuring temperature.

Neurologic examination documents responsiveness, cognition, and the presence of any focal deficits.

Laboratory, radiographic, and other ancillary data should be ordered to assess tissue and vital organ perfusion and to diagnose injury from trauma, find the source of infection with sepsis, or identify the cause of cardiac failure. A chest radiograph, ECG, finger-stick glucose measurement,CBC, urinalysis, serum electrolytes, and kidney and liver function tests are all indicated in the ED assessment. ABG are ordered for a base deficit calculation and to correlate arterial gas tensions (P_aO_2 and P_aCO_2) with those measured by pulse oximetry and capnography. Serum lactate measurement should be performed as early as possible in patients with suspected shock. Cardiac and abdominal bedside ultrasound scanning can screen for inadequate central venous volume, occult hemoperitoneum, abdominal aortic aneurysm, left ventricular failure, and cardiac tamponade. Consensus definitions of shock show the spectrum of hypoperfusion for the following three common causes of shock (Box 51-3):

1. Septic shock.Box 51 -4 provides a list of variables that can assist with detecting tissue hypoperfusion.
2. Hemorrhagic shock.A more useful approach defines hemorrhagic shock as being present when systemic hypoperfusion manifests as lactic acidosis with organ dysfunction.
3. Cardiogenic shock. Cardiogenic shock should be thought to be present whenever cardiac failure (ischemic, toxic, or obstructive) causes systemic hypoperfusion that manifests as lactic acidosis with organ dysfunction.

Box 51-3 Definitions and Criteria for Septic, Hemorrhagic, and Cardiogenic Shock

Septic Shock

SIRS

Two or more of the following:

1. Temperature >38℃ or <36℃
2. Heart rate >90 beats/min
3. Respiratory rate >20 breaths/min or P_aCO_2 <32 mmHg
4. White blood cell count >12,000/mm^3, <4000/mm^3, or >10% band neutrophilia

Severe Sepsis

SIRS with suspected or confirmed infection and associated with organ dysfunction or hypotension; organ dysfunction may include presence of lactic acidosis, oliguria, or altered mental status

Septic Shock

SIRS with suspected or confirmed infection with hypotension despite adequate fluid resuscitation; septic shock should still be diagnosed if vasopressor therapy has normalized blood pressure

Hemorrhagic Shock

Simple Hemorrhage

Suspected bleeding with pulse <100 beats/min, normal respiratory rate, normal blood pressure, and normal base deficit

Hemorrhage with Hypoperfusion

Suspected bleeding with base deficit <-4 mEq/L *or* persistent pulse >100 beats/min

Hemorrhagic Shock

Suspected bleeding with at least four criteria listed in Box 51-2

Cardiogenic Shock

Cardiac Failure

Clinical evidence of impaired forward flow of the heart,including presence of dyspnea, tachycardia, pulmonary edema,peripheral edema, or cyanosis

Cardiogenic Shock

Cardiac failure plus four criteria listed in Box 51-2

Box 51-4 Variables Indicating Tissue Hypoperfusion

Hypotension

Tachycardia

Low cardiac output

Mottled skin

Delayed capillary refill

Altered mental state
Hyperlactemia
Low mixed venous oxygen saturation
Low central venous oxygen saturation

MANAGEMENT

Monitoring Perfusion Status

In all patients with shock, HR, BP, and oxyhemoglobin saturation are continuously monitored. Cuff sphygmomanometer measurement of BP may be inaccurate in severe hypotensive states, and insertion of an arterial pressure monitoring line should considered.Urine output should be measured as an index of vital organ perfusion (0.5-1 mL/kg/hr in persons without preexisting renal disease).Patients with cardiac failure or renal failure may benefit from closer measurement of dynamic variables of fluid responsiveness that can be measured from an arterial line (such as stroke volume variation or stroke volume index) or a central venous line (CVP).

Quantitative Resuscitation

Quantitative resuscitation (also called *goal-directed therapy, goaloriented resuscitation*, or *hemodynamic optimization*) was first described in 1988.The *lactate clearance* refers to serial measurements of venous or arterial lactate and is calculated according to the following formula:

$$[(\text{Lactate}_{\text{initial}} - \text{Lactate}_{\text{delayed}})/\text{Lactate}_{\text{initial}}]\times 100$$

Lactate clearance has been shown to be equivalent to central venous oxygen saturation as an endpoint of early septic shock resuscitation. If the lactate concentration has not decreased by 10% to 20% 2 hr after resuscitation has begun, additional steps are undertaken to improve systemic perfusion. Resuscitation should continue until the lactate concentration drops below 2 mM/L.In such an approach, patients are resuscitated within the first 6 hr of care to achieve normalization of markers of preload (CVP) and perfusion (mean BP) and adequate oxygen delivery ($ScvO_2$ 70% or lactate clearance 10%) (Fig. 51-2). The most well-known quantitative resuscitation strategy, termed *early goal-directed therapy*, has also been found effective in patients with sepsis.

Ventilation

Rapid sequence intubation is the preferred method of airway control in most patients with refractory shock. Intubation prevents aspiration, increases oxygenation, treats acute respiratory failure, provides initial treatment for metabolic or hypercarbic acidemia, and protects the patient who will be sent to an uncontrolled environment (e.g., for tests). More important, if the patient has increased airway resistance (e.g., bronchospasm with anaphylaxis) or a decrease in lung compliance (e.g., pulmonary edema, ARDS), a more negative intrathoracic pressure must be generated to fill the lungs with each inspiration. Positive-pressure ventilation removes this impedance and can improve ventricular function and CO up to 30%.

Volume Replacement

The CVP is most often used to estimate right ventricular filling pressure.

Treating Specific Causes

Box 51-5 presents the general treatment approach for the three common causes of shock.

Box 51-5 Clinical Management Guidelines for Three Common Causes of Shock

Hemorrhagic Shock

- Ensure adequate ventilation and oxygenation.
- Provide immediate control of hemorrhage, when possible (e.g., traction for long bone fractures, direct pressure).
- Initiate judicious infusion of isotonic crystalloid solution (10-20 mL/kg).
- With evidence of poor organ perfusion and 30 min anticipated delay to hemorrhage control, begin PRBC infusion (5-10 mL/kg).
- With suspected central nervous system trauma or Glasgow Coma Scale score $<$9, immediate PRBC transfusion may be preferable as initial resuscitation fluid.
- Treat coincident dysrhythmias (e.g., atrial fibrillation with synchronized cardioversion).

Cardiogenic Shock

- Ameliorate increased work of breathing; provide oxygen and PEEP for pulmonary edema.

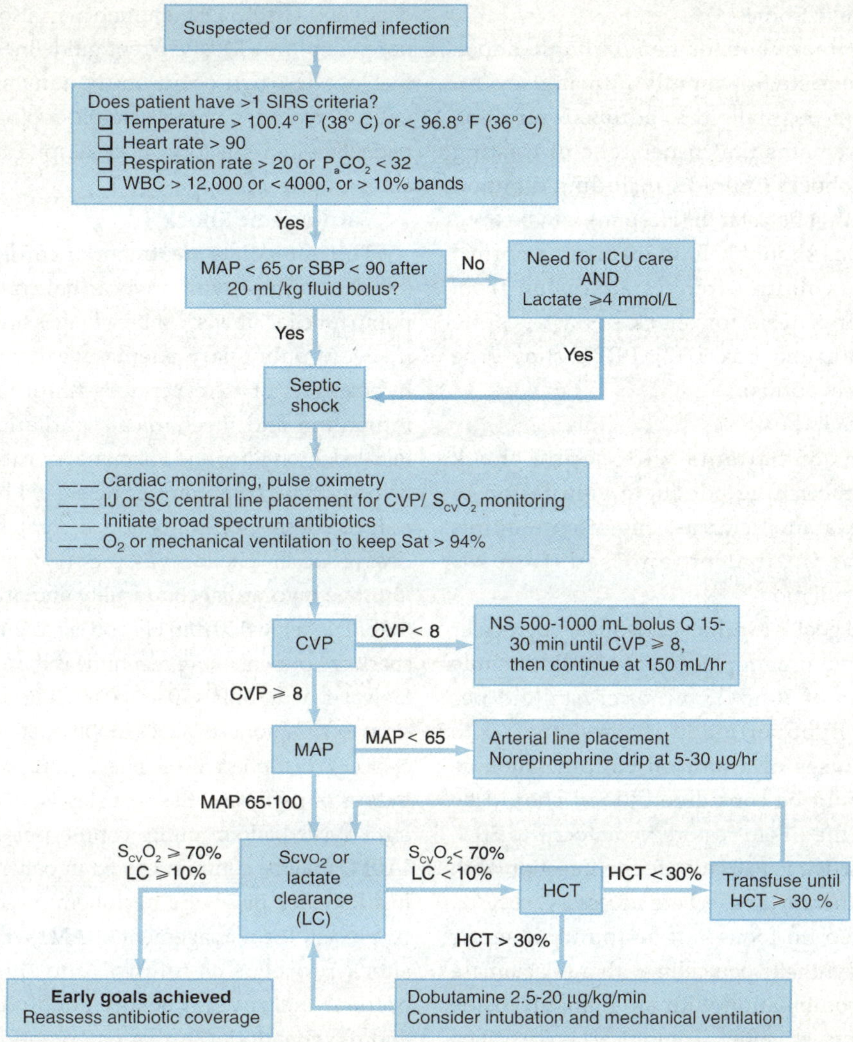

Fig. 51-2 Flow diagram outlining the protocol for quantitative resuscitation in treatment of patients with severe sepsis or septic shock. This protocol outlines specific hemodynamic and physiologic parameters the clinician should seek to achieve within the first 6 hr of care. This protocol is focused on resuscitation and should be used in conjunction with standard clinical care for patients with suspected infection, such as appropriate diagnostic studies to determine the focus of infection and appropriate antimicrobial agents to treat the infection.

- Begin vasopressor or inotropic support; norepinephrine (0.5 μg/min) and dobutamine (5 μg/kg/min) are common empirical agents.
- Seek to reverse the insult (e.g., initiate thrombolysis, arrange percutaneous transluminal angioplasty).
- Consider intra-aortic balloon pump counterpulsation for refractory shock.

Septic Shock

- Ensure adequate oxygenation; remove work of breathing.
- Administer 20 mL of crystalloid per kilogram or 5 mL of colloid per kilogram, and titrate infusion to adequate central venous pressure and urine output.
- Begin antimicrobial therapy; attempt surgical drainage or débridement.
- Begin PRBC infusion for hemoglobin <8 g/dL.
- If volume restoration fails to improve organ perfusion, begin vasopressor support; initial choice includes dopamine,infused at 5-15 μg/kg/min, or norepinephrine, infused at 0.5 μg/min.

Hemorrhagic Shock

Standard treatment for hemorrhagic shock historically consisted of rapidly infusing several liters of isotonic crystalloid in adults.Controlling hemorrhage remains the cornerstone of treating hemorrhagic shock. Colloids, including albumin and hydroxyethyl hetastarch (Hespan), can be used as well. Colloids should help to maintain a normal intravascular volume after retransfusion from hemorrhage.If criteria for shock persist despite crystalloid infusion (Box 51-2), PRBC should be infused (1-2 U in adults).

Septic Shock

Treatment of patients with septic shock begins by establishing adequate ventilation to correct hypoxia and acidosis.This often requires endotracheal intubation and sedation for mechanical ventilation.

The second goal is to achieve adequate ventricular filling. Initial volume replacement should include rapid infusion of 20 to 25 mL of crystalloid per kilogram. If hypoperfusion is persistent, 5 to 10mL/kg boluses of a natural colloid (such as albumin) should be considered.Blood should be transfused in the ED to restore hematocrit to 30%. The third directive is to eradicate the infection with antimicrobial therapy and, where necessary, surgical drainage.When no focus can be found in septic shock, a semisynthetic penicillin with a β-lactamase inhibitor, in combination with an aminoglycoside plus vancomycin, is a rational empirical choice. When neutropenia is suspected in a patient with sepsis syndrome, fatal septic shock can be cataclysmic. Septic shock refractory to volume restoration (urine output or BP remains low; lactate increases) requires vasopressor support. Norepinephrine (0.5-30 μg/min) is associated with improved efficacy and lower rates of adverse effects. Dobutamine may also be used with norepinephrine.Most current guidelines recommend that low-dose hydrocortisone be administered only to patients receiving chronic steroid replacement and in patients with refractory shock despite adequate fluid and vasopressor support.

Cardiogenic Shock

The immediate treatment of cardiogenic shock focuses on improving myocardial contractility and pump function. If work of breathing is tiring the patient, if severe pulmonary edema is causing significant hypoxemia, or if respiratory failure is imminent, intubation and mechanical ventilation should be initiated. Etomidate and ketamine have the least risk for hemodynamic compromise and should be used (but in reduced doses) for intubation, accompanied by a full dose of succinylcholine. Vasopressor or inotropic agents improve myocardial contractility and arteriolar tone.If the SBP is below 100 mm Hg and signs and symptoms of shock are present, norepinephrine is the agent of choice. However, if the SBP is 70 to 100 mm Hg and there are no signs or symptoms of shock, dobutamine is the agent of choice. When pharmacologic support fails to improve indices of perfusion, the next step is to initiate initiate intra-aortic balloon pump counterpulsation(IABPC). IABPC may be contraindicated in patients with aortic insufficiency or severe peripheral vascular disease. At present the management of AMI with cardiogenic shock proceeds as follows, and this constitutes optimal therapy: (1) ensure adequate ventilation and oxygenation, (2) treat emergent dysrhythmias, (3) initiate vasopressor or inotropic support, (4) administer aspirin if the patient is not allergic, and (5) initiate heparin anticoagulation and arrangement for emergent PCI.

(CHAI Yanfen)

Chapter 52

Sepsis Syndromes

KEY CONCEPTS

Sepsis is a progression of disease due to a dysregulated inflammatory cascade, leading to organ dysfunction and circulatory compromise in severe cases.

Elders, immunocompromised and neutropenic patients, and patients with multiple comorbidities are at increased risk for development of sepsis syndromes.

Treatment should focus on (1) improvement of tissue perfusion, (2) improvement of tissue oxygenation, (3) administration of appropriate antibiotics, and (4) early identification of infections requiring surgical management.

PERSPECTIVE

Background

Sepsis syndrome represents the body's host response to an infection.Tachycardia, tachypnea, fever, and immune system activation are common manifestations. If the body is unable to overcome this insult, cellular injury, tissue damage, shock, MOF, or death may ensue.

SIRS is defined as two or more of the following: tachycardia, tachypnea, hyperthermia or hypothermia, high or low white blood cell count, or bandemia; sepsis is the combination of infection plus SIRS; severe sepsis plus organ dysfunction; and septic shock is severe sepsis plus hypotension, defined as a SBP below 90 mm Hg, not responsive to a fluid challenge (Box 52-1).

Box 52-1 Definitions of Sepsis

Bacteremia (fungemia): presence of viable bacteria (fungi) in the blood, as evidenced by positive blood cultures

Systemic inflammatory response syndrome (SIRS): at least two of the following conditions: (1) oral temperature of >38℃or <35℃, (2) respiratory rate of >20 breaths/min or partial pressure of arterial carbon dioxide (P_aCO_2) of <32 mm Hg, (3) heart rate of >90 beats/min, (4) leukocyte count of >12,000/dL or <4000/dL or >10% bands

Sepsis: SIRS that has a proven or suspected microbial source

Severe sepsis: sepsis with one or more signs of organ dysfunction, hypoperfusion, or hypotension, such as metabolic acidosis, acute alteration in mental status, oliguria, or acute respiratory distress syndrome

Septic shock: sepsis with hypotension that is unresponsive to fluid resuscitation plus organ dysfunction or perfusion abnormalities as listed for severe sepsis

Multiple organ dysfunction syndrome: dysfunction of more than one organ, requiring intervention homeostasis

Culture-negative and culture-positive septic populations have similar outcomes in patients with similar severity of illness.Pneumonia, abdominal abscess with viscus perforation, and pyelonephritis are common primary causes of sepsis. Gram-positive organisms account for 25% to 50% of infections, gram-negative organisms for 30% to 60%, and fungi for 2% to 10%.

Elders and those with multiple comorbidities are overwhelmed more easily by systemic infection. Chemotherapy-induced neutropenia,acquired immunodeficiency syndrome, and steroid dependency increase susceptibility to sepsis. Increased use of indwelling devices contributes to the risk of systemic infection and sepsis.

Epidemiology

It is estimated that 571,000 cases of severe sepsis present to U.S. ED each year.Mortality rates from sepsis are estimated between 20% and 50%.The incidence of sepsis as a reason for hos-pitalization is rising disproportionately among elders compared with the young (Fig. 52-1).Respiratory and genitourinary infections are the most common causes of sepsis.

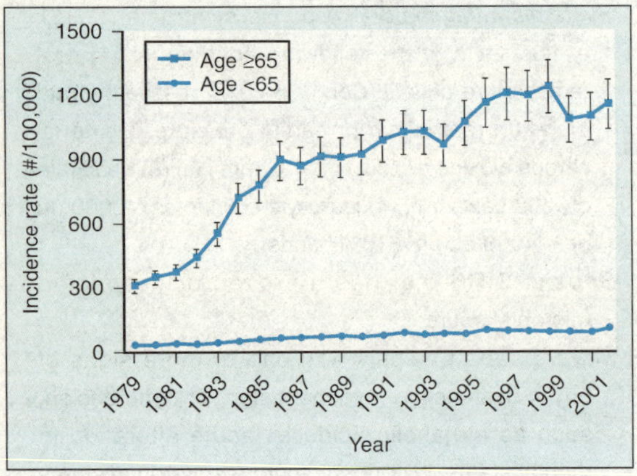

Fig. 52-1 Incidence of disease in young and old over time.

PRINCIPLES OF DISEASE

Pathophysiology

More than 30% of patients with sepsis do not have a definite microbiologic diagnosis.The initial host response is to mobilize inflammatory cells, particularly neutrophils and macrophages, to the site of infection. These inflammatory cells then release circulating molecules, including cytokines, which trigger a cascade of other inflamma-tory mediators that result in a coordinated host response.If these mediators are not appropriately regulated, sepsis will occur. In the setting of ongoing toxin release, a persistent inflammatory response occurs with ongoing mediator activation, cellular hypoxia, tissue injury, shock, MOF, and potentially death.

Mediators of Sepsis

Host response and pathogen characteristics are both important in the pathogenesis of sepsis. More than 100 discrete markers have been identified and attributed to the sepsis cascade.

The resulting host-pathogen interaction activates the inflammatory and coagulation cascades. The subsequent inflammatory signaling occurs through cytokines, chemokines, and other soluble mediators, including increased circulating levels of the interleukins interleukin (IL)-1, IL-6, and IL-8 and tumor necrosis factor alpha (TNF-α). Activation of the clotting cascade results in increased D-dimer levels and decreased circulating levels of protein C.

Coagulation and fibrinolytic components are proinflammatory, precipitating a worsening cycle of procoagulant and proinflammatory mediators. This cascade ultimately creates endorgan damage and DIC. If it is not effectively reversed, the process leads to cellular hypoxia, organ dysfunction, shock, and death.

The main proinflammatory cytokines are IL-1, TNF, and IL-8. The primary anti-inflammatory cytokines are IL-10, IL-6, transforming growth factor beta, soluble receptors to TNF, and IL-1 receptor antagonist (IL-1RA). If the resultant inflammatory response is adequate, the infection is controlled and cleared.If the response is deficient or excessive, however, a persistent and worsening cascade is produced, ultimately leading to shock, organ failure, and potentially death.

The hormone is stored in the pituitary gland and released in response to stressors such as pain, hypoxia, hypovolemia, and hyperosmolality.In severe sepsis, there is a brief rise in circulating vasopressin levels followed by a prolonged and severe suppression.Vasopressin has numerous physiologic effects, including vasoconstriction of the systemic vasculature, osmoregulation, and maintenance of normovolemia.

NO is a gas that has an important role in septic shock, regulating vascular tone by an indirect effect on smooth muscle cells. NO also contributes to platelet adhesion, insulin secretion, neurotransmission, tissue injury, and inflammation and cytotoxicity.Enhanced NO production is thought to contribute to the profound vasodilation found in patients in septic shock. NO seems to be a key mediator of sepsis.

In the setting of ongoing inflammatory activation, the mediators of sepsis continue to be produced and the cascade is perpetuated,the ultimate effect is a sequence of events starting with cellular dysfunction and ultimately leading to tissue damage, organ dysfunction, and death.

Organ System Dysfunction

The organ dysfunction that results from sepsis is central to the pathogenesis of the disease.The mortality rate was 9% for those patients with severe sepsis (sepsis plus organ dysfunction) and 28% for those with septic shock. The risk of death from sepsis approximately doubles for each organ that fails. The mortality rate for patients with no organ dysfunctions was 1%; rates for dysfunction of a single organ, two organs, three organs, and four or more organs were 6%, 13%, 26%, and 53%, respectively (Fig. 52-2B).

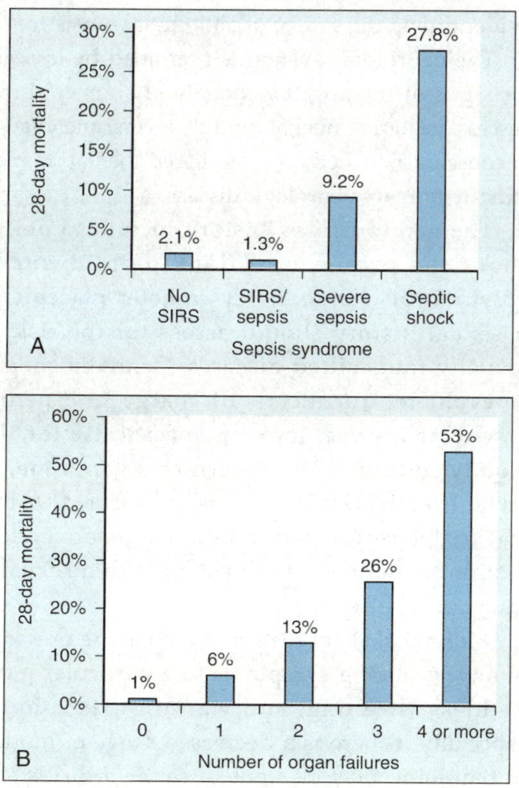

Fig. 52-2 Mortality rates by sepsis syndrome (A) and number of organ dysfunctions (B).

Neurologic

Patients with sepsis often display neurologic impairment manifested by altered mental status and lethargy, commonly referred to as septic encephalopathy. The incidence has been reported between 10% and 70%. The mortality rate in patients with septic encephalopathy is higher than that in septic patients without significant neurologic involvement.

Cardiovascular

Profound cardiovascular dysfunction is common with sepsis. The cardiovascular dysfunction and failure arise from both direct myocardial depression and distributive shock. Early in sepsis, a hyperdynamic state develops, characterized by increased cardiac output and decreased systemic vascular resistance.Much of the cardiovascular compromise from septic shock is reversible, and normal cardiovascular function usually returns within 10 d.

Pulmonary

The lung is an early victim of the inflammatory response to sepsis.Early infiltration with neutrophils, surfactant dysfunction, and edema later give way to monocyte infiltration and fibrosis. Significant right-to-left shunting, arterial hypoxemia, and intractable hypoxemia occur.

At the same time, airway resistance is increased and muscle function is impaired.ARDS is defined clinically (Box 52-2) and correlates with the pathologic finding of diffuse alveolar damage. The development of ARDS occurs 4 to 24 hr after radiographic abnormalities develop. Because of alveolar-capillary membrane damage, fluid accumulates in the alveoli.

Box 52-2 Definition of Acute Respiratory Distress Syndrome

- Impaired oxygenation, defined as a ratio of partial pressure of arterial oxygen to fractional inspired oxygen <200, irrespective of how much positive end-expiratory pressure is used
- Bilateral pulmonary infiltrates on frontal chest radiograph
- Pulmonary artery occlusion pressure ≤18 mm Hg or no clinical evidence of elevated left atrial pressures

Gastrointestinal

A shock state causes significant deleterious effects on a hollow viscus and its oxygen supply. A prolonged ileus accompanies hypoperfusion and persists beyond the perfusion deficit.

Solid organ involvement is also common.

Elevations in aminotransferases and bilirubin are common early in sepsis.Some of the mediators of sepsis are produced by the liver.

Endocrine

An absolute or relative adrenal insufficiency is common in sepsis.TNF-$\alpha$and corticostatin depress pituitary function. Other factors that may contribute to adrenal insufficiency in sepsis include decreased blood flow to the adrenal cortex, decreased pituitary function, and decreased pituitary secretion of adrenocorticotropic hormone due to severe stress.

Hematologic

Sepsis causes abnormalities in many parts of the coagulation system.Pathologic activation of the extrinsic (tissue factor dependent) pathway, protein C–protein S, and fibrinolysis lead to consumption of essential factors, causing DIC. The activation of the coagulation cascade produces fibrin deposition and microvascular thrombi.Tissue factor expression on monocytes is increased. This results in fibrin deposition and perhaps contributes to an increased incidence of MOF due to microvascular thrombi.

Protein C has been identified as an important modulator of both inflammation and coagulation in patients with sepsis.It is possible that protein C activation in early sepsis is impaired because of an inflammatory cytokine–mediated downregulation of thrombo-modulin. As a result, a consumptive coagulopathy ensues. This leads to increased fibrin deposition and a resulting upregulation of the fibrinolytic pathway as identified by low plasma levels of the fibrinolytic proteins and increased fibrin split products. This sequence of events leads to consumption of coagulation factors and DIC. In late sepsis, the fibrinolytic system is suppressed.

CLINICAL FEATURES

Symptoms and Signs

The septic patient manifests signs of systemic infection through tachycardia, tachypnea, hyperthermia or hypothermia, and hypotension. A septic patient will often have flushed skin with warm. The patient with an advanced shock state may appear mottled and cyanotic. Very early in the patient's presentation, vital sign changes such as tachycardia and tachypnea may be the only early indicators of sepsis.

Physical examination should also include detailed evaluation for focal infection, such as exudative tonsillitis, sinus tenderness, tympanic membrane injection, and crackles or dullness on lung auscultation.

The gastrointestinal system is the second most common source of sepsis. A history of abdominal pain, including its description, location, timing, and modifying factors, should be sought. Further history, including the time of the last bowel movement and the presence of nausea, vomiting, and diarrhea, should be noted.Looking for signs of peritoneal irritation, abdominal tenderness, and hyperactive or hypoactive bowel sounds, is critical in identifying the source of abdominal sepsis.

The neurologic system is examined by looking for signs of meningitis, encephalitis, or epidural abscess, including nuchal rigidity, fevers, and change in consciousness.Lethargy or altered mentation may indicate primary neurologic disease.

The genitourinary history includes queries about the presence of flank pain, dysuria, polyuria, discharge, Foley catheter placement. A sexual history should assess for the risk of sexually transmitted diseases. Genitalia should be evaluated for ulcers, discharge, and penile or vulvar lesions, looking specifically for the woody induration of Fournier's gangrene. A rectal examination should be performed. A red and friable cervix, cervical discharge, or cervical motion tenderness is consistent with a sexually transmitted disease.

Musculoskeletal history includes the presence of any localizing symptoms to a particular joint. Redness, swelling, and warmth over a joint, especially if there is a decreased range of motion in that joint, may be signs of septic arthritis and may mandate arthrocentesis. A patient should be completely exposed and the skin examined for evidence of cellulitis, abscess, wound infection, or traumatic injury.Back pain and fever are concerning for an epidural abscess. Local lymphadenopathy, swelling, and streaking should also be noted as signs of an advancing infection. Petechiae and purpura may represent a Neisseria meningitides infection or DIC.

The clinician should suspect endocarditis in the presence of a murmur or other stig-mata of endocarditis (e.g., splinter hemorrhages, Roth's spots, Janeway's lesions).

The Mortality in ED Sepsis (MEDS) prediction rule assigns point values to specific clinical characteristics (Table 52-1). The total score can be used to assess risk of death.

Table 52-1 Mortality in Emergency Department Sepsis (MEDS) Prediction Rule

RISK FACTOR	ODDS RATIO FOR DEATH	MEDS SCORE
Terminal illness (death within 30 days)	6.1	6 points
Tachypnea or hypoxia	2.7	3 points
Septic shock	2.7	3 points
Platelet count < 150,000/mm^3	2.5	3 points
Bands > 5%	2.3	3 points
Age > 65 years	2.2	3 points
Pneumonia	1.9	2 points
Nursing home resident	1.9	2 points
Altered mental status	1.6	2 points

RISK OF DEATH	TOTAL MEDS SCORE (% OF SEPSIS DEATHS
Very low	0-4 (1.1%)
Low	5-7 (4.4%)
Moderate	8-12 (9.3%)
High	13-15 (16.1%)
Very high	>15 (39%)

DIAGNOSTIC STRATEGIES

Hematology

WBC count is a marker of inflammation and activation of the inflammatory cascade. Leukocytosis is associated with infection; however, it is often insensitive and nonspecific. A bandemia (≥10% bands on a peripheral smear) is an imperfect indicator of infection.Platelets are an acute-phase reactant and may be elevated in the presence of infection. Conversely, a low platelet count is a significant predictor of bacteremia in patients with shock. Thrombocytopenia, elevated prothrombin time, elevated activated partial thromboplastin time(APTT), decreased fibrinogen, and increased fibrin split products are associated with DIC and severe sepsis syndrome.

Chemistry

Low bicarbonate level suggests acidosis and inadequate perfusion. An elevated AG acidosis in the setting of sepsis syndrome commonly represents lactic acidosis or DKA. Elevated serum creatinine concentration or decreased GFR signals renal dysfunction or failure, which indicates organ failure and a worse prognosis.

An elevated lactate level is associated with inadequate perfusion, shock, and poorer prognosis. Liver function tests can be used to identify liver failure or dysfunction. An elevated bilirubin level may suggest the gallbladder as a cause of sepsis. An elevated lipase level may represent pancreatitis as the cause of noninfectious SIRS.

Microbiology

Culture samples should be obtained before or soon after the administration of antibiotics in the patient with sepsis syndrome.

Special Procedures

A CVP line may guide fluid resuscitation, with a low CVP indicating the need for continued fluid repletion. The $ScvO_2$ monitor measures venous blood saturation,keeping the $ScvO_2$ greater than 70%. An arterial line can be useful for close monitoring of hypotensive patients.Swan-Ganz catheter for physiologic measurements may be useful in identifying the cause of shock and guiding fluid and inotropic therapy. Low systemic vascular resistance and high cardiac output are most commonly associated with sepsis.

Radiology

A chest radiograph should be obtained in all patients with suspected sepsis syndrome,bilateral infiltrates indicative of ARDS.

CT of superficial infections may be helpful to

further quantify the extent of infection and to identify abscesses. A CT scan of the abdomen and pelvis may identify abdominal or pelvic pathologic lesions. A head CT scan can identify septic emboli from endocarditis or increased intracranial pressure from a mass and should be considered before a lumbar puncture is performed. An abdominal ultrasound examination may be indicated for suspected cholecystitis, and a pelvic ultrasound examination for tuboovarian abscess or endometritis.MRI can be useful to identify soft tissue infection, such as necrotizing fasciitis or epidural abscess.

DIFFERENTIAL CONSIDERATIONS

SIRS is defined by hemodynamic and laboratory parameters alone, whereas sepsis must include a suspected infectious cause. Often, noninfectious sources can cause a syndrome that mimics sepsis; thus one must keep in mind a broad differential diagnosis when approaching these patients (Box 52-3).

Box 52-3 Differential Considerations for Sepsis and Septic Shock

Sepsis	Septic Shock
Dehydration	Hypovolemic shock
Acute respiratory distress syndrome	Acute blood loss
Anemia	Severe dehydration
Ischemia	Cardiogenic shock
Hypoxia	Pulmonary embolus
Congestive heart failure	Myocardial infarction
Vasculitis	Pericardial tamponade
Toxicologic	Tension pneumothorax
Poisonings	Vasogenic shock
Overdose	Anaphylaxis
Drug induced	Paralysis
Pancreatitis	Adrenal dysfunction
Hypothalamic injury	Environmental
Disseminated intravascular coagulation	Burn
Anaphylaxis	Heat exhaustion or stroke
Metabolic	Trauma
Hyperthyroidism	Blood loss
Diabetic ketoacidosis	Cardiac contusion
	Neuroleptic malignant syndrome

MANAGEMENT

The primary goal remains antimicrobial therapy and maintenance of adequate tissue oxygenation and perfusion.Initial resuscitation, including appropriate airway management, intravenous access, oxygen, early and appropriate antibiotics, and fluid resuscitation, remains the foundation on which new efforts may be applied.

The recommendation is for the use of goal-directed therapy (GDT) for all patients who have (1) suspected infection, (2) two or more SIRS criteria, and (3) evidence of hypoperfusion signified by either SBP of less than 90 mm Hg after 20 to 30 mL/kg fluid challenge or a lactic acid level greater than 4 mmol/dL (Fig. 52-3).

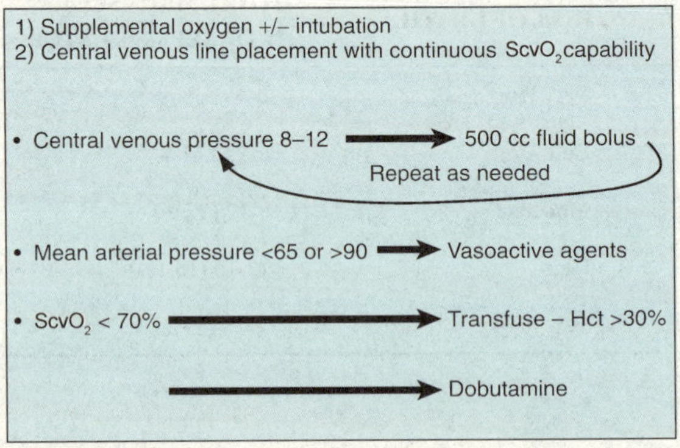

Fig 52-3. Summary of goal-directed therapy protocol.

Preload

The first step in GDT is to provide a proper filling pressure to ensure adequate cardiac preload. Patients with sepsis and septic shock required an average of 5 L of fluids in the first 6 hours of their resuscitation.The patients should receive crystalloid or colloid resuscitation to keep the CVP at a level of 8 to 12 mm Hg. In intubated patients with PPV, pathophysiologic principles support raising the target level to 12 to 16 mm Hg.

Perfusion Pressure

The next step in GDT is to maintain an adequate blood pressure. MAP should be kept between 60 and 90 mm Hg. If MAP is below 65 mm Hg in the presence of adequate preload, treatment with a vasopressor agent should be started; norepinephrine and dopamine are considered first-line agents.

Oxygen Delivery

The initial management of all critically ill patients should include supplemental oxygen with a goal to maintain a peripheral oxygen saturation of 95%.For patients with sepsis , a hematocrit between 27% and 30% has been reported to be most effective.

The therapeutic goal is to maintain $ScvO_2$ greater than 70% or to reduce lactate level by at least 10%. The patient has adequate oxygen-carrying capacity by transfusion of the patient to a hematocrit greater than 30%. If this is normalized and the patient is not tachycardic, dobutamine can be added to increase cardiac contractility and to increase CO, resulting in an overall improved oxygen delivery. The protocol should be run continuously with an effort toward normalization of the parameters during the entire resuscitation (Table 52-2).

Table 52-2 Management Recommendations for Hemodynamic Support

Basic Principles
Admission to intensive care unit
Arterial cannulation in patients with shock, although insertion may not be practical in the emergency department
Resuscitation to target tissue perfusion
Central venous or pulmonary arterial catheter placement to assess cardiac filling pressures
Fluid Resuscitation
Fluids are the primary modality to resuscitation
Colloids and crystalloids are equally effective
Invasive monitoring for patients not responding to initial resuscitation with target pulmonary capillary wedge pressure of 12 to 15 mm Hg[†]
Hemoglobin concentrations should be maintained above 8 to 10 g/dL

Continued

Vasopressor Therapy
Norepinephrine is the first-line agent in shock unresponsive to aggressive fluid resuscitation
Dopamine and phenylephrine are alternatives
Epinephrine is reserved for refractory hypotension
Routine low-dose (≤5 μg/kg/min) dopamine is not recommended[‡]
Vasopressin may be considered in refractory shock not responsive to aggressive fluid resuscitation and high-dose conventional vasopressors
Inotropic Therapy
Dobutamine is the first choice for patients with refractory low cardiac index
Dobutamine may improve cardiac index and organ perfusion, but empirical use is not recommended†
Vasopressors and inotropes can be titrated separately to maintain mean arterial pressure and cardiac output
Epinephrine and dopamine can be used as inotropes, but splanchnic perfusion may be compromised

Respiratory Support

Patients with "severe sepsis" required mechanical ventilation .Although there are no clear intubation guidelines, hypercapnia, persistent hypoxemia, airway compromise, and profound acidosis are valid indicators.

In addition to airway protection, intubation and mechanical ventilatory support provide PPV.Current recommendations are to maintain transalveolar pressures (measured as plateau pressures) below 35 cm H_2O because increased pressures are associated with VILI. Maintenance of relatively low transalveolar pressure with increasing end-expiratory pressure is an effective way to increase arterial oxygen delivery.

Cardiovascular Support

Fluid Resuscitation

Initial therapy for adults with septic shock should generally be 2 L of isotonic crystalloid. As much as 6 to 10 L of crystalloid may be required in the first 24 hr. Early GDT has been shown to be an effective way to guide fluid resuscitation and should be considered in all cases of septic shock. In less critically ill patients, fluid replacement should be titrated to clinical parameters such as heart rate, blood pressure, change in mental status, capillary refill, cool skin, and adequate urine output (0.5-1 mL/kg/hr). Normal saline and lactated Ringer's solution are equally effective and neither worsens lactic acidosis. Colloids are as effective as crystalloids.

Vasopressors

If appropriate fluid resuscitation has failed, vasopressor support may be required (Table 52-3). MAP of 65 mmHg has been recommended in otherwise healthy, normovolemic adult patients but must be correlated with other indicators of adequate perfusion, such as mental status and urine output. Patients with previously uncontrolled hypertension may require MAP of 75 mmHg or even higher.

Table 52-3 Dosing of Vasoactive Therapy

DRUG	DOSAGE
Dobutamine	5-15μg/kg/min
Dopamine	2-20μg/kg/min
Epinephrine	5-20μg/min
Norepinephrine	5-20μg/min
Phenylephrine	2-20μg/min

Fluid resuscitation remains the fundamental treatment option.Vasopressin alone has been shown to be ineffective compared with norepinephrine in the initial treatment of refractory septic shock. Epinephrine should be considered a supplemental agent if dopamine or norepinephrine is ineffective. Dobutamine should be used as the primary inotropic agent if myocardial dysfunction is evident.

Norepinephrine. Compared with dopamine in septic patients, norepinephrine increases GFR and urine output equally well. Recommended doses are 8 to 12 μg/min.

Dopamine. Dopamine is also often used for septic shock that is unresponsive to adequate volume expansion.Dosages higher than 20 μg/kg/min may produce significant vasoconstriction. Dopamine is most useful in patients who have depressed CO.

Phenylephrine. Phenylephrine is effective in restoring perfusion in patients with septic shock refractory to dopamine or dobutamine. Phenylephrine is less effective than norepinephrine in treatment of hypotension in septic patients. Phenylephrine does not impair cardiac and renal function and may be a good choice when significant tachyarrhythmia limits the use of other agents.

Epinephrine. As a result of all of the possible adverse effects of epinephrine, it is currently recommended only for those patients who are unresponsive to other vasopressors.

Vasopressin

In states of septic shock, there is an early surge of vasopressin followed by a profound drop in circulating vasopressin levels.This is the foundation for use of vasopressin as an adjunct therapy for patients with severe sepsis. Vasopressin should not be used as the sole initial therapy for refractory septic shock.

Inotropic Agents

Dobutamine

Dobutamine is a mixed alpha- and beta-agonist. In dosage ranges of dobutamine from 2 to 28 μg/kg/min, CI is increased at the expense of heart rate. In addition, decreased splanchnic blood flow is common. Dobutamine should be used in patients with depressed CI and persistent hypoperfusion in spite of adequate volume expansion and other vasopressor agents. In patients undergoing formal early GDT, when preload, perfusion pressure, and oxygen-carrying capacity have been normalized and a low $ScvO_2$ persists, dobutamine is used to increase CO and oxygen delivery.

Bicarbonate

Current consensus is that it should be reserved for severe acidemia (pH <7.0-7.2) as there may be a paradoxical decrease in intracellular pH as a result of diffusion of soluble carbon dioxide across the cell membrane.

Antibiotics

A neutrophil count of less than 500 cells/mm^3 should prompt empirical intravenous antibiotics in most chemotherapy patients.Early and appropriate antibiotic therapy should target the nidus of infection.If the patient's condition permits, appropriate culture specimens should be obtained before the administration of broad-spectrum antibiotics (Table 52-4).The results of initial microbiologic tests will help guide subsequent antibiotic treatment.With increasing rates of methicillin-resistant organisms, combinations that include nonpenicillin choices may be warranted.

Surgically correctable conditions, such as

intra-abdominal abscesses, perforated viscus, retained products of conception, or retained foreign body (such as a tampon), should be treated concurrently.

Table 52-4 Suggested Initial Antibiotic Management Pending Microbiologic Identification of Organism and Sensitivity

INFECTION	MODIFYING FACTORS	ANTIBIOTIC
Sepsis, unknown source	Immunocompetent	Antipseudomonal cephalosporin plusaminoglycoside or fluoroquinolone; orantipseudomonal penicillin plus aminoglycoside or fluoroquinolone; orcarbapenem plus aminoglycoside or fluoroquinolone
	Anaerobic infection	Add metronidazole or clindamycin to above regimen
	Methicillin-resistant Staphylococcus aureus(MRSA)	Add vancomycin to above regimen
	Neutropenia	Antipseudomonal penicillin plusaminoglycoside or fluoroquinolone; orcarbapenem plusaminoglycoside or fluoroquinolone
	Splenectomy	Cefotaxime orceftriaxone
	HIV infection	Ticarcillin-clavulanate plustobramycin
Pneumonia	Immunocompetent	Second- or third-generation cephalosporin plussecond-generation macrolide orfluoroquinolone
	Legionellasuspected	Azithromycin or fluoroquinolone or high-dose erythromycin
Abdominal infection	Immunocompetent	Ampicillin plusaminoglycoside plusmetronidazole
	Multidrug-resistant organism suspected	Ticarcillin-clavulanate or carbapenem; orpiperacillin-tazobactam plusaminoglycoside
	Urinary tract source	Fluoroquinolone; orthird-generation cephalosporin; orampicillin plusaminoglycoside
Cellulitis	Non-necrotizing fasciitis	Cefazolin ornafcillin
	MRSA possible	Vancomycin
	Necrotizing fasciitis (surgical drainage)	Ampicillin-sulbactam; orticarcillin-clavulanate; orpiperacillin plus aminoglycoside plusclindamycin; orcarbapenem
Intravenous catheter infection (remove catheter)	Outpatient acquired	Third-generation cephalosporin
	MRSA suspected	Add vancomycin
	Fungal infection	Amphotericin B
Cerebrospinal infection	Immunocompetent	Ceftriaxone plusvancomycin
	Elders or immunocompromised	Add ampicillin
Injection drug abuse	MRSA not suspected	Nafcillin plusaminoglycoside
	MRSA suspected	Vancomycin plusaminoglycoside

(SHOU Songtao)

SECTION 8

Pharmacotherapy of selected emergencies

Chapter 53

Antihypertensive medications

KEY CONCEPTS

Intravenous antihypertensive agents exert their effect either directly through receptor-mediated actions or indirectly through a decrease in production or release of endogenous vasoconstrictors.

The long-standing approach to acute antihypertensive therapy has been to target a maximal reduction in MAP of 20% to 25% within the first hour and a goal BP of 160/100 mm Hg by 2 to 6 hr.

Reductions in MAP exceeding 30% have been associated with more rapid symptom resolution and improved outcomes among patients with severe, acute hypertensive heart failure.

For the patients with aortic dissection,BP control to a specific target (SBP below 110 mmHg) is essential.

For acute ischemic stroke, AHA/ASA guidelines call for a BP reduction to below 185/110 mm Hg only when thrombolysis is planned. Otherwise, antihypertensive therapy is not indicated unless BP is greater than 220/120 mmHg, and even in such cases the goal is to decrease by approximately 15 % gradually, over the first 24 hr after onset.

Treatment of hypertensive encephalopathy should be directed toward initiation of immediate, aggressive antihypertensive therapy. Reductions in MAP of 30% to 40% may be needed. Symptom resolution is the best gauge of therapeutic effectiveness.

PERSPECTIVE

Existing intravenous antihypertensive agents exert their effect either directly through receptor-mediated actions or indirectly through a decrease in production or release of endogenous vasoconstrictors. The hemodynamic response to a specific medication or a class of medications is quite different (Table 53-1), thus the effects of antihypertensive medications can differ substantially.

Table 53-1 Hemodynamic Effect Profile of Common Intravenous Antihypertensive Medication

CLASSIFICATION	AGENT(S)	*Hemodynamic Effect* CARDIAC OUTPUT	SYSTEMIC VASCULAR RESISTANCE	CENTRAL VENOUS PRESSURE
Adrenergic inhibitors				
Alpha1-blockers	Phentolamine, urapidil	↑	↓	↑
Beta1-blockers	Esmolol, metoprolol	↓	↑ ↓	↑ ↓
Mixed alpha1/beta-blockers	Labetalol	↓	↓	↑ ↓
ACEI	Enalaprilat	↑ ↓	↓	↑ ↓
Calcium channel blockers				
Dihydropyridine	Clevidipine, nicardipine	↑	↓	↑ ↓
Nondihydropyridine	Diltiazem, verapamil	↓	↓	↑ ↓
Direct-acting vasodilators	Hydralazine	↑	↓	↑ ↓

Continued

CLASSIFICATION	AGENT(S)	Hemodynamic Effect: CARDIAC OUTPUT	SYSTEMIC VASCULAR RESISTANCE	CENTRAL VENOUS PRESSURE
Dopamine-1 receptor agonists	Fenoldopam	↑ ↓	↓	↑ ↓
Loop diuretics	Furosemide, bumetanide, torsemide	↑ ↓	↓	↓
Natriuretic peptide receptor agonists	Nesiritide	↑	↓	↓
Nitric oxide donors	Sodium nitroprusside, nitroglycerin, isosorbide dinitrate	↑	↓	↓

ACUTE BLOOD PRESSURE CONTROL

Although some oral (i.e., clonidine) or sublingual (i.e., captopril, nitroglycerin) medications are capable of this,patients who truly require acute lowering of BP benefit from the predictable, controlled effect of a parenteral agent.The long-standing approach to acute antihypertensive therapy has been to target a maximal reduction in MAP of 20% to 25% within the first hour and a goal BP of 160/100 mm Hg by 2 to 6 hr.

A general guide to intravenous antihypertensive therapy is provided in Table 53-2. According to the STAT (Studying the Treatment of Acute hypertension) registry, labetalol is the most common intravenous bolus medication used, and nitroglycerin is the infusion medication used most frequently for severe HTN in the ED.

An overview of respective treatment goals and relevant caveats for differing indications can be found in Table 53-3.

Table 53-2 User's Guide to Intravenous Antihypertensive Therapy

MEDICATION BY CLASS	BOLUS OR LOADING DOSE	INFUSION RATE	TIME TO ONSET	DURATION OF ACTION	COMMENTS
Adrenergic Inhibitors					
Phentolamine	5-15 mg q5min	0.2-0.5 mg/min	1-2 min	10-30 min	Avoid with coronary artery disease
Urapidil	12.5-50 mg q5min	9-30 mg/hr	1-2 min	2.5 hr	Not FDA approved
Esmolol	0.5-1 mg/kg × 1	50-300 μg/kg/min	1-2 min	20 min	
Metoprolol	5 mg q5min	None	10-30 min	5-8 hr	
Labetalol	20-80 mg q10min	1-2 mg/min	2-5 min	3-6 hr	Beta-blocker effects predominate(1 : 7)
ACE Inhibitor					
Enalaprilat	0.625-1.25 mg q15min	1-2 mg/hr	15-30 min	6-12 hr	May produce prolonged hypotension; avoid in pregnancy
Calcium Channel Blockers					
Clevidipine	None	2-32 μg/hr	1-2 min	1-5 min	Avoid with aortic stenosis and liver failure (hepatic metabolism)
Nicardipine	None	5-15 mg/hr	5-15 min	4-6 hr	Will decrease blood pressure but not often used for this indication
Diltiazem	0.25-0.35 mg/kg q15min	5-15 mg/hr	5-15 min	6 hr	
Verapamil	2.5-5 mg IV q15min	None	5-15 min	6 hr	

Continued

MEDICATION BY CLASS	BOLUS OR LOADING DOSE	INFUSION RATE	TIME TO ONSET	DURATION OF ACTION	COMMENTS
Direct-Acting Vasodilator					
Hydralazine	5-20 mg q30min	1.5-5 μg/kg/min	10-20 min	2-4 hr	Causes reflex activation of the sympathetic nervous system
Dopamine Antagonist					
Fenoldopam	None	0.1-0.3 μg/kg/min;titrate by 0.1 μg/kg	<5 min	30 min	Increases intraocular pressure; contains sodium metabisulfate—avoid in patient with sulfa allergy
Loop Diuretics					
Furosemide	40-240 mg q12hr	10-40 mg/hr	30-60 min	2-4 hr	Limited anithypertensive effect compared with other agents listed
Bumetanide	0.5-4 mg q12hr	None	30-60 min	2-4 hr	
Torsemide	10-20 mg q12hr	None	30-60 min	2-4 hr	
Natriuretic Peptide					
Nesiritide	2 μg/kg × 1	0.01 μg/kg/min	15 min	18 min	Indicated only for use in acute heart failure
Nitric Oxide Donors					
Sodium nitroprusside	None 1-2 mg q5min	0.25-10 μg/kg/min	Immediate	1-2 min	May cause precipitous drop in blood pressure with right ventricular ischemia or renal artery stenosis;bolus administration controversial;risk of cyanide toxicity with nitroprusside; avoid entire class in patients taking phosphodiesterase-5 inhibitors (e.g., sildenafil)
Nitroglycerin		5-200 μg/min	2-5 min	5-10 min	
Isosorbide dinitrate	3-4 mg q5min	1-10 mg/hr	2-5 min	5-10 min	

Table 53-3 Indication-Specific Approach to Management of Hypertensive Emergencies

INDICATION	GOALS OF TREATMENT	OPTIMAL AGENTS	ALTERATIVE THERAPY	CAVEATS
Acute coronary syndromes	Diminish cardiac workload and improve coronary artery perfusion	***Primary***: nitroglycerin ***Secondary***: metoprolol, laberalol	Esmolol, nicardipine	Routine use of intravenous beta-blocker therapy is controversoal.
Acute heart failure syndromes	Reduce impedance to forward flow and diminish cardiac workload	***Primary***: nitroglycerin, furosemide ***Secondary***: enalaprilat	Clevisipine, nicardipine, sodium nitroprusside	Intubation or noninvasive ventilatory support decreases preload and may drop BP. Enalaprilat may cause sustained hypotension. Though FDA approved, use of nesitride is controversial.
Aortic dissection	Reduce shear force and dP/dt	***Primary***: esmolol plus sodium nitroprusside ***Secondary***: labetalol	Esmolol plus (clevidipine or nicardipine), diltiazem, verapamil	Avoid beta-blockers if aortic regurgitation is present.

Continued

INDICATION	GOALS OF TREATMENT	OPTIMAL AGENTS	ALTERATIVE THERAPY	CAVEATS
Acute ischemic stroke	Reduce hemorrhagic conversion and edema while avoiding regional hypoperfusion	***Primary***: nicardipinw ***Secondary***: labetalol	Esmolol	Acute BP reduction is indicated only with planned fibrinolytic administration or when secondary target-organ dysfunction is involved.
Acute intracerebral hemorrhage	Reduce hematoma expansion and perihemat-omal edema	***Primary***: nicardipine ***Secondary***: labetalol	Esmolol	BP may decrease with pain management alone. Clevidipine is currently under investigation.
Hypertensive encep-halopathy	Decrease brain edema, reduce intracranial pressure, and improve autoregulatiory control	***Primary***: nicardipine ***Secondary***: labetalol	Esmolol, enalaprilat	Other causes of altered mental status should be considered in the workup.
Acute kidney injury	Decrease pressure in renal parenchyma and glomerular apparatus	***Primary***: fenoldopam ***Secondary***: clevidipine, nicardipine	Labetalol, sodium nitroprusside	Angiotensin-converting enzyme inhibitors and diuretics should be avoided.
Preeclampsia and eclampsia	Decrease intracranial pressure while maintaining placental perfusion	***Primary***: hydralazine ***Secondary***: labetalol	Nicardipine	Intravenous magnesium (6 g initially) is administered in all cases. Emergent cesarean section is definitive treatment.
Sympathetic crisis	Reduce alpha$_1$-adrenergic receptor-mediated vasoconstriction	***Primary***: phentolamine ***Secondary***: nitroglycerin	Fenoldopam, clevidi-pine, nicardipine, sodium nitroprusside	Benzodiazepines are first-line therapy when sympathetic crisis is caused by cocaine or amphetamines, Beta-blocker monotherapy (including labetalol) is contraindicated.

Acute Coronary and Acute Heart Failure Syndromes

In ACS complicated by HTN, the primary goal is a decrease in cardiac work and improved coronary artery perfusion. Reductions in MAP exceeding 30% have been associated with more rapid symptom resolution and improved outcomes among patients with severe, acute hypertensive heart failure.

To achieve such a profound decrease in MAP, higher doses of nitroglycerin (i.e., 1-2 mg by bolus or >250 μg/min) may be needed; and whereas sodium nitroprusside achieves a similar effect, it provides limited benefit over aggressive doses of nitroglycerin and has a number of added disadvantages, including the need for arterial line monitoring, risk of cyanide toxicity, and potential for compound photodegradation. All nitrates should be used with caution in patients who have taken a PDE5 inhibitor such as sildenafil (Viagra) or tadalafil (Cialis) within the preceding 24 to 48 hr as this can lead to a persistent hypotensive episode. ACEI are well toleratedin such patients and have been associated with rapid symptom improvement in patients with hypertensive heart failure. Enalaprilat can be administered by intravenous bolus or infusion and is the preferred ACEI in the setting of acute heart failure, but cautious dosages (0.625-1.25 mg per dose up to a maximum of 2.5 mg over 30 min) are recommended as the drug is long acting. Given their short half-life, third- and fourth-generation intravenous dihydropyridine calcium channel blockers (i.e., nicardipine and clevidipine) are emerging as potential alternatives. Labetalol and other intravenous agents with inhibitory beta adrenergic effects, such as metoprolol, should be avoided in the early stages of treatment.

Aortic Dissection

For the patients with aortic dissection,BP control to a specific target (SBP below 110 mm Hg) is essential.This is best accomplished by decreasing heart rate and SV through administration of a rapid-acting intravenous beta-blocker such as esmolol. It is important that beta blocker therapy be initiated before vasodilation. Once beta blockers have been initiated, agents such as sodium nitroprusside, nicardipine, or clevidipine can be rapidly titrated to reduce SBP as low as can be tolerated (and ideally to below 120 mm Hg) within 30 min. Diltiazem and verapamil may also be used.

Acute Stroke Syndromes

For acute ischemic stroke, the current American Heart Association/American Stroke Association (AHA/ASA) guidelines call for a BP reduction to below 185/110 mm Hg only when thrombolysis is planned. Otherwise, antihypertensive therapy is not indicated unless BP is greater than 220/120 mmHg, and even in such cases the goal is to decrease by approximately 15 % gradually, over the first 24 hr after onset. In contrast, for acute intracerebral hemorrhage, the 2010 AHA/ASA guidelines state that "aggressive" reduction is warranted when SBP exceeds 200 mm Hg or MAP exceeds 150 mm Hg, and more modest decreases are indicated (target BP 160/90 mm Hg or MAP 110 mm Hg) when lesser elevations (SBP >180 mm Hg or MAP >130 mm Hg) are present.

Several ongoing prospective trials should help clarify residual questions surrounding BP control in acute stroke, present evidence-based recommendations can be summarized as follows: (1) administration of antihypertensive therapy in the ED for a suspected ischemic cause should be avoided, unless thrombolysis is planned; and (2) aggressive BP reduction should be initiated in the setting of acute intracranial hemorrhage, targeting SBP between 160 and 180 mm Hg within the first few hours of arrival. Both labetalol and nicardipine appear to maintadequate cerebral perfusion while producing generalized reductions in vascular resistance and have emerged as the favored therapies in the setting of acute stroke syndromes. Nicardipine may offer some advantage over labetalol as it results in a more rapid achievement of BP goals. Nimodipine, an oral dihydropyridine calcium channel blocker, is specifically indicated for patients with subarachnoid hemorrhage. Esmolol may also be used. Sodium nitroprusside can cause an increase in intracranial pressure.

Hypertensive Encephalopathy

Once alternative causes of altered mentation have been ruled out, therapy should be directed toward initiation of immediate, aggressive antihypertensive therapy. Reductions in MAP of 30% to 40% may be needed. Symptom resolution is the best gauge of therapeutic effectiveness.

Sodium nitroprusside is often used as primary treatment for hypertensive encephalopathy patients. This may be worsened by the relative increase in ICP known to occur with sodium nitroprusside therapy. Similar effects may also occur with hydralazine, and unless BP is completely refractory to other therapy, it is best to avoid use of nitroprusside or hydralazine. In contrast, nicardipine and labetalol produce an even reduction in resistance across vascular beds and have become the agents of choice for patients with hypertensive encephalopathy.

Acute Kidney Injury

When antihypertensive therapy is indicated, fenoldopam, a potent dopamine 1A receptor agonist, is preferred. Enalaprilat should be avoided as it produces differential effects on the precapillary and postcapillary glomerular vascular bed. Peripheral-acting calcium channel blockers, such as clevidipine and nicardipine are acceptable first-line alternatives to fenoldopam. Other agents, including labetalol and sodium nitroprusside, may also be used.

Preeclampsia and Eclampsia

Whereas delivery is the definitive treatment, BP control is a critical part of early management. Preeclampsia and eclampsia represent an overwhelming of cerebral autoregulation, and rapid BP reduction is essential. The threshold for intervention, therefore, is set lower than with other hypertensive emergencies (i.e., SBP exceeding 160 mm Hg).

Magnesium sulfate is considered first-line

therapy for all cases of preeclampsia and eclampsia. Hydralazine and labetalol by intravenous bolus are equally effective. Nicardipine is a reasonable alternative and may produce a more profound decrease in BP than labetalol.

Sympathetic Crises

Hyperadrenergic states can result from endogenous sources of catecholamine excess and they are triggered by intake of exogenous substances that interfere with norepinephrine metabolism, such as cocaine, amphetamines, and tyraminecontaining foods. The net result is a cardiostimulatory and vasopressor response that manifests clinically as tachycardia and marked HTN.

When BP is persistently elevated and end-organ compromise is present, antihypertensive treatment will be needed. Phentolamine is considered first-line therapy. Nitroglycerin can also be used and is specifically indicated for patients with associated chest pain and suspected coronary artery vasospasm. Other agents, including fenoldopam, clevidipine, nicardipine, and sodium nitroprusside, are acceptable alternatives. A shortacting beta-blocker such as esmolol is ideal for controlling heart rate .Consequently, intravenous labetalol is susceptible to a similar differential response and should be used with caution in the setting of catecholamine excess.

CHRONIC ANTIHYPERTENSIVE THERAPY

A listing of most currently available monotherapy and combined antihypertensive therapy agents is provided in Table 53-4. Although the JNC 7 recommends initial treatment with thiazide diuretics for virtually all patients, ACEI or angiotensin receptor blockers are acceptable first-line alternatives, particularly in those with a history of diabetes or cardiac comorbidities. Beta-blockers are used in patients whose therapy with other agents has been maximized without adequate BP control. Of note, most patients with stage Ⅱ HTN will require multiple agents to control their BP. Anxiolytic or analgesic medication administration accompanied by resumption of chronic oral antihypertensive therapy is more rational and beneficial.

Table53-4 Summary of Oral Agents Available for Management of Chronic Hypertension

AGENT BY CLASS	TRADE NAME(S)	USUAL DOSE RANGE, TOTAL MILLIGRAMS PER DAY, AND INTERVAL	COMMON SIDE EFFECTS AND COMMENTS
Diuretics (Common)			Short-term: increase cholesterol and glucose levels
Thiazides			
Chlorothiazide	Diuril	125-500 qd	Biochemical abnormalities: decreasepotassium, sodium, and magnesium levels, increase uric acid and calcium levels
Chlorthalidone	Hygroton	12.5-50 qd	
Hydrochlorothiazide (HCTZ)	HydroDIURIL, Microzide, Esidrix	12.5-50 qd 2-4 qd	
Polythiazide	Renese	1.25-5 qd	Rare: blood dyscrasias, photosensitivity, pancreatitis, hyponatremia
Indapamide	Lozol, Mykrox Zaroxolyn	0.5-1 bid or tid	
Metolazone		2.5-5 qd	
Loop			
Bumetanide	Bumex	0.5-4 bid or tid	
Furosemide	Lasix	40-240 bid or tid	
Torsemide	Demadex	20-100 qd or bid	
Potassium-Sparing			Hyperkalemia may occur
Amiloride hydrochloride	Midamor	5-10 qd	
Triamterene	Dyrenium	25-100 qd	

Continued

AGENT BY CLASS	TRADE NAME(S)	USUAL DOSE RANGE, TOTAL MILLIGRAMS PER DAY, AND INTERVAL	COMMON SIDE EFFECTS AND COMMENTS
Mineralocorticoid Receptor Antagonists			
Spironolactone	Aldactone	25-100 qd	
Eplerenone	Inspra	50-100 qd or bid	
Adrenergic Inhibitors			Postural hypotension
Central Alpha-Agonists			Sedation, dry mouth, bradycardia, withdrawal hypertension
Reserpine		0.05-0.25 qd	
Clonidine hydrochloride	Catapres	0.2-1.2 bid or tid	
	Catapres-TTS	0.1-0.3 weekly	
Guanabenz acetate	Wytensin	4-8 bid	
Guanfacine hydrochloride	Tenex	0.5-2 qd	
Methyldopa	Aldomet	250-1000 bid	
Alpha$_1$-Blockers			Hepatitis and lupus-like syndrome
			Postural hypotension
Doxazosin mesylate Postural hypotension	Cardura	1-16 qd	
Prazosin hydrochloride	Minipress	2-20 bid or tid	
Terazosin hydrochloride	Hytrin	1-20 qd	
Beta-Blockers			Bronchospasm, bradycardia, heart failure; may mask insulin-induced hypoglycemia
Acebutolol	Sectral	200-800 qd	Less serious: impaired peripheral circulation, insomnia, fatigue, exercise intolerance, hypertriglyceridemia (except agents with sympathomimetic activity)
Atenolol	Tenormin	25-100 qd or bid	
Betaxolol	Kerlone	5-20 qd	
Bisoprolol fumarate	Zebeta	2.5-10 qd	
Metoprolol tartrate	Lopressor	50-300 bid	
Metoprolol succinate	Toprol-XL	50-300 qd	
Nadolol	Corgard	40-320 qd	
Nebivolol hydrochloride	Bystolic	5-20 qd	
Penbutolol sulfate	Levatol	10-20 qd	
Pindolol	Visken	10-60 bid	
Propranolol hydrochloride	Inderal	40-480 bid	
Timolol maleate	Inderal LA	40-480 qd	
	Blocadren	20-60 bid	
Mixed Alpha$_1$-/Beta-Blockers			Postural hypotension, bronchospasm
Carvedilol	Coreg	6.25-50 bid	
Labetalol hydrochloride	Normodyne, Trandate	200-1200 bid	
Direct Vasodilators			Headaches, fluid retention, tachycardia
Hydralazine hydrochloride	Apresoline	50-300 bid	
Minoxidil	Loniten	5-100 qd	Lupus syndrome
			Hirsutism
Calcium Channel Blockers (CCB)			Conduction defects, worsening of systolic dysfunction, gingival hypertrophy
Nondihydropyridines			
Diltiazem hydrochloride	Cardizem SR, Cardizem CD,	50-300 bid	
	Dilacor XR, Tiazac	5-100 qd	
Verapamil hydrochloride	Isoptin SR, Calan SR	90-480 bid	Constipation
	Verelan, Covera-HS	120-480 qd	

Continued

AGENT BY CLASS	TRADE NAME(S)	USUAL DOSE RANGE, TOTAL MILLIGRAMS PER DAY, AND INTERVAL	COMMON SIDE EFFECTS AND COMMENTS
Dihydropyridines			Pedal edema, flushing, headache, gingival hypertrophy
Amlodipine besylate	Norvasc	2.5-10 qd	
Felodipine	Plendil	2.5-20 qd	
Isradipine	DynaCirc	5-20 bid	
Nicardipine	DynaCirc CR	5-20 qd	
Nifedipine	Cardene SR	60-90 bid	
Nisoldipine	Procardia XL, Adalat CC	30-120 qd	
	Sular	20-60 qd	
Angiotensin-Converting Enzyme Inhibitors (ACEI)			Common: cough Rare: angioedema, hyperkalemia, rash, loss of taste, leukopenia
Benazepril hydrochloride	Lotensin	5-40 qd or bid	
Captopril (G)	Capoten	25-150 bid or tid	
Enalapril maleate	Vasotec	5-40 qd or bid	
Fosinopril sodium	Monopril	10-40 qd or bid	
Lisinopril	Prinivil, Zestril	5-40 qd	
Moexipril	Univasc	7.5-15 qd or bid	
Perindopril	Aceon	4-8 qd or bid	
Quinapril hydrochloride	Accupril	5-80 qd or bid	
Ramipril	Altace	1.25-20 q or bid	
Trandolapril	Mavik	1-4 qd	
Angiotensin Ⅱ Receptor Blockers (ARB)			Angioedema (very rare), hyperkalemia
Candesartan	Atacand	8-32 qd	
Eprosartan	Tevetan	400-800 qd or bid	
Losartan potassium	Cozaar	25-100 qd or bid	
Valsartan	Diovan	80-320 qd	
Irbesartan	Avapro	150-300 qd	
Olmesartan	Benicar	20-40 qd	
Telmisartan	Micardis	20-80 qd	
Direct Renin Inhibitors			Rare angioedema, hyperkalemia (especially with ACEI use), hypotension, diarrhea, rash, renal stones
Aliskiren	Tekturna	150-300 qd	
Fixed Dose Combinations ***ACEI + Diuretic***			Side effect profile of combination tablets is similar to individual components,but the overall incidence is greatly diminished
Benazepril + HCTZ	Lotensin HCT	5/6.25, 10/12.5, 20/12.5, 20/25 qd	
Captopril + HCTZ	Capozide	25/15, 25/25, 50/15, 50/25 qd	
Enalapril + HCTZ	Vaseretic	5/12.5, 10/25 qd	
Lisinopril + HCTZ	Prinzide, Zestoretic	10/12.5, 20/12.5, 20/25 qd	
Moexipril + HCTZ	Uniretic	7.5/12.5, 15/12.5, 15/25 qd	
Quinapril + HCTZ	Accuretic	10/12.5, 20/12.5 qd	
Perindopril + indapamide			
ARB + Diuretic			
Irbesartan + HCTZ	Avalide	150/12.5, 300/12.5, 300/25 qd	
Losartan + HCTZ	Hyzaar	50/12.5, 100/25 qd	
Olmesartan + HCTZ	Benicar HCT	20/12.5, 40/12.5, 40/25 qd	

Continued

AGENT BY CLASS	TRADE NAME(S)	USUAL DOSE RANGE, TOTAL MILLIGRAMS PER DAY, AND INTERVAL	COMMON SIDE EFFECTS AND COMMENTS
Telmisartan + HCTZ	Micardis HCT	40/12.5, 80/12.5, 80/25 qd	
Valsartan + HCTZ	Diovan HCT	80/12.5, 160/12.5, 160/25 qd	
Beta-Blocker + Diuretic			
Atenolol + chlorthalidone	Tenoretic	50/25, 100/25 qd	
Bisoprolol + HCTZ	Ziac	2.5/6.25, 5/6.25, 10/6.5 qd	
Metoprolol + HCTZ	Lopressor HCT	50/25, 100/25, 100/50 qd	
Timolol + HCTZ	Timolide	10/25 qd	
CCB + ACEI			
Amlodipine + benazepril	Lotrel	2.5/10, 5/10, 5/20 qd	
Felodipine + enalapril	Lexxel	5/2.5, 5/5 qd	
Felodipine + ramipril	Triapin Mite Triapin	2.5/2.5 qd 5/5 qd	
Verapamil + trandolapril	Tarka	180/2, 240/1, 240/2, 240/4 qd	
CCB + ARB			
Amlodipine + olmesartan	Azor	5/20, 5/40, 10/20, 10/40 qd	
Amlodipine + telmisartan	Exforge Twynsta	5/160, 5/320, 10/160, 10/320 qd 5/40, 5/80, 10/40, 10/80 qd	
Renin Inhibitor + Other			
Aliskiren + HCTZ	Tekturna HCT	150/12.5, 150/25, 300/12.5, 300/25 qd	
Aliskiren + amlodipine	Tekamlo	150/5, 150/10, 300/5, 300/10 qd	
Aliskiren + amlodipine + HCTZ	Amturnide	150/5/12.5, 300/5/12.5, 300/5/25, 300/10/12.5, 300/10/25 qd	
Aliskiren + valsartan	Valturna	150/160, 300/320 qd	
Diuretic Combinations			
Amiloride + HCTZ	Moduretic	5/50 qd	
Triamterene + HCTZ	Dyazide, Maxzide	37.5/25, 75/50 qd	

(CHAI Yanfen)

Chapter 54

Antiarrhythmic Agents

KEY CONCEPTS

Medications used to treat dysrhythmias are classified into four major categories on the basis of their electrophysiologic effects

All antidysrhythmics can cause "prodysrhythmic effects."

CLASSIFICATION OF ANTIDYSRHYTHMIC DRUGS

Medications used to treat dysrhythmias are classified into four major categories on the basis of their electrophysiologic effects (Box 54-1). Other agents fall outside this classification system and are discussed separately.

Box 54-1 Classification of Antidysrhythmic Drugs

Class Ⅰ

Sodium (fast) channel blockers. Slow depolarization with varying effects on repolarization. These "membrane-stabilizing" drugs have prominent antiectopic effects.

Class ⅠA

Moderate slowing of depolarization and conduction. Prolong repolarization and action potential duration.

Procainamide

Quinidine

Disopyramide

Class ⅠB

Minimally slow depolarization and conduction. Shorten repolarization and action potential duration.

Lidocaine

Phenytoin

Tocainide

Mexiletine

Class ⅠC

Markedly slow depolarization and conduction. Prolong repolarization and action potential duration.

Flecainide

Encainide

Lorcainide

Propafenone (shares properties with class IA agents)

Vernakalant (atrial specific, investigational)

Class Ⅱ

Beta-adrenergic blockers

Propranolol

Esmolol

Metoprolol

Atenolol

Class Ⅲ

Antifibrillatory agents. Prolong action potential duration and refractory period duration with antifibrillatory properties.

Bretylium (historical significance)

Amiodarone

Dofetilide

Ibutilide

Sotalol

Dronedarone

Azimilide

Class Ⅳ

Calcium (slow) channel blockers

Verapamil

Diltiazem

Miscellaneous

Digitalis

Magnesium sulfate

Adenosine

Class Ⅰ agents exert their major effects on the fast Na^+ channels, resulting in membrane stabilization. The subclasses ⅠA, ⅠB, and ⅠC are distinguished on the basis of differential effects on depolarization, repolarization, and conduction.

Class Ⅱ agents are the beta-adrenergic antagonists, which depress SA node automaticity and slow AV node conduction. Class Ⅲ agents prolong repolarization and refractory period duration, predominantly via their effects on K^+ channels. Class Ⅳ agents are the Ca^{2+} channel blockers, which slow conduction through the AV node and suppress other calcium-dependent dysrhythmias. Other agents important in the emergency treatment of dysrhythmias include magnesium sulfate, digitalis, and adenosine.

All antidysrhythmics can cause "prodysrhythmic effects." This occurs most often in patients with existing structural heart disease and in patients receiving new or higher doses of antidysrhythmic agents. The class Ⅰ and Ⅲ agents are associated with prodysrhythmic effects in up to 15% of patients.

Class Ⅰ Agents

Class ⅠA Agents

Class ⅠA agents slow conduction through the atria, AV node, and His-Purkinje system and suppress conduction via accessory pathways. Class IA agents also exhibit anticholinergic and mild negative inotropic effects. Procainamide is the most commonly used class IA agent in the emergency treatment of ventricular and supraventricular dysrhythmias. Intravenous procainamide is administered at a rate of 20 to 30 mg/min in stable patients until the dysrhythmia is terminated, hypotension occurs, or the QRS complex widens (to 50% of the pretreatment width), or up to a total dose of 18 to 20 mg/kg (12 mg/kg if CHF is present).

Class ⅠB Agents

Class ⅠB agents slow conduction and depolarization less than other class Ⅰ agents, and they shorten repolarization rather than prolonging it. Class ⅠB agents have little effect on accessory pathway conduction. Lidocaine is the sole class IB agent used in emergency rhythm management. Lidocaine is useful for suppressing dysrhythmias from enhanced automaticity such as VT. Lidocaine also suppresses SA and AV node function and is associated with asystole in the setting of myocardial ischemia.

Class ⅠC Agents

The class ⅠC agents profoundly slow depolarization and conduction and have pronounced antidysrhythmic properties. Up to 15% of patients treated with class ⅠC agents experience new or increased ventricular dysrhythmias. Class ⅠC agents are approved only for oral use.

Flecainide

Flecainide is used in the treatment of SVT and certain forms of VT outside the setting of acute ischemia. Initiation of oral therapy requires continuous ECG monitoring. Long term use of flecainide in those with a previous MI is associated with an increased risk of fatal dysrhythmia.

Propafenone

Propafenone shares properties with both class ⅠA and ⅠC agents, with intermediary effects on sodium channels. It also possesses some beta-adrenergic and calcium channel-blocking properties. Propafenone is used for the oral treatment of atrial fibrillation and ventricular dysrhythmias. It has a lower observed prodysrhythmic rate at therapeutic doses.

Class Ⅱ Agents

Class Ⅱ agents suppress SA node automaticity and slow conduction through the AV node. Class Ⅱ agents are well suited to control the ventricular rate in patients with Af and AF. Beta-blockers can terminate AVNRTs. In the setting of acute myocardial ischemia, beta-blockers play a role in preventing ventricular dysrhythmias. Side effects of beta-blockers include bronchospasm, bradycardia, hypotension, and CHF. All beta-blockers are active at both $beta_1$ and $beta_2$ receptors (Table 54-1) to varying degrees. Those with more prominent beta1 effects are said to be cardioselective. Relative contraindications to the use of beta-blockers include asthma or COPD, advanced CHF, bradycardia or heart block beyond first-degree, and third-trimester pregnancy.

Esmolol

Esmolol is a beta1-selective agent attractive in the emergency setting because of its rapid onset of action and short elimination half-life (min). An intravenous bolus of 500 μg of esmolol per kg followed by a continuous infusion starting at 50 μg/kg/min is a common starting approach, with titration to need and effect.

Metoprolol

Metoprolol is available in oral and intravenous preparations. Metoprolol (5-10 mg IV every 10-15 min titrated to response) will slow atrial and nodal fast rhythms.

Table 54-1 Cardiac and Respiratory Beta-Adrenergic Receptors and Responses to Pharmacologic Manipulation

RESPONSE TO RECEPTORS	LOCATION	STIMULATION	ANTAGONISM
$Beta_1$	Heart	Increased heart rate and ectopy	Decreased heart rate and ectopy
		Increased contractility	Decreased contractility
$Beta_2$	Airway (smooth muscle)	Decreased tone (relaxation)	Increased tone (contraction)
	Peripheral vasculature	Decreased tone (relaxation)	Increased tone (contraction)

Class Ⅲ Agents

All class Ⅲ agents prolong the refractory period by blocking K^+ channels, and they have variable effects on the QT interval. In general, class Ⅲ agents are alternatives to the class Ⅰ agents for the treatment of many ventricular and atrial dysrhythmias.

Bretylium

Bretylium was once the most commonly used class Ⅲ agent, but its hemodynamic side effects were unfavorable.

Amiodarone

Amiodarone is approved for the treatment of both ventricular and supraventricular dysrhythmias. In addition to features in common with all class Ⅲ agents, amiodarone has numerous other effects, including actions that are similar to those of class ⅠA, class Ⅱ, and class Ⅳ agents.

The serum half-life of amiodarone is 25 hr after a single intravenous dose and up to 50 d during long-term oral use. The acute side effects of amiodarone are primarily limited to hypotension, bradycardia, and heart failure (Box 54-2). Rates of prodysrhythmia are relatively low . Long-term amiodarone use, however, is associated with significant extracardiac side effects, including irreversible lung and thyroid disease. Amiodarone alters the pharmacokinetics of numerous other drugs, including digoxin and warfarin.

Ibutilide

Ibutilide has a unique mechanism of action characterized by induction of a slow inward Na^+ current, thereby prolonging the refractory period. Intravenous ibutilide is approved for cardioversion of Af and AF. Ibutilide is associated with QT interval prolongation, and polymorphic VT is more common than with amiodarone although still relatively rare.

Box 54-2 Adverse Effects of Amiodarone

Acute Effects
- Hypotension
- Slowing of heart rate
- Decreased contractility

Long-Term Effects

Common
- Corneal deposits
- Photosensitivity
- Gastrointestinal intolerance

Less Common
- Hyperthyroidism
- Heart failure
- Pulmonary toxicity, fibrosis
- Hypothyroidism
- Bradycardia
- Prodysrhythmic effect

Drug Interactions

Increase Levels
- Phenytoin
- Procainamide
- Warfarin
- Digoxin
- Flecainide

Sotalol

Sotalol is beta-adrenergic receptor blocker with type Ⅲ antidysrhythmic properties via inhibition of K^+ channels. It is used orally for suppression of supraventricular and ventricular dysrhythmias.

Dofetilide

Dofetilide is a pure class Ⅲ agent that blocks K^+ efflux, increasing the refractory period. It is approved for chemical cardioversion and maintenance of sinus rhythm in patients with Af or AF, but because of its prodysrhythmic effects, it has limited usefulness.

Dronedarone

Structurally related to amiodarone, dronedarone displays class Ⅲ properties plus those of other antidysrhythmic classes. The incidence of polymorphic VT associated with dronedarone is very low. Dronedarone is approved for oral use to maintain sinus rhythm in patients with Af or AF but is contraindicated in patients with severe or recent heart failure decompensation.

Class Ⅳ Agents

Class Ⅳ agents block the slow Ca^{2+} channels, slowing

conduction within the AV node and suppressing the SA node to a lesser degree. Their primary use is in patients with SVT. Of the two commonly used class Ⅳ agents, diltiazem is more frequently used for ventricular rate control in patients with Af or AF.

All class Ⅳ agents are associated with peripheral vasodilation. Verapamil has the least effect on peripheral vascular tone, and diltiazem has an effect between that of verapamil and purely peripherally acting calcium channel blockers, such as nifedipine. Class Ⅳ drugs should not be used in patients with second- or third-degree AVB.

Diltiazem

Intravenous diltiazem 0.25 to 0.35 mg/kg over 2 min controls the ventricular response rate in 90% of patients with Af and is associated with minimal hypotension. If the IV bolus is successful, a continuous infusion (5-15 mg/hr initially, titrated to need) or an oral dose (60-90 mg initially) will help sustain the response.

Verapamil

Verapamil terminates or controls the ventricular response rate in 80 to 90% of tachycardic rhythms. Intravenous verapamil is given at a dose of 0.1 mg/kg over 1 to 2 min. In elderly patients or those with preexisting borderline hypotension (SBP of 90-110 mm Hg), a smaller dose (0.05 mg/kg, or 2.5 mg increments) is preferred.

Miscellaneous Agents

Digoxin

Digoxin can behave as an excitant, a depressant, or both. Excitant effects of digoxin have to do with enhanced automaticity and triggered activity, particularly at high therapeutic or toxic doses. At the same time, digoxin slows AV node conduction at therapeutic doses via lengthening of the refractory period.

Digoxin (0.25-0.5 mg IV) can control the ventricular rate in patients with SVT, including Af and AF. Side effects of digoxin are listed in Box 54-3 and are aggravated by hypokalemia, hypercalcemia, hypomagnesemia, increased catecholamines, and acid-base disturbances.

Magnesium

Magnesium can aid control of many tachydysrhythmias. Magnesium (1-2 g IV) plays a central role in terminating torsades de pointes and as an aid in VT therapy. A side from these indications, magnesium is considered at best an adjunctive, second- or third- line agent in other settings.

Box 54-3 Adverse Effects of Digitalis

Common Effects
- Gastrointestinal intolerance (nausea, vomiting, abdominal pain, diarrhea, anorexia)
- Fatigue
- Drowsiness
- Visual color disturbances
- Headache
- Depression
- Apathy

Less Common Effects
- Psychosis
- Cardiac symptoms
- Heart block
- Increased ectopy
- Combined block and ectopy (multifocal atrial tachycardia with block or complete atrioventricular block with accelerated junctional rhythm, usually in overdose setting)
- Ventricular tachycardia

Adenosine

Adenosine is a naturally occurring purine nucleoside used for the termination of narrow-complex tachydysrhythmias. Administered as an intravenous bolus, adenosine causes an abrupt slowing of AV conduction in both anterograde and retrograde pathways. Adenosine usually has an onset of action of 5 to 20 s and a duration of effect of 30 to 40 s. Except in rare cases of catecholamine-induced ventricular dysrhythmias, adenosine has little or no effect on infranodal conduction. Adenosine is often used as a diagnostic agent in patients with wide complex tachydysrhythmias when the cause is unclear. An initial dose of 6 mg as a rapid bolus for adults weighing 50 kg or greater is recommended. If no response is seen within 1 to 2 min, the second dose is doubled (12 mg) and administered. If no effect is seen after a final 12 mg dose, the rhythm should be reassessed and another agent used. Side effects include flushing, dyspnea, chest pressure, nausea, headache, dizziness, transient bradycardia or heart block, and hypotension. Asystole can occur but is usually transient.

Similarly, some narrow-complex tachydysrhythmias that terminate with adenosine will recur later given the short duration of action.

(CHAI Yanfen)

Chapter 55

Drug Therapy in Pregnancy

KEY CONCEPTS

1% to 3% of birth defects'etiology are thought to be due to pharmaceutical or environmental agents.

The impact of exposure on the pregnancy depends on the age of the fetal. During the time of organogenesis (days 21–56 of fetal life), the fetus is much more vulnerable to toxic insults.

The CNS develops during the 10th to 17th weeks of pregnancy. Exposures during this period may affect neurologic development and subsequent function.

Because fetal pH is slightly more alkalotic than maternal pH, weak organic acids (e.g., salicylate) may become ion trapped in the fetal circulation, increasing fetal exposure.

Certain medications, such as anticonvulsants, warfarin derivatives, NSAID, sulfonamides, fluoroquinolones, ACEI, and oral hypoglycemic agents, are known teratogens or cause potential toxic effects in the newborn and should be avoided, if possible, during pregnancy.

PERSPECTIVE

Medication use during pregnancy is extremely common. In a worldwide survey of more than 14,000 patients, WHO reported that more than 86% of women used at least one prescription drug while pregnant. About 3% to 5% of all live birth affected by major birth defects. While most of birth defects'etiology remained to be unknown, 1% to 3% of these are thought to be due to pharmaceutical or environmental agents. Why one pregnancy would be affected and not another remains to be elucidated. Any chemical, pharmacologic, environmental, or mechanical agent which can cause deviant or disruptive development of the conceptus is called a teratogen. The definition includes functional impairment, growth restriction, and congenital malformations, which may range from subtle neurobehavioral effects to devastating physiologic effects and physical deformities, including fetal death. Highly teratogenic medications seem to be few in number, estimated at well below 50 agents (Box 55-1).

Box 55-1 Drugs and Agents Considered Human Teratogens and Developmental Toxins

Alkylating agents (e. g.,busulfan, chlorambucil,cyclophosphamide)	Ionizing radiation
Aminopterin and methotrexate*	Isotretinoin (systemic)
Amiodarone	Lead
Aminoglycosides (streptomycin and others)	Lithium
Androgens	Methimazole
ACEI	Methylene blue
Carbamazepine	Methylmercury
Carbon monoxide	Misoprostol
Chlorobiphenyls	Nonsteroidal antiinflammatory gents
Cocaine	Paramethadione,trimethadione
Corticosteroids	Phenytoin
Coumarin derivatives	Polychlorinated biphenyls
Danazol	Progestins
Diethylstilbestrol	Quinine
Ergotamine	Statins
Ethanol (in large doses)	Tetracycline
Fluconazole (in high doses)	Thalidomide
Iodine	Tobacco
	Trimethadione
	Valproic acid

It's tedious and often flawed to establish teratogenicity. Because of ethical reasons, we can only perform animal research instead of controlled prospective human studies to determining risk initially, but it isn't always applicable to humans. So we can only collect much of our current knowledge on teratogenicity from case reports, case-control studies, or cohort studies, which are inherently weak in establishing a causal relationship. A multitude of confounding factors may often complicate these reports, so it's difficult to make the determination of a causal link between a specific exposure and malformations. The outcome of pregnancy can be influenced by the genetic background of the fetus, timing and duration of the exposure, environmental factors, multiple exposures, nutritional deficits, maternal illness, and illicit drug use, and so on. In order to understand the connection between the outcome of a pregnancy and an associated in utero exposure, we need large population studies. Finally, as in the case of diethylstilbestrol, teratogenicity may not be apparent for years after birth.

Classification of Teratogenic Risk

Depending on the strength of evidence for its safety or teratogenicity (Box 55-2), the United States. FDA assigns one of five letters, A, B, C, D, and X, to the drug , aiding physicians in determining the teratogenic potential of a particular medication. Many clinicians believe that the classification system conveys the incorrect impression that there is a gradation of reproductive risk from exposure across categories (i.e., that risk increases from A to B to C to D to X) and that the drugs within a given category present similar reproductive risks. In addition, using this classification, more than 90% of newly drugs approved in the United States were assigned an undetermined teratogenic risk, class C.

Box 55-2 FDA Classification:Teratogenic Risk of Drugs

Class A: Controlled studies have shown no risk. Adequate well-controlled studies in pregnant women have failed to show risk to fetus.

Class B: No evidence exists of risk for humans. Animal studies show risk or are negative, but no studies in human had been done.

Class C: Use may engender risk for fetus. Human studies are lacking, and animal studies may be positive or lacking. Potential for benefit may outweigh potential for harm.

Class D: Positive evidence of risk is based on studies or postmarketing data. Potential for benefit may outweigh potential for harm.

Class X: Drugs are contraindicated in pregnancy on the basis of human or animal studies or postmarketing reports that indicate benefit is clearly outweighed by risk.

PRINCIPLES OF DISEASE

The fetus may be affected by drugs via a variety of mechanisms. Some drugs may alter the availability of substrates, such as vitamins, glucose, oxygen, and amino acids, needed for normal nutrition and growth. Others may directly affect cellular growth and differentiation. The impact of exposure on the pregnancy depends on the age of the fetal. During the time of organogenesis (days 21–56 of fetal life), the fetus is much more vulnerable to toxic insults. Owing to major body organs are formed during this period, exposure at this time may result in major anatomic defects. Exposure after the period of organogenesis may not have an impact on organogenesis, but it may affect the growth and development of the fetus. The CNS develops from 10th to 17th weeks of pregnancy, so that exposures during this period may affect neurologic development and subsequent function.

Drug Transfer across the Placenta

Drug transfer across the placenta occurs most commonly by simple passive diffusion or by protein transport. Maternal and fetal circulation is separated by a thin layer of trophoblastic cells. Molecular size, ionic state, lipid solubility, and extent of protein binding, all of them may affect the capacity of drugs transfer across the placenta. If the molecular mass of a drug is less than 5 kDa, it will be readily diffuse. A drug in the form of anionic can diffuse through the lipid layer more readily than that in the form of ionized. Free drug diffuses more readily than drug that bound to plasma proteins. Since fetal pH is slightly more alkalotic than maternal pH, weak organic acids (e.g., salicylate) may become ion trapped in the fetal circulation, with increasing fetal exposure.

Drug Transfer during Lactation

For the most part, drugs and substances that are ingested or injected by the mother diffuse passively into milk and then back into the maternal circulation for excretion. Many factors may affect the amount of drug diffusing into milk. Lipid-soluble and nonionic substances diffuse more readily, and high protein bound substances diffuse less readily. The neonate usually can detoxify a substance without adverse effect no matter if it's concentrated in maternal milk or not, and only a few drugs pose a serious danger to a breast-feeding infant. Only in rare situations of known drug toxicity to the infant and in all cases of maternal critical illness, we advocate interrupt breast-feeding. Table 55-1 summarizes the compatibility of medications and their effects in pregnancy and lactation.

DRUG THERAPY DURING PREGNANCY

In fact, the health of fetus is closely related to the health of mother. Physicians should not withhold lifesaving medications from pregnant patients because of a reported risk to the fetus and should resuscitate pregnant patients according to advanced life support guidelines. Any agent prescribed by physicians should presents maternal benefits outweighing the risks to the fetus. Therapeutic medications for asthma, arrhythmias, status epilepticus, life-threatening overdoses and HIV infection are included in this category. When a pregnant or lactating woman have to take some drugs, physicians must weigh the benefits of treatment against the inherent risks of treatment or disease, consider the pharmacokinetics of the drug during pregnancy and lactation. Then, they should choose a drug in relatively safety instead of those remain unclified whether it's harmful to fetal. They also should strictly control the dosage and administration of a drug, choose the minimum dose and stop it timely.

Analgesic Agents

Acetaminophen

Acetaminophen (paracetamol) is widely used during pregnancy. It is safe throughout pregnancy and no association was found between it and congenital malformations. In fact, in a population-based case-control study, when acetaminophen was used for febrile illnesses in the first trimester, it may decrease the risk of certain craniofacial malformations. During lactation, only a small amount of acetaminophen is excreted into breast milk, and the amount that does get through is tolerated by the neonate's sulfhydration pathway, so the acetaminophen can be safe. However, in overdose situations, there may be an increase in the incidence of spontaneous abortion and fetal demise, especially when antidote treatment with N-acetylcysteine was delayed.

Aspirin

In early studies, association was found between aspirin and an increased risk of perinatal and neonatal bleeding, increased risk of postmaturity, prolonged labor, low birth weight, neonatal hypoglycemia, neonatal metabolic acidosis and neonatal death. However, a number of recent meta-analyses in human failed to demonstrate a teratogenic effect of aspirin, although there was a trend toward a slightly increased incidence of gastroschisis (a defect in the abdominal wall through which abdominal contents protrude) when used NSAID including aspirin in the first trimester. Furthermore, in the Perinatal Antiplatelet Review of International Studies (PARIS) Collaboration, low doses of aspirin were actually found to be beneficial and to reduce the risk of preeclampsia, premature birth and adverse perinatal outcomes. During the lactation, aspirin can be excreted into breast milk. As aspirin is associated with Reye's syndrome, we don't advocate breast-feeding when it was taken.

Nonsteroidal Anti-Inflammatory Drugs

NSAID are prostaglandin synthesis inhibitors, they can block blastocyst implantation and may therefore inhibit conception. When NSAID are used in the first trimester, they can increase the risk of spontaneous abortions, and also can slightly increase the risk of cardiac septal defects, oral clefts, and gastroschisis. When they are used in the third trimester, NSAID inhibit labor and have been used as tocolytic agents for premature labor. Association was found between use of NSAID in the latter period of pregnancy and a number of negative effects on the neonate, most notably premature closure of the ductus arteriosus, leading to neonatal pulmonary hypertension and death. Other negative effects include increased incidence of fetal periventricular hemorrhages, fetal nephrotoxicity, oligohydramnios, and neonatal gastrointestinal hemorrhage. So non-aspirin NSAID should be avoided in the first trimester and the latter period of pregnancy. NSAID seems to be safe during lactation.

Opiate Analgesics

In general, short-term, episodic use of opiates such as oxycodone, hydrocodone, morphine and fentanyl appear safe in pregnancy. But their use near term may lead to severe respiratory depression of the neonate. Besides, long-term use of opiates is discouraged in general because it may result in fetal addiction, low birth weight, and neonatal abstinence syndrome. The characteristics of neonatal abstinence syndrome are CNS hyperirritability and autonomic nervous system dysfunction and a higher mortality in the offspring. The short-term use of opiates appears to be safe during lactation, but we should closely monitor nursing infants' respiratory depression.

Anesthetics, Sedative-Hypnotics, and Neuromuscular Blocker

One of the indications of General anesthetics, sedative-hypnotics, and neuromuscular blockers is RSI. For procedural sedation, we can also use some anesthetics and sedative-hypnotics. Most of the data regarding the use of these agents during pregnancy have been obtained from animal studies and from retrospective human data. No association was found between the agents and congenital malformations.

Anesthetics

Etomidate. Etomidate is an ultra-short-acting hypnotic agent that is commonly used for procedural sedation or RSI. No reports on developmental effects of etomidate in animal researches have been published. So it is in human. However, pregnant women were found to have significant reductions in serum cortisol concentrations 1 hour after delivery if they undergoing cesarean section with etomidate. It's unclear why it happened. Breast-feeding seems to be viable, because etomidate is excreted in milk in very small amounts and decreases rapidly.

Ketamine. Ketamine is a rapidly acting dissociative anesthetic that is commonly used in pediatric procedural sedation and may be used in RSI. It is frequently used in obstetrics and no reports on fetal development malformations have been published. Ketamine has a dose-dependent oxytocic effect and in high doses (>2 mg/kg), it may result in uterine tetany, increased maternal blood pressure, heart rate and an increased neonatal muscle tone. There are also some reports on neonatal depression have been published. No published data on breast-feeding were found. Ketamine may remain in breast milk for 12 hr, so the American Academy of Pediatrics (AAP) considers breast-feeding is viable when it is used after this time.

Midazolam. Midazolam is a short-acting benzodiazepine commonly used in procedural sedation or RSI. In most animal researches, no association was found between fatal exposure to midazolam and the risk of congenital defects even when high doses are used. However, in human, the safety of midazolam in the first and second trimesters of pregnancy remains to be unknown, because there are no data about it. Benzodiazepines do not appear to result in malformations in human observational studies. Neonates exposed to midazolam at term may exhibit signs of respiratory depression and decreased muscle tone. The AAP considers midazolam use during lactation of concern because there are few data addressing the issue. Numbers of studies reported that midazolam may remain in breast milk for 8 hr after maternal ingestion.

Propofol. Propofol is a rapidly acting sedative anesthetic that is commonly used in RSI and procedural sedation. In animal researches, there are no association between its use and malformations. But there are still no data on its use in the first and second trimesters of pregnancy in humans. Although high doses are used at term can result in neonatal respiratory and CNS depression, its use at term seems to be safe. Propofol is excreted in breast milk in negligible amounts 24 hr after its use, so it seems that breast-feeding is viable.

Thiopental. Thiopental is an ultra-short-acting barbiturate that may be used during RSI or for status epilepticus. Even in high doses, no reports on congenital defects of thiopental in animal researches have been published. Similarly, no association was found between its use and an increase in congenital anomalies in humans. Thiopental is excreted in milk in concentrations that are too low to be pharmacologically significant and is considered compatible with breast-feeding.

Neuromuscular Blockers

Nondepolarizing Neuromuscular Blocking Agents. Rocuronium and vecuronium are nondepolarizing neuromuscular blocking agents indicated for RSI. The association between the effect of these agents and organogenesis is remain to be unknown. Since the maternal dose crosses the placenta very little, these agents are not thought to pose a significant teratogenic risk. Furthermore, according to the manufacturers, no association was found between increase in congenital anomalies and small laboratory animals which were injected with rocuronium daily. Although very little of either drug is excreted in milk because of their chemical properties, women are not expected to breast-feed while taking neuromuscular blockers.

Depolarizing neuromuscular Blocking Agents. Depolarizing neuromuscular blocking agents, such as Succinylcholine, are used in RSI for its rapid onset of action and short duration of paralysis. Data on its use in early pregnancy in human is limited, but it seems that there are no association between its use and congenital defects. In addition, it appears to have no effect on the newborn, except in rare cases of neonates with pseudocholinesterase deficiency. As occurs in adults with the same condition, newborns with cholinesterase deficiency exhibit prolonged respiratory depression and paralysis. No data on breast-feeding was found, but it may be safe as succinylcholine is hydrolyzed quickly.

Sedative-Hypnotics

Benzodiazepines. Benzodiazepines are indicated for RSI, acute seizures or alcohol withdrawal, and sedation of the acutely agitated patient. During pregnancy, using benzodiazepines in short-term seems to be safe. We found association between its use during the first trimester of pregnancy and the increased risk of oral clefts in some case reports. But in an observational study based on the Swedish medical birth registry, no such association was found. Neonates may exhibit signs of toxicity, including apnea, cyanosis, unresponsiveness, hypotonia, poor feeding and withdrawal symptoms characterized by irritability and tremulousness, resulting from their exposure to benzodiazepines. Owing to the reported risk of apnea, monitoring the effects of exposed to benzodiazepines through breast-feeding closely is needed.

Anticoagulants and Thrombolytics

Warfarin.

Warfarin (Coumadin) is a known human teratogen. About 4% to 5% of exposed fetuses may affected by birth defects. Using warfarin during the 6 to 9 w of pregnancy is at highest risk for birth defects, and the severity of the defects seems to be dose dependent. The fetal warfarin syndrome has been linked to multiple abnormalities, such as hypoplasia of the nasal bones, midline dysplasia including agenesis of the corpus callosum, optic atrophy and blindness, mental retardation, seizures, and stippling of the bones with scoliosis and shortening of limbs. Breast-feeding seems to be viable, because warfarin is so highly protein bound that only a little can be secreted into milk. However, when breast-feeding premature infants, warfarin may associates with an increased risk for intraventricular hemorrhage. So, breast-feeding is not recommended in that case.

Heparin.

Unfractionated heparin is a highly charged heterogeneous molecule with a molecular mass between 5 and 35 kDa. Because heparin can't across the placenta, it does not present a direct risk to the fetus. In early reports, the use of heparin for the prevention or treatment of venous thromboembolism during pregnancy is associated with an increased risk of prematurity, stillbirth, and fetal hemorrhage. But, recently reports have a different opinion that the increased risks previously associated with heparin were determined to be related to underlying maternal condition rather than heparin. When anticoagulation during pregnancy is required, heparin is considered the agent of choice. Sometimes, its use may result in osteopenia and immune-mediated thrombocytopenia and maternal hemorrhage at delivery. Monitoring these adverse effects of exposed to heparin carefully is needed for patients. Because of its chemical properties of high molecular weight, heparin is not excreted in breast milk. However, breast-feeding is not recommended in critically ill patients.

LMWH may be used during pregnancy and in the postnatal period for therapeutic or prophylactic anticoagulation. All currently available LMWH products have been used safely during pregnancy.

Thrombolytic Agents

Thrombolytic agents, such as alteplase, reteplase, urokinase, and streptokinase, have been used successfully in pregnant women who suffered from life-threatening pulmonary embolus or AMI. So far, no reports on the teratogenic effects of thrombolytic agents were published. However, maternal hemorrhage occurred when alteplase or urokinase was used during the intrapartum period. Most thrombolytics' half-life is short, so breast-feeding may be safe.

Antidotes

N-Acetylcysteine.

N-Acetylcysteine is a mucolytic agent, and few study on its teratogenic effects have been reported. In some studies, pregnant patients who overdose on acetaminophen were treated successfully in the same manner as nonpregnant patients without untoward effects. Owing to N-Acetylcysteine has been used in neonates without untoward effects, breast-feeding may be viable during lactation, though the data is limited.

Deferoxamine.

The indications of deferoxamine include iron toxicity occurring from iron overdose or from multiple transfusions in thalassemia patients. Association was found between it and developmental effects on ossification in some animal models. Data on human is limited, but it seems not to affect the fetus. No reports on the effects of deferoxamine on the nursing infant were published, but it is probably compatible.

Digoxin Immune Fragment

The indications of digoxin immune fragment (Fab) therapy include life threatening digitalis overdose and preeclampsia. Data on the use of digoxin immune Fab during pregnancy is limited, only a few case reports were found. A conclusion on the effects of DIG Fab cannot be made based on these reports. Thus in cases of life threatening digitalis overdose with arrhythmias, the benefits of treatment of the mother outweigh the risk to the fetus. The amount of drug diffusing into milk is not large, so it seems to be safe during lactation.

Dimercaprol

Dimercaprol or British antilewisite is a chelating agent, and the indications of it include acute mercury, lead, arsenic, gold poisoning, and Wilson's disease. Data on human is limited. However, it is teratogenic in mice and has been linked to increased mortality, growth restriction, cleft facial features, cerebral herniation, and abnormal digits in mice. In certain cases of heavy metal poisoning, the maternal benefits of dimercaprol use outweigh its potential risks to the unborn fetus. Heavy metals poisoning patients is not allowed to breast-feed.

Flumazenil

Flumazenil is a benzodiazepine antagonist. It has not been linked to teratogenic effects in animals and data on humans are limited. Whether use it in pregnancy and lactation or not depends on the potential maternal benefit compared with possible risks to the fetus and nursing infant. As the half-life of Flumazenil is short, breast-feeding may be safe after a few hours.

Fomepizole

Fomepizole is a competitive inhibitor of alcohol dehydrogenase, and the indication of it includes methanol and ethylene glycol poisoning. No data on its use during pregnancy neither in animals nor in humans. So, its safety during pregnancy remains to be unknown. In cases of toxic alcohol poisoning, the benefits of treatment of the mother outweigh the possible risks to the fetus or nursing infant. During these situations, using ethyl alcohol may be considered and breast-feeding is not recommended.

Hydroxycobalamin

Hydroxycobalamin is a vitamin B_{12} derivative and the indication of it is cyanide toxicity. No data on its use during pregnancy in humans. But in cyanide poisoning, benefits of its use can outweigh any risk to the fetus. No associations were found between hydroxycobalamin and developmental abnormality in animal researches. Breast-feeding is not recommended during cyanide poisoning, but hydroxycobalamin, like its related compounds, is considered compatible with breast-feeding.

Methylene Blue

The indication of methylene blue is methemoglobinemia. In the past, it's also used to identify twins and detect rupture of the membranes. However, an association was found between its use and hemolytic disease in the newborn, hyperbilirubinemia, and deep blue staining of the newborn. It also has been linked to an increased incidence of intestinal obstruction and atresia in the newborn. During acute severe methemoglobinemia, breast-feeding is not recommended, but the effects of methylene blue on the nursing infant are expected to be minimal.

Naloxone

The indication of naloxone is severe respiratory depression in opiate overdose. Because it can readily cross the placenta, its use during pregnancy may result in increase of fetal wakefulness, fetal movement and heart rate, as well as effects attributable to antagonism of fetal endorphins. However, no data on reproductive abnormalities were found. In addition, its use in opiate addicted mothers may precipitate withdrawal in both mother and term fetus. Breast-feeding seems to be safe.

Physostigmine

Physostigmine is an anticholinesterase agent, and the indication of it is severely anticholinergic poisoning associated with delirium. Data on its use during pregnancy is limited. And no association between physostigmine and fetal development was found. However, use of physostigmine at term may decrease Apgar scores at 1 and 5 min mildly. Breast-feeding is not recommended during anticholinergic poisoning, but physostigmine is considered compatible with breast-feeding.

Pralidoxime

Pralidoxime can reactivate cholinesterase, so the indication of it is organophosphate/cholinergic poisoning. Data on its use during pregnancy is limited. And no association was found between pralidoxime and fetal development. In cases of organophosphate poisoning, the benefits to the mother generally outweigh the possible risk to the fetus. Breast-feeding is not recommended during cholinergic poisoning.

Pyridoxine

Pyridoxine is a vitamin. Both good maternal health and good fetal development need it. The indications of it include isoniazid poisoning and gyromitrin mushroom poisoning. Its use has been advocated by some for nausea and vomiting of pregnancy, gestational hypertension, and diabetes. No association was found between pyridoxine and any adverse developmental effects. Breast-feeding seems to be safe.

Succimer

Succimer is a heavy metal chelator, and the indications of it include lead, arsenic, mercury, and cadmium poisoning. In animal researches, association was found between it and congenital defects. Succimer can adversely affect zinc and copper metabolism in animal models. There are only few case reports on its use in human pregnancy were published, and no conclusions had be drawn on its teratogenic effects. Though no data on its use during lactation was found, breast-feeding is not recommended during heavy metal poisoning.

Antimicrobial Agents

Pregnant women who suffered from infections may be adversely affected. Both pregnancy outcomes and fetal development may be influenced. Infections can result in spontaneous abortion if they occur in the first trimester. And infections also can result in preterm labor and delivery if they occur in the second or third trimester. However, pregnancy also can be adversely affected by antimicrobial agents. For example, aminoglycosides have been linked to nephrotoxic and ototoxic in both the mother and her offspring, tetracyclines have been linked to dental staining of the developing fetus, and lincosamides have been linked to skeletotoxic. Besides, antimicrobial agents also have the potential to adversely affect neonate, such as direct effects on the neonate, changes in bowel flora, diarrhea, and potential interference with culture results. During pregnancy, the penicillins, cephalosporins, and macrolide antibiotics are the first choice for infections unless these have failed to control the infection or in cases of severe maternal intolerance to these drugs. The age of the pregnancy, severity of infection, and maternal tolerance for the drug used all have influence on the choice of antimicrobial therapy. Many drugs also are secreted into breast milk.

Antibiotics

Aminoglycosides. Aminoglycosides, such as gentamicin, streptomycin, tobramycin and neomycin, should be avoided during pregnancy. These drugs readily cross the placenta and their use in pregnancy has been linked to fetal ototoxicity and nephrotoxicity. Reports on ototoxicity of kanamycin and streptomycin in the mother and her offspring have been published. However, aminoglycosides seem to have no structural teratogenic effect in humans. No association was found between exposure to gentamicin, streptomycin, tobramycin, or neomycin in utero and either ototoxicity or nephrotoxicity. Because aminoglycosides can only be secreted in milk of small amounts and poorly absorbed from the gastrointestinal tract, breast-feeding may be safe.

Cephalosporins. No controlled studies on the safety of the first- to fourth-generation cephalosporins' use during pregnancy have been reported. However, they may be safe. Some cephalosporins' use may interfere with culture results if a neonatal fever workup is required. Besides, some cephalosporins can secret in milk.

Chloramphenicol. Chloramphenicol is a broad-spectrum antibiotic with excellent blood-brain barrier penetration. Relationship has been found between the use of chloramphenicol and bone marrow suppression and aplastic anemia, which may be fatal. However, in many developing countries, it remains to be the first choice for meningitis. Outside of these complications, its use during pregnancy seems to be safe except at term. Association was found between its use at term and the development of cardiovascular collapse (the "gray baby" syndrome) in a neonate. So, its use at term is forbidden. Although no data on its safety during lactation was found, breast-feeding is not advocated because of its complications.

Clindamycin. No association was found between clindamycin and birth defects. Besides, in animal models, no association was found between clindamycin and congenital abnormalities in the offspring. The American Academy Of Pediatrics(AAP) considers breast-feeding to be safe. However, other agencies don't agree with that, as rare association was found between clindamycin and bloody diarrhea in the nursing infant.

Fluoroquinolones. Association between fluoroquinolones and numerous toxic effects on bone and cartilage growth was found in animal models. And its use during pregnancy, especially during the first trimester is not encouraged. A number of observational studies, however, failed to demonstrate such a toxic effect on the human fetus. Besides, a recent meta-analysis found no increase in the rates of spontaneous abortions, birth defects, prematurity, or low birth weight when fluoroquinolones were used in the first trimester. The AAP considers ciprofloxacin to be compatible with breast-feeding because breast-fed infant plasma levels are low. Data on other quinolones are inconsistent, suggesting that it's better to avoid using in lactation.

Linezolid. An indication of linezolid is methicillin-resistant Staphylococcus aureus infection. Association between linezolid and embryonic death, decreased weight, and abnormalities in cartilage and ossification was found in animal models. But in human, reported data is limited. Only when the maternal benefits outweigh possible risks to the fetus can we use it in pregnancy. Linezolid can secret in milk, but only a small amount of it can reach the nursing infant, implying that breast-feeding might be safe.

Macrolides. No well-controlled studies on effects of erythromycin, azithromycin and clarithromycin on fetus were reported, but they seem to be safe for use in pregnancy and lactation. Some reports have associate erythromycin with pyloric stenosis, however, these studies were not controlled. Association was found between the estolate salt of erythromycin and development of hepatotoxicity in pregnant women, so, its use during pregnancy should be forbidden. Association was found between clarithromycin and an increased risk of fetal and embryonic death and congenital malformations in animal models. However, no association was found in humans so far. In addition, a prospective controlled multicenter study comparing the outcomes of pregnancies exposed to new macrolides (including clarithromycin) to matched controls did not find any differences in the types or patterns of malformations between the two groups. Azithromycin is not likely to be excreted in large amounts in milk, so it may be the first choice for lactating mothers.

Metronidazole. The indications of metronidazole include anaerobic infections, amebiasis, Clostridium difficile infection, and bacterial vaginoses. Data on the use of metronidazole during pregnancy are mixed. Metronidazole is mutagenic and carcinogenic in mice, thus, many physicians avoid prescribing it during pregnancy. However, a number of studies did not reveal any increased incidence of congenital malformations when metronidazole was used in the first trimester. Furthermore, no untoward effects were found when metronidazole was frequently used during the second and third trimesters to treat bacterial vaginosis. Because of its potential mutagenic and carcinogenic effects in rats and its slow elimination from infants, it is not recommended for use during lactation.

Nitrofurantoin. Nitrofurantoin is indicated in urinary tract infections. It seems to be safe throughout pregnancy except near term. However, in a population-based multicenter case-control study, association was found between its use in the first trimester and a number of congenital abnormalities, including anencephaly, microcephaly, hypoplastic left heart, atrial septal defects, and craniofacial clefts. Besides, there are rare reports of hemolytic anemia in the newborn when the drug is used near term.

Penicillins. The first- to fourth-generation penicillins and their derivatives (including procaine, benzathine, clavulanate, sulbactam, and tazobactam) are considered safe for use in pregnancy, as is oral probenecid. Breast-feeding seems to be safe, however, their use may interfere with culture results in the workup of neonatal fever.

Sulfonamides. The indications of sulfonamides include uncomplicated urinary tract infections and Pneumocystis jiroveci (formerly known as Pneumocystic carinii) pneumonia. Another use of sulfonamides is in the treatment of methicillin-resistant S. aureus. In this circumstance, sulfamethoxazole is combined with trimethoprim, presumably to improve antimicrobial efficacy. Both of them are folate antagonist and have traditionally been contraindicated in pregnancy because of association was found between them and an increased risk of neural tube defects and other congenital abnormalities, such as cleft palate. According to a number of observational studies, association was found between trimethoprim-sulfamethoxazole in the first trimester and an increased risk of cardiovascular and urinary tract malformations in the offspring. Furthermore, using sulfonamides near term can result in kernicterus. Because they theoretically compete with bilirubin for protein-binding sites, leaving large amounts of free bilirubin to diffuse, be deposited in the infant's brain, and cause kernicterus. Thus, it should be avoided. However, this complication has not been reported in neonates yet, presumably because free bilirubin is effectively cleared by the placental circulation. In contradistinction, kernicterus has occurred in newborns exposed to sulfonamides after birth. Only a small amount of drug diffusing into milk and a healthy neonate can generally tolerate it. However, in ill or premature infants and in infants with hyperbilirubinemia or glucose-6-phosphate dehydrogenase deficiency, they are contraindicated.

Tetracyclines. The indications of tetracycline include infections with atypical bacteria, Yersinia pestis infection, and anthrax. It readily crosses the placenta and reaches the fetus. Association between tetracycline and the development of fatal fatty liver was clarified in pregnant women, including fetal genitourinary anomalies, inguinal hernias, and limb abnormalities. It also chelates calcium, causing abnormalities in bone growth and staining of decidual teeth. Thus, tetracycline is contraindicated during pregnancy. Because of tetracycline binds to breast milk calcium, only a small amount reaches the nursing infant, and it may be used for short periods (<10 d) during breast-feeding.

Doxycycline also readily crosses the placenta. It does not bind to calcium and is less associated with stained teeth than tetracycline is. In addition, no association was found between it and an increase in any type of congenital malformation However, doxycycline is not advocated for long-term use in lactation. Doxycycline does not bind to breast milk calcium, so the amount of drug reaches the nursing infant is larger than tetracycline, which could theoretically increase its side effects in the newborn.

Vancomycin. An indication of vancomycin is methicillin-resistant S.aureus and C. difficile infection. No association was found between it and birth defects in animals or in humans. Reports of auditory abnormalities and renal insufficiency in neonates of mothers treated with vancomycin are believed to be false positives because these abnormalities were resolved on retesting. Vancomycin can be secreted in breast milk, however, gastrointestinal tract can't absorb it well. Data on its effects on nursing infant remain to be known.

Antifungal Medications

Nystatin is the drugs of choice for mucocutaneous fungal infections during pregnancy and lactation. It has a long safety profile during pregnancy and lactation. It is poorly absorbed from skin, mucous membranes, and the gastrointestinal tract. Although no association between clotrimazole, miconazole, and ketoconazole and major birth defects was found, they are considered second-line treatment of fungal infections in pregnancy. In one case-control study, they have been linked to a minor increase in the incidence of hypoplastic left ventricle. In addition, ketoconazole is teratogenic in rats. When fluconazole was used in large doses (>400 mg/d), it is teratogenic. In that situation, association was found between fluconazole and an increased incidence of craniofacial and cardiovascular defects in offspring and multiple abnormalities of the skeleton and cartilage. However, when it was used in lower doses or with single-dose (150 mg) therapy for vaginal candidiasis, same association can hardly be identified. Ketoconazole, fluconazole, and itraconazole are excreted into breast milk. On the basis of the safe use of ketoconazole in neonates and the lack of negative reports, it is considered compatible with breast-feeding.

Antituberculous Agents

Tuberculosis places the mother and fetus at greater risk if it is untreated with antituberculous medications. Isoniazid, ethambutol, and rifampin cross the placenta, but in a review of antituberculous treatment during pregnancy, they have not been associated with major congenital malformations. Although association between rifampin and hemorrhagic disease of the newborn was found, it remains to be recommended as first-line therapy for treatment of pregnant women. All of them seem to be safe during lactation.

Antiviral Agents

Antiherpetic Drugs. Acyclovir is a purine analogue, and a indication of it is herpesvirus infections. Valacyclovir is rapidly metabolized to l-valine and acyclovir, the active metabolite. Acyclovir readily crosses the placenta in human, and acyclovir is concentrated in fetal circulation in larger amounts than in maternal circulation. No association was found between acyclovir or valacyclovir and congenital malformations or adverse effects on the offspring. During pregnancy, intravenous acyclovir is the first choice for life-threatening maternal herpes simplex virus infections, such as disseminated disease, herpes encephalitis, and varicella pneumonia, which brings a maternal mortality of 44% if untreated Neither acyclovir nor valacyclovir is indicated for the treatment of non–life-threatening genital herpes infection in pregnant women. Because there are only little data on famciclovir 's use during pregnancy have been reported, it is not advocated in pregnancy. Acyclovir is concentrated in milk, in which levels may be higher than in plasma. No reports on adverse outcomes in infants of mothers taking acyclovir or in infants treated with acyclovir for disseminated herpes have been published, thus, it seems to be safe in lactation.

Anti-Influenza Drugs. Affected by influenza in pregnancy may result in an increase in morbidity and mortality. No association was found between M2 ion channel inhibitors such as amantadine and rimantadine, and improved maternal and pregnancy outcomes. Similarly, no association was found between improved maternal and pregnancy outcomes and neuraminidase inhibitors, such as oseltamivir and zanamivir, . However, in human, association was found between amantadine and various malformations including cardiac defects. Besides, amantadine appears teratogenic and embryonic in rats. In a cohort study, no association was found between both class of anti-influenza drugs and an increase in malformations or stillbirths. However, association was found between them and an increase in the incidence of necrotizing colitis in premature newborns exposed to either of these classes of drugs. Oseltamivir seems to be compatible with breast-feeding.

Anti-HIV Drugs. The indication of Anti-HIV drugs is immediately after a needle-stick injury or sexual contact with an infected individual. No association was found between these agents' use during pregnancy and birth defects. However, the mutagenesis, carcinogenesis and their long-term effects on the liver, heart and reproductive system of these drugs remain to be elucidated.

In animal and human researches, association was found between didanosine, lamivudine, stavudine, zidovudine, and zalcitabine and a small risk of structural malformations and mitochondrial dysfunction in the developing fetus, but, no association was found between birth defects and protease inhibitors, such as ritonavir and nelfinavir. However, even if a negative association is proven, the risk of morbidity and mortality from HIV infection far outweighs the risk of toxicity of most of these substances. When indicated, the benefits of treatment outweigh the drugs'toxicities, so treatment should not be withheld. In addition, zidovudine has been shown to significantly reduce vertical and perinatal transmission of HIV from the mother to the fetus. Because of the risk of postnatal HIV transmission through milk, breast-feeding is not recommended by the Centers for Disease Control and Prevention.

Cardiovascular Agents

Antidysrhythmics

Arrhythmias are usual complications of pregnancy. Most are benign and have good prognosis, while a few are fatal. Electrical cardioversion can be used for unstable tachycardias and medication for the stable tachycardias .When antidysrhythmics are chosen, the drug's side effects shoud be taken into account to protect the mother and the fetus.

Adenosine. Adenosine is natural in the human body and have a quick metabolic rate. It can be used safely throughout pregnancy to terminate the maternal supraventricular and fetal tachycardia. Adenosine is safe in lactation.

Amiodarone. Iodine in amiodarone may cause congenital goiter and transient neonatal hyperthyroidism or hypothyroidism. Moreover, amiodarone has been associated with many congenital abnormalities, such as cardiac structural abnormalities, growth restriction, and developmental delay. So the FDA has approved amiodarone for a Pregnancy Category D classification. We should weigh the advantages and disadvantages when amiodarone is used during pregnancy. Refractory cases of supraventricular or ventricular tachycardias in the mother and incessant tachycardias in the fetus maybe the indications. Because the high concentration of iodine in amiodarone can excrete into milk, amiodarone should be avoided in nursing mothers.

Digoxin and Quinidine. Congenital defects has not been reported when Digoxin and quinidine are used in humans or animals. Digoxin and quinidine can be safely used during pregnancy and lactation. They are first-line agents for the treatment of significant maternal dysrhythmias. Overdoses of these drugs may led to premature labor, spontaneous abortions.

Lidocaine. Lidocaine rapidly passes through the placental barrier and becomes ion trapped in the fetus. There is no evidence that use of lidocaine during early pregnancy may lead to any abnormal fetal development. However, overdose is linked to neonatal CNS depression, apnea, hypotonia, seizures, and bradycardia. Lidocaine is considered compatible with breast-feeding. As a whole, lidocaine is a weak base.

Procainamide. Clinical practices have shown procainamide can be used successfully and safely during pregnancy to terminate stable wide-complex tachyarrhythmias. It has not been linked to abnormal fetal development and appears good tolerance with short-term use Procainamide and its metabolite have appeared in breast milk, therefore, procainamide should be avoided in nursing mothers.

Flecainide. Flecainide's structure is similar to procainamide's and is a class IC antiarrhythmic agent Although flecainide has been associated with fetal hyperbilirubinemia, hepatotoxicity, and loss of fetal heart rate variability, clinical practices have indicated that flecainide is safe in termination of maternal and fetal tachycardia as long as it was used properly. Experiments on animal have found that flecainide might cause birth deformities in some animal species, including cardiac and musculoskeletal abnormalities. Flecainide can passes through the placental barrier, but the concentrations of flecainide in milk are not toxic to infants. Some authorities considers flecainide compatible with breast-feeding despite limited experience.

Ibutilide. As a class III antiarrhythmic,Ibutilide is used to terminate atrial fibrillation and flutter. The data is limited in terms of its successful and safe use during latter pregnancy in humans. In animals, ibutilide is proved to be teratogenic and associated with cardiac septal defects as well as skeletal dysgenesis, especially in high-dose administration. We should weight the advantages and disadvantages when ibutilide is used during pregnancy and chose the proper case with caution.

Sotalol. Sotalol has been used during pregnancy to effectively and safely cure atrial arrhythmias and hypertension. It has also been successfully used to terminate fetal atrial tachycardias. Teratogenic effects have not been found in animals. Bradycardia which usually persists for 24 hr in the newborn is the most common side effect. Sotalol can go into milk, but does not appear to led to the nursing infant's bradycardia or hypotension. Some authorities consides Sotalol compatible with breast-feeding.

Antihypertensives

Hypertension is a common complication in pregnency, and about 12% of pregnant woman complicate with hypertension, especially in the third trimester. In the United States, hypertension accounts for 16% of maternal deaths. According to the JNC guidelines, IV labetalol may be used effectively and safely to cure hypertensive emergencies in pregnancy.

Angiotensin-Converting Enzyme Inhibitors. In animals, ACEI increase the rate of stillbirths. In human, ACEI led to the most significant adverse fetal effects including oligohydramnios, anuria, renal agenesis, increased risk of stillbirth, intrauterine growth restriction, fetal skull abnormalities, pulmonary hypoplasia, respiratory distress syndrome and fetal and neonatal hypotension. FDA has approved ACEI for a Pregnancy Category D classification. Some authorities consider captopril and enalapril compatible with breast-feeding.

Angiotensin* Ⅱ *Receptor Antagonists. Angiotensin Ⅱ receptor antagonists has been reported to cause fetal abnormalities similar to the abnormalities seen with ACEI, including renal agenesis, neonatal anuria, oligohydramnios, intrauterine growth restriction, persistent patent ductus arteriosus, abnormal ossification. The use in any stage of pregnancy should be avoided. The data on their safety in lactation remains limited.

Beta-Blockers. Beta-blockers have not been associated with fetal malformations and have proved to be safe with short-term use. They have been considered a first-line medications of hypertension in pregnancy. Beta-Blockers,especially acebutolol, atenolol,and propranolol have adverse fetal effects of intrauterine growth restriction and a low placental weight. If pregnant woman use beta-blockers near term,persistent beta blockade in the newborn may occurs. Nonselective beta-blockers, such as propranolol, also have side effects of neonatal hypoglycemia, respiratory depression,and hyperbilirubinemia in the newborn. These adverse effects are less common in cardioselective beta-blocker, such as atenolol or metoprolol. Esmolol is a common short-acting beta-blocker used to terminate maternal supraventricular dysrhythmias and hypertension during surgery,but has been linked to fetal bradycardia, neonatal bradycardia and hypotension, and severe fetal distress . The action of Beta-blockers on the nursing infant is complicated. Close observation their adverse effects on infant is recommended.

Calcium Channel Blockers. Clinical practice has demonstrated that calcium channel blockers may be used without risk for the treatment of supraventricular arrhythmias and hypertension in pregnant women. Intravenous verapamil has also been used for the treatment of fetal tachycardia,while intravenous nicardipine has been used to control preeclampsia. In addition, some calcium channel blockers, such as nifedipine and diltiazem, have been used as tocolytic agents. Animal experimental researches have demonstrated that use of calcium channel blockers during early pregnancy was associated with a dose-dependent increase in embryonic mortality and skeletal abnormalities. But these abnormalities have not been seen in human. Some side effects of calcium channel blocker include maternal hypotension, tachycardia, and fetal distress, especially significant when sublingual nifedipine or intravenous nicardipine is administrated. Some authorities consider these drugs compatible with breast-feeding.

Hydralazine is a direct-acting smooth muscle relaxant used to treat hypertension with rapid onset of action.Becaue of the common side effects of maternal hypotension, placental abruption and neonata. It is no longer recommended as a first-line but a second-line agent in the treatment of hypertensive emergency in pregnancy. Hydrochlorothiazide is considered compatible with breast-feeding by the American Academy of Pediatrics.

Diuretics. Diuretics generally are not recommended for pregnancy-induced hypertension because of their maternal hypovolemia adverse effects. Animal experimental researches have found loop diuretics such as furosemide associated with fetal renal and skeletal abnormalities. These effects have not been seen in humans, but a slightly increased risk of hypospadias has been described. The only role for pregnant use of furosemide is pulmonary edema secondary to congestive heart failure. Furosemide can pass into breast milk but is considered compatible with breast-feeding by the American Academy of Pediatrics. Thiazide diuretics have adverse effects of hypoglycemia, electrolyte abnormalities, meconium staining in neonates when given near term, and even increase perinatal mortality in some cases. In addition, thiazide diuretics may directly inhibit the smooth muscle and led to uterine inertia. Thiazide diuretics are considered compatible with breast-feeding.

Nitrates. Animal researches have demonstrated that nitroglycerin may cause fetal harm, but current researches in humans do not show any major adverse effects on the fetus or neonate. As a rapidly and short-acting agent, nitroglycerin appears safe and effective in the treatment of intrapartum fetal distress due to uterine hyperactivity. For the treatment of hypertensive emergencies in pregnancy nitroprusside has the same benefit and risk as in general population. Long-term and large doses use of nitroprusside may result in cyanide toxicity and severe metabolic acidosis. Nitroprusside readily passes through the placental barrier, and the concentration in fetus is twice as much as that in mother. Therapeutic doses do not appear to make the fetus poisoned, because we have optimal agents with safety and effectiveness such as labetalol, nitroprusside is considered the last resort. Data in terms of its safe use during lactation is limited, and breast-feeding is not recommended.

Vasopressors

Vasopressors should be initiated in shock pregnancy only after adequate fluid resuscitation has been achieved. Vasopressors has the capability of increasing uterine and makes a reduction in placental blood flow. Therefore, the indications, benefits and risks should be taken into account when it is used in pregnant women .Regarding its safety characteristic, phenylephrine appears to be the optimal agent in the treatment of circulatory shock during pregnancy.

Dobutamine. Dobutamine is an non-digitalis positive inotropic drug that is indicated in cardiac dysfunction caused by various origin. Animal and clinic trials have not found dobutamine associated with any adverse effects on fetus or neonate.

Dopamine. Dopamine has specific agonist action on dopamine receptors ,besides agonist action on alpha- and beta-adrenoceptors. Recent studies do not reveal low-dose dopamine may improve mortality or renal function. In clinical practices, dopamine has been used in pregnant women complicating shock, including spinal shock due to spinal anesthesia. Dopamine has been found to decrease uterine vascular flow, but fetal adverse effects have not been observed in animal studies. The data on the safety during breast-feeding remains limited, and breast-feeding is not recommended during critical illness.

Epinephrine. Epinephrine has been commonly used in the treatment of severe anaphylaxis, refractory shock and status asthmaticus. Epinephrine has been associated with fetal anoxic injury, intracranial hemorrhage, and increased incidence of inguinal hernias. The data on the safety during breast-feeding remains limited.

Norepinephrine. Experimental researches on animal have found norepinephrine may led to vascular and skeletal abnormalities. Meanwhile, it reduces placental blood flow and cause fetal anoxia, and increased the incidence of cerebral hemorrhage. The data on the safety during breast-feeding remains limited, but breast-feeding with norepinephrine use is not recommended.

Ephedrine and Phenylephrine. Ephedrine and phenylephrine have been used effectively in the treatment of pregnant shock from any cause. The incidence of adverse effects such as tachycardia, maternal gastric intolerance and fetal acidosis in ephedrine is more common than in phenylephrine. Phenylephrine has taken the place of ephedrine in shock during pregnancy.

Endocrine Agents

Diabetes Medications

Diabetes mellitus may greatly increase incidence of congenital malformations in multiple organ systems. It is also closely related to an increase in perinatal morbidity. On the other hand, hypoglycemia is also associated with adverse pregnancy outcomes, therefore, glycemic control in pregnancy should be achieved in a accurate manner.

Insulin. Insulin can not cross through the placenta barrier. It is thoughted to be the safe agent for diabetes mellitus types 1 and 2 in pregnancy.

Sulfonylureas. Sulfonylureas are considered to be possibly more teratogenic and less effective than insulin in the control of gestational diabetes. Meanwhile, sulfonylureas have been related to neonatal hypoglycemia when used in pre-delivery women. Generally, the information about their use during pregnancy is limited. A randomized clinical study has demonstrated that glyburide was as effective and safe as insulin during pregnancy. Duo to high protein binding rate, glyburide and glipizide are not likely to pass into breast milk, but monitoring glucose in nursing infants is sensible.

Metformin. Severe adverse effects including metabolic acidosis and hepatotoxicity have been confirmed in adults taking metformin. Fetal malformations in animals has not been observed. In a clinical research about women taking metformin for polycystic ovary disease, major birth defects was not found. In addition, metformin does not easy to result in neonatal hypoglycemia, a common sulfonylureas-induced complication. Metformin is considered compatible with breast-feeding. Due to its potential severe effects in adults and its excretion into milk, it should be used with caution in lactating mothers.

Thyroid Medications

Maternal hyperthyroidism is related to series of pregnant complication, including spontaneous abortion, preterm labor, placental abruption and maternal congestive heart failure. Maternal hyperthyroidism also increased the risk of some related disease in offspring, such as intrauterine growth restriction, intrauterine fetal death and neonatal goiter.

Propylthiouracil. PTU has been used during pregnancy to prevents the synthesis of thyroxine and prevents the peripheral conversion of T_4 to T_3.PTU has been associated with transient goiter and hypothyroidism of the newborn, but it scarely led to congenital defects. Methimazole and carbimazole also used for hyperthyroidism in pregnancy have been associated with abnormal development of the skin. PTU may goes into breast milk in negligible amounts and is considered compatible with breast-feeding.

Iodides. Iodides are used for hyperthyroidism crisis. They are quickly absorbed by the fetal thyroid gland and lead to fetal hypothyroidism and goiter.

Levothyroxine. Several risks including spontaneous abortion, intrauterine growth restriction, placental abruption, and fetal demise have been confirmed in hypothyroidism pregnancy. Hypothyroidism has been related to severe neurologic impairment of the offspring. Levothyroxine is a synthetic formulation of naturally thyroxine T_4, which has been used for the treatment of hypothyroidism during pregnancy. Adverse effects on the offspring has not been found when levothyroxine is used in pregnant women.

Gastrointestinal Agents

Antacids

H_2 Receptor Antagonists. H_2 Receptor Antagonists are commonly used during pregnancy. H_2 Receptor Antagonists have not been associated with congenital malformation, and proved to be safe for the nursing infant.

Proton Pump Inhibitors. Proton Pump Inhibitors have not been demonstrated relating to any increased risk for major congenital birth defects, spontaneous abortions, or preterm delivery in a meta-analysis. Proton pump inhibitors including esomeprazole, lansoprazole, pantoprazole and rabeprazole, are commonly used during pregnancy. Researchers have discovered proton pump inhibitors might increase the incidence of gastrointestinal, hepatic and thyroid cancers in animals. Data regarding proton pump inhibitors on human nursing infants remains limited.

Antiemetic Medications

Phenothiazines. Metoclopramide, prochlorperazine and promethazine are classified as phenothiazines that have been commonly used in the treatment of nausea and vomiting of pregnancy. Current evidence does not support an association with major congenital abnormalities. Phenothiazines may go into breast milk and cause sedation and other untoward effects in neonates. Therefore, they should be cautiously used in nursing mothers by the recommendations of American Academy of Pediatrics.

Serotonin 5-HT$_3$ Receptor Antagonists. Serotonin 5-HT$_3$ receptor antagonists, such as dolasetron, granisetron and ondansetron have not been found associated with any fetal malformations. The AAP considers these agents compatible with breast-feeding.

Neurologic Agents

Anticonvulsants

Anticonvulsants have a generally teratogenic effect, and congenital malformations occurred in 30% of exposed pregnancies. The longer and the more pregnant women use anticonvulsants, the higher risks for birth defects will be. Valproate is related to the most frequent and serious adverse effects on the mothers and fetus compared with phenytoin, carbamazepine, and lamotrigine . On the other hand, in some cases, seizures control during pregnancy may outweigh anticonvulsants' negative effecte. Because generalized seizures during pregnancy are associated with an increased risk of spontaneous abortion and fetal hypoxia. Monotherapy and the lowest dose of anticonvulsant are recommended. Dividing of the daily dose to decrease peak plasma levels is sensible. Gradual increase of the dosage is often required to maintain adequate seizure control.

Classic Anticonvulsants. The classic anticonvulsants are teratogenic, and the FDA has approved them for the Pregnancy Category D classification . Carbamazepine has proved associated with an increased risk of craniofacial defects, neural tube defects, and developmental delay. Phenobarbital has proved associated with a slightly increased risk of congenital heart disease and cleft lip or palate, and its prolonged use during pregnancy may led to neonatal withdrawal. Phenytoin has been associated with the fetal hydantoin syndrome including several characteristic. Those are craniofacial abnormalities including cleft lip and palate, impaired growth, varying degrees of ossification abnormalities of the extremities and digits, delayed neurologic development and multiple cardiovascular anomalies. The fetal hydantoin syndrome occurs in 5% to 10% of pregnancies that taking phenobarbita. Valproic acid has been linked to multiple facial anomalies, congenital heart disease, strabismus, and neural tube defects.

Carbamazepine, phenobarbital and phenytoin have also been linked to coagulation disorders of the neonates, presumably due to placental transport inhibition of vitamin K. Carbamazepine, phenytoin, and valproic acid may present in breast milk, and the low concentration in breast milk make them compatible with breast-feeding. However, as phenobarbital has proved associated with neonatal sedation and respiratory depression, it is not considered compatible with breast-feeding.

Newer Anticonvulsants. Lamotrigine, levetiracetam and topiramate are known as newer anticonvulsants. They have been associated with a mildly increased incidence of major birth defects including oral clefts, skeletal abnormalities, and hypospadias. The risks of these birth defects increase with the number of used anticonvulsants. But these findings have not been seen in two studies comparing the newer anticonvulsants. These newer anticonvulsants also appeared to have a good toleration in the nursing infant, except for topiramate, which caused excess sedation and incresed the incidence of respiratory depression.

Migraine Medications

Ergot Alkaloids. Ergotamine and dihydroergotamine have been commonly used in the treatment of migraines. Some animal experimental researches have demonstrated they were associated with intrauterine growth restriction, probably because of reductions in uteroplacental blood flow. Although ergotamine and dihydroergotamine have not been associated with teratogenic effects, due to their oxytocic effects, they are contraindicated in pregnancy. Ergotamine and dihydroergotamine may be secreted into breast milk and cause ergot poisoning of the nursing infant. Therefor ,they are also contraindicated in breast-feeding.

Triptans. The triptans are selective serotonin agonists, have been effectively used in the treatment of vascular headaches, such as migraines and cluster headaches. They have been associated with teratogenic in some animal researches, but recent data in humans demonstrate they are safety during pregnancy. Sumatriptan may secrete into breast milk, but the low concentration in breast milk makes it compatible with breast-feeding.

Respiratory Agents

Antihistamines

Antihistamines have been commonly and

safely used in the treatment of allergic reactions, nausea and vomiting during pregnancy. The familiar antihistamines include chlorpheniramine, diphenhydramine, doxylamine, hydroxyzine, and meclizine First-generation antihistamines are not recommended during breast-feeding due to their inhibiting lactation. In addition, serious CNS adverse effects, including seizures, have been reported in neonates, especially the premature, when mothers receive antihistamines. The newer generation antihistamines, such as cetirizine and loratadine, prove safe during pregnancy and may be used for the treatment of severe allergies. These drugs may secrete into human milk, but in the case of loratadine, very small amounts enter the neonatal body. The AAP recommends these drugs compatible with breast-feeding.

Asthma Medications

Asthma during pregnancy increases the incidence of neonatal death, low-birth-weight , preeclampsia, infants preterm birth, and small for-gestational-age infants. Poorly controlled asthma may also make the mother have a increasing rate of chorioamnionitis, hypertensive disorders of pregnancy, cesarean section, and prolonged hospitalization stay. Better asthma control has been associated with an less complications and improved outcome. Beta-adrenergic medications, including terbutaline, albuterol, and metaproterenol, have been commonly used in the treatment of asthma. They have also been used during the last trimester to treat premature labor. Albuterol is the most common medication and is the treatment of choice in asthma during pregnancy. Albuterol appears safe even with long-term use, and it is compatible with breast-feeding.

None of the beta-adrenergic medications has been associated with fetal or congenital malformations, except some have been related to significant cardiovascular and metabolic effects, which have a transient feature and a good fetal toleration. Transient hyperglycemia followed by insulin secretion secondary to beta-agonists may also occur, resulting in neonatal hypoglycemia, especially in diabetic pregnant women. Significant maternal and fetal arrhythmias may also occur when terbutaline is used intravenously or orally in pregnant women. Maternal pulmonary edema and death have been reported. The FDA has disapproved its use in preterm labor because safer beta$_2$-agonists and tocolytic agents are available. Long-acting beta-agonists also prove safe during pregnancy.

Animal experimental researches have not found ipratropium may cause birth deformities. However, data regarding its safety in human pregnancy remains limited. Ipratropium is compatible with breast-feeding. Major birth effects or perinatal complications have not been found in the pregnant women taking cromolyn sodium. Cromolyn sodium is compatible with breast-feeding.

Corticosteroids

Corticosteroids have been commonly used in pregnant women for the treatment of various illnesses, such as allergy, asthma, and autoimmune diseases. Inhaled corticosteroids are mainly used in the maintenance treatment of asthma during pregnancy, oral and intravenous corticosteroids are the mainstay of therapy for acute exacerbations of asthma. Generally, they are not associated with human teratogens. However, they may mildly increase the incidence of orofacial clefts when oral steroids are used during the first trimester. Moreover, their use in the third trimester may increases the incidence of preterm delivery, preeclampsia, low birth weight, congenital adrenal hyperplasia and neonatal cataracts. Prednisone is considered safe during breast-feeding. Data on the safety of leukotriene antagonists in pregnancy remains limited.

Decongestants

Decongestants including phenylpropanolamine and pseudoephedrine, may strongly contract the blood vessel and result in placental ischemia. Therefore, they are not recommended during pregnancy. Increased incidence of abnormalities, such as gastroschisis and intestinal atresia, may occurs if phenylpropanolamine or pseudoephedrine is used in early pregnancy, even though the risk is low. Pseudoephedrine may secrete into breast milk in small quantities, and is considered compatible with breast-feeding.

Table 55-1 Summary of Medication Safety in Pregnancy and Lactation

MEDICATION	PREGNANCY	LACTATION
Analgesic agents		
Acetaminophen or paracetamol	Safe (B)	Safe
Nonsteroidal anti-inflammatory drugs (NSAID)		
Salicylate	Not recommended (D)	Safe for short-term use
Other NSAID	Not recommended (D)	Safe
Opiates: Most opiates are considered safe for short-term use but are all reclassified in category D if used for prolonged periods or if used in high doses at term (due to respiratory depression in newborn). Do not use opiates combined with aspirin or NSAID.		
Morphine—short-term use	Safe (C)	Safe
Fentanyl—short-term use	Safe (C)	Safe
Methadone	Safe (B/C)	Safe
Meperidine—short-term use	Safe (C)	Safe
Codeine	Possible risk (C)	Not advised if longer than 2 d
Oxycodone—short-term use	Safe (C)	Probably safe
Hydrocodone—short-term use	Safe (C)	Probably safe
Hydromorphone—short-term use	Safe (B)	Probably safe
Oxycodode—short-term use	Safe (B)	Probably safe
Antibiotics: Use of antibiotics near term may interfere with culture results in neonates.		
Penicillins		
First-generation penicillins: penicillin G, benzathine penicillin, bicillin, penicillin VK	Safe (B)	Safe
Second-generation penicillins: oxacillin, dicloxacillin, nafcillin	Safe (B)	Safe
Third-generation penicillins: ampicillin, ampicillin-sulbactam, amoxicillin, amocillin-clavulanate	Safe (B)	Safe
Fourth-generation penicillins: ticarcillin, ticarcillin-clavulanate, piperacillin, piperacillin-tazobactam, carbenicillin	Safe (B)	Probably safe
Cephalosporins		
First generation: cephalexin, cefazolin, cefadroxil	Safe (B)	Safe
Second generation: cefuroxime, cefaclor, cefoxitin, cefprozil	Safe (B)	Safe
Third generation: cefdinir, cefotaxime, ceftazidime, ceftriaxone, cefpodoxime, ceftizoxime	Safe (B)	Probably safe
Chloramphenicol: *Do not* use at term because it can cause "gray baby syndrome."	Safe until term (C)	Possible toxicity
Macrolides		
Erythromycin: *Do not* use estolate salt.	Safe (B)	Safe
Azithromycin	Safe (B)	Safe
Clarithromycin	Probably safe (C)	Probably safe
Sulfonamides: May cause kernicterus in newborn if given in third trimester.	Not recommended near term (C)	Safe, except in premature infants or infants with G6PD deficiency or hyperbiliru-binemia

Continued

MEDICATION	PREGNANCY	LACTATION
Quinolones		
First generation: nalidixic acid	Moderate risk (C)	Safe
Second generation: ciprofloxacin, norfloxacin, ofloxacin	Small risk (C)	Probably safe
Third generation: levaquin	Small risk (C)	Probably safe
Fourth generation: gatifloxacin, moxifloxacin	Small risk (C)	Probably safe
Aminoglycosides	Not recommended (D)	Safe
Clindamycin	Safe (B)	Safe
Vancomycin	Safe (B)	Safe
Linezolid: Maternal benefit may outweigh risks to fetus or embryo.	Unknown (C)	Safety unknown
Tetracyclines	Not recommended (D)	Not recommended
Nitrofurantoin: May cause hemolytic anemia in newborn if used in third trimester.	Safe (B), except in third trimester	Probably safe
Metronidazole	Contraindicated in first trimester, safe in second and third trimesters (B)	Not recommended
Antifungals		
Nystatin	Safe (B/C)	Safety unknown
Clotrimazole	Safe (B/C)	Safety unknown
Ketoconazole	Probably safe (C)	Probably safe
Fluconazole	Not recommened in high doses (C)	Safe
Terbinafine	Low risk (B)	Not recommended
Antituberculous medications in general present a maternal benefit that is much greater than the fetal or embryonic risk and may be prescribed during any stage of pregnancy when indicated.		
INH	Safe (C)	Probably safe
Rifampin	Probably safe (C)	Probably safe
Ethambutol	Safe (C)	Probably safe
Antiviral agents		
Antiherpetic medications		
Acyclovir	Safe (B)	Safe
Valacyclovir	Safe (B)	Safe
Famciclovir	Small risk (B)	Potentially toxic
Anti-influenza agents		
Amantadine	Possible risk (C)	Safety unknown
Oseltamivir	Safe in animals (C)	Safety unknown
Anti-HIV medications in general present a maternal benefit that is much greater than the fetal or embryonic risk and may be prescribed during any stage of pregnancy when indicated.		

Continued

MEDICATION	PREGNANCY	LACTATION
Reverse transcriptase inhibitors		
Zidovudine	Caution in first trimester (C)	Not recommended
Lamivudine	Caution in first trimester (C)	Not recommended
Didanosine	Caution in first trimester (B)	Not recommended
Tenovir	Caution in first trimester (B)	Not recommended
Indinavir	Caution in first trimester (C)	Not recommended
Protease inhibitors		
Ritonavir	Caution in first trimester (B)	Not recommended
Nelfinavir	Caution in first trimester (B)	Not recommended
Anticoagulants		
Warfarin	Contraindicated	Safe
Heparin	Safe (B)	Safe
Low-molecular-weight heparin	Safe (B)	Safe
Thrombolytics: Benefits to the mother generally outweigh the risk to the fetus.		
Alteplase	Safe (C)	Probably safe
Reteplase	Safe (C)	Probably safe
Urokinase	Safe (B)	Probably safe
Streptokinase—no human data	Safe in animals (C)	Hold breast-feeding
Tenectaplase—no human data	Safe in animals (C)	Hold breast-feeding
Anticonvulsants: Benefits to the mother outweigh the risks to the fetus and embryo. Monotherapy is recommended. Use of highly teratogenic anticonvulsants is recommended in refractory cases only.		
Carbamazepine	Teratogen (D)	Probably safe
Valproic acid	Teratogen (D)	Probably safe
Phenobarbital	Not recommended (D)	Not recommended
Phenytoin	Teratogen (D)	Safe
Lamotrigine	Small risk in animals (C)	Not recommended
Levetiracetam	Small risk in animals (C)	Safety unknown
Topiramate	Small risk in animals (C)	Safety unknown
Gabapentin	Small risk in animals (C)	Probably safe
Sedative-hypnotics		
Benzodiazepines: Results are inconsistent. There may be a small risk of abnormalities. In the acute short-term treatment of status epilepticus, agitated delirium, and alcohol or benzodiazepine withdrawal, benefits to the mother outweigh risks to the fetus or embryo. Not recommended for long-term use.		
Diazepam—low risk in first and third trimesters	Safe acutely; unsafe for chronic use (D)	Potential toxicity
Lorazepam—low risk in first and third trimesters	Safe acutely; unsafe for chronic use (D)	Potential toxicity
Chlordiazepoxide—low risk in first and third trimesters	Safe acutely; unsafe for chronic use (D)	Potential toxicity

Continued

MEDICATION	PREGNANCY	LACTATION
Oxazepam—low risk in first and third trimesters	Safe acutely; unsafe for chronic use (D)	Potential toxicity
Midazolam—low risk in first and third trimesters	Safe acutely; unsafe for chronic use (D)	Potential toxicity
Barbiturates		
Methohexital	Safe (C)	Safety unknown
Thiopental	Safe (C)	Safety unknown
Ketamine: Risk mainly with high doses close to delivery.	Safe (B)	Probably safe after 12 hr
Propofol	Safe (B/C)	Not recommended
Etomidate	Safe (B/C)	Probably safe
Paralytic agents		
Depolarizing agents		
Succinylcholine	Low risk, especially around delivery (C)	Probably safe
Nondepolarizing agents		
Rocuronium	Limited data (C)	Probably safe
Vecuronium	Limited data (C)	Probably safe
Antiarrythmics: In cases of refractory arrhythmias, the benefits to the mother may outweigh risks to the fetus or embryo.		
Adenosine	Safe (C)	Safe
Amiodarone	Not recommended (D)	Contraindicated
Digoxin—caution in third trimester (oxytocic)	Safe (C)	Safe
Disopyramide	Caution in third trimester (B)	Probably safe
Encainide	Limited data (C)	Probably safe
Flecainide	Limited data (C)	Not recommended
Quinidine	Safe (C)	Not recommended
Procainamide	Safe (C)	Not recommended
Ibutilide	Risk in animals	Not recommended
Lidocaine	Safe (B)	Probably safe
Sotalol	Probably safe (C)	Not recommended
Antihypertensives		
Angiotensin antagonists		
Angiotensin-converting enzyme inhibitors	Not recommended (D)	Some are safe
Angiotensin Ⅱ receptor antagonists	Not recommended (D)	Safety unknown
Beta-blockers		
Labetalol	Probably safe (C)	Probably safe
Atenolol	Caution in second and third trimesters (D)	Potential toxicity

Continued

MEDICATION	PREGNANCY	LACTATION
Esmolol	Caution in third trimester (C)	Safety unknown
Metoprolol	Caution in second and third trimesters (D)	Potential toxicity
Propranolol	Caution in second and third trimesters (D)	Probably safe
Calcium channel blockers		
Diltiazem—tocolytic	Probably safe (C)	Probably safe
Verapamil	Probably safe (C)	Probably safe
Amlodipine	No data (C)	No data
Nifedipine—not sublingual	Probably safe (C)	Probably safe
Diuretics: Caution for dehydration and electrolyte abnormalities.		
Furosemide	Low risk (C)	Probably safe
Bumetanide	Low risk (C)	Probably safe
Ethacrynic acid	Low risk (B)	Probably safe
Torsemide	Low risk (B)	Probably safe
Hydrochlorothiazide—contraindicated in gestational HTN	Safe (B)	Safe
Nitrates		
Nitroprusside	Some risk (C)	Potential toxicity
Nitroglycerin	Probably safe (C)	Probably safe
Vasodilators		
Hydralazine	Safe (C)	Safe
Alpha effectors		
Clonidine	Caution in third trimester (C)	No data
Other		
Methyldopa	Safe (B)	Safe
Fenoldopam	No data (B)	No data
Medications used in the treatment of asthma, allergies, and upper respiratory infection: For asthmatic patients, maternal benefits outweigh risks to fetus or embryo.		
Beta-adrenergics considered safe for short-term use		
Epinephrine	Risk (C)	Potential toxicity
Metaproterenol	Safe (C)	Probably safe
Salmeterol	Limited data (C)	Probably safe
Albuterol	Safe (C)	Probably safe
Terbutaline	Low risk (C)	Probably safe
Anticholinergic agents		
Ipratropium	Safe (B)	Probably safe

Continued

MEDICATION	PREGNANCY	LACTATION
Mast cell stabilizers		
Cromolyn sodium	Safe (B)	Probably safe
Leukotriene inhibitors		
Zafirlukast	Risk (B)	No data
Zileuton	Risk (C)	Not recommended
Montelukast	Risk (B)	No data; probably compatible
Corticosteroids safe for short-term use: Human data suggest an increased risk of orofacial clefts.		
Prednisolone	Risk (C)	Safe
Prednisone	Risk (C)	Safe
Methylprednisolone	Risk (C)	Safe
Antihistamines		
Chlorpheniramine	Safe (B)	Not recommended
Diphenhydramine	Safe (B)	Not recommended
Dimenhydramine	Safe (B)	Not recommended
Doxylamine	Safe (B)	Not recommended
Hydroxyzine	Risk (C)	Not recommended
Meclizine	Safe (B)	Not recommended
Cetirizine	Probably safe (B)	Not recommended
Fexofenadine	Class C	Safe
Loratadine	Probably safe (B)	Safe
Decongestants		
Pseudoephedrine	Risk (C)	Probably safe
Antiemetics		
Dopamine antagonists		
Promethazine	Safe (C)	Not recommended
Prochlorperazine	Safe (C)	Potential toxicity
Metoclopramide	Safe (B)	Potential tocxicity
5-HT_3 antagonists—generally safe		
Dolasetron	Low risk (B)	Probably safe
Granisetron	Low risk (B)	Probably safe
Ondansetron	Safe (B)	Probably safe
Medications used in the treatment of diabetes		
Insulin	Safe (B)	Safe
Sulfonylureas		
Glipizide	Low risk (C)	Probably safe. Caution: Nursing infants should be monitored.

Continued

MEDICATION	PREGNANCY	LACTATION
Glyburide	Low risk (C)	Probably safe. Caution: Nursing infants should be monitored.
Metformin	Moderate risk (C)	Probably safe
Pioglitazone	Moderate risk (C)	Probably safe
Rosiglitazone	Moderate risk (C)	Probably safe
Antacids		
H_2 blockers		
Famotidine	Low risk (B)	Probably safe
Ranitidine	Safe (B)	Probably safe
Nizatidine	Low risk (B)	Probably safe
Cimetidine	Safe (B)	Safe
Proton pump inhibitors		
Omeprazole	Low risk (C)	Safety unknown
Esomeprazole	Low risk (B)	Safety unknown
Lansoprazole	Low risk (B)	Safety unknown
Pantoprazole	Low risk (B)	Safety unknown
Antidotes and toxicology: When indicated, the benefits to the mother will outweigh the possible risks to the fetus.		
Antidote: acetaminophen overdose		
N-acetylcysteine	Safe (B)	Safe
Universal antidote		
Charcoal	Safe (B)	Safe
Antidote: iron toxicity		
Deferoxamine	Probably safe (C)	No data
Antidote: digitalis		
DIG Fab	No data (C)	No data
Antidote: benzodiazepines		
Flumazenil	No data (C)	No data
Antidote: toxic alcohols		
Fomepazole	No data (C)	No data
Antidote: cyanide poisoning		
Hydroxycobalamine	Safe (B)	Safe
Antidote: methemoglobinemia		
Methylene blue	Risk noted (C)	Not recommended
Antidote: narcotics		
Naloxone	Safe (B)	Safe

Continued

MEDICATION	PREGNANCY	LACTATION
Universal antidote		
PEG-ELS	Safe (B)	Safe
Antidote: anticholinergics		
Physostigmine	No data	No data
Antidote: organophosphates		
Pralidoxime	No data	No data
Antidote: isoniazid overdose		
Pyridoxine	Safe (B)	Safe
Antidote: lead poisoning		
Succimer	No data	No data

G6PD, glucose-6-phosphate dehydrogenase; PEG-ELS, polyethylenegycol-electrolyte lavage solution.

(CAO Yu)

REFERENCES

1. American College of Emergency Physicians: Emergency ultrasound guidelines. Ann Emerg Med 2009; 53: 550-570.
2. Roth D, et al: Accuracy of noninvasive multiwave pulse oximetry compared with carboxyhemoglobin from blood gas analysis in unselected emergency department patients. Ann Emerg Med 2011;58: 74-79.
3. Bair AE, Caravelli R, Tyler K, Laurin EG: Feasibility of the preoperative Mallampati airway assessment in emergency department patients. J Emerg Med 2010; 38: 677-680.
4. Mort TC, Waberski BH, Clive J: Extending the preoxygenation period from 4 to 8 mins in critically ill patients undergoing emergency intubation. Crit Care Med 2009; 37: 68-71.
5. Wong E, Ng YY: The difficult airway in the emergency department. Int J Emerg Med 2008; 1: 107-111.
6. Martin LD, Mhyre JM, Shanks AM, Tremper KK, KheterpalS: 3,423 emergency tracheal intubations at a university hospital: Airway outcomes and complications. Anesthesiology 2011; 114: 42-48.
7. Jagoda AS, Bruns JJ Jr: Elevated intracranial pressure. In: Walls RM, Murphy MF, Luten RC, eds. Manual of Emergency Airway Management ,4th ed. Philadelphia: Lippincott, Williams & Wilkins/Wolters Kluwer Health; 2012: 395-366.
8. Nouira S, et al: Noninvasive pressure support ventilation and CPAP in cardiogenic pulmonary edema: A multicenter randomized study in the emergency department. Intensive Care Med 2011; 37: 249-256.
9. Morris AC, et al: Reducing ventilator associated pneumonia in intensive care: Impact of implementing a care bundle. Crit Care Med 2011; 39: 2218-2224.
10. Gajic O, et al: Early identification of patients at risk of acute lung injury: Evaluation of lung injury prediction score in a multicenter cohort study. Am J Res pir Crit Care Med 2011; 183: 462-470.
11. Kagawa E, et al: Outcomes of extracorporeal membrane oxygenation inadult patients with refractory shock and cardiac arrest. Circulation 2010; 122: A271.
12. Gruenewald M, et al: Visual evaluation of left ventricular performance predicts volume responsiveness early after resuscitation from cardiac arrest. Resuscitation 2011; 82: 1553-1557.
13. Berg RA, et al: Part 5: Adult basic life support: 2010 American Heart Association Guidelines for Cardiopulmonary Resuscitation and Emergency Cardiovascular Care. Circulation 2010; 122(Suppl 3): S685-S705.
14. Neumar RW, et al: Part 8: Adult advanced cardiovascular life support: 2010 American Heart Association Guidelines for Cardiopulmonary Resuscitation and Emergency Cardiovascular Care. Circulation 2010; 122(18 Suppl 3): S729-S767.
15. Neumar RW, et al: Post-cardiac arrest syndrome. Circulation 2008; 118: 2452-2483.
16. Rossetti AO, Oddo M, Logroscino G, Kaplan PW: Prognostication after cardiac arrest and hypothermia: A prospective study. Ann Neurol 2010; 67: 301-307.
17. Gillies MA, et al: Therapeutic hypothermia after cardiac arrest: A retrospective comparison of surface and endovascular cooling techniques. Resuscitation 2010; 81: 1117-1122.
18. Tang AS, et al: Cardiac-resynchronization therapy for mild-to-moderate heart failure. N Engl J Med 2010; 363: 2385-2395.
19. Al-Majed NS, McAlister FA, Bakal JA, Ezekowitz JA: Meta-analysis: Cardiac resynchronization therapy for patients with less symptomatic heart failure. Ann Intern Med 2011; 154: 401.
20. Packer DL, et al: ICDs: Evidence, guidelines, and glitches. Heart Rhythm 2011; 8: 800.
21. Rossaint R, et al: Management of bleeding following major trauma: An updated European guideline. Crit Care 2010; 14: R52.
22. Bhuiya F, Pitts S, McCaig L: Emergency department visits for chest pain and abdominal pain: United

States, 1999-2008. NCHS Data Brief 2010; 43: 1.

23. Rostoff P, et al: Electrocardiographic prediction of acute left main coronary artery occlusion. Am J Emerg Med 2007; 25: 852.
24. Haissaguerre M, et al: Sudden cardiac arrest associated with early repolarization. N Engl J Med 2008; 358: 2016-2023.
25. Bhuiya F, Pitts S, McCaig L: Emergency department visits for chest pain and abdominal pain: United States, 1999-2008. NCHS Data Brief 2010; 43: 1.
26. Fromm RE: Cardiac troponins in the intensive care unit: Common causes of increased levels and interpretation. Crit Care Med 2007; 35: 584.
27. Agewall S, Giannitsis E, Jernberg T, Katus H: Troponin elevation in coronary vs. non-coronary disease. Eur Heart J 2011; 32: 404-411.
28. Anderson JL, et al: ACC/AHA 2007 guidelines for the management of patients with unstable angina/non–ST-elevation myocardial infarction: A report of the American College of Cardiology/American Heart Association Task Force on Practice Guidelines. J Am Coll Cardiol 2007; 50: e1.
29. Hiratzka LF, et al: 2010 ACCF/AHA/AATS/ACR/ASA/SCA/SCAI/SIR/STS/SVM guidelines for the diagnosis and management of patients with thoracic aortic disease: Executive summary. A report of the American College of Cardiology Foundation/American Heart Association Task Force on Practice Guidelines, American Association for Thoracic Surgery, American College of Radiology, American Stroke Association, Society of Cardiovascular Anesthesiologists, Society for Cardiovascular Angiography and Interventions, Society of Interventional Radiology, Society of Thoracic Surgeons, and Society for Vascular Medicine. Circulation 2010; 121: e266-e369.
30. Wen D, Zhou XL, Li JJ, Hui RT: Biomarkers in aortic dissection. Clin Chim Acta 2011; 412: 688-695.
31. Fan QK, et al: Evaluation of D-dimer in the diagnosis of suspected aortic dissection. Clin Chem Lab Med 2010; 48: 1733-1737.
32. Cooper L: Myocarditis. N Engl J Med 2009; 360: 1526.
33. Nihoyannopoulos P, Dawson D: Restrictive cardiomyopathies. Eur J Echocardiogr 2009; 10: 23-33.
34. Lloyd-Jones D, et al: Heart Disease and Stroke Statistics—2010 Update. A Report From the American Heart Association. Circulation 2010; 121: e1.
35. Quinn RR, et al: The 2010 Canadian Hypertension Education Program recommendations for the management of hypertension: Part I—blood pressure measurement, diagnosis and assessment of risk. Can J Cardiol 2010; 26: 241.
36. Nishijima DK, Paladino L, Sinert R: Routine testing in patients with asymptomatic elevated blood pressure in the ED. Am J Emerg Med 2010; 28: 235.
37. Hackam DG, et al: The 2010 Canadian Hypertension Education Program recommendations for the management of hypertension: Part 2—therapy. Can J Cardiol 2010; 26: 249.
38. Tan HL, Spekhorst HHM, Peters RJG, Wilde AAM: Adenosine induced ventricular dysrhythmias in the emergency room. Pacing Clin Electrophysiol 2011; 24: 450-455.
39. Stiell IG, Macle L, CCS Atrial Fibrillation Guidelines Committee: Canadian Cardiovascular Society Atrial Fibrillation Guidelines 2010: Management of recent-onset atrial fibrillation and flutter in the emergency department. Can J Cardiol 2011; 27: 38-46.
40. Scheuermeyer FX, Grafstein E, Heilbron B, Innes G: Emergency department management and 1 year outcomes of patients with atrial flutter. Ann Emerg Med 2011; 57: 564-571.
41. Bui AL, Horwich TB, Fonarow GC: Epidemiology and risk profile of heart failure. Nat Rev Cardiol 2011; 8: 30.
42. Lam LL, et al: Meta-analysis: Effect of B-type natriuretic peptide testing on clinical outcomes in patients with acute dyspnea in the emergency setting. Ann Intern Med 2010; 153: 728.
43. Kociol RD, et al: Troponin elevation in heart failure prevalence, mechanisms, and clinical implications. J Am Coll Cardiol 2010; 56: 1071.
44. Cinar O, et al: Can mainstream end-tidal carbon dioxide measurement accurately predict the arterial

carbon dioxide level of patients with acute dyspnea in ED. Am J Emerg Med 2012; 30: 358-361.
45. Gori CS, Magrini L, Travaglino F, Di Somma S: Role of biomarkers in patients with dyspnea. Eur Rev Med Pharmacol Sci 2011; 15: 229.
46. Cibinel GA, et al: Diagnostic accuracy and reproducibility of pleural and lung ultrasound in discriminating cardiogenic causes of acute dyspnea in the emergency department. Intern Emerg Med 2012; 7: 65-70.
47. National Asthma Education and Prevention Program Expert Panel: Report 3: Guidelines for the Diagnosis and Management of Asthma. NIH Publication No. 08-5846. Washington, DC: U.S. Department of Health and Human Services, National Institutes of Health, National Heart, Lung and Blood Institute; 2007.
48. Courtney DM, et al: Clinical features from the history and physical examination that predict the presence or absence of pulmonary embolism in symptomatic emergency department patients: Results of a prospective, multicenter study. Ann Emerg Med 2010; 55: 305-315.
49. Kline JA, Corredor DM, Hogg MM, Hernandez J, Jones AE: Normalization of vital signs does not reduce the probability of acute pulmonary embolism in symptomatic emergency department patients. Acad Emerg Med 2012; 19: 11-17.
50. Pollack CV, et al: Clinical characteristics, management, and outcomes of patients diagnosed with acute pulmonary embolism in the emergency department: Initial Report of EMPEROR (Multicenter Emergency Medicine Pulmonary Embolism in the Real World Registry). J Am Coll Cardiol 2011; 57: 700-706.
51. Moore CL, Copel JA: Point-of-care ultrasonography. N Engl J Med 2011; 364: 749-757.
52. Wilkerson RG, Stone MB: Sensitivity of bedside ultrasound and supine anteroposterior chest radiographs for the identification of pneumothorax after blunt trauma. Acad Emerg Med 2010; 17: 11-17.
53. Harper SJ, Cheslyn-Curtis S: Acute pancreatitis. Ann Clin Biochem 2011; 48: 23.
54. Bharwani N, Patel S, Prabhudesai S, Fotheringham T, Power N: Acute pancreatitis: The role of imaging in diagnosis and management. Clin Radiol 2011; 66: 164.
55. Barkun AN, et al: International consensus recommendations on the management of patients with nonvariceal upper gastrointestinal bleeding. Ann Intern Med 2010; 152: 101-113.
56. Singri N, Ahya SN, Levin ML: Acute renal failure. JAMA 2003; 289: 7473.
57. Bosch X, Poch E, Grau JM: Rhabdomyolysis and acute kidney injury. N Engl J Med 2009; 361: 62.
58. American Diabetes Association: Standards of medical care in diabetes—2011. Diabetes Care 2011; 34: S11-S62.
59. Waugh N, et al: Newer agents for blood glucose control in type 2 diabetes: Systematic review and economic evaluation. Health Technol Assess 2010; 14: 1-248.
60. Buckley MS, Leblanc JM, Cawley MJ: Electrolyte disturbances associated with commonly prescribed medications in the intensive care unit. Crit Care Med 2010; 38(Suppl): S253-S264.
61. Kraut JA, Madias NE: Metabolic acidosis: Pathophysiology, diagnosis and management. Nat Rev Nephrol 2010; 6: 274.
62. Huy N, et al: Cerebrospinal fluid lactate concentration to distinguish bacterial from aseptic meningitis: A systemic review and meta-analysis. Crit Care 2010; 14: R240.
63. Crystal SC, Robbins MS: Epidemiology of tension-type headache. Curr Pain Headache Rep 2010; 14: 449-454.
64. Friedman BW, et al: Treating headache recurrence after emergency department discharge: A randomized controlled trial of naproxen versus sumatriptan. Ann Emerg Med 2010; 56: 7-17.
65. Kessler C, Tristano J, De Lorenzo RA: The emergency department approach to syncope: Evidence-based guidelines and prediction rules. Emerg Med Clin North Am 2010; 28: 487.
66. Serrano LA, et al: Accuracy and quality of clinical decision rules for syncope in the emergency department: A systematic review and meta-analysis. Ann Emerg Med 2010; 56: 362.
67. Koita J, Riggio S, Jagoda A: The mental status examination in emergency practice. Emerg Med Clin

North Am 2010; 28: 439-451.
68. Martindale JL, Goldstein JN, Pallin DJ: Emergency department seizure epidemiology. Emerg Med Clin North Am 2011; 29: 15-27.
69. Huff JS, Fountain NB: Pathophysiology and definitions of seizures and status epilepticus. Emerg Med Clin North Am 2011; 29: 1-13.
70. Furie KL, et al: Guidelines for the prevention of stroke in patients with stroke or transient ischemic attack: A guideline for healthcare professionals from the American Heart Association/American Stroke Association. Stroke 2011; 42: 227-276.
71. Morgenstern LB, et al: Guidelines for the management of spontaneous intracerebral hemorrhage: A guideline for healthcare professionals from the American Heart Association/American Stroke Association. Stroke 2010; 41: 2108-2129.
72. Lees KR, et al: Time to treatment with intravenous alteplase and outcome in stroke: An updated pooled analysis of ECASS, ATLANTIS, NINDS, and EPITHET trials. Lancet 2010; 375: 1695-1703.
73. Stromberg C, Johansson G, Adolfson A: Acute abdominal pain: Diagnostic impact of immediate CT scanning. World J Surg 2007; 31: 2347.
74. Mell MW, et al: Effect of early plasma transfusion on mortality in patients with ruptured abdominal aortic aneurysm. Surgery 2010; 148: 955-962.
75. Thompson AR, Cooper JA, Ashton HA, Hafez H: Growth rates of small abdominal aortic aneurysms correlate with clinical events. Br J Surg 2010; 97: 37-44.
76. Oyasiji T, Angelo S, Kyriakides TC, Helton SW: Small bowel obstruction: Outcome and cost implications of admitting service. Am Surg 2010; 76: 687-691.
77. Levine MR, Gorman SM, Young CF, Courtney DM: Clinical characteristics and management of wound foreign bodies in the ED. Am J Emerg Med 2008; 26: 8.
78. Bernard SA, et al: Prehospital rapid sequence intubation improves functional outcome for patients with severe traumatic brain injury: A randomized controlled trial. Ann Surg 2010; 252: 959-965.
79. American College of Emergency Physicians: Role of the Emergency Physician in Injury Prevention and Control for Adult and Pediatric Patients, 2012. Available at www.acep.org/Content.aspx?id=29820. Accessed April 12, 2011.
80. Hausfater P, et al: Elevation of cardiac troponin I during nonexertional heat-related illnesses in the context of a heatwave. Crit Care 2010; 14: R99.
81. Pease S, et al: Early organ dysfunction course, cooling time and outcome in classic heatstroke. Intensive Care Med 2009; 35: 1454-1458.
82. Luks AM, et al: Wilderness Medical Society consensus guidelines for the prevention and treatment of acute altitude illness. Wilderness Environ Med 2010; 21: 146-155.
83. Lakosha H, Tremblay F, De Becker I: High-voltage electrical trauma to the eye. Can J Ophthalmol 2009; 44: 605.
84. Celebi A, et al: Myocardial infarction after an electric shock: A rare complication. Cardiol J 2009; 16: 362.
85. Ramati A, et al: Alteration in functional brain systems after electrical injury. J Neurotrauma 2009; 26: 1815.
86. Jamaty C, et al: Lipid emulsions in the treatment of acute poisoning: A systematic review of human and animal studies. Clin Toxicol (Phila) 2010; 48: 1-27.
87. Rentsch KM: Laboratory diagnostics in acute poisoning: Critical overview. Clin Chem Lab Med 2010; 48: 1381-1387.
88. Wu AH: Limitations of point-of-care testing in the ED or ICU: A role for regional centralized toxicology laboratories. Clin Pharmacol Ther 2010; 88: 295-298.
89. Tenore PL: Advanced urine toxicology testing. J Addict Dis 2010; 21: 436-448.
90. Roberts DM, et al: Enhanced elimination in acute barbiturate poisoning—a systematic review. Clin Toxicol (Phila) 2011; 49: 2.
91. McMartin KE: Antidotes for alcohol and glycol toxicity: Translating mechanisms to treatment. Clin

Pharmacol Ther 2010; 88: 400.
92. Anz AW, et al: Management of venomous snakebite to the extremities. J Am Acad Orthop Surg 2010; 18: 749.
93. McGarth T, Hamilton R: Hyperbaric oxygen in the treatment of venomous snakebite. Undersea Hyperb Med 2010; 37: 393.
94. Ruha AM, Curry SC, Albrecht C, Riley B: Late hematologic toxicity following treatment of rattlesnake envenomation with Crotalidae polyvalent immune Fab antivenom. Toxicon 2011; 57: 53.
95. Jones AE, et al: Lactate clearance vs central venous oxygen saturation as goals of early sepsis therapy: A randomized clinical trial. JAMA 2010; 303: 739-746.
96. Jones AE, Puskarich MA: Sepsis-induced tissue hypoperfusion. Crit Care Nurs Clin North Am 2011; 23: 115-125.
97. Puskarich MA, et al: Association between timing of antibiotic administration and mortality from septic shock in patients treated with a quantitative resuscitation protocol. Crit Care Med 2011; 39: 2066-2071.
98. Gaieski DF, et al: Impact of time to antibiotics on survival in patients with severe sepsis or septic shock in whom early goal-directed therapy was initiated in the emergency department. Crit Care Med 2010; 38: 1045-1053.
99. Levy MM, et al: The Surviving Sepsis Campaign: Results of an international guideline-based performance improvement program targeting severe sepsis. Crit Care Med 2010; 38: 367-374.
100. Vasu TS, et al: Norephinephrine or dopamine for septic shock: Systematic review of randomized clinical trials. J Intensive Care Med 2012; 27: 172-178.
101. Shepard TH: Catalog of Teratogenic Agents, 13th ed. Baltimore: Johns Hopkins University Press; 2010.
102. Briggs GG, et al: Drugs in Pregnancy and Lactation: A Reference Guide to Fetal and Neonatal Risk, 9th ed. Baltimore: Lippincott Williams & Wilkins; 2011.

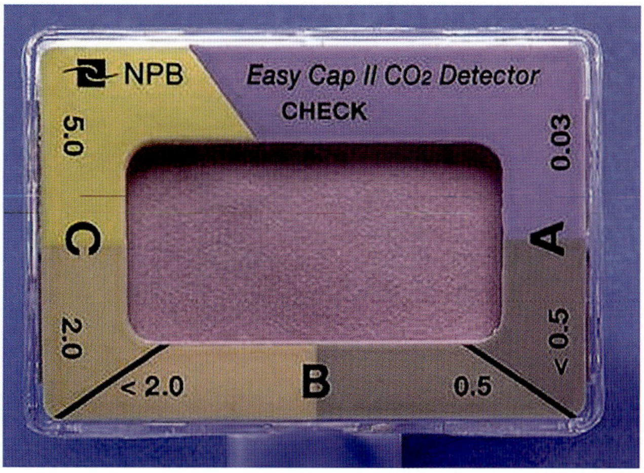

Fig. 3-4 $ETCO_2$ detector before application.

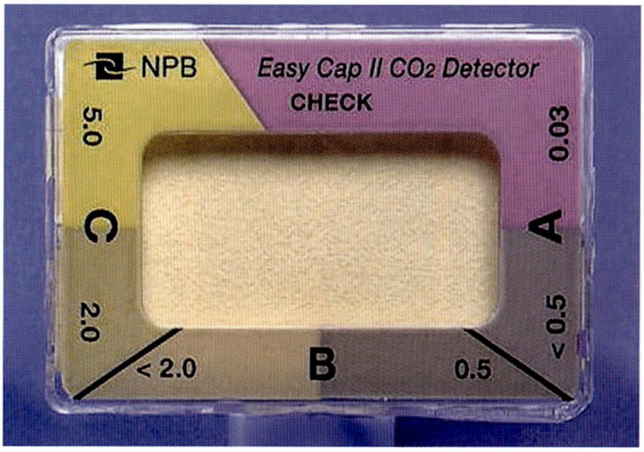

Fig. 3-5 Positive detection of CO_2 turns the indicator yellow, indicating tracheal placement of the endotracheal tube.

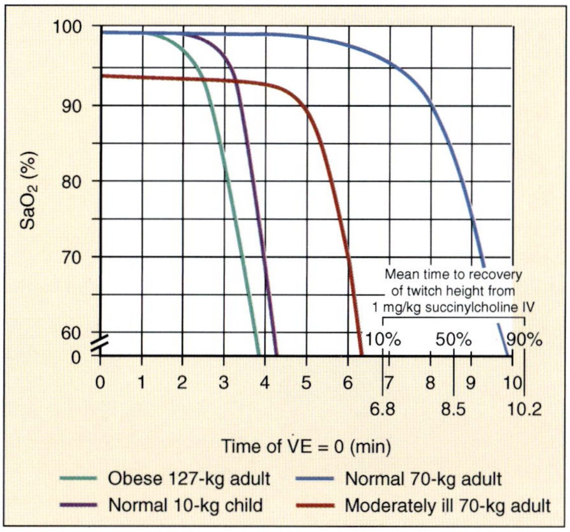

Fig. 3-10 Desaturation time for apneic, fully preoxygenated patients.

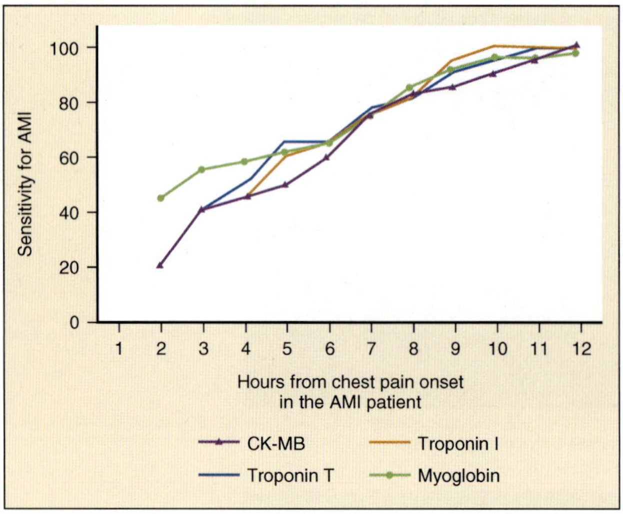

Fig. 10-20 Serum marker sensitivity relative to the time of onset of chest pain in the patient with AMI.

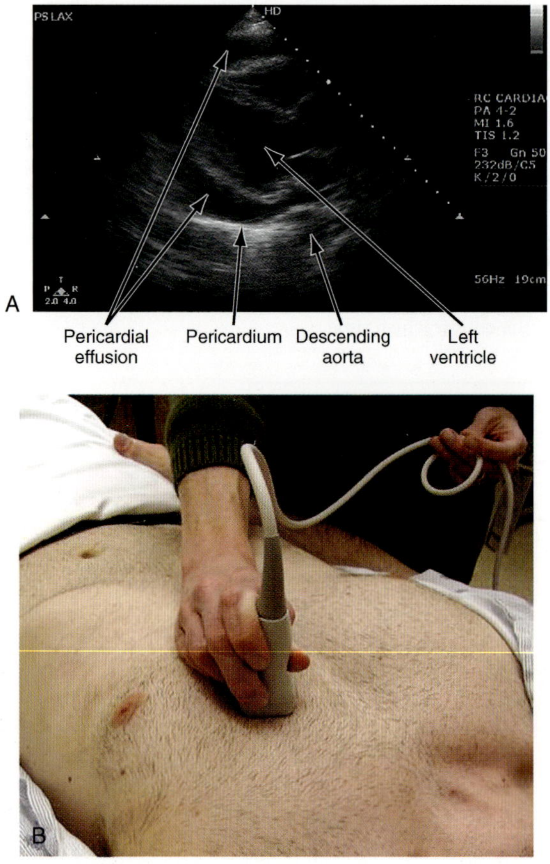

Fig. 12-2 A, Bedside ultrasound showing a pericardial effusion. B, The proper technique for ED ultrasound of pericardial effusion.

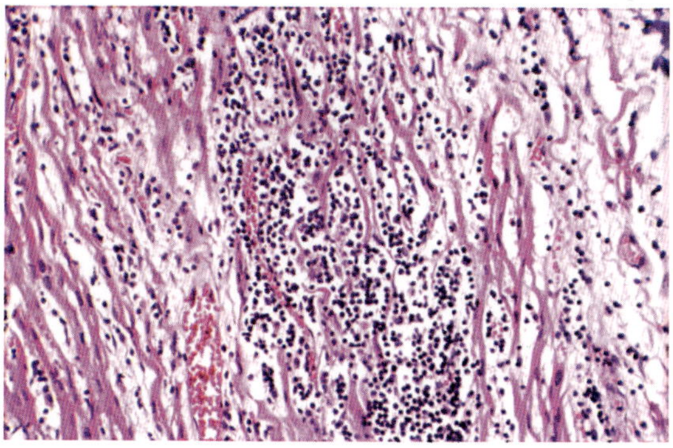

Fig. 12-4 Myocardial biopsy specimen showing myocarditis.

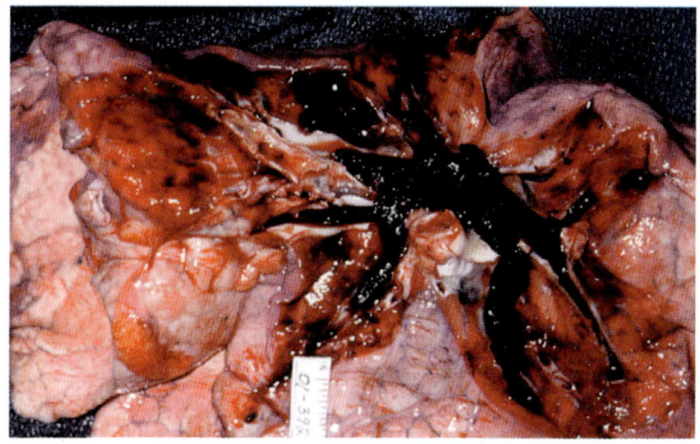

Fig. 20-1 Massive PE on autopsy.

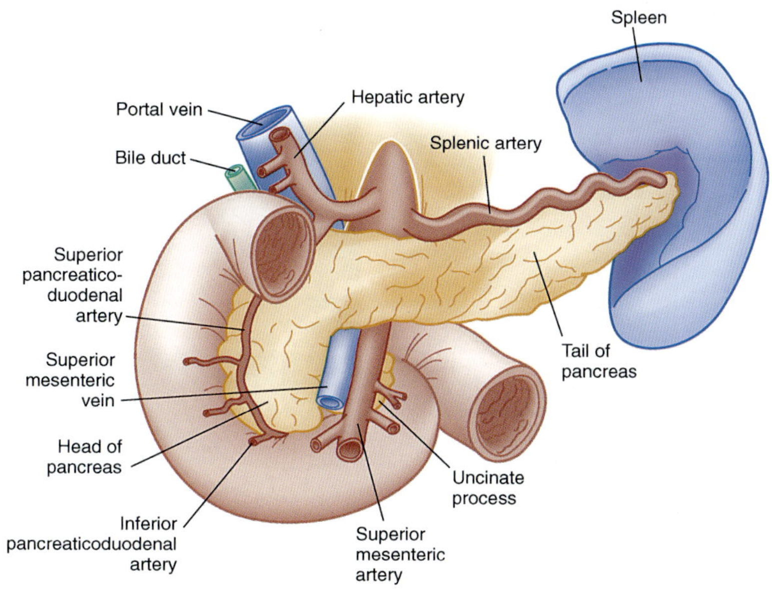

Fig. 22-1 Diagrammatic representation of the pancreas, anterior view.

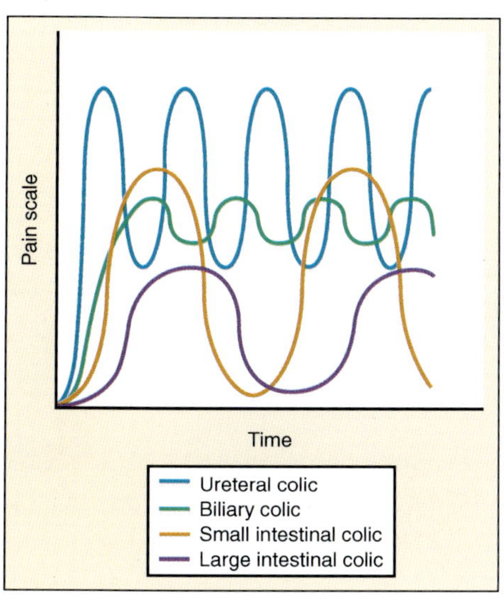

Fig. 35-3 The characteristics of colicky AAP.

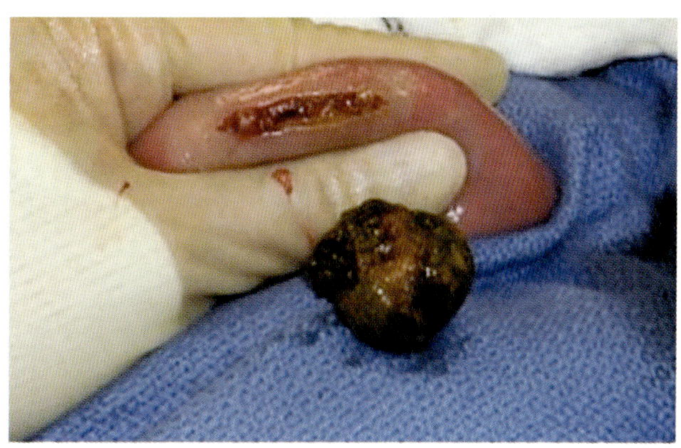

Fig. 37-2 Gallstone ileus of the small intestine at laparotomy.

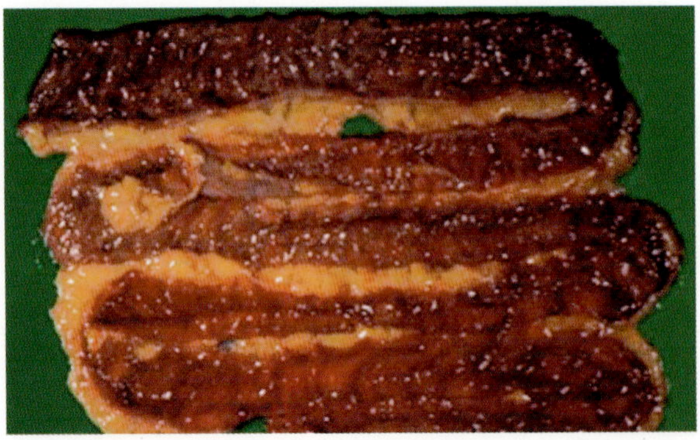

Fig. 37-4 Gross pathologic image of intestinal ischemia and infarction.

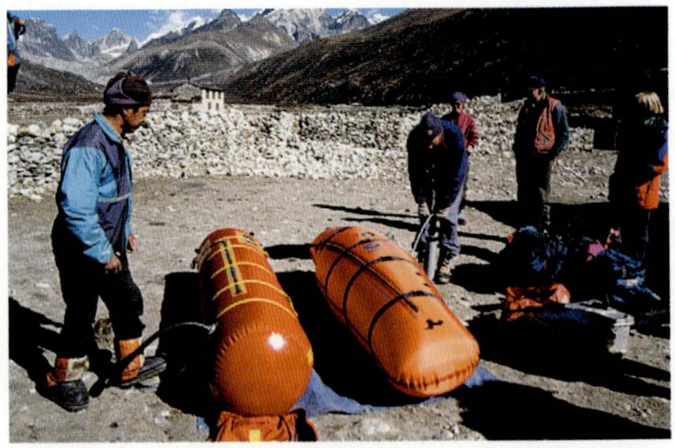

Fig. 42-4 Gamow bag (*left*) and Certec bag (*right*): lightweight, portable hyperbaric chambers.

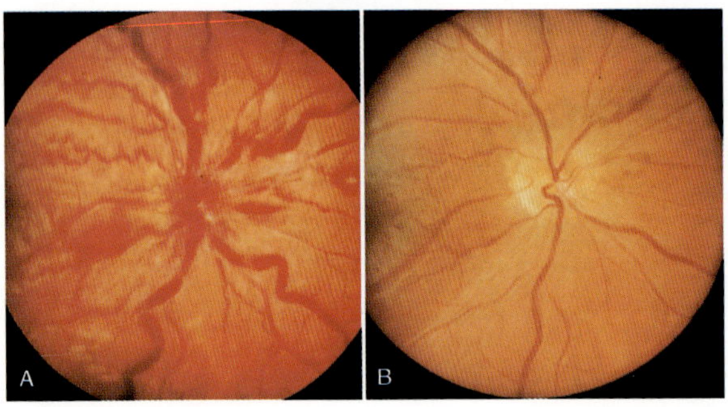

Fig. 42-6 High-altitude retinal hemorrhages. A, Acute. B, After 1 week of resolution.

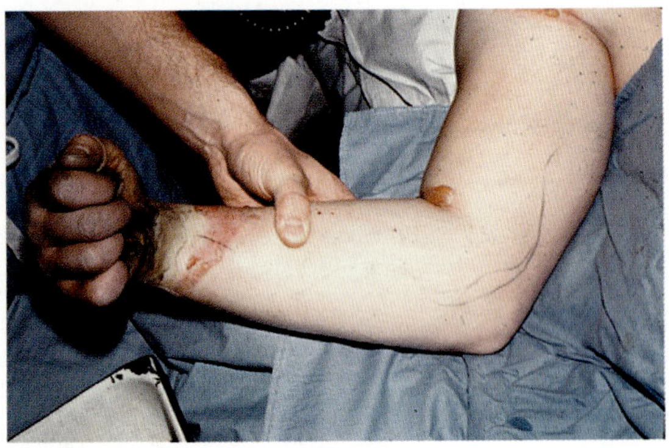

Fig. 44-1 Kissing burn.

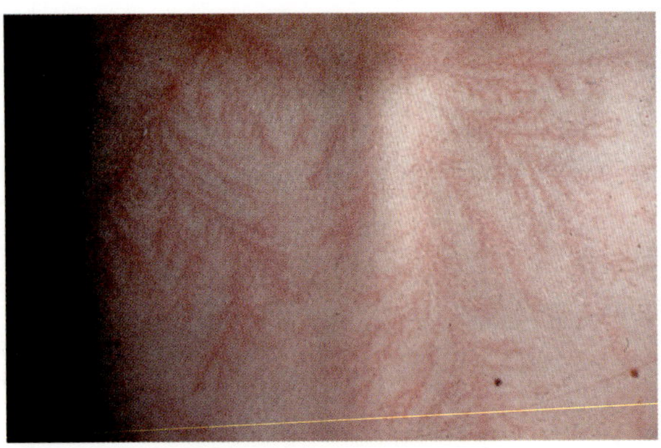

Fig. 44-2 Feathering burn.

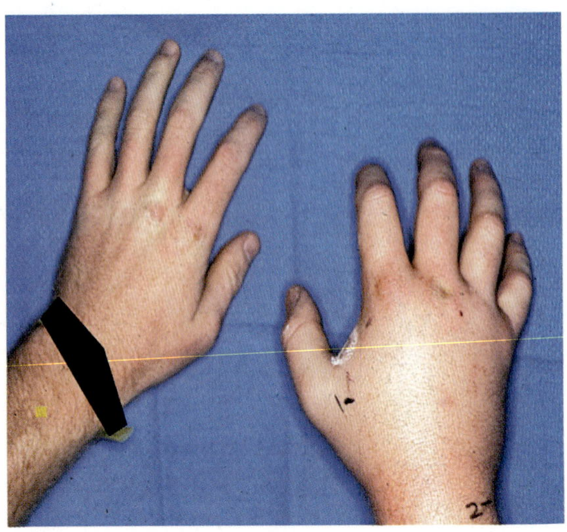

Fig. 50-3 Northern copperhead (Agkistrodon contortrix mokasen) bite on right hand with normal left hand for comparison.